Basic Histology

Many of the illustrations in this book were prepared with financial aid from the
Fundação de Amparo à Pesquisa do Estado de São Paulo.

Basic Histology

3rd Edition

LUIS C. JUNQUEIRA, MD

Professor of Histology & Embryology
Institute of Biomedical Science
University of São Paulo, Brazil

Honorary Research Associate in Biology
Harvard College, Boston

Formerly Research Associate
Medical School, University of Chicago

JOSÉ CARNEIRO, MD

Professor of Histology & Embryology
Institute of Biomedical Science
University of São Paulo, Brazil

Formerly Research Associate
Department of Anatomy
Medical School, McGill University
Montreal, Canada

Formerly Visiting Associate Professor
Department of Anatomy
Medical School, University of Virginia
Charlottesville, Virginia

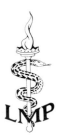

Los Altos, California 94022   **LANGE Medical Publications**

A Concise Medical Library for Practitioner and Student

Current Medical Diagnosis & Treatment 1980 (annual revision). Edited by M.A. Krupp and M.J. Chatton. 1116 pp.	1980
Current Pediatric Diagnosis & Treatment, 6th ed. Edited by C.H. Kempe, H.K. Silver, and D. O'Brien. 1122 pp, *illus.*	1980
Current Surgical Diagnosis & Treatment, 4th ed. Edited by J.E. Dunphy and L.W. Way. 1162 pp, *illus.*	1979
Current Obstetric & Gynecologic Diagnosis & Treatment, 2nd ed. Edited by R.C. Benson. 976 pp, *illus.*	1978
Review of Physiological Chemistry, 17th ed. H.A. Harper, V.W. Rodwell, and P.A. Mayes. 702 pp, *illus.*	1979
Review of Medical Physiology, 9th ed. W.F. Ganong. 618 pp, *illus.*	1979
Review of Medical Microbiology, 14th ed. E. Jawetz, J.L. Melnick, and E.A. Adelberg. 593 pp, *illus.*	1980
Review of Medical Pharmacology, 6th ed. F.H. Meyers, E. Jawetz, and A. Goldfien. 762 pp, *illus.*	1978
Basic & Clinical Immunology, 3rd ed. Edited by H.H. Fudenberg, D.P. Stites, J.L. Caldwell, and J.V. Wells. About 775 pp, *illus.*	1980
Clinical Cardiology, 2nd ed. M. Sokolow and M.B. McIlroy. 718 pp, *illus.*	1979
General Urology, 9th ed. D.R. Smith. 541 pp, *illus.*	1978
General Ophthalmology, 9th ed. D. Vaughan and T. Asbury. 410 pp, *illus.*	1980
Correlative Neuroanatomy & Functional Neurology, 17th ed. J.G. Chusid. 464 pp, *illus.*	1979
Principles of Clinical Electrocardiography, 10th ed. M.J. Goldman. 415 pp, *illus.*	1979
Handbook of Obstetrics & Gynecology, 7th ed. R.C. Benson. 808 pp, *illus.*	1980
Physician's Handbook, 19th ed. M.A. Krupp, N.J. Sweet, E. Jawetz, E.G. Biglieri, R.L. Roe, and C.A. Camargo. 758 pp, *illus.*	1979
Handbook of Pediatrics, 13th ed. H.K. Silver, C.H. Kempe, and H.B. Bruyn. 735 pp, *illus.*	1980
Handbook of Poisoning: Prevention, Diagnosis, & Treatment, 10th ed. R.H. Dreisbach. 578 pp.	1980

Table of Contents

Preface

The third edition of *Basic Histology* represents the authors' continuing effort to present in compact but amply illustrated format the foundations of histology for medical students and others in the biologic sciences. Again we emphasize cellular biology as the most fundamental approach to the study of tissue physiology.

We have been most gratified by the success this book has achieved since the first appearance of the English language edition in 1975. We gratefully acknowledge our dependence on our readers' suggestions for changes and additions in the ongoing effort to keep up to date with advances in the field.

We are very glad to be able to say that in preparing this new edition we have had the assistance of Bruce Lipton, PhD, Associate Professor of Anatomy at the University of Wisconsin–Madison. Dr Lipton has reviewed every word of our revisions, making further revisions as required, and has worked closely with our publishers in California to make certain that *Basic Histology* is up to date and accurate in all important respects. We look forward to a continued close relationship with this young scientist and scholar in future editions of this work.

As the third edition goes to press we are pleased to be able to announce that an Italian edition has been published and that translations are going forward in French, German, Japanese, Serbo-Croatian, Dutch, and Indonesian.

—LCJ
—JC

June, 1980

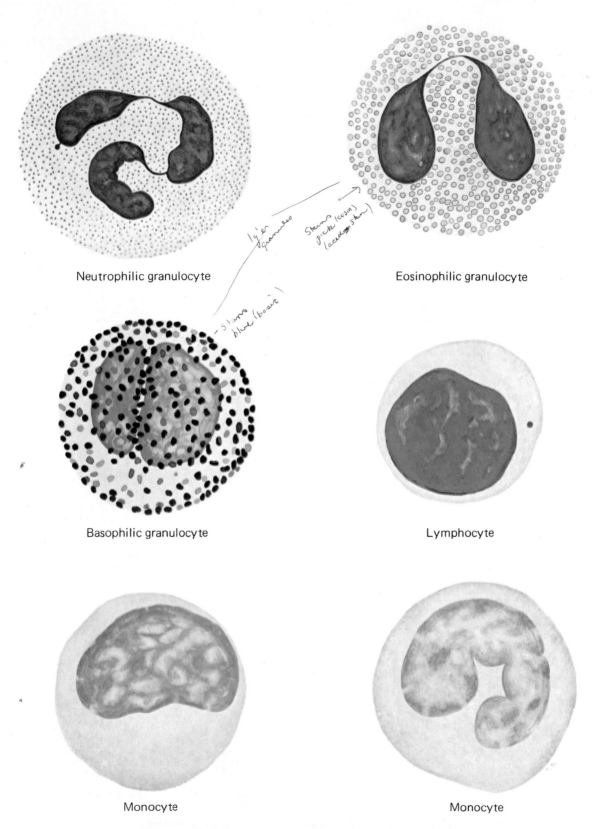

Neutrophilic granulocyte

Eosinophilic granulocyte

Basophilic granulocyte

Lymphocyte

Monocyte

Monocyte

The 5 Types of Human Leukocytes. (See Fig 13—5.)

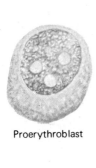

Proerythroblast

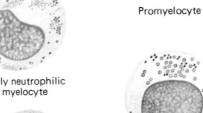

Myeloblast

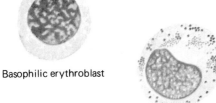

Basophilic erythroblast

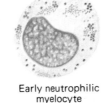

Early neutrophilic
myelocyte

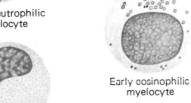

Promyelocyte

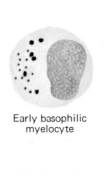

Early basophilic
myelocyte

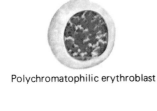

Polychromatophilic erythroblast

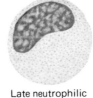

Late neutrophilic
myelocyte

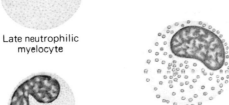

Early eosinophilic
myelocyte

Normoblast

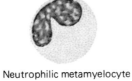

Neutrophilic metamyelocyte

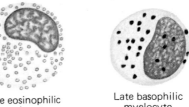

Late eosinophilic
myelocyte

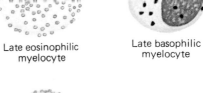

Late basophilic
myelocyte

Reticulocyte

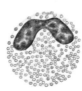

Neutrophil with
band-shaped nucleus

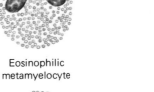

Eosinophilic
metamyelocyte

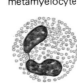

Erythrocyte

Mature neutrophil

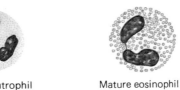

Mature eosinophil

Mature basophil

Stages of Development of Erythrocytes and Granulocytes. (See Fig 14—3.)

Familiarity with the tools and methods of any branch of science is essential for proper understanding of the subject. Some of the more common methods used to study cells and tissues and the principles involved in these methods will be reviewed here: units of measurement, preparation of tissues for examination, optical microscopy, phase contrast microscopy, polarizing microscopy, electron microscopy, radioautography, examination of living cells and tissues, differential centrifugation, and problems in interpretation of tissue sections.

The most important units of measurement used in histology are given in Table 1–1. At a recent international conference, it was recommended that the Ångström unit (Å; 10^{-10} meter) be abandoned in favor of the **nanometer** (nm, 10^{-9} meter) and that the nanometer be used in place of the **millimicron** (mμ, 10^{-9} meter). In this book, the nanometer will be used in place of the Ångström unit (1 nm = 10 Å). The **micron** (μ) is now called a **micrometer** (μm), with value (10^{-6} meter) unchanged.

layers of tissues or transparent membranes of living animals (eg, the mesentery, the tail of a tadpole, the wall of a hamster's cheek pouch) can be observed in the microscope. In such instances, it is possible to study these structures for long periods and under varying physiologic or experimental conditions. If a permanent slide preparation is desired, small fragments of these thin structures can be fixed, spread on a glass slide, stained and mounted with resin, and examined under the microscope. In most cases, however, tissues must be sliced into thin sections before they can be examined. These sections are cut by precision fine cutting instruments called **microtomes,** and the organ or tissue must be fixed and prepared for sectioning. (See Table 1–2.)

The ideal microscope tissue preparation would of course be preserved with suitable chemicals so that the tissue on the slide would have the same structure and chemical composition as it has in the body. This is sometimes possible but, as a practical matter, seldom feasible, and artifacts resulting from the preparation process are almost always present.

Table 1–1. Units of measurement used in light and electron microscopy.*

SI Unit*	Symbol and Value
Micron (micrometer)	μ (μm) = 0.001 mm, 10^{-6} m
Millimicron (nanometer)	mμ (nm) = 0.001 μm, 10^{-9} m
Ångström	Å = 0.1 nm, 10^{-10} m

*The preferred SI *(Système International)* units (in parentheses) will be used throughout this book.

PREPARATION OF TISSUES FOR MICROSCOPIC EXAMINATION

The most common procedure used in the study of tissues is the preparation of permanent histologic slides that can be studied with the aid of the optical microscope. Under the optical microscope, tissues are examined by transillumination. Since tissues and organs are usually too thick for transillumination, technics have been developed for obtaining thin, translucent sections. In some cases, very thin

Table 1–2. Stages through which the tissues must pass before paraffin impregnation. (The next steps are microtome sectioning, staining, and mounting.)

Stage	Purpose	Duration
1. Fixation in simple or compound fixatives (Bouin's, Zenker's formalin)	To preserve tissue morphology and chemical composition	About 12 h, according to the fixative and the size of the piece of tissue
2. Dehydration in graded concentrated ethyl alcohol (70% up to 100% alcohol)	To remove cell water	6–24 h
3. Clearing in benzene, xylene, or toluene	To impregnate the tissues with a paraffin solvent	1–6 h
4. Embedding in melted paraffin at 58–60 C	Paraffin penetrates all intercellular spaces and even into the cells, making the tissues more resistant to sectioning	½–6 h

Fixation

In order to avoid tissue digestion by enzymes (autolysis) or bacteria and to preserve physical structure, pieces of organs should be promptly and adequately treated prior to or as soon as possible following removal from the animal's body. This treatment—**fixation**—usually consists of submerging the tissues in chemical substances or perfusing them with those substances in order to preserve as much as possible of their morphologic and chemical characteristics.

The chemical substances used to fix tissues are called **fixatives.** Some fixatives (eg, mercuric chloride, picric acid) promote the precipitation or clumping of proteins. Others (eg, formalin, glutaraldehyde) promote coagulation but not coarse precipitation of proteins. All fixatives have both desirable and undesirable effects. The goal of combining the desirable effects and minimizing the undesirable ones has led to the development of several mixtures. The most commonly used mixtures are **Bouin's fluid,** composed of picric acid, formalin (a saturated solution—37% by weight of formaldehyde gas in water), acetic acid, and water; and **Zenker's formalin (Helly's fluid),** containing formaldehyde, potassium dichromate, mercuric chloride, and water. The simple fixatives most commonly used are a 10% solution of formalin in saline and a 2–6% solution of buffered glutaraldehyde.

The chemistry of the process involved in fixation is complex and not well understood. However, formaldehyde and glutaraldehyde are known to react with the amine groups (NH_2) of tissue proteins. In the case of glutaraldehyde, the fixing action is reinforced by the fact that it is a dialdehyde and can cross-link.

In view of the high resolution afforded by the electron microscope, greater care is necessitated in fixation in order to preserve ultrastructural detail. Toward that end, a double fixation procedure, using a buffered glutaraldehyde solution first, followed by a second fixation in buffered osmium tetroxide, has become a standard procedure in preparations for fine structural studies.

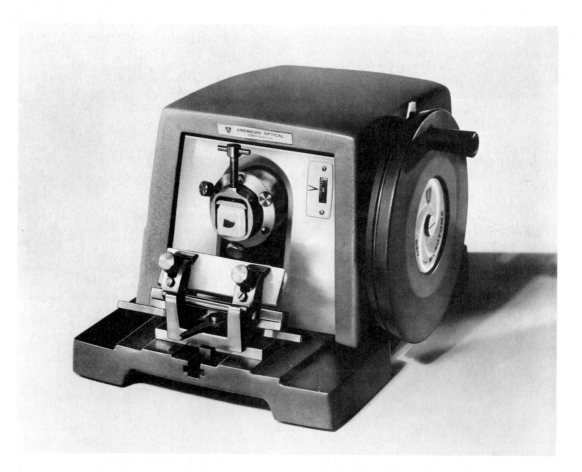

Figure 1–1. Microtome for paraffin-embedded tissues. Rotation of the drive wheel—seen with a handle on the right side of the instrument—moves the tissue block holder up and down. Each turn of the drive wheel advances the specimen holder a controlled distance, generally 3–8 μm, and the block strikes the knife edge, cutting the sections. The sticky paraffin sections adhere to each other, producing a ribbon which is collected and fixed on a slide. (Courtesy of American Optical Corp.)

Embedding

In order to be able to obtain thin sections with the microtome, tissues must be infiltrated after fixation with a substance that will impart a firm consistency necessary for cutting. This can be gelatin, celloidin, paraffin, resins, or other plastic materials.

Paraffin is used routinely for light microscopy; resins of the epoxy type (Epon or Araldite) are more commonly employed for electron microscopy.

The process of embedding or tissue impregnation is usually preceded by 2 main steps: **dehydration** and **clearing.** The water of the fragments to be embedded is first extracted by bathing successively in a graded series of mixtures of ethanol with water (usually from 70% to 100% ethanol). The ethanol is then replaced by a lipid solvent. (In paraffin embedding, the solvent used is xylene or benzene.) As the tissues become impregnated with the solvent, they usually become transparent in a step called **clearing.** Once the tissue is impregnated with the solvent, it is placed in melted paraffin in the oven, usually at 58–60 C. The heat causes the solvent to evaporate, and the space becomes filled with paraffin. Tissues to be embedded for electron microscopy are also dehydrated in ethanolic solutions. However, instead of using the lipid solvents as in paraffin embedding, the tissues are subsequently infiltrated with plastic solvents such as propylene oxide. These solvents are miscible with and later replaced by plastic solutions (eg, Epon, Araldite) hardened by means of cross-linking polymerizers or heat. This is the infiltration or embedding procedure.

The small blocks of paraffin containing the tissues are then sectioned by the steel blade of the microtome to a thickness of 3–8 μm* (Fig 1–1). The sections are laid out on warm water and transferred to glass slides. For electron microscopy, much thinner sections are necessary (0.02–0.1 μm); embedding is therefore performed in a hard epoxy plastic. The blocks thus obtained are so hard that glass or diamond knives are usually necessary to section them. Since the electron beam in the microscope cannot penetrate glass, the extremely thin plastic sections are collected on small metal (usually etched copper) screens. Those portions of the sections spanning the holes in the mesh of the screen can be examined in the microscope.

Immersion of tissues in lipid solvents such as benzene or xylene dissolves the tissue lipids, which is an undesirable effect when these compounds are studied. To prevent this, a **freezing microtome** has been devised in which the tissues are hardened at low temperatures in order to provide the rigidity necessary to permit sectioning. The freezing microtome—and its more elaborate and efficient successor, the **cryostat**—permit sections to be obtained quickly without going through the embedding procedure described above. They are often

*For investigative work this may vary from 1–20 μm.

used in hospitals, for they allow rapid study of pathologic specimens during surgical procedures. They are also effective in the histochemical study of very sensitive enzymes or small molecules, since freezing does not inactivate enzymes and hinders the diffusion of small molecules.

Staining

With few exceptions, most tissues are colorless, so that observing them unstained in the light microscope is difficult. Methods of staining tissues have therefore been devised that not only make various tissue components conspicuous but also permit distinctions to be made among them. This is done by using mixtures of dyes which stain tissue components more or less selectively. Most dyes used in histologic studies behave like acidic or basic compounds and have a tendency to form electrostatic (salt) linkages with ionizable radicals of the tissues. Tissue components that stain more readily with basic dyes are termed **basophilic;** those with an affinity for acid dyes are termed **acidophilic.**

Examples of basic dyes are toluidine blue and methylene blue. Hematoxylin behaves in the manner of a basic dye, ie, it stains the tissues basophilically. The main tissue components that ionize and react with basic dyes do so because of acids in their composition (nucleoproteins and acid mucopolysaccharides). Acid dyes (eg, orange G, eosin, acid fuchsin) stain mostly the basic components present in cytoplasmic proteins. The basic or acid character of a dye usually explains the staining reaction on a chemical basis, but a physical basis is sometimes also present.

Of all dyes, the combination of hematoxylin and eosin (H&E) is most commonly used. Many other dyes are used in different histologic procedures. Although they are useful in visualizing the different tissue components, they usually provide no insight into the chemical nature of the tissue being studied.

Besides tissue staining with dyes, impregnation with such metals as silver and gold is a much used technic, especially in the study of the nervous system. Table 1–3 summarizes some staining technics used in preparing microscope slides.

Since the electrons in the beam of an electron microscope are not of wavelengths in the visible spectrum, colored dyes are not applicable in fine structural studies. In view of their ability to scatter or absorb electrons, heavy metal salts such as lead citrate and uranium acetate are the primary stains used in electron microscopy.

THE LIGHT MICROSCOPE

With the light microscope, stained preparations are usually examined by transillumination.

Table 1—3. Examples of staining technics commonly used in histology.

Technics	Components	Nucleus	Cytoplasm	Collagen	Elastic Fibers	Reticular Fibers
H&E	Hematoxylin and eosin	Blue	Pink	Pink	Irregular	. . .
Masson's trichrome	Iron hematoxylin, acid fuchsin, Ponceau 2R, light green	Black	Red	Green	. . .	Green
Weigert's elastic stain	Resorcin and fuchsin, HCl, hematoxylin, Ponceau's picric acid, glacial acetic acid	Gray	Yellow	Red	Black	. . .
Silver impregnation for reticular fibers	Silver salt solution	. . .	. . .	Dark brown	. . .	Black

The microscope is composed of both mechanical and optical parts. The mechanical components are illustrated in Fig 1–2. The optical components consist of 3 systems of lenses: condenser, objective, and ocular. The **condenser** projects a cone of light to illuminate the object to be observed. (The role of the condenser is usually underestimated because it does not contribute to the magnification; however, its proper use influences the quality of the image observed.) The **objective** lens enlarges the object and projects its image in the direction of the ocular lens. The **ocular** lens further amplifies this image and projects it onto the viewer's retina or onto a screen or photographic plate. The degree of total magnification is obtained by multiplying the magnifying power of the objective and ocular lenses.

Resolution

The critical factor in obtaining a good image with the microscope is the resolution, which is the

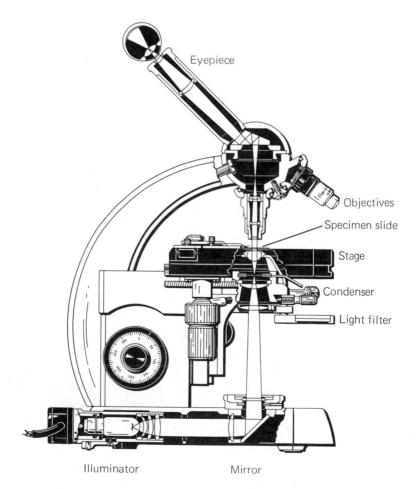

Figure 1 –2. Schematic drawing of a student's light microscope showing its main components and the pathway of light from the source (substage lamp) to the eye of the observer. (Courtesy of Carl Zeiss Co.)

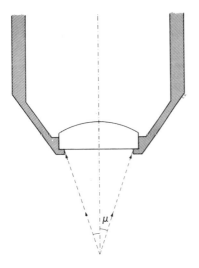

Figure 1–3. Drawing of the light beam which enters the objective lens to show the semiangle of aperture (μ) from which the numerical aperture can be calculated.

resolving power and is only of value when accompanied by a high resolution capacity. The resolving power of a microscope depends mainly on its objective lens. The ocular lens only enlarges the image obtained by the objective; it does not improve resolution. Thus, high magnification with low resolution gives blurred images of little value.

Numerical Aperture

One of the main characteristics of an objective lens is its numerical aperture (NA), for resolution is a function of NA and of the light wavelength employed (Fig 1–3). NA can be defined as the smallest refractive index (n)* observed between the microscopic preparation and the objective multiplied by the sine of the semiangle of aperture of the lens (μ): NA = n × sine μ (Fig 1–3).

The resolution of an objective can be defined by the equation:

$$R = \frac{K \times \lambda}{NA}$$

where K is a constant of 0.61 and λ is the wavelength. Resolution is directly proportionate to the wavelength used and inversely proportionate to the NA. To calculate the resolution when working with white light, a wavelength of 0.55 μm is most often used. This corresponds to yellowish-green, a color to which the human eye is very sensitive. Fig 1–4 is an example of the importance of resolution in microscopy.

smallest distance between 2 particles that can be distinguished from each other. For example, 2 particles will appear distinct if they are separated by a distance of 0.3 μm and the microscope has a resolution factor of 0.2 μm. However, if the same particles are examined with a microscope that has a resolution factor of only 0.5 μm, they will appear as a single point. The resolving power of the best light microscopes is approximately 0.2 μm.

The quality of an image—its clarity and richness of detail—depends on the microscope's resolving power. The **magnification** is independent of its

*The refractive index is a measure of the optical density of an object. A light wave traverses an object readily or otherwise depending on the object's optical density.

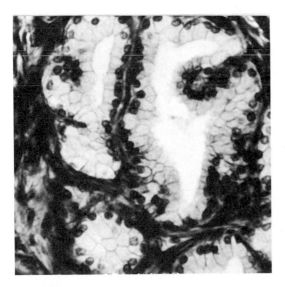
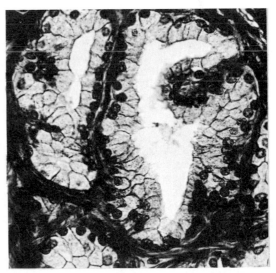

Figure 1–4. Photomicrographs of the same microscopic field at the same magnification (× 350) but with objectives of different numerical apertures (NA). The photomicrograph on the left was made with an objective of NA = 0.22; the one on the right was made with an objective of NA = 1.0. Dog prostate gland stained by Masson's trichrome stain. Observe that the picture at right (NA = 1.0) shows more detail and is sharper than the one on the left.

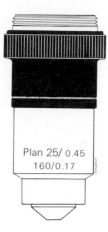

Figure 1–5. Drawing of an objective with the following characteristics: magnification × 25, NA = 0.45, planachromatic, corrected for 160 mm tube and for 0.17 mm coverslips.

An objective lens system often has several numbers engraved on it (Fig 1–5). The first number (upper left) refers to the enlargement; to its right is the NA. The number on the left in the second line is the tube length in millimeters; the number on the right indicates the thickness (in millimeters) of the coverslip for which the objective is corrected. The thickness of the coverslip is important in dry field examination, but when oil immersion is used the oil equalizes the refractive index of the light path between the coverslip and the objective, and the thickness between the usual limits of the coverslip becomes irrelevant.

Objective & Ocular Lenses

Objective and ocular lenses are formed by systems of lenses put together in order to achieve partial correction of their individual defects (aberrations). Although a perfect lens system has not been developed, it is possible to devise objective lenses with increasing optical perfection.

Three common aberrations are as follows:

A. Chromatic Aberration: This type of aberration occurs because spherical lenses bring light of shorter wavelength into focus closer to the retina than light of longer wavelength. Consequently, several slightly separate images of the object are formed and details are blurred. In the **achromatic** lens system, this aberration is corrected to a large extent.

B. Spherical Aberration: In spherical aberration, the quality of the image is hindered because the optical properties of the center of a lens are somewhat different from those of its periphery. In **apochromatic** objective lens systems, complete correction of chromatic and spherical aberrations has been achieved.

C. Curvature of Field: Lenses with this aberration produce an image in which the central field is

in focus while the peripheral field is out of focus or vice versa. **Planar** lenses are corrected to provide "flat field" focus, in which the entire field is in focus.

PHASE CONTRAST MICROSCOPY

Unstained biologic specimens are usually transparent and difficult to view in detail since all parts of the specimen have almost the same optical density. Consequently, another form of microscopy—**phase contrast microscopy**—has been developed that produces in vivo visible images from transparent objects (Fig 1–6).

Phase contrast microscopy is based on the fact that light passing through media with different re-

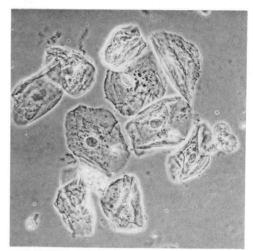

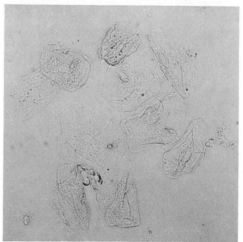

Figure 1–6. Desquamated cells from the oral mucosa. (Unstained fresh preparation.) The top photomicrograph was taken with the phase contrast microscope; the bottom photomicrograph with the standard light microscope. × 300.

fractive indexes slows down and changes direction. Within the cell, different organelles—such as the nuclei, mitochondria, and secretion granules—exhibit different refractive indexes and consequently alter the light passing through them. This forms phase differences between 2 adjoining regions. These phase differences are—by means of a special optical system—transformed into differences of light intensity so that the image becomes visible (Fig 1–6). The examination of fresh tissue or living cells has been facilitated by the development of phase contrast microscopy.

THE POLARIZING MICROSCOPE

When light passes through certain substances or body tissues, it divides in a way that produces 2 light rays from one. This is called **polarization**. It occurs with substances whose atoms have a periodic arrangement. Whether or not this arrangement is apparent, these substances are **crystalline (birefringent)**. Substances that do not belong to the crystalline group are **amorphous (monorefringent)**.

The velocity with which light travels through amorphous substances is always the same regardless of the direction. Therefore, the substance has only one refractive index. In crystalline substances, light velocity changes according to the direction of propagation; from one light ray, 2 refracted rays result. They are polarized rectilinearly, ie, the direction of light vibration follows a determinate direction.

Crystalline calcium carbonate (calcite) is highly birefringent. The **ordinary** ray follows the law of isotropic substances (Descartes' law); the **extraordinary** ray follows slightly different laws.

In the polarizing microscope, the properties of the extraordinary ray are utilized whereas those of the ordinary ray are not. This is achieved with the use of the Nicol prism, made from calcite and balsam. The Nicol prism permits only the passage of rectilinearly polarized light; the ordinary ray is eliminated by total reflection.

Sheets of **Polaroid film** are most often used at present. They contain special organic compounds so disposed that ordinary vibration is totally absorbed, resulting in a uniform field superior to that provided by the Nicol prism.

If this polarized light is transmitted to a second Nicol prism or Polaroid plate similar to the first, it does not pass through when the main axes of the 2 prisms or plates are crossed. In any other position, light is transmitted with greater or lesser intensity.

Principle of the Polarizing Microscope

The polarizing microscope contains a rotating stage with 2 polarizing elements: one located under the stage—the **polarizer**—and the other located above it, adjacent to the eyepiece on the **analyzer**.

The polarizer and the analyzer are placed so that their main axes are perpendicular, thus preventing the appearance of light in the eyepiece. When the stage contains an amorphous object, there is no light because the light rays are not modified. However, when a crystalline or birefringent object is placed on the stage, light appears with greater or lesser intensity in the microscope field, depending on the orientation of the analyzer. The usual test is to rotate the specimen to find the points of maximum and minimum brightness.

With the polarizing microscope it is therefore possible to distinguish between monorefringent and birefringent substances. With birefringent substances, it is now possible to discern their internal arrangement and their orientation at the submicroscopic level.

Although the birefringence observed in biologic specimens is generally weak, such crystalline or semicrystalline substances as bone tissue, cellulose walls, structures with linear symmetry (collagen, muscle fibers, nerve fibers, cilia, flagella), and structures with radial symmetry (starch granules, lipid droplets) can be easily studied by making use of this principle.

ELECTRON MICROSCOPY

The principle upon which electron microscopy is based can be understood by referring to the following equation (used above to calculate the resolution in the light microscope):

$$R = \frac{K \times \lambda}{NA}$$

where K is a constant of 0.61. The wavelength (λ) of an electron beam accelerated by 60 kV is approximately 0.005 nm, which gives a very high theoretic resolution. In practice, however, a resolution of 1 nm in tissue sections is considered to be quite satisfactory. This by itself permits enlargements to be obtained up to 200 times greater than those achieved with the light microscope.

The electron microscope functions on the principle that a beam of electrons can be deflected by electromagnetic fields in a manner similar to light deflection in glass lenses. Electrons are produced by high-temperature heating of a metallic filament (cathode) in a vacuum. The electrons emitted are then submitted to a difference of potential of approximately 60–100 kV or more between the cathode and the anode (Fig 1–7). The anode has the shape of a metallic plate with a small hole in its center. Electrons are accelerated from the cathode to the anode. Some of these particles pass through the central orifice of the anode, forming a constant

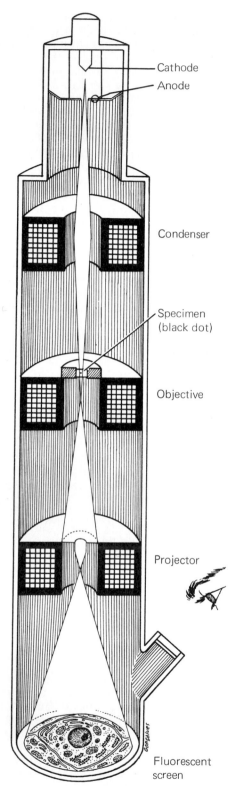

Figure 1 –7. Pathway of the electron beam in the electron microscope. The ultrathin section is placed just over the objective electromagnetic lens. The image is projected on a fluorescent screen and observed directly or through a × 10 magnifying optical system.

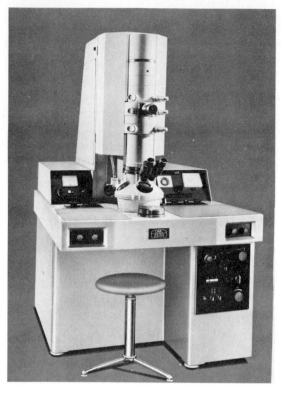

Figure 1 –8. Photograph of the Zeiss model EM 9A electron microscope. (Courtesy of Carl Zeiss Co.)

stream (or beam) of electrons. This beam is deflected by electromagnetic lenses in a way roughly analogous to that which occurs in the optical microscope. Thus, the condenser focuses the beam at the object plane and the objective forms an image of the object. The image obtained is further enlarged by 1–2 projecting lenses and is finally projected on a fluorescent screen or photographic plate (Figs 1–7 and 1–8).

Differences Between Electron & Light Microscopes

In contrast to what happens in the light microscope, the enlargement produced by the objective in the electron microscope is fixed (or unvariable). The enlargements are produced by changes in the magnetic field of the projecting "lenses," which are analogous to the "zoom" ocular lens in the light microscope.

Because electrons are easily scattered or absorbed by the object, one must use very thin sections of tissue—usually 0.02–0.1 μm. Another characteristic of the electron microscope is that the electrons are scattered or absorbed by portions of the object with high molecular weight, whereas in the light microscope light is absorbed by stained structures. The scattered electrons are absorbed by the aperture of the objective lens (usually a diameter of 25–100 μm). The aperture filters out the scattered electrons that thus do not contribute to image formation. The structures that scatter electrons thus appear in the fluorescent screen as dark bodies (electron-dense regions). The capacity to scatter electrons depends on the molecular weight (and therefore the density) of a given particle. Heavy metals (eg, uranium, lead) are therefore used to impregnate tissue sections; they increase contrast and permit better images.

Limitations in the Use of the Electron Microscope

The nature of the electron beam requires that work with the electron microscope be done in high vacuum with very thin sections. These conditions preclude the use of living material. Additionally, the action of an electron beam on an object can damage it and can produce unwanted changes in tissue structures. Electron microscopy is a rapidly developing field, however. Recent advances include the use of high-voltage (500,000–1,000,000 V) electron microscopes in which the high speed of acceleration of the electrons in the beam allows the penetration and consequently the visualization of relatively thick plastic sections (1–5 μm). The development of a phase (Crewe) electron microscope

has permitted direct visualization of atoms. Other recent advances in electron microscopy include instruments that provide higher resolution and the use of live specimens.

PROBLEMS IN THE INTERPRETATION OF TISSUE SECTIONS

During the study and interpretation of stained tissue sections in microscope preparations, it should be remembered that the observed product is the end result of a series of processes which considerably distort the image observable in the living tissue, mainly through shrinking and retraction. As a consequence of these processes, the spaces frequently seen between the cells and other tissue components are artifacts. Furthermore, there is a tendency to think in terms of only 2 dimensions when examining thin sections, whereas in actuality the structures from which the sections are made have 3 dimensions. In order to understand the architecture of an organ, it is therefore necessary to study sections made in different planes and to reason accordingly (Fig 1–9).

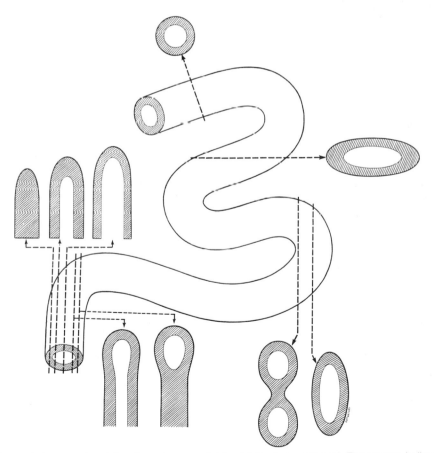

Figure 1–9. Some of the aspects a tube-shaped organ might exhibit when sectioned. The arrows indicate what is seen under the microscope in each particular section plane.

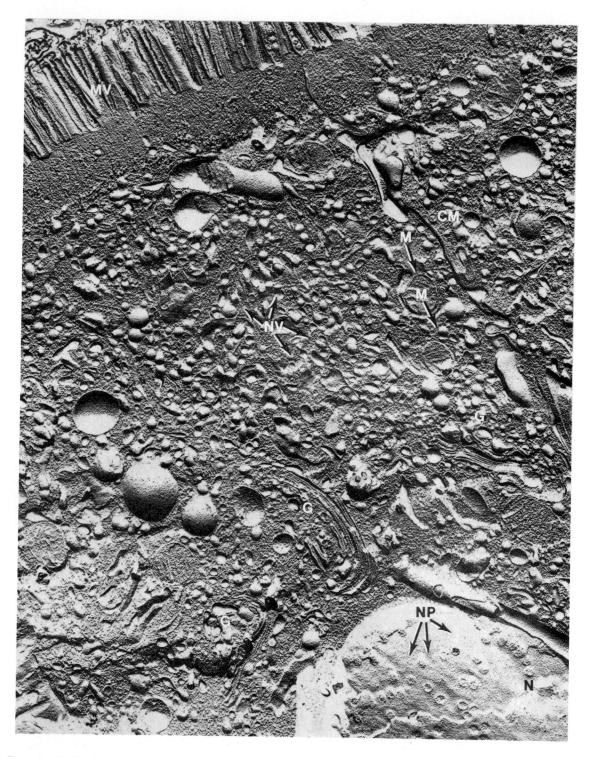

Figure 1–10. Electron micrograph of a mouse intestinal epithelial cell. This picture was obtained by a process called freeze etching. It consists of freezing a fragment of tissue to very low temperatures and fracturing it with a sharpened metal blade. The fractured surface is kept at low temperature in a vacuum environment. A portion of the water in the surface thus sublimates, giving a bas-relief effect (etching). A replica of this surface is then obtained by covering it with a layer of platinum and carbon. In this picture, one can observe in material that has not been submitted to the processes of embedding and sectioning the presence of the various cell components described by classic transmission electron microscopy, eg, microvilli (MV), cell membrane (CM), mitochondria (M), Golgi apparatus (G), nucleus (N), nuclear pores (NP), and nuclear vesicles (NV). × 24,000. (Courtesy of LS Staehelin.)

The **serial sectioning technic** is often used in the study of organ and tissue structure. In this technic, sequential serial sections of a whole organ or an organ fragment are prepared and studied. By analysis of each section in the sequence in which it was prepared, information on the 3-dimensional architecture of the organ can be gained.

Another difficulty in the study of microscope preparations is the impossibility of differentially staining all tissue components on only one slide. It is therefore necessary to examine several preparations stained by different methods before a general idea of the composition and structure of any type of tissue can be obtained.

FREEZE FRACTURE & FREEZE ETCHING

The technic of freeze fracture, combined with freeze etching, is a new development in electron microscopy that permits examination of tissues without fixation and embedding. Although it is not free of artifacts, this technic is useful for verifying the results obtained with the conventional technic in which ultrathin sections of fixed tissue are examined under the electron microscope. The freeze fracture technic confirmed what we already knew about cell ultrastructure and has furnished new information regarding the structure of the cell membrane and associated structures.

The technic of cell fracture consists of freezing a fragment of tissue at very low temperatures and then fracturing it with a sharp metal blade. The fractured tissue is kept at low temperature in a high-vacuum environment. During this step the water sublimates, leaving a dehydrated surface of the fractured tissues. Still in a vacuum environment, a replica of this surface is obtained by deposition of a layer of carbon. Over the carbon replica, a layer of a heavy metal (gold, platinum) is deposited at an angle, thus giving a shadowed aspect when viewed with the electron microscope. After the deposition of carbon and heavy metal, the whole assembly is brought to normal atmospheric pressure; the tissue is destroyed, usually by a strong acid. The replica is then placed over a copper grid of the same type used in standard electron microscopy. Fig 1–10 shows the replica of a freeze-fractured mouse intestinal epithelial cell in which most cell organelles can be seen, thus confirming their structure as shown by conventional transmission electron microscopy.

SCANNING ELECTRON MICROSCOPY

A variant of electron microscopy called scanning electron microscopy, in use since 1963, permits 3-dimensional analysis of surfaces. The scanning electron microscope possesses a deflection layer between the electromagnetic lens and the object, which causes a deflection of the electron beam so that it is incident upon the object, and scans point by point, in a sequence with determined time. The electrons do not pass through the object because of its thickness and because of a coating formed by the deposition of heavy metal (eg, gold) on its surface. In this way, the electron beam—called the primary beam—is reflected. Secondary electrons are created and are caught by special detectors that make electrical signals which are then transferred to a television tube. The tube gives a 3-dimensional image of the object's surface.

A scanning electron micrograph illustrating the surface of the oocyte before and after fertilization and the initial stages of the formation of a morula is shown in Fig 24–16.

RADIOAUTOGRAPHY

Radioautography permits the localization of radioactive substances in cells or tissues by means of the effect of emitted radiation on photographic emulsions. Silver bromide crystals present in the emulsion act as microdetectors of radioactivity. In radioautography, tissue sections obtained from animals previously treated with radioactive compounds are covered with photographic emulsion by dipping mounted specimens in a glass container filled with a warmed mixture of gelatin and silver bromide (Fig 1–11). The slide, now covered with this thin layer of emulsion, is then dried and stored in a light-proof box in a refrigerator. After different exposure times depending on the experiment and the radioactive element, the slides are developed photographically and examined. All silver bromide crystals hit by radiation are reduced to small black granules, which indicate the existence of radioactivity in the structures in contact with these granules. The location and amount of radiation are thus determined, and the quantity of silver granules is proportionate to the intensity of the radioactivity present. The tissue is then stained with regular stains and the preparation is mounted in resin and covered with a coverslip. This procedure can be employed in electron microscopy by using thin sections of resin-embedded radioactively-labeled tissue. In this type of radioautography, the granules usually appear as short, coiled filaments (Fig 1–12).

In light microscopy, radioautography permits distinction of radioactive particles that are 1 μm

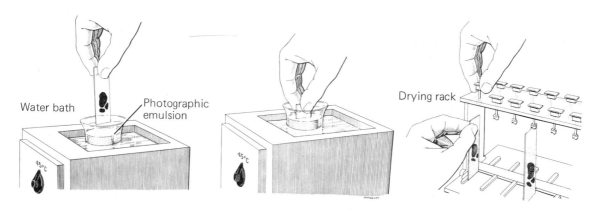

Water bath   Photographic emulsion   Drying rack

Figure 1–11. Radioautographs are usually made by dipping labeled tissues fixed on slides in photographic emulsion. All steps shown above are made in the darkroom under a dark red safelight.

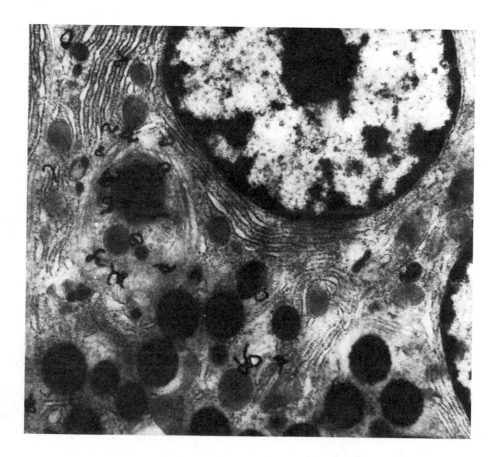

Figure 1–12. Radioautograph observed under the electron microscope. Section of pancreas of a rat killed 20 minutes after a labeled injection of ^{3}H-tryptophan. The coiled black filaments appear in the developed photograph emulsion, indicating radioactive spots in the cell. Silver deposits, which appear as dots under the light microscope, usually exhibit a coiled structure under the electron microscope. Radioactivity is mainly concentrated in the granular endoplasmic reticulum and in the secretory granules. × 5000. (Courtesy of A Sesso.)

apart. It therefore has a resolving power (or resolution) of 1 μm; in electron microscopy, this resolution is increased 5–10 times.

Radioautography is often used to study important dynamic biologic phenomena. As soon as it became possible to synthesize radioactive isotopes of normal metabolites with the aid of carbon 14 (^{14}C) and tritium (^{3}H), it was possible to study not only different metabolic pathways in tissue specimens but also the speed with which metabolic processes occurred. For example, the metabolism of proteins and nucleic acids can be studied by injecting labeled amino acids and nucleosides into animals. In both cases, the precursors are incorporated within the tissues and cells into protein or nucleic acids and can be localized and quantitated with the aid of radioautography. If a fixed unit of time is used in the experiments, it is possible to estimate the speed of the metabolic process under study. The metabolism of proteins, carbohydrates, lipids, and nucleic acids has been localized and analyzed using this procedure. Specific examples include localization of the site and time of DNA synthesis in the nucleus and in mitochondria as well as the sulfation of glycoproteins at the Golgi apparatus of the goblet and fibroblast cells.

EXAMINATION OF LIVING CELLS & TISSUES

Living cells from the body of an animal can be suspended in an appropriate liquid (saline solution, serum) and examined under the light microscope. Such cells, however, will soon die by a process known as autolysis if they are not provided with an appropriate medium and gaseous atmosphere (described on p 40).

Prolonged study of living cells and tissues can be achieved by culturing them in solutions that contain the necessary nutrients to keep them alive. The culture medium should be changed frequently since the nutrients become depleted and toxic products of metabolism accumulate. Rigorous aseptic technic is necessary during the process of cell cultivation in order to avoid contamination of the culture medium.

The first culture media used consisted of blood plasma and an extract from embryonic tissues, and the composition of the fluid was complicated and difficult to control. Synthetic media of rigidly defined chemical composition are now available. In preparing cultures, the cells can be dispersed mechanically or by prior treatment with enzymes such as trypsin or collagenase.

Once isolated, the cells can be cultivated in a suspension or spread out on a culture plate surface to which they can adhere as a single layer of cells (Fig 1–13).

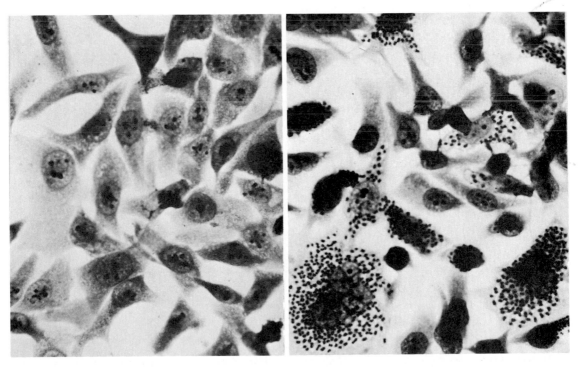

Figure 1–13. Photomicrographs of chicken fibroblasts grown in tissue culture. ***Left:*** Normal cells. ***Right:*** Fibroblasts infected by *Trypanosoma cruzi*. Giemsa staining was used. × 340. (Courtesy of S Yoneda.)

Organs can also be cultured, starting from the respective embryonic rudiments. For example, a small bone can be maintained in a culture and allowed to grow. This technic permits study of the factors that influence the development of the organs in conditions much simpler than those that exist inside the living organism. The term organ culture means primarily the culture of fragments of organs maintained in conditions such that the architecture of the organ is kept intact.

Cultures have been used for the study of the metabolism of normal and cancerous cells. This technic is most useful in experiments with viruses that proliferate only in the interior of cells. Some protozoa have also been studied in tissue culture to observe their development inside the cytoplasm (Fig 1–13).

In cytogenetic research, tissue cultures permit the study of mitoses and of chromosomes in human cells. Determination of human karyotypes (the number and morphology of an individual's chromosomes) is accomplished by the short-term cultivation of blood lymphocytes or of skin fibroblasts. In examining these cells during mitotic division, one can detect anomalies in the number and morphology of the chromosomes, thus perhaps establishing the diagnosis of certain diseases caused by these anomalies.

THE ISOLATION & STUDY IN VITRO OF PURE CELL STRAINS

Recently, new technics have been developed that permit the isolation of pure fractions of one cell type, such as the pancreatic acinar cell, the liver cell, and the parietal cell of the stomach. In the body these cells are mixed with other cell types, and this hinders their biochemical and cytophysiologic study. Isolated cancer cells, which are usually mixed with blood vessels and connective tissue cells, can now be studied in pure cell preparations.

All methods used are based on the enzymatic digestion of the cellular and extracellular components that bind cells together. The most used enzymes are proteases, collagenase, and hyaluronidase. The incubation of tissue with these enzymes loosens the cells, and they are then separated by weak shearing forces (agitation, pipetting, etc). The cell suspension with different cell types is then purified by centrifugal fractionation or by gravity sedimentation. This last procedure consists of gently depositing a cell suspension on the surface of a gradient of albumin. The cells slowly settle in the solution of albumin, stopping at different heights according to their density.

These methods will permit a much more accurate study of the biology of some cell types.

DIFFERENTIAL CENTRIFUGATION

Differential centrifugation is the physical process by which centrifugal force is used to separate organelles and cellular inclusions as a function of the sedimentation coefficient of each one. The sedimentation coefficient of a particle depends on its size, form, and density and on the viscosity of the medium. If a cell is subjected to an adequate centrifugal force, the organelles inside the cell will be distributed in different layers (Fig 1–14). In each layer, one finds only one type of organelle, and its position inside the cell depends on its coefficient of sedimentation.

By means of the technic of centrifugation, any cellular organelle can be isolated and its chemical composition and its functions determined in vitro.

Differential centrifugation is achieved by subjecting a suspension of cellular elements obtained by a process called **homogenization** to the action of different centrifugal forces (Fig 1–15).

The organ or tissue from a recently killed ani-

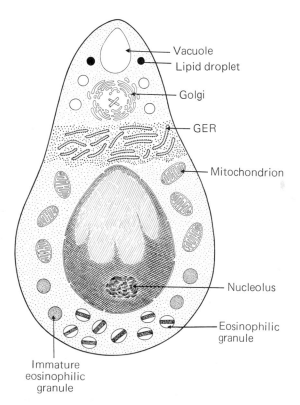

Figure 1–14. Stratification seen in an immature eosinophil after centrifugation. Cell components of higher density (eosinophilic granules, nucleus) accumulate at the bottom of the cell, whereas lighter organelles (Golgi, granular endoplasmic reticulum [GER]) are displaced to the opposite side. (Redrawn and reproduced, with permission, from Bessis in: The Cell. Vol 5. Brachet J, Mirsky AE [editors]. Academic Press, 1961.)

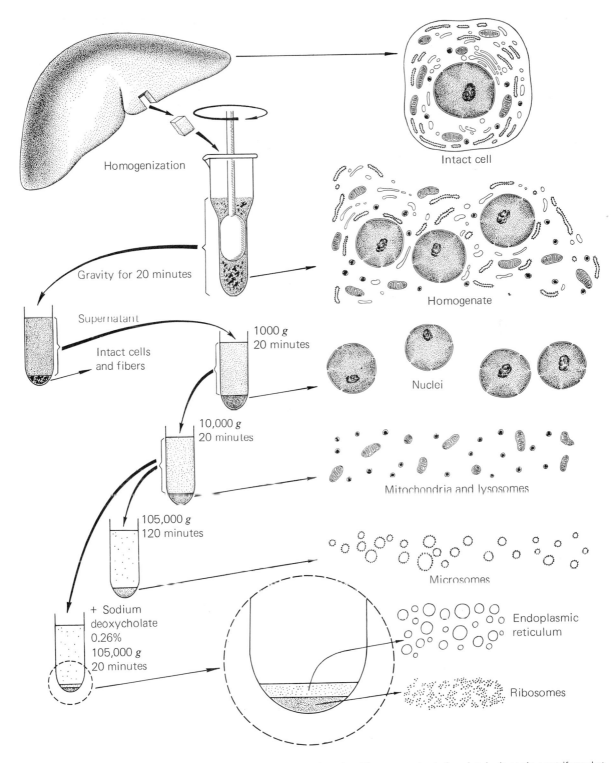

Figure 1–15. Isolation of cell constituents by differential centrifugation. The supernatant of each tube is again centrifuged at higher speeds. The drawings at right show the cellular organelles at the bottom of each tube after centrifugation. Centrifugal force is expressed by *g*, which is equivalent to the force of gravity (1000 *g* means a force 1000 times stronger than that of the gravitational field). (Redrawn and reproduced, with permission, from Bloom W, Fawcett DW: *A Textbook of Histology,* 9th ed. Saunders, 1968.)

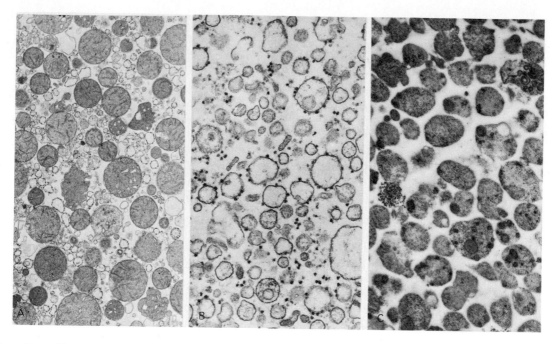

Figure 1–16. Electron micrographs of 3 cell fractions isolated by density gradient centrifugation. *A:* Mitochondrial fraction, contaminated with microsomes. × 13,000. *B:* Microsomal fraction. × 42,500. *C:* Lysosomal fraction. × 25,000. (Courtesy of P Baudhuin.)

mal is cut into very small fragments, which are then immersed in an appropriate solution. Sucrose in an 0.25 M concentration is often used, but the density and viscosity of the medium can vary.

The fragments of the organ with the solution of sucrose are placed in a homogenizer, usually consisting of a glass cylinder within which is a rod that turns with great velocity (Fig 1–15). The fragments of the tissues are crushed by the friction of the rod on the wall of the cylinder, breaking the cell membranes and liberating the organelles and the inclusions into the solution.

After homogenization is complete, the suspension is allowed to rest for a few minutes so that the fibers of connective tissue, large cell remnants, and intact cells can settle out. The supernatant is then centrifuged, and the more dense particles (organelles or inclusions) sediment first. The supernatant from each centrifugation is subjected again to greater centrifugal force, thus separating out the different cellular components, in decreasing order of their density, as shown in Fig 1–15.

An improvement in the technic of differential centrifugation is centrifugation against a gradient, or **zonal centrifugation.** The gradient consists of a sucrose solution whose concentration (density) is maximal at the bottom of the tube and minimal at the top, with a gradual increase in concentration from top to bottom. The homogenate is placed on top of this stabilized gradient and centrifuged. The particles penetrate the gradient, but do so only to a

level where an equilibrium exists between the action of the centrifugal force and the tendency of the particle to float. This technic permits one to obtain purer fractions of organelles.

In contrast to the continuous gradient just described, one can use a discontinuous gradient, which is made up of superimposed zones whose density decreases from one zone to the other, starting from the bottom and proceeding to the top of the centrifuge tube.

All of the stages of the technics described are carried out at a temperature slightly higher than the freezing point in order to combat the action of enzyme systems that would disrupt the organelles during the separation.

Control of the purity of the fractions thus obtained is carried out with the light microscope (for nuclei, mitochondria, and secretory granules), with the electron microscope (for ribosomes, microsomes, etc) (Fig 1–16), or with chemical methods. For example, the fraction that contains the lysosomes can be identified by the quantity of acid phosphatase, an enzyme usually found in these particles, while the fraction containing the nuclei can be identified by the quantity of DNA present in it.

The isolation of cellular components by differential centrifugation represents a great technical advance and allows the detailed study of cellular components that have been obtained in a relatively pure state, ie, nuclei, nucleoli, mitochondria, granular endoplasmic reticulum, ribosomes, secretory granules, and pigment granules. An example of the application of this method is the study of the physiology of mitochondria; after much discussion, it was established by the isolation of these organelles and confirmed in vitro that they are responsible for the processes of liberation of energy and for storage of ATP.

● ● ●

References

Allfrey V: The isolation of subcellular components. In: *The Cell*. Vol 1. Brachet J, Mirsky AE (editors). Academic Press, 1960.

Baker JR: *Cytological Technique*, 4th ed. Methuen, 1960.

Baserga R, Malamud D: *Autoradiography: Techniques and Application*. Harper & Row, 1969.

Caro LG: High resolution autoradiography. In: *Methods in Cell Physiology*. Vol 1. Prescott DM (editor). Academic Press, 1964.

Everhart TE, Hayes TL: The scanning electron microscope. Sci Am 226:54, Jan 1972.

Hayat MA. *Principles and Techniques of Electron Microscopy*. Vol 1. Van Nostrand Reinhold, 1970.

Humason GL: *Animal Tissue Techniques*. Freeman, 1962.

Kopac MJ: Microsurgical studies on living cells. In: *The Cell*. Vol 1. Brachet J, Mirsky AE (editors). Academic Press, 1960.

Kopriwa BM, Leblond CP: Improvements in the coating technique of radioautography. J Histochem Cytochem 10:269, 1962.

Lillie RD: *Histopathologic Technique and Practical Histochemistry*, 2nd ed. Blakiston, 1954.

McManus JFA, Mowry RW: *Staining Methods: Histologic and Histochemical*. Hoeber, 1960.

Parker RC: *Methods of Tissue Culture*, 3rd ed. Hoeber, 1961.

Rogers AW: *Techniques of Autoradiography*, 2nd ed. Elsevier, 1973.

Salpeter MM, Bachmann L: Assessment of technical steps in electron microscope autoradiography. In: *The Use of Radioautography in Investigating Protein Synthesis*. Leblond CP, Warren KB (editors). Academic Press, 1965.

2 | Histochemistry & Cytochemistry

The chemistry of tissues and cells is studied by both microscopic and chemical analytic methods. Chemical substances in tissues and cells can be identified by chemical reactions that produce insoluble colored compounds—observed with the light microscope—or electron scattering of precipitates that can be observed with the electron microscope. In Perls's reaction, for example, potassium ferrocyanide reacts with ferric ions in the tissues to produce an insoluble dark blue precipitate of ferric ferrocyanide.

In addition to the chemical reactions that take place in the tissues, other methods—chiefly physical ones—are frequently used. Examples are interference microscopy, which permits determination of the mass of cells or tissues; and microspectrophotometry, which permits, by means of ultraviolet light, localization and quantitation of DNA and RNA in the cells.

BASIC HISTOCHEMICAL & CYTOCHEMICAL PRINCIPLES

For a histochemical reaction to be recognized as valid and meaningful, it must fulfill the following basic requirements:

(1) The substances being analyzed must not diffuse out of their original sites. This problem is easily solved when macromolecules (eg, DNA, proteins) are analyzed. However, when the substance is soluble in the fixative used or in the medium where the reaction is taking place—as in the case of urea and glycogen and of sodium, potassium, or chloride ions—special care must be exercised in the interpretation of the results. Fixatives should preserve the structure of the cell and prevent diffusion of compounds to be studied. For example, the fixatives used to study lipids should not contain lipid solvents, and acid fixatives should not be used in technics for identifying calcium phosphate since calcium phosphate is soluble in an acid medium. The fixatives most commonly used are formaldehyde (formalin) for light microscopic and glutaraldehyde for electron microscopic histochemical procedures.

(2) The product of the reaction should be insoluble and colored or electron-scattering. Insolubility prevents diffusion of the product of the reaction into the fluid reagent or its spread to a different site in the specimen. A colored or electron-scattering product can be studied with the light or electron microscope.

(3) The method employed should be specific for the substance or chemical groups being studied.

(4) The procedure must not denature or block reactive groups.

In some histochemical reactions, the intensity of color produced is directly proportionate to the concentration of the substance being analyzed. The concentration of the substances under study can be determined by **histophotometry.** This procedure is carried out in a histophotometer, a combination microscope and spectrophotometer. By measuring the light absorbed by small areas of a cell or a tissue, it is possible to quantitate chemical substances in this region. This method has recently been much improved by the introduction of scanning devices that analyze with great precision the optical density of the images produced by the cytochemical method and relay the information to a computer that processes the results. This method is of great importance for it permits the analysis of a specific cell type in tissues that present various cell types, a frequent occurrence in nature.

SOME EXAMPLES OF HISTOCHEMICAL METHODS FOR SUBSTANCES OF BIOLOGIC INTEREST

Ions

A. Iron: When sections of tissues containing ferric ions (Fe^{3+}) are incubated in a mixture of potassium ferrocyanide and hydrochloric acid, the ions can be detected by the formation of a highly insoluble, dark blue precipitate of ferric ferrocyanide (Perls's reaction). This method not only allows localization in the tissues of cells that catabolize hemoglobin but also permits diagnosis of diseases in which deposits of iron occur in the tissues.

B. Phosphates: Phosphates are demonstrated by reacting with silver nitrate. The silver phosphate formed is, in the following phase of the reaction, reduced by hydroquinone, thus forming a black precipitate of reduced silver (Fig 2–1). This reaction is frequently used to study bone and the ossification process because the only insoluble phosphate found abundantly in the body is calcium phosphate, which is present in large amounts in bone tissue.

Lipids

Lipids are best revealed with dyes that are more soluble in them than in the medium in which they are dissolved.

In this process, frozen sections are immersed in alcoholic solutions saturated with the appropriate dyes. The stain then migrates from the alcohol to the cellular lipid droplets. The dyes most commonly used for this purpose are Sudan IV and Sudan black; they confer on lipids red and black colors, respectively (Fig 2–2).

Additional methods used for the localization of cholesterol and its esters, phospholipids, and glycolipids are useful in the diagnosis of metabolic diseases in which intracellular accumulations of different kinds of lipids occur.

Nucleic Acids

A. Deoxyribonucleic Acid (DNA): DNA is studied chiefly with Feulgen's reaction, a method that starts with the hydrolysis of DNA by hydrochloric acid. This process separates purine bases from sugar, promoting the formation of aldehyde groups in deoxyribose. The free aldehyde groups then react with the Schiff reagent (basic fuchsin bleached by sulfurous anhydride), producing an insoluble red substance. By using this staining procedure in conjunction with histophotometry, it is possible to quantitate the content of DNA in the nuclei of cells.

B. Ribonucleic Acid (RNA): RNA can be identified in tissues by virtue of its great affinity for basic stains (basophilia)—eg, it stains intensely with toluidine blue or methylene blue. Since RNA is not the only basophilic substance in the tissue, it is necessary to incubate a control slide with ribonuclease, an enzyme that destroys RNA. Any structure that loses its basophilia as a result of pretreatment with ribonuclease is considered to contain RNA.

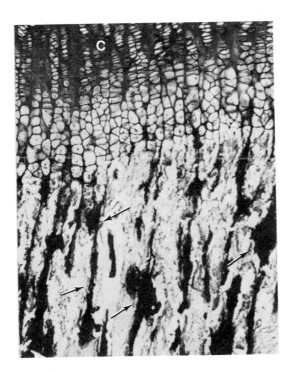

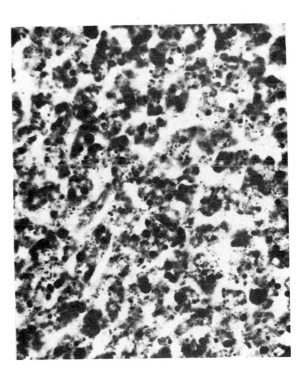

Figure 2–1. Photomicrograph of a section from the epiphysis of an undecalcified bone treated with silver nitrate and subsequently reduced by hydroquinone. The black precipitate in the ossified tissue (arrows) indicates the presence of calcium phosphate. Nonreacting cartilage tissue (C) lies in the upper portion of the section. × 120.

Figure 2–2. Photomicrograph of a section of puppy liver stained by Sudan black. Observe the stained intracellular lipid droplets. × 200.

Proteins

Reactions for nonspecific demonstration of proteins in tissues and cells are based chiefly on methods of identifying amino acids. Localization and, sometimes, quantitation of proteins in tissues can be done by means of reactions that produce a color with tyrosine (Millon reaction), tryptophan (tetrazotized benzidine; Fig 2–3), and arginine (Sakaguchi reaction). The Sakaguchi reaction is used frequently in the study of the distribution of basic proteins in nuclei (eg, histones and protamines, which are both rich in arginine). There are also methods for studying the abundant SH and SS groups of certain proteins such as keratin.

Polysaccharides

Polysaccharides in the body occur either in a free state or combined with proteins. In the combined state, they constitute an extremely complex heterogeneous group. A ubiquitous polysaccharide in the body not bound to protein is **glycogen,** which can be demonstrated by the periodic acid-Schiff (PAS) reaction. The PAS reaction, based on the oxidative action of periodic acid (HIO_4) on 1,2-glycol groups present in the glucose residues, gives rise to aldehyde groups as shown in the following equation:

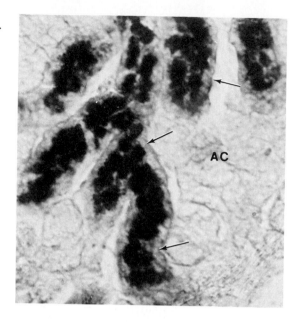

Figure 2–3. Section of mouse submandibular gland stained by the tetrazotized benzidine method for proteins containing tryptophan. The acinar cells (AC) show no reaction; the tubules (arrows) are filled with strongly reacting secretory granules. (Courtesy of LC Bruschi.)

$$\text{Glucose moiety in glycogen} \quad + HIO_4 \longrightarrow \quad \text{Aldehyde moiety}$$

As in Feulgen's reaction, these aldehyde groups react with bleached fuchsin (Schiff's reagent), producing a new complex compound having an insoluble purple or magenta color. This can be seen in the light microscope, and we call such substances PAS-positive. Since other PAS-positive substances occur in cells, the specificity of this reaction depends on pretreatment with a glycogenolytic enzyme (eg, salivary amylase). Structures that stain intensely with the PAS reaction but fail to do so after pretreatment with amylase are considered to contain glycogen. Using this method, glycogen can be demonstrated in normal liver and striated muscle. It also permits the diagnosis of several diseases in which abnormal intracellular accumulations of glycogen are observed.

A variety of anionic, unbranched long chain polysaccharides composed of aminated monosaccharides (amino sugars) constitute the **glycosaminoglycans** (formerly known as mucopolysaccharides). These substances contain chains of repeating units of amino sugars. Complexes of covalently bound glycosaminoglycans inserted at regular intervals along a protein core comprise the **proteoglycans.** In proteoglycans, which are significant constituents of connective tissue matrices (see Chapters 5 and 7), the carbohydrate moieties constitute the major component of the molecule. The term **glycoprotein** is currently used to designate macromolecules of protein containing lesser amounts of carbohydrate that are not in the form of regular repeating units, as are the proteoglycans. Glycoproteins such as thyroglobulin present in thyroid gland and gonadotropins of the pituitary contain a high proportion of protein. Other glycoproteins with a low protein content, such as those produced by some epithelial cells, are identified as **mucous substances.** Some glycoproteins contain no acid groups (ie, neutral glycoproteins); others have limited amounts of carboxyl or sulfate radicals (ie, acid mucous substances). The carbohydrate moiety of proteoglycans and glycoproteins containing sulfate and carboxyl groups react strongly with the alcian blue dye (Figs 2–4 and 2–5). Neutral glyco-

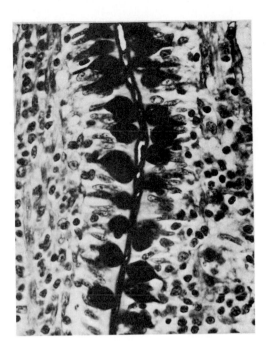

Figure 2 –4. Photomicrograph of an intestinal villus stained by alcian blue. The goblet cells stain intensely because of their high content of glycosaminoglycans. × 400.

proteins can be identified in tissue sections by the fact that they react with the PAS method but are not digested by prior incubation with a glycogenolytic enzyme. Using specific enzymes that digest proteoglycans and some glycoprotein components, one can distinguish these substances in tissue sections.

Catecholamines

The fact that formaldehyde reacts with catecholamines to produce fluorescent compounds makes it possible to localize epinephrine (adrenaline) and norepinephrine (noradrenaline) in tissue. This method is founded on the observation that ring hydroxylated phenylethylamines, indolealkylamines, and their corresponding amino acids are converted to fluorescent complexes in the presence of relatively dry formaldehyde vapor at 60–80 C. This reaction has been helpful in studying the distribution of catecholamines and their precursors in neuronal pathways, cell bodies, and nerve endings.

Enzymes

Many histochemical methods are used to reveal and identify enzymes. When unstable enzymes are studied, sections of frozen, unfixed material must be used. However, many enzymes may retain

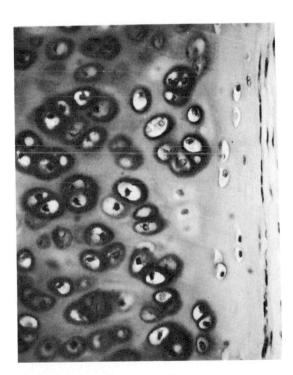

Figure 2 –5. Photomicrograph of a section of hyaline cartilage stained with PAS and alcian blue. The region of the matrix close to the cartilage cells contains an abundance of acidic proteoglycans and stains blue with the alcian method. The rest of the matrix contains neutral glycoproteins which stain red using the PAS method.

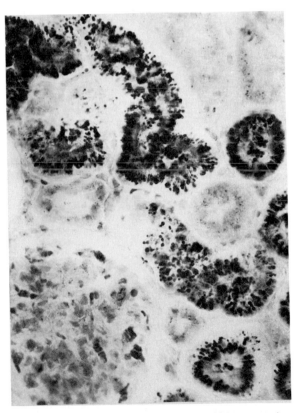

Figure 2 –6. Photomicrograph of a rat kidney section treated by the lead acid phosphatase method. The lysosomes stain intensely as dark granules present in the proximal convoluted tubule cells. × 400.

their activity in tissues fixed with aldehyde fixatives such as formalin or glutaraldehyde. Most enzymatic histochemical procedures are based on the production of intensely stained or electron-dense precipitates at the site of enzymatic activity. Three examples of enzymes that can be demonstrated by either the light or the electron microscope are described below:

A. Acid Phosphatase: One method of demonstrating acid phosphatase activity consists of incubating formalin-fixed tissue sections in a solution containing sodium glycerophosphate and lead nitrate buffered to pH 5.0. The enzyme hydrolyzes the glycerophosphate, liberating the phosphate ion that reacts with lead nitrate to produce an insoluble, colorless precipitate of lead phosphate at the site of the enzymatic activity. In a second step, the preparation is immersed in a solution of ammonium sulfide that reacts with the colorless lead phosphate to produce a black precipitate of lead sulfide. This method permits the localization of this enzyme's activity and is frequently used to demonstrate **lysosomes,** cytoplasmic organelles that contain acid phosphatase (Figs 2–6 and 2–7).

B. Dehydrogenases: These enzymes remove hydrogen from one substrate and transfer it to another. There are many different dehydrogenases

in the body; they play an important role in several metabolic processes and can be distinguished by means of the substrate on which they act. The histochemical demonstration of dehydrogenases consists of incubating nonfixed tissue sections in an adequate substrate containing **tetrazole,** a weakly stained, soluble H^+ acceptor. The enzyme transports hydrogen from the substrate to tetrazole and reduces it to an intensely stained insoluble compound called **formazan,** which precipitates at the site of the enzymatic activity. By this method, succinate dehydrogenase—a key enzyme in the citric acid (Krebs) cycle—can be localized in mitochondria (Fig 2–8).

C. Peroxidase: This enzyme, which is present in several types of cells, promotes the reduction of certain substrates with the transfer of hydrogen ions

$$
\begin{array}{ccccccccc}
& & OH & & & & & & O \\
OH & & | & & & & & & \| \\
| & + & R & + & Peroxidase & \rightarrow & 2H_2O & + & R \\
OH & & | & & & & & & \| \\
& & OH & & & & & & O \\
\end{array}
$$

Hydrogen   Substrate   Insoluble and
peroxide   electron-dense
                                                                 precipitate

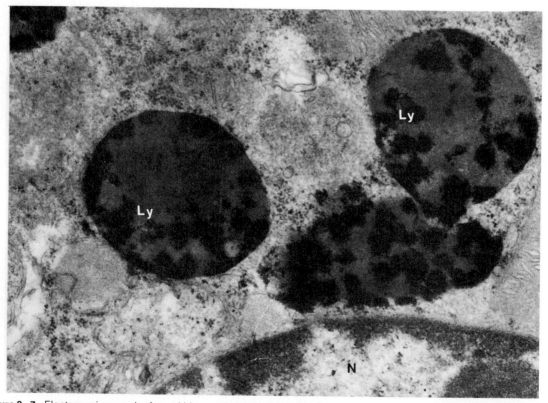

Figure 2–7. Electron micrograph of a rat kidney cell previously treated by the Gomori method for acid phosphatase. The 3 dark, rounded structures above the nucleus (N) are lysosomes (Ly). The denser heterogeneous precipitate within these structures is the lead phosphate that scatters the electrons. The information in this electron micrograph is equivalent to that in the light micrograph illustrated in Fig 2–6. (Courtesy of E Katchburian.)

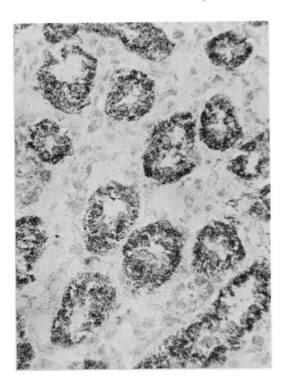

Figure 2–8. Photomicrograph of a frozen section of fresh, unfixed kidney previously incubated in succinate plus monotetrazole (MTT). The dark precipitate seen in the tubules indicates the activity of succinate dehydrogenase. × 400. (Courtesy of AGE Pearse.)

to hydrogen peroxide, forming molecules of water.

In this method, sections of adequately fixed tissue are incubated in a solution containing hydrogen peroxide and 3,3'-diaminoazobenzidine. In the presence of peroxidase, the latter compound is oxidized, resulting in an insoluble colored precipitate that permits the localization of peroxidase activity in the optical and electron microscopes. Since the enzyme is extremely active, it produces an appreciable amount of insoluble precipitate in a short time, making this procedure a very sensitive histochemical assay.

FLUORESCENCE MICROSCOPY

This technic is based on the fact that when certain fluorescent substances are stimulated by light of a proper wavelength, they emit light with a longer wavelength. In fluorescent microscopy, tissue sections are usually stimulated with ultraviolet light so that the emission is in the visible portion of the spectrum. The fluorescent substances appear as brilliant shiny particles on a dark background. In this procedure, a microscope with a strong ultraviolet light source is used. Special filters that

eliminate ultraviolet light are employed to protect the observer's eyes.

Fluorescent Compounds

Some naturally fluorescent substances are normal constituents of cells, eg, vitamin A, vitamin B_2, and porphyrins. Other fluorescent compounds that have an affinity for tissues and cells are used as fluorescent stains. Acridine orange is most widely used because it can combine with DNA and RNA. When observed in the fluorescent microscope, the DNA–acridine orange complex emits a yellowish-green light whereas the RNA–acridine orange complex emits a reddish-orange light. Thus it is possible to identify and localize nucleic acids in the cells (Fig 2–9). Since cancer cells usually contain larger amounts of RNA than normal cells, acridine orange can be used to identify them in smears obtained from patients.

Fluorescent spectroscopy is a method of analyzing the light emitted by a fluorescent compound in a spectroscope. It can be used to characterize several compounds present in cells and is of particular importance in the study of catecholamines.

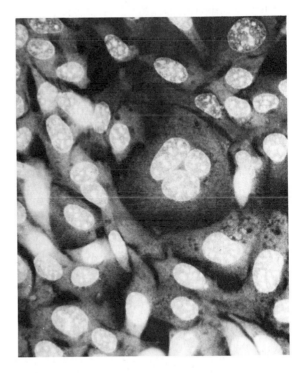

Figure 2–9. Photomicrograph of kidney tissue culture from an embryonic hamster transformed by simian virus 40, stained with acridine orange and photographed with the fluorescent microscope. A green fluorescence (shown as white in photo) appears in the regions containing DNA (nucleus); a reddish-orange color (shown as gray) is characteristic of the RNA-rich cytoplasm. In the center is a giant cell. Reduced from × 750. (Courtesy of A Geraldes and JMV Costa.)

Chapter 2. Histochemistry & Cytochemistry

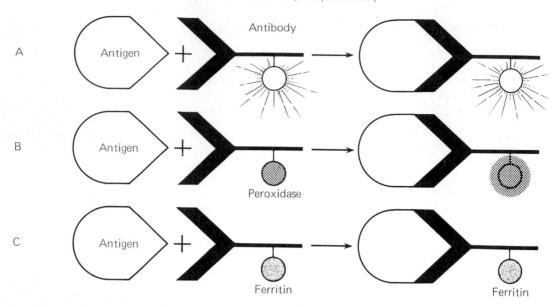

Figure 2–10. Three current methods of labeling and identifying specific proteins by immunocytochemistry. *A:* The antibody is coupled to a fluorescent compound. After incubation, the sections containing the antigen exposed to the labeled antibody solution are studied in the fluorescent microscope. *B:* The antibody is coupled to peroxidase. After the antigen-antibody reaction, the section is submitted to the histochemical method for peroxidase and studied with the light or electron microscope (see text). *C:* The antibody is coupled to ferritin. After the antigen-antibody reaction, this material is studied with the electron microscope, in which the electron-dispersing iron atoms of ferritin can be visualized.

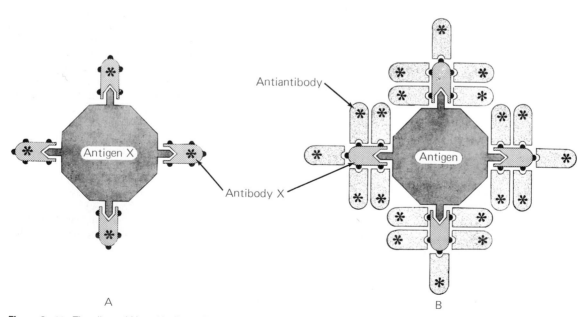

Figure 2–11. The direct *(A)* and indirect *(B)* technics of immunofluorescence. In the direct technic, fluorescently-tagged antibody binds to the antigen present in the cells. Observe that in this hypothetical case each antigen molecule binds only 4 antibody molecules. In the indirect technic, nonfluorescent antibody is first bound to the antigen, and fluorescent antiantibody (also called fluorescent immunoglobulin) then binds itself to the antibody. Because each antibody molecule binds 5 molecules of fluorescent antiantibody, the indirect procedure is more sensitive in that each antigen molecule indirectly binds 20 fluorescent antibody molecules.

IMMUNOCYTOCHEMISTRY

Specific amino acids or reactive groups can be identified by conventional cytochemical methods, but these technics cannot localize specific proteins. The fluorescent antibody method has proved most useful in localizing specific proteins and certain other macromolecules. This test is based on the reaction of the body when exposed to foreign substances called **antigens** or **immunogens.** The body will respond by producing **antibodies** that react specifically and bind strongly to the antigen and result in neutralization of the foreign substance. Antibodies are proteins of the globulin group (immunoglobulins) that appear in plasma and tissue fluids after antigen injection. Their production enables the organism to oppose invasion by foreign microorganisms and to eliminate certain proteins and other foreign matter not recognized as self. **Immunocytochemistry** is based on the coupling of immunoglobulins to substances that render them visible in the microscope without causing loss of biologic activity of the antibody. Since the labeled immunoglobulins bind specifically to their antigens, these compounds permit localization of specific antigens in tissue specimens. When a solution containing labeled antibodies is incubated with a tissue section containing the antigen, the antibodies bind specifically to the antigens, whose location can now be visualized in either the light or electron microscope.

Three methods of labeling antibodies are frequently used (Fig 2–10):

(1) **Coupling with fluorescent compounds:** This permits one to identify the site of specific antigens using a fluorescence microscope.

(2) **Coupling with an enzyme:** This permits detection of the labeled antibody by conventional enzyme cytochemistry. The enzyme most often used is peroxidase, which can be detected by the method described above, using either the light or electron microscope.

(3) **Coupling to an electron-scattering compound that can be detected in the electron microscope:** An iron-rich protein called **ferritin** is often used as an antibody marker. In the electron microscope, the location of electron-dense ferritin-bound antibodies can be easily identified.

There are both direct and indirect methods for antigen localization by immunocytochemistry.

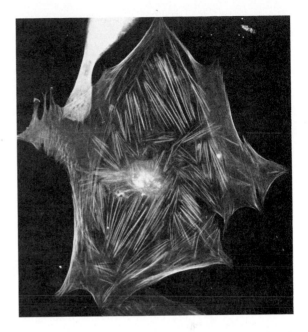

Figure 2–12. Actin fibrils composed of aggregates of actin filaments in the cytoplasm of a cultured human fibroblast preincubated in fluorescent actin antibody. (Reproduced, with permission, from E Lazarides: J Cell Biol 65:545, 1975.)

(1) **Direct method:** Sections of a tissue suspected of containing an antigen (protein X) are incubated with a labeled antibody to X, and the antibody will specifically combine with X. The excess antibodies are washed off, and the tissue is processed according to the methods outlined above (Fig 2–11A). The location of the antigen is then detected in either the light or electron microscope.

(2) **Indirect method:** In this method, the antibodies against protein X are not labeled but simply applied directly to the tissue section.

The antibody molecules, if prepared by injecting protein X into a rabbit, are in turn capable of binding labeled goat antibodies prepared against rabbit immunoglobulins. Thus, when the section is flooded with labeled goat antibodies against rabbit immunoglobulins, the location of the original protein X can be visualized. This technic has the advantage of considerably increasing the sensitivity of the method (Fig 2–11B).

• • •

References

Barka T, Anderson PJ: *Histochemistry: Theory, Practice, and Bibliography.* Hoeber, 1963.

Chayen T, Bitensky L, Butcher RG: *Practical Histochemistry.* Wiley, 1973.

Coons AH: Fluorescent antibody methods. In: *General Cytochemical Methods.* Danielli JF (editor). Academic Press, 1958.

Glick D: *Techniques of Histo- and Cytochemistry: A Manual of Morphological and Quantitative Micromethods for Inorganic, Organic and Enzyme Constituents in Biological Materials.* Interscience, 1949.

Harper HA, Rodwell VW, Mayes PA: *Review of Physiological Chemistry,* 17th ed. Lange, 1979.

Hayat MA: *Electron Microscopy of Enzymes.* Vols 1, 2, and 3. Van Nostrand Reinhold, 1973.

Lison L: *Histochimie et Cytochimie Animale: Principes et Méthodes.* 2 vols. Gauthier-Villars, 1960.

Nakane PK: Application of enzyme-labeled antibody methods for the ultrastructural localization of hormones. In: *Recent Progress in Electron Microscopy of Cells and Tissues.* Yamada E & others (editors). University Park Press, 1976.

Pearse AGE: *Histochemistry: Theoretical and Applied.* Churchill, 1973.

Pollister AW, Ornstein L: The photometric chemical analysis of cells. In: *Analytical Cytology,* 2nd ed. Mellors RC (editor). McGraw-Hill, 1959.

Scarpelli DG, Kanczak NM: Ultrastructural cytochemistry: Principles, limitations and applications. Int Rev Exp Pathol 4:55, 1965.

Thaer AA, Sernetz M (editors): *Fluorescence Techniques in Cell Biology.* Springer-Verlag, 1973.

Wisse E & others (editors): *Electron Microscopy and Cytochemistry: Proceedings of the Second International Symposium, Drienerlo, The Netherlands.* American Elsevier, 1973.

Zugibe FT: *Diagnostic Histochemistry.* Mosby, 1970.

Mammalian tissue is made up of 3 distinct components: cells, intercellular substance, and tissue fluid. The cells comprise the greater part of the body and are its basic morphologic and functional unit.

CELLULAR FUNCTIONS & DIFFERENTIATION

During the process of evolution, the cells of metazoan organisms gradually became modified and specialized, resulting in increased efficiency of function. Through phylogenetic development, undifferentiated primitive cells exhibiting several functional activities, each with little efficiency, were transformed into a series of differentiated cells that were collectively able to perform some specific functions with much greater efficiency. This process of cell specialization is known as **cell differentiation.**

For example, the muscle cell during its differentiation elongates into a spindle-shaped cell that synthesizes and accumulates myofibrillar proteins. The resulting cell, called a muscle fiber, acts to efficiently convert chemical energy into contractile force. Another example is the pancreatic cell, which becomes specialized to synthesize and secrete digestive enzymes.

Morphologic modifications during differentiation are understandably accompanied by chemical changes, and the quantitative synthesis of one or more specific proteins by each differentiated cell type characterizes this process. Examples are the synthesis of the proteins actin and myosin by the muscle cell or of several digestive enzymes by the acinar pancreatic cells. Cellular functions involving specialized cells in the body are listed in Table 3–1.

Cells are not always restricted to carrying out one function; more commonly, cells are capable of performing 2 or more functions. Thus, the cells of the proximal convoluted tubules of the kidney not only transport ions but also reabsorb metabolites and digest proteins. Similarly, the intestinal epithelial cells reabsorb metabolites and synthesize diges-

Table 3–1. Cellular functions in specialized cells.

Function	Specialized Cell(s)
Movement	Muscle cell
Conductivity	Nerve cell
Synthesis and secretion of enzymes	Pancreatic acinar cells
Synthesis and secretion of mucous substances	Mucous gland cells
Synthesis and secretion of steroids	Some adrenal gland, testis, and ovary cells
Ion transport	Cells of the kidney and salivary gland ducts
Intracellular digestion	Macrophages and some white blood cells
Transformation of physical and chemical stimuli into nervous impulses	Sensory cells
Metabolite absorption	Cells of the intestine, kidney, etc

tive enzymes (proteins) such as disaccharidases and peptidases (see Chapter 16).

It will be seen that the morphology of the cell varies according to its functions.

CELL COMPONENTS

The cell is composed of 2 basic parts: **cytoplasm** and **nucleus.** Individual cytoplasmic components are usually not clearly visible in common hematoxylin and eosin-stained preparations; the nucleus, however, appears intensely stained dark blue or black (Fig 4–1).

Cytoplasm

The outermost component of the cytoplasm, separating it from its extracellular environment, is the plasma membrane (plasmalemma). The cytoplasm is composed of a matrix in which are embedded several structures classified into 3 groups: organelles, inclusions, and other components. The structures known as organelles are present in all eukaryotic cells, are enclosed in a membrane, and contain enzymes that participate in cellular meta-

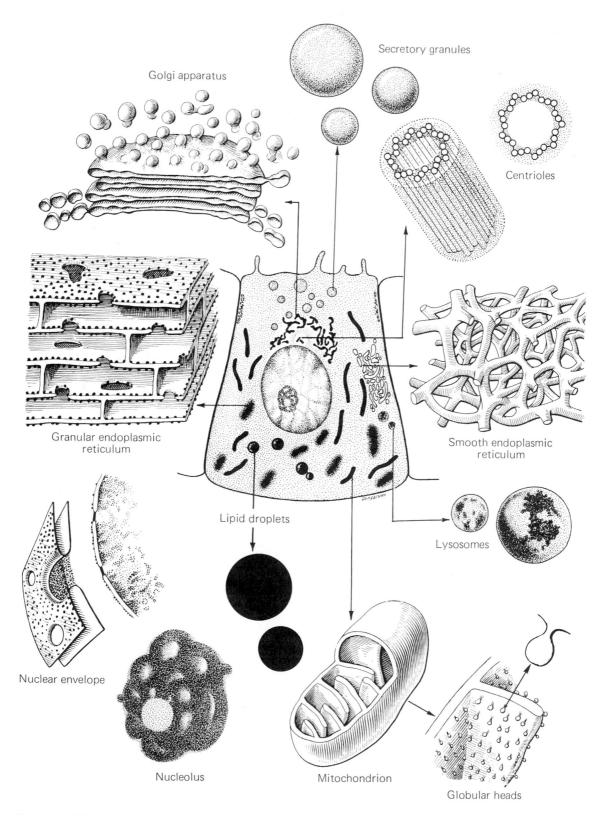

Golgi apparatus

Secretory granules

Centrioles

Granular endoplasmic
reticulum

Smooth endoplasmic
reticulum

Lipid droplets

Lysosomes

Nuclear envelope

Nucleolus

Mitochondrion

Globular heads

Figure 3 –1. Diagram showing a hypothetical cell in the center as seen with the light microscope. It is surrounded by its various structures as seen with the electron microscope. (Redrawn and reproduced, with permission, from Bloom W, Fawcett DW: *A Textbook of Histology,* 9th ed. Saunders, 1968.)

bolic activity. They are permanent components of the cytoplasm. Examples include the endoplasmic reticulum, the mitochondria, the Golgi apparatus, and the lysosomes. The inclusions generally are temporary components of certain cells and usually are accumulations of pigment, lipids, proteins, or carbohydrates that may or may not be enclosed in a membrane. The other components cannot be classified as one of the 2 preceding classes and have different structures and functions. They are not enclosed in a membrane and do not participate directly in cellular metabolism. This group comprises the centriole, microtubules, and microfilaments.

Plasma Membrane

All eukaryotic cells are enveloped by a limiting membrane composed of phospholipids, protein, and, to a lesser extent, polysaccharides. The cell membrane (plasmalemma) functions as a selective barrier that regulates the passage of certain materials into and out of the cell. In addition, membranes may **facilitate** the transport of specific materials through this limiting barrier. Membranes also carry out a number of specific recognition and regulatory functions, to be discussed later.

Cell membranes range from 7.5 to 10 nm in thickness and consequently are visible only in the electron microscope. Micrographs reveal that the plasmalemma—and, for that matter, almost all other organellar membranes—exhibit a trilaminar structure after fixation in osmium (Fig 3–2). Based on the universality of this appearance, this 3-layered structure has been designated **unit membrane.**

Membrane phospholipids (eg, lecithin, cephalin) consist of 2 long, nonpolar (hydrophobic) hydrocarbon chains bound to a bulbous, charged (hydrophilic) peptide head. Within the membrane, the lipids are presumably most stable when organized

into a double layer with their hydrophobic (nonpolar) chains directed toward the center of the membrane and their charged hydrophilic heads directed outward (Fig 3–2). The trilaminar appearance of membranes in the electron microscope is apparently due to the deposition of reduced osmium on the hydrophilic portions on each side of the lipid bilayer. Some of the lipids, known as glycolipids, possess polysaccharide chains that extend outward from the surface of the cell membrane (Fig 3–4, top).

The proteins, which constitute a major molecular constituent of membranes (> 50% w/w), can be divided into 2 groups. **Integral proteins** represent a class of proteins that are directly incorporated within the lipid bilayer, while **peripheral proteins** exhibit a more loose association with membrane surfaces. The loosely bound peripheral proteins can be easily extracted from cell membranes, while integral proteins can only be extracted by drastic methods.

From freeze-fracture electron microscopic studies, it appears that many integral proteins are distributed as globular molecules intercalated among the lipid molecules. Some of the smaller proteins are partially embedded in the lipid bilayer, so that they may extend outward from either the outer or inner surfaces. Other proteins are large enough to extend across the 2 lipid layers and protrude from both membrane surfaces. Some of the proteins that completely cross the membrane are believed to provide for a channel through which water-soluble substances, such as ions, can pass back and forth between the extracellular and intracellular compartments. The existence of such protein channels replaces the necessity for the so-called membrane pores postulated by cell physiologists to account for the data generated by permeability experiments. Other proteins, which may possess lipid (lipoproteins) or carbohydrate

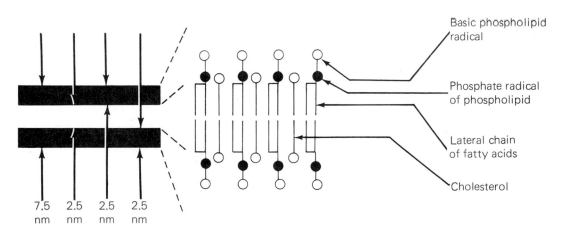

Figure 3–2. The ultrastructure *(left)* and molecular structure *(right)* of the cell membrane. The dark lines at left represent the 2 dense layers observed in the electron microscope due to deposition of osmium in the hydrophilic portions of the lipid molecules.

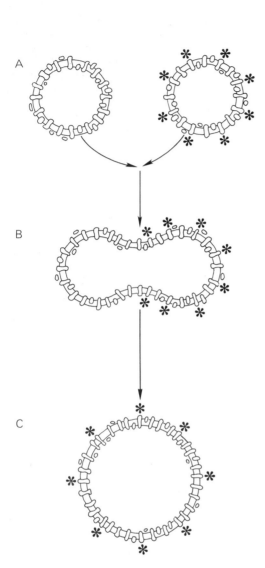

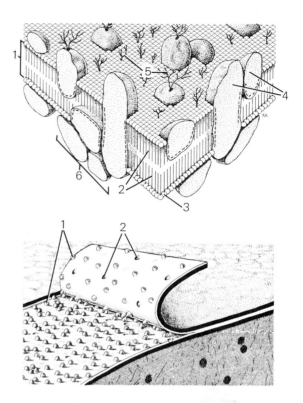

Figure 3 –4. *Top:* Ultrastructure of the cell membrane. The membrane consists of a bimolecular lipid layer (1) with protein molecules (4) nested in it. Hydrophobic regions of the lipids consist of linear arrays (2), while hydrophilic portions exhibit a globular morphology (3). Some proteins cross the bilipid layer while others are partially embedded. Carbohydrate chains (5) are bound to lipids and proteins present on the outer surface. On the inner surface, cytoplasmic proteins (6) are bound to proteins embedded within the lipid. The dotted regions within the proteins represent areas that contain hydrophobic amino acids which interact and bind with the lipids and consequently anchor these proteins within the membrane. *Bottom:* Membrane cleavage occurs when a cell is frozen and fractured (cryofracture). Observe that some of the membrane proteins (1) remain bound to one surface, whereas others remain on the opposite surface. For every protein particle that bulges on one surface, a corresponding depression (2) appears within the opposite surface. In the frozen tissue, hydrophilic bonds are more rigid and stable, while the hydrophobic lipid interactions remain more fluid. Consequently, cleavage occurs in this region because the lipid layers are bound by the weaker hydrophobic bonds. The study of these protein particles by cryofracture contributed significantly to our knowledge of cell membranes. (Modified and reproduced, with permission, from Krstić RV: *Ultrastructure of the Mammalian Cell.* Springer-Verlag, 1979.)

Figure 3 –3. Experiment demonstrating the fluid nature of proteins within the cell membrane. The plasmalemma is shown as 2 parallel lines (representing the lipid portion) in which proteins are embedded. Some of these particles are characteristic of the cell at top right and are identified by asterisks. In this experiment, 2 different types of cells derived from tissue cultures (one with a fluorescent marker [right] and one without) are fused (A → B) owing to the action of Sendai virus. Minutes after the fusion of the membranes, the fluorescent marker of the labeled cell spreads to the entire surface of the fused cells and finally covers it uniformly (C).

(glycoproteins) side chains, are arranged as mosaics within the cell membrane (Fig 3–4).

Integration of the proteins within the lipid bilayer is the result of hydrophobic interactions between the lipids and nonpolar (hydrophobic) regions on the surface of the membrane proteins (Fig 3–4, top). However, the integral proteins are not bound rigidly in place and are able to move by gliding within the cell membrane. Under certain circumstances, these proteins can accumulate at one region of the plasma membrane, forming a localized **cap** of proteins. This process, called **capping,** has been observed in several cell types and appears to be a general phenomenon. Experiments have also revealed that some membrane protein movement is not random but is probably controlled by intracellular mechanisms involving the participation of microtubules and microfilaments. Figure 3–3 illustrates an experiment that demonstrates the fluidity of integral proteins within the cell membrane. The above-described "mosaic" disposition of membrane proteins, in conjunction with the fluid nature of the lipid layer, constitutes the basis of the presently accepted **fluid mosaic model** for membrane structure as illustrated in Fig 3–4.

The transfer of material into the cell by passive or active transport is not followed by visible morphologic changes. Substances may also enter the cell by processes visible in the electron microscope. When the ingestion of discrete amounts of fluid occurs, the process is called **pinocytosis,** which is of 2 types: In one type, small vesicles bud from the plasma membrane, invaginate into the cytoplasm,

and lose contact with it (Figs 4–17 and 4–19). In a second type, large vesicles are formed by elevation of membrane extensions (Fig 12–4). The term **phagocytosis** is usually restricted to mean ingestion of particles such as bacteria. **Endocytosis** is a general term that refers to the visible entry of substances into the cell and comprises both pinocytosis and phagocytosis. **Exocytosis** is the extrusion of material from the cell, as occurs in gland cells. In exocytosis, fusion occurs between the cell membrane and the membrane surrounding the vesicle leaving the cell.

The structures of other membranes (nuclear envelope, endoplasmic reticulum, Golgi apparatus, secretory granules, and lysosomes)—although not identical—are similar to those of the plasma membrane. The structural and functional differences observed are at present being actively investigated. Chemical differences have been noted, and structural differences have been associated with the presence of different structural proteins, lipids, enzymes, and receptors on them.

Cellular Communication

It has been shown that many cells within tissues of both vertebrates and invertebrates are not independent and isolated units but have intercellular communications, permitting the free interchange of ions and larger molecules. This occurs by means of specialized junctions present between membranes of neighboring cells. This communication phenomenon has been studied by the following technics:

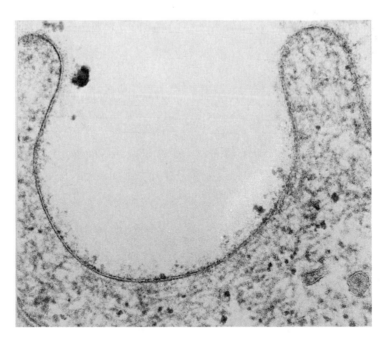

Figure 3 –5. Electron micrograph of a section of the surface of an epithelial cell, showing the unit membrane with its 2 dark lines limiting a clear band. On the surface of the membrane is a layer of granular material forming the cell coat. × 100,000.

A. Following the intracellular microinjection of stains or fluorescent compounds by means of micropipettes, the injected compound gradually passed to neighboring cells and then to still other cells.

B. By inserting microelectrodes into neighboring cells, it was shown that an electric current can pass between cells with very slight loss of voltage (Fig 3–6). The curves registered for the electrical impulse (curve I) were compared with tracings from the 3 microelectrodes (curves II, III, and IV). Analysis led to the following conclusions:

1. The electrical stimulus is transmitted with no loss of its intensity to an electrode inserted in the same cell. The cell cytoplasm is a good conductor and does not hinder the flow of the stimulus (curve II).

2. When the electrical impulse is applied to cell 2, it is not registered in cell 1 (curve IV). This indicates that the plasma membranes between cells 1 and 2 offer high resistance.

3. When the electrical impulse is applied to cell 2, the stimulus registered in the electrode inserted in cell 3 is almost the same (curve III) as the one observed in the electrode of cell 2 (curve II), where the total impulse was measured initially and within the cell (curves I and II). This is due to low resistance between cells 2 and 3 and suggests that there is communication between these cells.

Careful measurements show that the resistance between communicating cells can be 1000 times lower than between noncommunicating cells. These results are important because they demonstrate that most tissues are not merely an aggregate of independent cells but function as an integrated unit. Cellular communication appears during embryogenesis and is probably important in the coordination of intrauterine development. The structure responsible for this type of communication is called the **gap junction** or **nexus** (Figs 3–7 and 3–8). In this structure, the plasma membranes of adjoining cells are closely apposed but separated by a space or gap 2 nm wide. Evidence strongly suggests that gap junctions comprise an array of parallel hol-

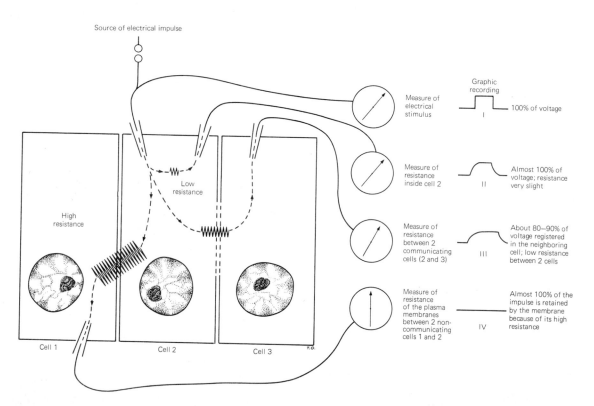

Figure 3 –6. Experiments measuring the electrical conductivity between cells with or without communication. Cells 1 and 2 do not communicate, whereas cells 2 and 3 do. In cell 2, two microelectrodes were inserted. One is connected simultaneously to a stimulator (generator of electrical impulse) and to a measuring device. The other electrode is connected to a registering electrode and measures the current that crosses the cell cytoplasm. Electrodes were also inserted in cells 1 and 3 to measure the current that passes from cell 2 to cell 1 and from cell 2 to cell 3. Graphs obtained from the electrical stimulations are shown to the right of the figure. The upper graph expresses the total impulse measured by the electrode to the left of cell 2. The second graph shows only a very small lowering of the current due to the resistance of the cytoplasm. The third and fourth graphs show that most of the current (80–90%) passes from cell 2 to cell 3 while practically no current crosses the membranes that separate cell 2 from cell 1. Cells 2 and 3 have a special junction that lowers the membrane's resistance. This does not occur between cells 1 and 2.

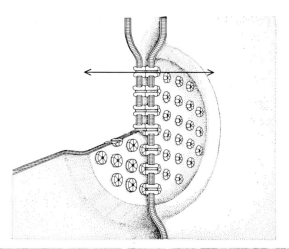

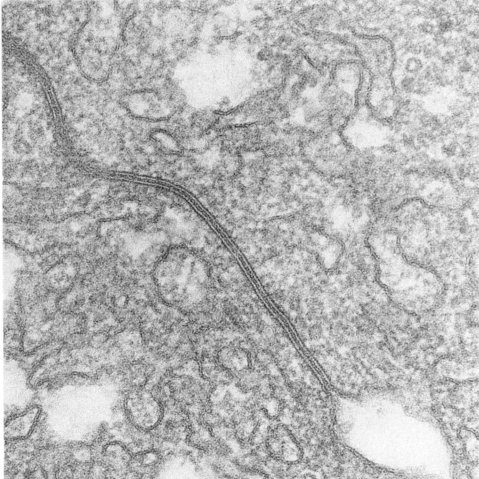

Figure 3 –7. Gap junction between 2 rat liver cells. At the junction, 2 apposed membranes are separated by an electron-dense space or gap 2 nm wide. In the upper portion (oblique view) is a model of a gap junction depicting the structural elements that allow the exchange of nutrients and signal molecules between cells without loss of material into the intercellular space. The communicating "pipes" are formed by pairs of abutting particles, which are in turn composed of 6 dumbbell-shaped protein subunits that span the lipid bilayer of each cell membrane. The channel passing through the cylindric bridges is about 2 nm in diameter, limiting the size of the molecules that can pass through it. Unlike the tight junction, fluids and tracers in the intercellular space can permeate the gap junction by flowing around the protein bridges. (Illustration at top is from Staehelin LA, Hull BE: Junctions between living cells. Sci Am 238:41, May 1978. Copyright © 1978 by Scientific American, Inc. All rights reserved. Illustration at bottom is × 193,000. Courtesy of MC Williams.)

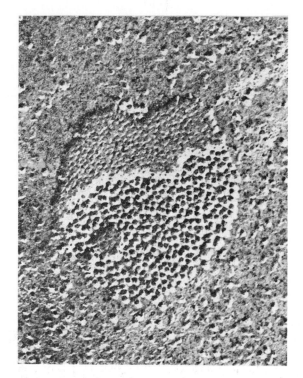

Figure 3 –8. Gap junction as seen on cryofracture preparation. It appears as a plaquelike agglomeration of intramembrane protein particles. (Courtesy of A Pinto da Silva.)

low tube-like protein structures that traverse the closely bound membranes of 2 adjoining cells (Fig 3–7). Gap junctions have been isolated by differential centrifugation, and their proteins are being actively studied. The junctions have been observed in many tissues such as cardiac muscle, smooth muscle, liver, kidney, thyroid, skin, urinary bladder, pancreas, and adrenals.

Gap junctions can be rapidly formed between previously isolated cells. Metabolic inhibitors—especially those blocking oxidative phosphorylation—can inhibit the formation of junctions or undo junctions already present between cells. This suggests that the maintenance of intracellular junctions is an active process dependent on energy production. In addition, it is probable that calcium ions and a specific glycoprotein complex at the cell surface are needed to establish junctions between cells.

Mitochondria

Mitochondria are present in all eukaryotic cells. They are organelles that transform with high efficiency the chemical energy of the metabolites present in cytoplasm into available energy that is easily accessible to the cell. This energy is stored in a class of substances that are rich in energy. These substances, typified by adenosine triphosphate (ATP), promptly release energy when required by the cell to perform any type of work, whether it be

of osmotic, mechanical, electrical, or chemical nature. The mitochondria are spherical or filamentous particles 0.1–0.5 μm wide that can attain a length of up to 10 μm. Their distribution in cells varies. They tend to accumulate in parts of the cytoplasm where metabolic activity is more intense, such as at the apical ends of ciliated cells (Fig 4–11), in the middle piece of spermatozoa (Fig 23–4), or at the base of ion-transferring cells (Fig 4–17). In instances where they are not polarized, they have a tendency to be oriented along the long axis of cylindric or long cells, or radially on round cells.

Cells contain great numbers of mitochondria—an estimated 2500 in one liver cell—but always in a characteristic number for that cell. The mitochondria are composed mainly of protein. Lipids are present to a lesser degree, along with small quantities of DNA and RNA. Like most cell components, mitochondria have a short life span, and their proteins are constantly being renewed. The average half-life of mitochondrial proteins in rat liver cells is 10 days. The ultrastructure of mitochondria varies with the organ and species from which the tissue is obtained for examination. In addition, different fixation procedures may greatly alter mitochondrial morphology.

Mitochondria generally have a characteristic structure under the electron microscope (Figs 3–1 and 3–9). They are composed of an external membrane and an internal membrane, and the latter projects folds into the interior of the mitochondria, giving rise to the **cristae.** These membranes surround 2 spaces—one outer space between the 2 membranes, called the intracristal space, and one within the internal membrane penetrated by the cristae. Filling the space between the cristae is a fine granular matrix of variable electron density. Most mitochondria have flat, shelflike cristae in their interiors (Figs 3–1 and 3–9) though steroid secretors (eg, adrenal and gonadal cells; see Chapter 4) frequently contain tubular cristae (Fig 4–26). The cristae increase the internal surface area of the mitochondria, and it is on this surface that enzymes of the oxidative phosphorylation and electron transport systems are located. The membrane-bound enzymes are organized into a particulate fringe lining the matrix side of the inner membrane. Using specific staining procedures on osmotically stressed isolated mitochondria, the ADP to ATP phosphorylation enzymes are seen to exist as globular proteins connected to the membrane via cylindric stalks. The other electron transport enzymes are found embedded within the membrane. Enzymes for the Krebs and fatty acid cycles are found to reside within the matrix space.

The number of mitochondria and the number of cristae in each mitochondrion are proportionate to the rate of metabolism of the cells. Thus, cells with a high rate of metabolism (eg, cardiac muscle or kidney tubule cells) have abundant mitochondria with a large number of closely packed cristae, whereas others with low metabolism have few mitochondria with short cristae.

Between the cristae is an amorphous **matrix** rich in protein and some DNA. In a great number of cell types, the mitochondrial matrix also exhibits rounded electron-dense granules rich in cations such as calcium and magnesium. Although their function is not completely understood, the granules are apparently related to the mitochondrion's ability to concentrate cations.

The DNA isolated from the mitochondrial matrix has been shown to have a circular structure. DNA strands are synthesized within the mitochondrion, and their duplication is independent of nuclear DNA. Particles resembling ribosomes are present, as well as many mitochondria-specific types of RNA (ribosomal, messenger, and transfer). These observations are consistent with the finding of unique mitochondrial proteins within the matrix

of this organelle. This extranuclear genetic system is related to the synthesis of some—but not all—of the mitochondrial proteins. For example, mitochondrial DNA has been shown to code for structural proteins and enzymes of the inner membrane (eg, cytochrome oxidase), whereas nuclear DNA codes for most of the matrix and outer membrane proteins.

Metabolites within the cell are utilized within mitochondria by the catalytic activity of the enzymes of the citric acid (Krebs) cycle, and the energy liberated in this process is captured through oxidative phosphorylation. The end product of these reactions is the high-energy compound ATP. In addition, CO_2 and water are concurrently produced. The dense mitochondrial matrix is considered to be the site of most of the enzymes that participate in this production of ATP.

The initial degradation of proteins, carbohy-

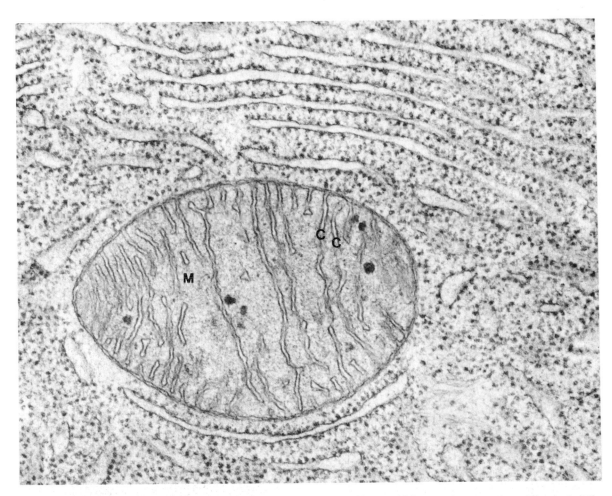

Figure 3 –9. Electron micrograph of a section of pancreas. A mitochondrion—with its membranes, cristae (C), matrix (M), and dense granules—is clearly visible. In vitro and in vivo experiments have shown that the morphology of mitochondria changes with their functional activity. Thus, when oxidative phosphorylation is stimulated, the space between the external and internal membranes swells with a condensation of the mitochondrial matrix. It is believed that this swelling may play an important role in transport mechanisms occurring in the cell. Surrounding the mitochondrion is a typical endoplasmic reticulum with ribosomes. × 50,000. (Courtesy of KR Porter.)

drates, and fats is carried out in the cytosol or matrix—that portion of the cell outside the mitochondria. The ultimate metabolic end product of these extramitochondrial metabolic pathways is acetyl-CoA, which then enters the mitochondria. Within the mitochondria, acetyl-CoA combines with oxaloacetate to form citric acid. Within the citric acid cycle, there are several reactions of decarboxylation producing CO_2, and 5 pairs of hydrogen atoms are removed by specific reactions of oxidation catalyzed by dehydrogenases. The H atoms react ultimately with oxygen to form H_2O. The **electron transport system,** which is known to be located in the mitochondrial internal membrane, by virtue of the action of cytochromes a, b, and c and coenzyme Q, as well as cytochrome oxidase, possesses mechanisms to capture released energy at 3 points by formation of ATP from ADP and phosphate. Under aerobic circumstances, the combined activity of extramitochondrial glycolysis and the citric acid cycle as well as the electron transport system gives rise to 38 molecules of ATP per mole of glucose. This is 19 times the energy obtainable under anaerobic circumstances, when only the glycolytic pathway can be utilized.

Origin & Evolution of Mitochondria

New mitochondria originate from preexisting mitochondria by accretion of material, causing growth and subsequent division of the organelle. During mitosis, an equal division of the mitochondria occurs between parent and daughter cell.

The fact that mitochondria present a circular DNA molecule and respiratory enzymes in their membranes, as in bacteria, has led to speculation regarding the evolutionary origin and history of this organelle. It has thus been proposed that mitochondria evolved from an ancestral prokaryote which became adapted to a symbiotic life within the host eukaryotic cell. The fact that the processes of protein synthesis in mitochondria are much more similar to those occurring in bacteria than in eukaryotes gives weight to this opinion. Thus, certain antibiotics such as chloramphenicol inhibit both mitochondrial and bacterial protein synthesis and have no effect on cytoplasmic protein synthesis.

Endoplasmic Reticulum & Ribosomes

This organelle appears as flattened, rounded, or tubular vesicles that frequently anastomose with one another in a network form. The disposition of these vesicles varies considerably from cell to cell and also in different parts of one particular cell. There are 2 types of endoplasmic reticulum— granular (rough) and agranular (smooth). Endoplasmic reticulum appears very early in embryonic development and varies in appearance and size with the functional state of the cells.

The membranes of the endoplasmic reticulum are frequently continuous with the nuclear envelope membrane. These membranes are usually arranged in the form of flattened cisternae stacked in parallel (especially in cells that synthesize and segregate proteins), and they convey the impression of reservoirlike formations. Small membranous "transfer" vesicles, a second component of this organelle, represent the vehicle for transfer of materials from the cisternae of endoplasmic reticulum to the Golgi apparatus.

The membranes of the **granular (rough) endoplasmic reticulum** have **ribosomes** attached to their external surfaces (Figs 3–1 and 3–9). These are small, electron-dense particles, 15–20 nm in diameter, attached to the outer surfaces of the membranes. They are composed of RNA and protein and are responsible for the basophilia seen in the cytoplasm of cells. There are 2 classes of ribosomes: one type found in the prokaryotes, chloroplasts, and mitochondria and the other in the cytoplasm of eukaryotic cells. Both classes of ribosomes are composed of 2 different-sized subunits that are synthesized in the nucleoli. Ribosomes can appear as isolated granules free in the cytoplasm or linked in groups called **polysomes.** Polysomes or **polyribosomes** (Fig 3–10A) are groups of ribosomes held together by a common strand of messenger RNA. The polysomes may adhere to the surface of the endoplasmic reticulum or may exist free in the cytoplasm. In the adherent state, they form the granular endoplasmic reticulum present in cell types that primarily synthesize proteins for export from the cytosol. This separation of proteins occurs in several cell types (such as fibroblasts and plasma cells) wherein the synthesized proteins are injected through the membrane of the endoplasmic reticulum and remain segregated in the interior of that structure (Fig 3–10B). The carbohydrate portion of secreted glycoproteins is synthesized by enzymes incorporated within the membranes of the endoplasmic reticulum and Golgi apparatus. In many cells, protein synthesis occurs in the endoplasmic reticulum, while the polysaccharides are added in the Golgi apparatus. Therefore, besides participating in protein synthesis, granular endoplasmic reticulum also has a function in the synthesis of glycoproteins.

In cell types in which the proteins produced remain in the cytosol and are consequently not segregated from the cytoplasm, the polysomes appear free in the cytoplasm and are not attached to membranes of the endoplasmic reticulum. These proteins are not segregated within the endoplasmic reticulum and can be observed permeating the cytoplasm. For example, the immature red blood cell (erythroblast) synthesizes hemoglobin and retains it within the cytosol. (These concepts are summarized in Figs 3–10A and 3–10B.)

The ribosomes, which are intensely basophilic, react with such basic stains as methylene blue and toluidine blue because of the constituent RNA that reacts as polyanions owing to the presence of phosphate groups. Thus, the sites in cytoplasm that stain

A
Free polysome showing protein
synthesis with no segregation

B
Bound polysomes showing protein
synthesis with segregation

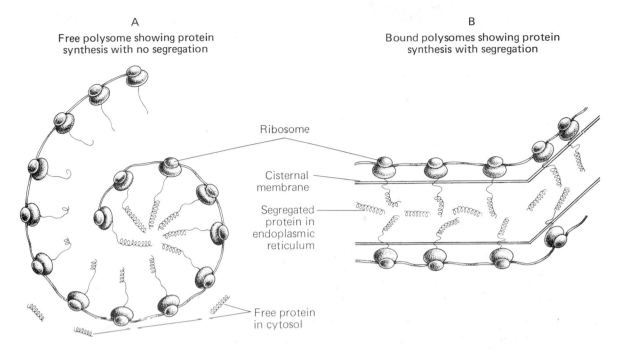

Ribosome

Cisternal
membrane

Segregated
protein in
endoplasmic
reticulum

Free protein
in cytosol

Figure 3–10. This diagram illustrates (in *A*) the concept expressed in the text that cells synthesizing proteins (represented here by spirals) that are to remain within the cytosol display (free) polysomes (nonadherent to the endoplasmic reticulum). In *B,* where the proteins are segregated in the reticulum and may eventually be extruded from the cytoplasm (exportation proteins), not only do the polysomes adhere to the membranes of granular endoplasmic reticulum but also the proteins produced by them are injected into the interior of the organelle across its membrane. In this way, the proteins—especially enzymes such as ribonucleases and proteases, which could have undesirable effects on the cytoplasm—are separated from it.

with these dyes are usually rich in ribosomes. These basophilic regions in cytoplasm were described in the 19th century and were named according to the cell studied. In glandular cells, they were known as **ergastoplasm;** in neurons, as **Nissl bodies;** and in other cells as **basophilic bodies** or **components.** Although the ribosomes are below the resolution of the light microscope, they can be visualized indirectly because of their staining characteristics.

The term **microsome** as used in cytology and biochemistry denotes vesicles generated by fragmentation of the granular endoplasmic reticulum during the process of homogenization that precedes differential centrifugation. The fusion of membrane fragments of the ruptured endoplasmic reticulum forms small vesicles which may have ribosomes. These microsomes can then be isolated by means of differential centrifugation. It is now possible to fractionate the microsomes further and separate the membranous component from the ribosomes (Figs 1–14 and 1–15).

There are no ribosomes attached to the membrane of the **smooth** or **agranular endoplasmic reticulum.** This organelle, very abundant in the liver cell, is composed entirely of membranes that generally appear as profusely anastomosing tubules or flat cisternae (Fig 3–1). The smooth and the granular endoplasmic reticulum intercommunicate (Fig 3–11); there are also intercommunications between smooth endoplasmic reticulum and the nuclear envelope. Smooth endoplasmic reticulum not only exhibits a diverse morphologic appearance in different cell types but is also associated with a variety of functional specializations. For example, in cells that synthesize steroids, smooth endoplasmic reticulum is abundant and contains enzymes essential for the synthesizing process (Figs 4–26 and 4–27). It is also responsible for the conjugation, oxidation, and methylation processes employed by the cell to neutralize or detoxify certain hormones and noxious substances. Smooth endoplasmic reticulum participates in the contraction processes of muscle cells, where it appears in a special form called **sarcoplasmic reticulum** that is involved with the sequestration and release of calcium ions. It is also involved in the synthesis of the glycogen in liver cells, where the enzyme glucose-6-phosphatase is found within its membranes.

Golgi Apparatus

This organelle, which is present in almost all cells, appears as a group of piled-up flat vesicles with peripheral dilatations (Figs 3–1 and 3–11). Some authors also include in the Golgi apparatus the small "transfer vesicles" derived by a budding process from the smooth and granular endoplasmic

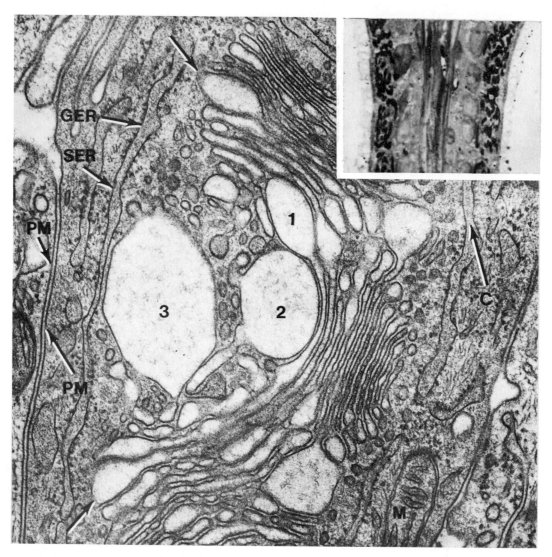

Figure 3 –11. Electron micrograph of a Golgi apparatus of a mucous cell. To the right is a cisterna (C) of the granular endoplasmic reticulum containing granular material. Close to it are small vesicles containing this material. In the center are flattened and piled up cisternae of the Golgi apparatus. Dilatations can be observed running out from the ends of the cisternae. These dilatations gradually detach themselves from the cisternae and fuse, forming the secretory granules (1, 2, and 3). PM is the plasma membrane of 2 neighboring cells. Near the membrane is an endoplasmic reticulum with a smooth section (SER) and a granular (rough) section (GER). × 30,000. *Inset:* The aspect of the Golgi apparatus as seen in 1 μm sections of epididymis cells impregnated by silver. × 1200.

reticulum. The Golgi apparatus usually occupies a finite and fixed area in the cytoplasm of most cells. In nerve or liver cells, it is clearly seen as interconnected groups of scattered flattened vesicles throughout the cytoplasm (Fig 3–12). The size and development of this organelle are variable from cell to cell and also change with the type of activity of the cell.

The Golgi apparatus plays a role in the process of synthesis, concentration, and storage of secretory products of most glandular cells. The proteins synthesized in granular endoplasmic reticulum are transferred to the Golgi apparatus, probably with the aid of the **transfer vesicles.** Within the vesicles, proteins migrate to and fuse with the Golgi body, where they are collected and condensed into relatively large, dense particles and enclosed by a membrane to form secretory granules. The Golgi apparatus is a polarized structure in that its outer surface (also called **immature face**) receives the transfer vesicles while the secretory granules develop and pinch off from the opposite inner surface (**mature face**).

Radioautographic studies using sulfur-35 (^{35}S) reveal that in cells which elaborate sulfated glycoproteins, the Golgi apparatus is the site of sulfation.

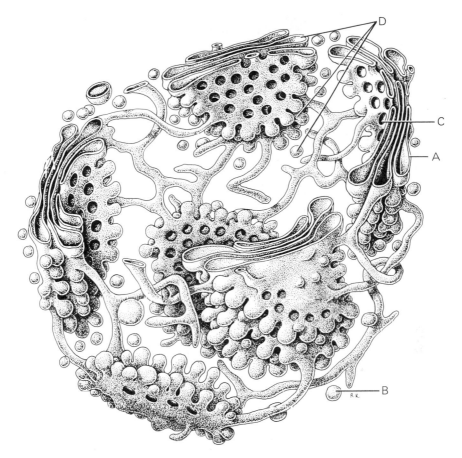

Figure 3 –12. Three-dimensional representation of the Golgi apparatus. This organelle consists of stacks of flattened membranous sacs. Within each stack, the cisternal sacs are not interconnected at the **forming face** (A, convex surface). New cisternae grow by assimilating membranes and contents of small transfer vesicles (B). At the **maturing face** of the Golgi (C), old cisternae are eliminated as a result of the formation and "pinching off" of secretory granules (D). (Reproduced, with permission, from Krstić RV: *Ultrastructure of the Mammalian Cell.* Springer-Verlag, 1979.)

Similar experiments performed with labeled galactose and glucose indicate that the Golgi apparatus is also the site of the addition of polysaccharide to proteins during the formation of glycoproteins.

Lysosomes

Lysosomes are membrane-bound vesicles that contain a variety of lytic enzymes whose main function is related to intracytoplasmic digestion. Lysosomes are present in almost all cells but are particularly abundant in cells exhibiting phagocytic activity (eg, macrophages, white blood cells). Although the nature and activity of lysosomal enzymes varies depending on the cell type being studied, the most common are acid phosphatase, ribonuclease, deoxyribonuclease, cathepsins (A, B, and C), sulfatases, and β-glucuronidase. Generally, lysosomal enzymes are active at acid pH.

Lysosomes are usually spherical, range in diameter from 0.2 to 0.5 μm, and present a uniformly granular appearance in electron micrographs (Fig 3–14). The enveloping single unit membrane serves to separate the lytic enzymes from the cytoplasm, an important role in that it prevents the lysosomal enzymes from attacking and digesting cytoplasmic organelles.

Lysosomal enzymes are apparently synthesized in the rough endoplasmic reticulum and subsequently transferred to the Golgi apparatus, wherein the enzymes are modified and packaged into vesicular lysosomes. These small vesicles containing the inactive enzymes are identified as **primary lysosomes** (Fig 3–14).

In cells carrying out intracellular digestion, extracellular substances are taken into the cell via phagocytosis or pinocytosis. Through these processes, ingested substances are trapped within membrane-bound vesicles known as **phagosomes.** The membranes of primary lysosomes fuse with the phagosome membrane, which results in the release of the lytic enzymes and their subsequent mixing with the phagocytosed material. The phenomenon of intracellular digestion takes place within this new vacuole, which is called the **secondary lysosome**

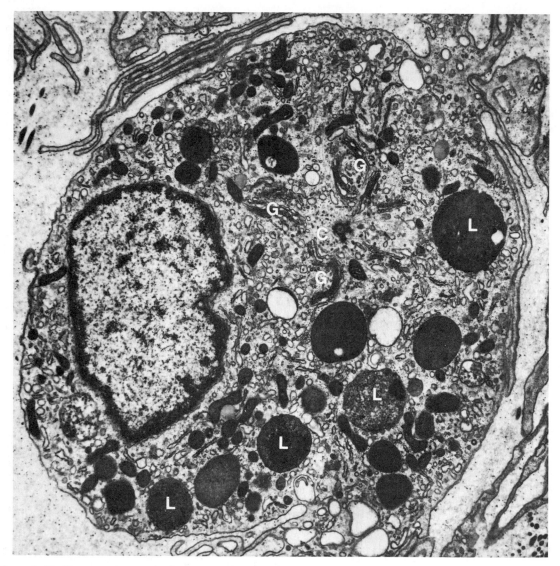

Figure 3–13. Electron micrograph of a mesenteric macrophage. Observe the presence of abundant cytoplasmic extensions. In the center is a centriole (C) surrounded by Golgi cisternae (G). Secondary lysosomes (L) are abundant. × 15,000.

(Figs 3–13, 3–15, and 3–16). Secondary lysosomes are usually spherical and can be recognized in the electron microscope by virtue of their heterogeneous electron-dense matrix. In addition, secondary lysosomes can be identified histochemically by assays that detect the presence of lytic enzymes (eg, acid phosphatase) within the vacuoles (Fig 2–7).

Following digestion of the contents of the secondary lysosome, the catabolites diffuse through the limiting membrane and enter the cytoplasm. The remaining undigestible compounds are retained within the vesicle and constitute the so-called **residual bodies.** In most cases, the residual bodies migrate to and fuse with the plasmalemma, thus releasing their contents into the extracellular space. However, in certain cells (eg, neurons, heart muscle, hepatocytes), the residual bodies are not released but are stored in the cytoplasm as **lipofuscin** or **age pigment.**

Another function of the lysosomes concerns the turnover of cytoplasmic organelles. Under certain conditions, organelles or portions of the cytoplasm may become membrane-bound. Primary lysosomes fuse with this structure and initiate the lysis of the enclosed cytoplasm (Fig 3–16). The resulting secondary lysosomes are known as **autophagosomes.** The digested products of this hydrolysis are probably recycled by the cell to permit renewal, rearrangement, and reconstruction of the cytoplasm. In certain pathologic conditions, or when cellular damage occurs, the lysosomes may rupture, release their enzymes, and ultimately destroy the cell from within. This event is recognized as **autolysis.**

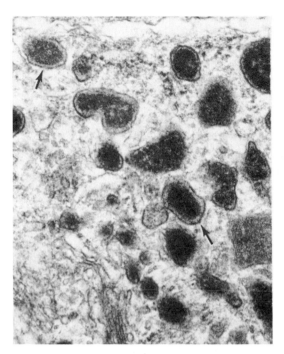

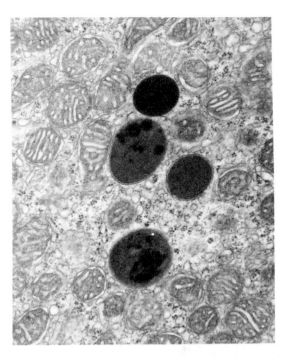

Figure 3 –14. Electron micrograph of the cytoplasm of a macrophage showing primary lysosomes (arrows) characterized by uniform granular content and surrounding membrane. × 45,000.

Figure 3 –15. Electron micrograph showing 4 dark secondary lysosomes surrounded by numerous mitochondria.

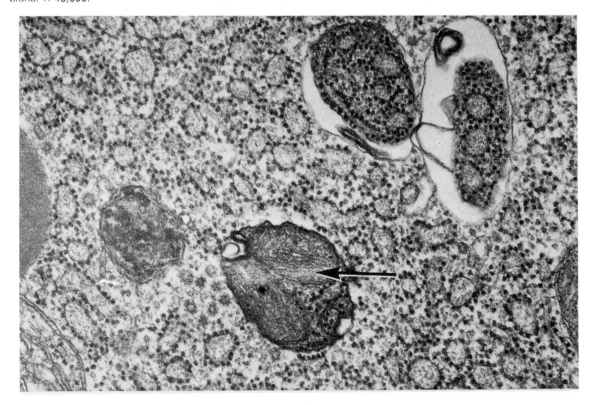

Figure 3 –16. Section of a pancreatic acinar cell showing autophagosomes. *Above:* Two portions of the granular endoplasmic reticulum segregated by a membrane. *Below:* An autophagosome containing mitochondria (arrow) plus granular endoplasmic reticulum. *Left:* Probably a secondary lysosome with undigestible material, also called a residual body.

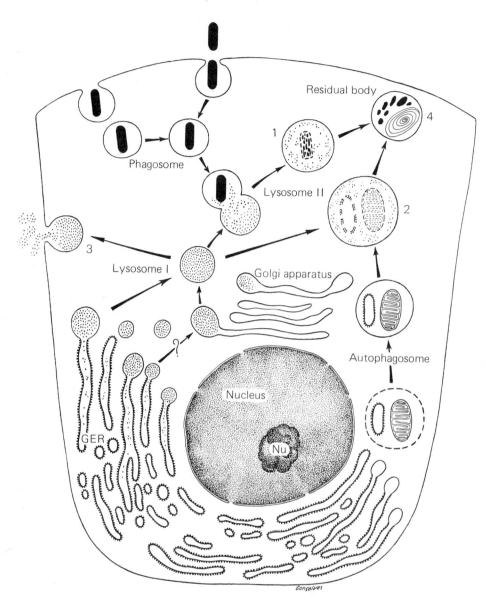

Figure 3 –17. Present concepts of the functions of the lysosomes. Synthesis occurs in the granular endoplasmic reticulum (GER). Participation of the Golgi apparatus in lysosome formation is discussed in the text. *1* and *2:* Lysosome participation in intracellular digestion. *3:* Extrusion and extracellular action of lytic enzymes. *4:* A residual body.

In some cases, primary lysosomes are eliminated from the cell, in which case their enzymes act in the extracellular milieu. An example is the destruction of bone matrix by collagenase synthesized and released by osteoclasts. This type of reaction might play a significant role in an inflammation or injury response. Several possible pathways relating to lysosome activities are schematically illustrated in Fig 3–17.

Lysosomes play an important part in the metabolism of certain substances in the human body and consequently many diseases have been ascribed to deficiencies of lysosomal enzymes. Thus, in **metachromatic leukodystrophy**, there is an

intracellular accumulation of sulfated cerebrosides caused by a deficiency of lysosomal sulfatase. In most of these diseases, a specific lysosomal enzyme is absent, and the digestion of certain substances (glycogen, cerebrosides, gangliosides, sphingomyelin, etc) does not occur. As a result of the accumulation of these substances, there is a subsequent interference with the normal function of the cells.

Peroxisomes or Microbodies

Recently it has been possible to isolate another cytoplasmic organelle from liver by differential centrifugation. This peroxisome (or microbody) (Fig

3–23) is slightly smaller than a mitochondrion, has a single boundary membrane and in some species contains a characteristic electron-dense central core. This organelle is quite widespread and has been identified in protozoa and in plant and animal cells. The peroxisomes are known to have high catalase, urate oxidase, and D-amino acid oxidase activities in their matrices. It seems probable that peroxisomes participate in several different metabolic processes. In vertebrates, they may be related to the oxidation of D-amino acids produced by bacteria in the digestive tract and absorbed by the body.

MICROTUBULES, MICROFILAMENTS, & INTERMEDIATE FILAMENTS

In addition to the membrane-bound organelles, the cytoplasmic matrix exhibits a complex network consisting of microtubules, microfilaments, and intermediate filaments (Fig 3–18). These structural proteins not only provide for the form and shaping of cells but also play an important role in cytoplasmic and cellular movement.

Microtubules

Within the cytoplasmic matrix of most eukaryotic cells are rod- or pipelike organelles known as microtubules. Generally, they have an outer diameter of 24 nm consisting of a dense wall 5 nm thick and a less dense (possibly hollow) core 14 nm wide. Microtubule lengths are variable, and individual tubules have often been observed to attain lengths of several micrometers (Figs 3–18 to 3–21). Normally, a clear zone, probably composed of mucopolysaccharides, isolates the tubules from the adjacent cytoplasm. Occasionally, arms or bridges are found linking 2 or more tubules together (Fig 3–21).

Microtubules are composed of proteinaceous subunits known as **tubulin** (Figs 3–19 and 3–21). Tubulin, a heterodimer, is a molecule consisting of 2 nonidentical monomers designated α and β tubulins. Both tubulins have a molecular weight of about 60,000, and amino acid analysis of the relatively close primary structure of these proteins suggests that α and β tubulins evolved from a single prototubulin.

Under appropriate conditions either in vivo or in vitro, tubulin subunits polymerize into typical microtubules. Using special staining procedures, tubulin appears to organize into **protofilaments** that run parallel to the length of the tubule. A total of 13 protofilaments generally comprise the wall of a microtubule (Figs 3–19 and 3–21).

Microtubule growth, via subunit polymerization, generally occurs at one terminal end of existing tubules. This end is frequently referred to as a **nucleation site.** If colchicine, vinblastine, or podophyllotoxin (antimitotic alkaloids that bind tubulin) is incorporated at this site, microtubule growth will be blocked. In studies with purified tubulins, new tubule formation can occur only in the presence of cell extracts that contain "rings," structures with a greater diameter than that of microtubules. These rings, considered to be **nucleating centers** or "seeds" for tubule assembly, represent coiled tubulin protofilaments.

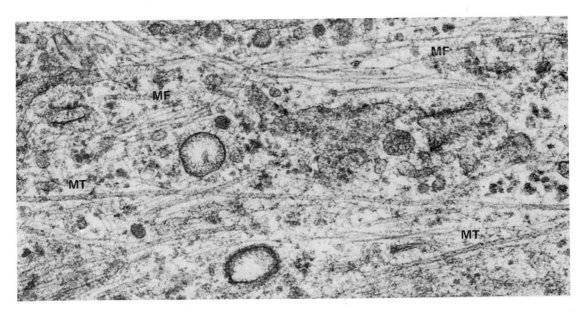

Figure 3 –18. Electron micrograph of rat fibroblast cytoplasm. Observe the microfilaments (MF) and microtubules (MT). × 60,000. (Courtesy of E Katchburian.)

Modulation in microtubule number and length is believed to reflect the alteration of a tubulin monomer-polymer equilibrium. New tubule formation or increase in length of existing tubules would result from the polymerization of free monomers. The dissolution or shortening of tubules would return subunits to the monomer pool (Fig 3–21).

Within the cytoplasm, microtubules may exist in states ranging from an apparently random distribution to highly complex organized subcellular structures. Functions attributed to microtubules are usually based on 2 criteria: (1) the process must be sensitive to the pharmacologic agents known to interact with tubulin, and (2) morphologic data (numbers and orientation of tubules) must be sufficient to implicate tubules with a given cellular process.

Microtubules have been considered to play a significant role in the development and maintenance of cell form based on the observation that tubules in intact cells or from cell-free preparations are normally quite straight and never exhibit oblique bends. These observations suggest that microtubules have a rigid nature and lend support to the implication that they serve as a cytoskeletal element. Morphologic studies indicate a structural role, since microtubules are usually present in a proper orientation either to effect development of or to maintain a given cellular asymmetry. In addition, procedures known to disrupt microtubules generally result in the loss of this cellular asymmetry.

Microtubules have also been implicated as playing a major role in the intracellular transport of other organelles. Time lapse cinematography of living cells reveals a significant movement and redistribution of cytoplasmic components (eg, mitochondria, vesicles). Examples include axoplasmic transport in neurons, melanin dispersion in pigment cells, chromosome movements along the mi-

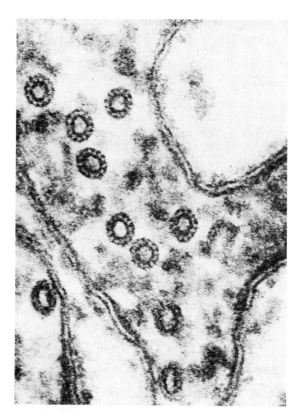

Figure 3 –19. Section of a Sertoli cell of the testicle of *Rana polypedatus*. This material was fixed with glutaraldehyde containing tannic acid. This compound makes the dimers of the microtubules visible, and they are here shown in cross section of the microtubules. Each dimer appears as small white dots surrounded by a dark collar. × 247,000. (Courtesy of V Mizuhira.)

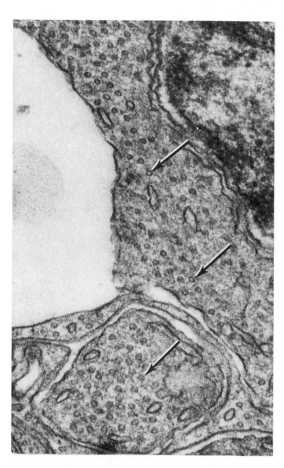

Figure 3 –20. Electron micrograph of a section of a photosensitive retinal cell of a monkey. Observe the accumulation of transversely sectioned microtubules (arrows). Reduced slightly from × 80,000.

totic spindle, and vesicle movements between the endoplasmic reticulum and Golgi and between the Golgi and the cell membrane. In each of these examples, movement is directly related to the elaboration and presence of complex microtubule networks, and such activities are suspended if microtubules are disrupted.

Microtubules also provide the basis for several complex cytoplasmic organelles, including centrioles, cilia, and flagella. **Centrioles** are cylindric structures (0.15 μm in diameter and 0.3–0.5 μm in length) primarily composed of highly organized microtubules (Fig 3–21). Each centriole is composed of 9 sets of microtubule triplets arranged in the fashion of a "pinwheel." The tubules are so close together that adjacent tubules share a common wall. A single pair of centrioles is normally found in nondividing cells. In each pair, the long axes of the centrioles are at right angles to each other. Prior to cell division, each centriole duplicates itself, and the resulting 2 pairs move to opposite sides of the cell and become organizing centers for the developing mitotic spindles (Fig 3–37).

Centrioles duplicate by the growth of a **procentriole** that forms on the surface of, and at right angles to, the original centriole. At first, the procentriole consists of 9 single tubules; later, 9 pairs of tubules arise in close association, with the original tubules completing the centriolar organization.

In nondividing cells, the centriole pairs are usually found in a juxtanuclear position and in association with the Golgi body. Associated with the centrioles are dense **pericentriolar bodies** from which microtubules seem to arise, suggesting that these bodies represent nucleation centers for tubule formation. The pair of centrioles in conjunction with the Golgi apparatus constitute the **cytocenter** of the cell. This complex—and associated microtubule arrays—are apparently related to the transport and distribution of vesicles and secretory granules associated with protein synthesis.

Cilia and **flagella** are motile processes that have a highly organized microtubule core and extend from the surface of many different cell types. Ciliated cells usually possess a large number of cilia that range from 2 to 10 μm in length. Flagellated cells normally have only one or 2 flagella, which range in length from 100 to 200 μm. Cilia and flagella both have a diameter of 0.3–0.5 μm and possess the same complexly organized core of microtubules.

This core consists of 9 pairs of microtubules surrounding 2 central tubules. This sheaf of filaments, possessing the characteristic "9+2 pattern," is called an **axoneme.** The 9 peripheral pairs of **doublets** share a common wall of 2–3 protofilaments. The central pair of tubules are separated from one another and are enclosed within a **central sheath.** Adjacent doublets are linked to each other via protein bridges called **nexins** and are also linked to the central sheath by radial spokes. The tubule

units of each doublet are identified as subfibers **A** and **B.** Subfiber A is essentially a complete microtubule with 13 protofilaments, while subfiber **B** has only 10 or 11 protofilaments. Extending from the surface of subfiber A are pairs of arms that are molecules of an ATPase enzyme known as **dynein** (Fig 3–21).

At the base of each cilium or flagellum is a **basal body.** A basal body is essentially identical to a centriole except at its basal end, which has a complex central organization resembling a cartwheel. At the apical end of the basal body, the 9 triplets converge into the 9 doublets of the ciliary or flagellar axoneme. In developing cilia or flagella, the basal bodies act in some way as a template to control the assembly of the axoneme subunits.

Recent experimental investigations show that the undulating motion exhibited by cilia and flagella is propagated by sliding of adjacent doublets within the axoneme. This sliding mechanism is mediated by the dynein (ATPase) arms that extend from subfiber A of each doublet. It is currently thought that the dynein on the subfiber A of one doublet binds to and "walks along" the surface of subfiber B of the adjacent doublet.

Microfilaments

Contractile activity in skeletal muscle primarily results from an interaction between 2 proteins: **actin** and **myosin.** In muscle, actin is present as a thin (5–7 nm diameter) filament composed of globular subunits organized into a double-stranded helix. In the last few years, structural and biochemical studies reveal that actin constitutes 10–15% of the total protein of *all* cells examined. In nonmuscle cells, actin is usually present in the form of microfilament (5–7 nm diameter) networks. The microfilaments in nonmuscle cells are equated to skeletal muscle actin on the basis of comparisons that consist of the following: (1) Structural analyses: Actin and microfilaments have the same dimensions and globular structure. (2) Biochemical studies: Molecular weights, peptide maps, and amino acid analyses of both actin and microfilaments (nonmuscle) are almost identical. (3) Functional studies: Microfilaments resemble actin in their ability to (a) bind heavy meromyosin (an enzymatically produced subunit of myosin) in an "arrowhead" configuration; (b) act as an enzyme cofactor for myosin ATPase; and (c) assemble into macromolecular threadlike aggregates that will contract in the presence of myosin and ATP.

Biochemical analyses reveal that nonmuscle cells normally contain several species of actin, with some actins differing only in regard to a single amino acid substitution. The close similarities of actin within a given cell, as well as between cells of far-ranging species on the evolutionary scale, attest to the highly conserved nature of this protein. The differences in amino acid composition appear to be related to specific functional and stability charac-

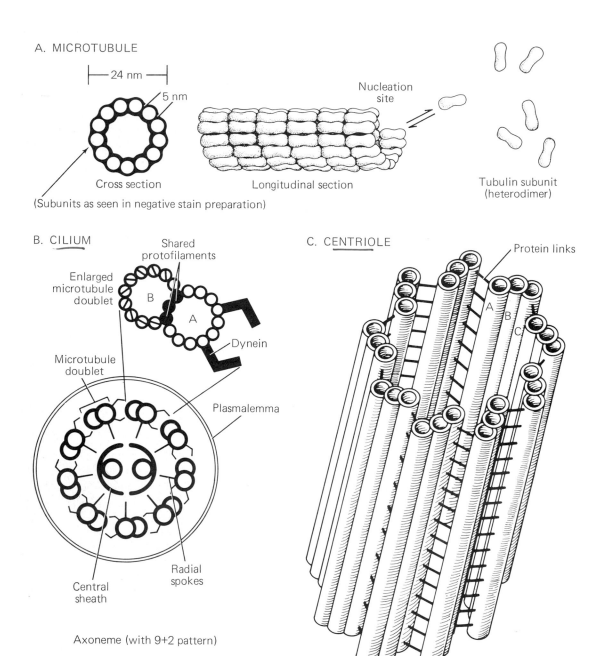

A. MICROTUBULE

├── 24 nm ──┤

5 nm

Cross section

(Subunits as seen in negative stain preparation)

Longitudinal section

Nucleation site

Tubulin subunit (heterodimer)

B. CILIUM

Shared protofilaments

Enlarged microtubule doublet

B

A

Dynein

Microtubule doublet

Plasmalemma

Central sheath

Radial spokes

Axoneme (with 9+2 pattern)

C. CENTRIOLE

Protein links

A

B

C

Figure 3 –21. Schematic representation of microtubules, cilium, and centriole. **A:** Microtubules as seen in the electron microscope following fixation with tannic acid in glutaraldehyde. The unstained tubulin subunits are delineated by the dense tannic acid. Cross sections of tubules reveal a ring of 13 subunits, while in longitudinal section the tubules appear to be composed of 13 linear "protofilaments." Changes in microtubule length are related to the addition or loss of individual tubulin subunits. **B:** A cross section through a cilium reveals a core of microtubules called an **axoneme.** The axoneme consists of 2 central microtubules surrounded by 9 microtubule doublets. In the doublets, microtubule A is complete and consists of 13 subunits, while microtubule B shares 2–3 protofilaments with A. When activated, the dynein arms link adjacent tubules and provide for the sliding of tubules in the presence of ATP. **C:** Centrioles consist of 9 microtubule triplets linked together in a pinwheellike arrangement. In the triplets, microtubule A is complete and consists of 13 subunits, whereas tubules B and C share tubulin subunits. Under normal circumstances, these organelles are found in pairs with the centrioles disposed at right angles to one another.

teristics of the various actins found within a cell. Within cells, microfilaments can be organized in many different forms: (1) In skeletal muscle, they assume a paracrystalline array integrated with thick (16 nm) myosin filaments (2) In most cells, microfilaments are present as a thin sheath just beneath the plasmalemma. These filaments appear to be associated with membrane activities such as endo- and exocytosis and contraction of microvilli (fingerlike projections on some cell surfaces). (3) In cells expressing migratory activity, microfilaments are often found as an irregular lattice matrix at the leading end of the cell as well as constituting the primary structural component of migratory (filopodial) processes. (4) Microfilaments are intimately associated with a number of cytoplasmic organelles, vesicles, and granules. The filaments are believed to play a role in moving and shifting cytoplasmic components (cytoplasmic streaming). (5) Microfilaments form a "purse string" ring of filaments whose constriction results in the cleavage of mitotic cells. (6) In most cells, microfilaments are found scattered in what appears to be an unorganized fashion within the cytoplasm. It is currently thought that such actin networks provide a "cytoskeleton" or structural framework within the cell (Fig 3–25).

While actin filaments in muscle cells are structurally stable, microfilaments in nonmuscle cells are readily able to dissociate and reassemble. Microfilament polymerization appears to be under the direct control of minute changes in Ca^{2+} and cAMP levels. In view of the ability to assemble and disassemble these filaments, cells can precisely control the distribution and concomitantly the functional activity of microfilaments in the cytoplasm.

Presumably, most microfilament-related activities depend upon the simultaneous presence of **myosin,** a protein that binds actin. The structure and activity of the "thick" myosin filaments are described in the section on muscle tissues. A soluble form of myosin has been isolated from most motile nonmuscle cells. The myosin apparently functions by complexing with the microfilaments forming contractile "actomyosin." The myosin in normal preparations is not evident in electron micrographs but may be visualized utilizing special procedures that alter the ionic balance, pH, or temperature of the cell before fixation. Myosin-actin interactions are described in detail in the discussion of the muscle tissue.

There are 3 examples showing that actin may function in the absence of myosin: (1) Actin containing microvilli are able to contract without myosin being present. (2) Some acrosomes (processes of sperm that aid in fertilization) consist of an actin core which provides for the growth and structural framework of the acrosome in the absence of myosin. (3) Pure actin solutions can undergo "gelation," which in the cytoplasm would provide for a structural cytoskeleton matrix.

Intermediate Filaments

Recent ultrastructural investigations reveal that 3 major filamentous structures are present in almost all eukaryotic cells. In addition to the microtubules and microfilaments, cells contain a class of intermediate-sized filaments, also known as **tonofilaments,** with a diameter of 8–10 nm. These filaments have been considered to be involved with the "slow" component of axoplasmic transport, as a smooth muscle cytoskeletal component, in pigment granule movement, as a junctional complex structural element, and with cell spreading.

Most studies show that intermediate filaments are not chemically related to microtubules and microfilaments, although all 3 filament types are structurally integrated within the cytoplasmic matrix. One recent investigation suggested that intermediate filaments possess an actin core, since, following brief trypsinization, the filaments bind heavy meromyosin, a functional assay normally used to identify actin.

Cytoplasmic Inclusions

These are usually transitory components of the cytoplasm, composed mainly of accumulated metabolites or deposits of varied nature. The ac-

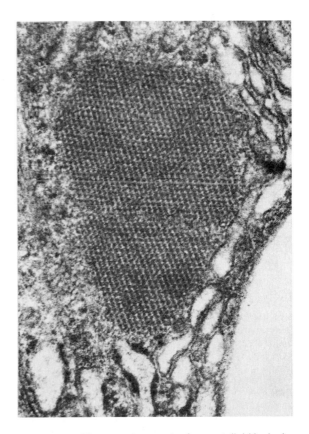

Figure 3 –22. Electron micrograph of a crystalloid inclusion body from a human adrenal cell. Most of these inclusions are composed of proteins. (Courtesy of M Magalhães.)

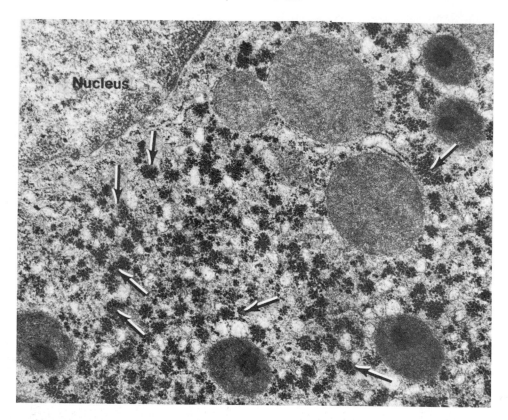

Figure 3 —23. Electron micrograph of a section of a liver cell showing glycogen inclusions appearing as accumulations of electron-dense particles (arrows). The dark structures with a dense core are peroxisomes. × 30,000.

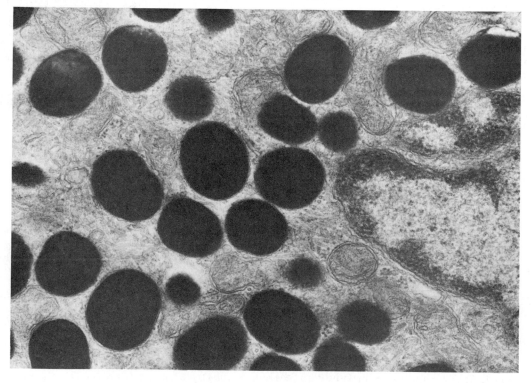

Figure 3 —24. Section of a melanophore. The nucleus is shown at right. The cytoplasm is full of dense, membrane-bound melanin granules. Mitochondria are also numerous. × 20,000.

cumulated metabolites occur in several forms, one of them being lipid droplets present in adipose tissue and liver cells. Carbohydrate accumulations are also visible in several cells in the form of glycogen. After impregnation with lead salts, this substance appears as collections of coarse, irregular, electron-dense particles (Fig 3–23). Proteins are stored in glandular cells as secretory granules; these are periodically released into the extracellular medium. In some cells, protein crystalloids of unknown significance have been described (Fig 3–22).

Deposits of colored substances—**pigment**—are often found in cells (Fig 3–24). They may be synthesized by the cell (eg, in the skin melanocytes) or may come from outside the body (eg, vitamin A). One of the most common pigments is **lipofuscin,** a yellowish-brown substance that increases in quantity in cells with age. Its chemical constitution is complex. It is believed that granules of lipofuscin derive from secondary lysosomes and represent de-posits of undigested substances. Another widely distributed pigment, **melanin,** is abundant in the epidermis of the skin and in the pigment layer of the retina in the form of dense, intracellular, membrane-bound granules.

Matrix or Cytosol

Very little is known about the composition of the matrix, which is the basic component of cytoplasm. It is believed to consist mainly of large enzymatic or nonenzymatic protein molecules linked (or not linked) to carbohydrates, mineral salts, and other absorbed soluble substances. Recent evidence suggests that the matrix has a high content of the protein actin. This protein is probably responsible for the sol-gel transformations that normally occur in the cytoplasm and form a diffuse and thin 3-dimensional network when in the gel phase (Fig 3–25).

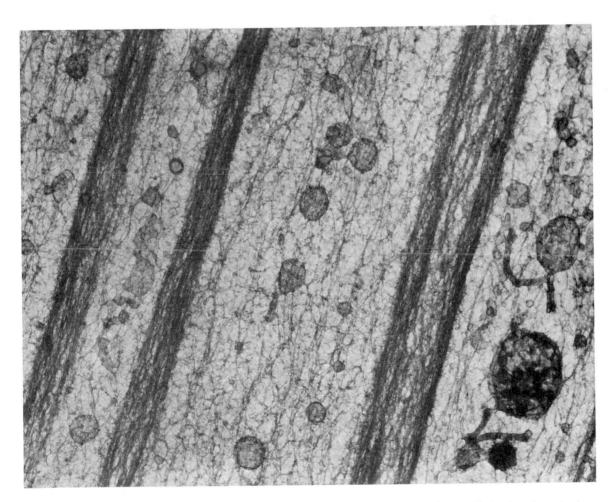

Figure 3 –25. High voltage electron micrograph of a thick section of a human tissue culture cell showing the cytoplasm formed by a 3-dimensional network of thin filaments. The dark lines crossing the figure are bundles of filaments present in elongating cells. (Courtesy of KR Porter.)

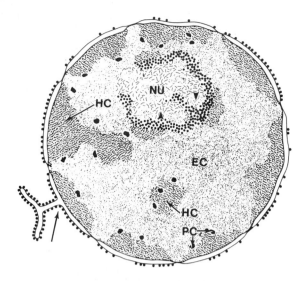

Figure 3 –26 (at left). Structure of a nucleus. The nuclear envelope merges with the endoplasmic reticulum (arrow). HC, heterochromatin; EC, euchromatin. The dark heavy dots (PC) are perichromatin granules. In the nucleolus (NU), fibrillar and granular portions can be distinguished. The portions of heterochromatin surrounding the nucleolus form the **nucleolus-associated chromatin.** Portions of euchromatin appear interspersed with nucleolar material (arrowhead).

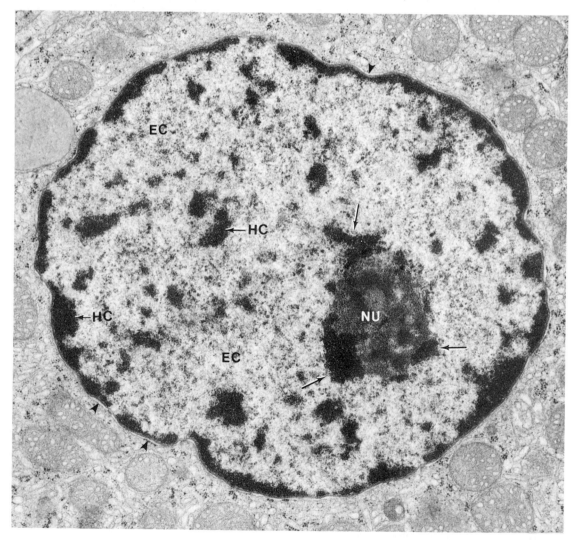

Figure 3 –27. Electron micrograph of a nucleus. HC, heterochromatin; EC, euchromatin. Arrows point to nucleolus (NU). Arrowheads show perinuclear cistern. (Courtesy of J James.)

THE NUCLEUS

The nucleus of the cell appears as a rounded or elongated structure, usually in the center of the cell. In mammalian tissues, its diameter usually varies between 5 and 10 μm. The nucleus is composed of the nuclear envelope, chromatin, the nucleolus, and nucleoplasm (Fig 3–26).

Nuclear Envelope

A nuclear "membrane" can be observed under the light microscope as a thin membrane surrounding the nucleus. Under the electron microscope, however, the nucleus is surrounded by a double-layered structure consisting of 2 parallel unit membranes 40–70 nm apart, providing for a perinuclear space called **perinuclear cistern.** This structure is called the **nuclear envelope.** What is actually seen in the light microscope as the nuclear "membrane" is mainly a layer of heterochromatin that lines and binds to the internal surface of the nuclear envelope (Figs 3–27 and 3–28). Ribosomes are frequently attached to the outer membrane, and this portion of

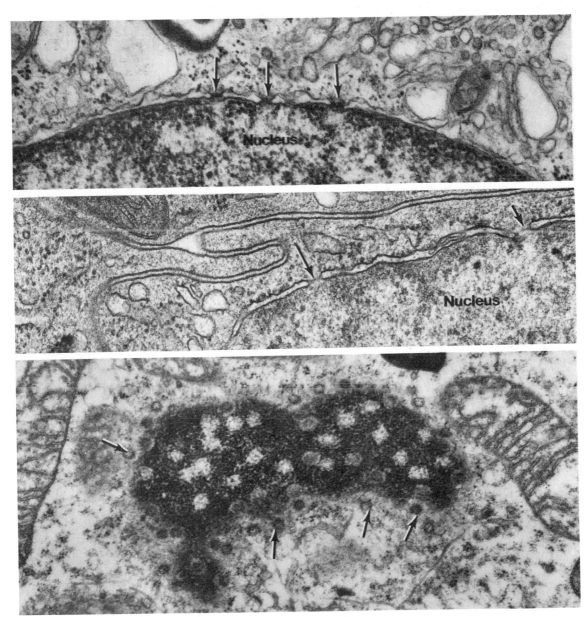

Figure 3 –28. Electron micrographs of nuclei showing their envelopes composed of 2 membranes and the nuclear pores (arrows). The 2 upper pictures are of transverse sections. The lower one is of a tangential section. Observe that the pores are closed by a diaphragm that appears as dense rounded structures in the lower picture (arrows). Chromatin, frequently condensed below the nuclear envelope, is not usually seen in the pore regions. × 80,000.

the nuclear envelope is sometimes continuous with the granular endoplasmic reticulum (Fig 3–26). When covered with ribosomes, the nuclear envelope functions as granular endoplasmic reticulum, synthesizing polypeptide chains and segregating them in the perinuclear cistern between its 2 membranes. Around the nuclear envelope, at sites where the inner and outer membranes fuse, there are circular gaps, the **nuclear pores,** that provide pathways between the nucleus and the cytoplasm. The structures of these pores vary with the cell being studied (Figs 3–26, 3–28, and 3–30). The pores are not open but are bridged by an electron-dense membrane forming a single-layered diaphragm of basic protein. This monolayer structure is thinner than the membranes comprising the nuclear envelope. The permeability of the nucleus to molecules is variable, but all pores are permeable to some macromolecules.

Chromatin

Two types of chromatin can be distinguished with the electron microscope (Figs 3–26 and 3–27). **Heterochromatin,** which is electron-dense and appears as coarse granules or patches, is visible in the light microscope after appropriate staining. **Euchromatin** is visible only in the electron microscope and assumes the form of a loose network of fine fibrils below the resolution of the light microscope. The proportion of heterochromatin to euchromatin provides for the light to dark appearance of nuclei in light and electron microscopic tissue sections. The intensity of nuclear staining resulting from the chromatin is frequently used to differentiate and identify different tissues and cell types in the light microscope. Consequently, the morphology of chromatin in cell nuclei is mentioned throughout this book with respect to the study and identification of cells and tissues.

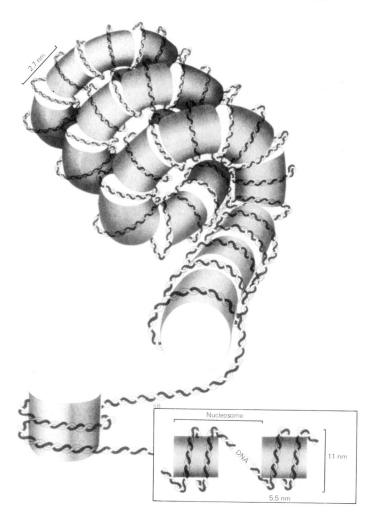

Figure 3 –29. Chromatin is composed of repeating units of small particles visible with the electron microscope in suitable preparations. These units **(nucleosomes)** contain a core of histones. DNA surrounds these particles in helical formation and binds them together. The strands that grossly resemble a necklace form a superhelix. (Reproduced, with permission, from Bradbury EM: La chromatine. La Recherche 9:466, 1978.)

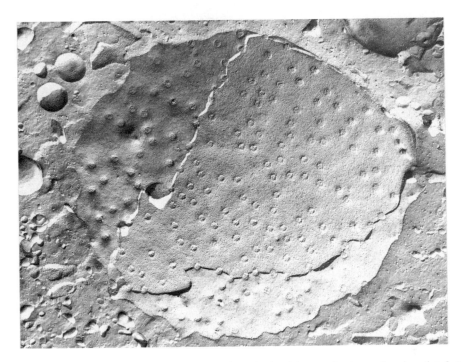

Figure 3 –30. Electron micrograph of rat intestine preparation obtained by cryofracture, showing the 2 membranous components of the nuclear envelope and the nuclear pores. (Courtesy of A Pinto da Silva.)

Chromatin is composed mainly of coiled strands of DNA bound to basic proteins (histones); its structure is schematically presented in Fig 3–29. Chromatin DNA represents the major form of DNA in the cell and consequently carries most of the genetic information. Within the chromatin, the messenger, ribosomal, and transfer ribonucleic acids (mRNA, rRNA, and tRNA), as well as their precursors, are synthesized.

The nucleoprotein of chromatin is coiled, and the degree of coiling varies during cell activity. The chromatin pattern of a nucleus has been considered a guide to the cell's activity. In lightly staining nuclei (with few heterochromatin clumps), more DNA surface is available for the transcription of genetic information. In darkly staining nuclei, less surface is available as a result of the coiling of DNA. In general, cells with light nuclei are more active than those with condensed, dark nuclei.

Careful study of the chromatin of mammalian cell nuclei has revealed the presence of a heterochromatin mass frequently observed in female cells but not in male cells. This chromatin clump is the **sex chromatin.** It was first observed in nerve cells obtained from female cats and is present in cells of most mammals, including humans. This heterochromatin mass is one of the pair of X chromosomes that exists in female cells. It remains tightly coiled and is visible during interphase, while the other X chromosome is uncoiled and not visible. The coiling of this chromosome explains why it is easily stained and can be observed with the light microscope.

Evidence suggests that the coiled X chromosome comprising the sex chromatin is genetically inactive. The male has one X chromosome and one Y chromosome as sex determinants; the X chromosome is dispersed, and therefore no sex chromatin is visible. In human epithelial cells, sex chromatin appears as a small granule attached to the nuclear membrane. The cells lining the internal surface of the cheek are frequently used to study sex chromatin. Blood smears are also often used, in which case the sex chromatin appears as a drumsticklike appendage to the nuclei of the neutrophilic leukocytes (Fig 3–31).

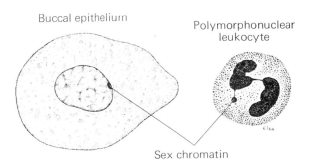

Buccal epithelium

Polymorphonuclear leukocyte

Sex chromatin

Figure 3 –31. Morphology of sex chromatin in human mouth epithelium and in a polymorphonuclear leukocyte. In the epithelium, it appears as a small, dense granule adhering to the nuclear envelope. In the leukocyte, it has a drumstick shape.

* = Barr body

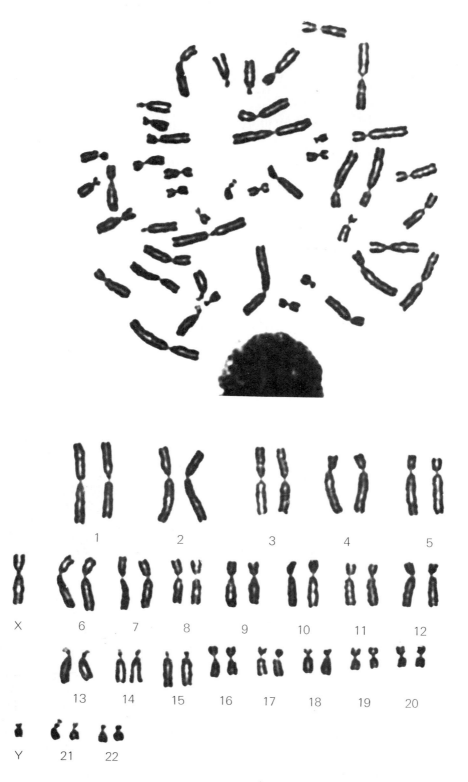

Figure 3 –32. *Above:* Photomicrograph of chromosomes of a human cell obtained during metaphase. *Below:* The chromosomes grouped according to their morphologic characteristics. (Courtesy of G Gimenez-Martin.)

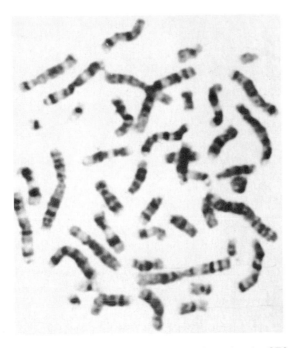

Figure 3 –33. Human karyotype preparation using the GTG banding technic (*G* bands by *Trypsin* and *Giemsa* stain). Each chromosome has a particular pattern of banding, permitting identification of individual chromosomes. × 2000. (Courtesy of A Wajntal.)

The study of sex chromatin has wide applicability in medicine because it permits analysis of genetic sex in doubtful cases (hermaphroditism, pseudohermaphroditism). It is essential for the study of other anomalies involving the sex chromosomes—eg, Klinefelter's syndrome, in which testicular abnormalities, azoospermia, and other symptoms are associated with the presence of XXY chromosomes in the cell.

The study of chromosomes of animals, and particularly of humans, made considerable progress after the discovery of methods of inducing cells to divide, then arresting mitotic cells during metaphase and subsequently causing cellular rupture, which permits the separation, detailed observation, and analysis of the chromosomes. Mitosis can be induced by phytohemagglutinin and can be arrested by colchicine. Rupture of cells is brought about by initial immersion in a hypotonic solution, causing swelling, after which cells are flattened and broken between a glass slide and a coverslip. The pattern of chromosomes obtained with a human cell after staining is illustrated in Figs 3–32 and 3–33. In addition to the 2 sex chromosomes X and Y, it is customary to group the remaining chromosomes according to their morphologic characteristics in 22 successively numbered pairs (Fig 3–32).

Up until recently, recognition of individual chromosomes was not possible because different chromosomes of the same karyotype often had the same general morphology. The development of technics that reveal segmentation of chromosomes in transverse, differentially stained bands made it possible not only to identify individual chromosomes but also to study in detail phenomena of genetic deletion and translocation. These technics are based mainly on the appearance of transverse bands in chromosomes previously treated with saline or enzyme solution and stained with fluorescent dyes or Giemsa's blood staining technic (Fig 3–33). (See Chapter 13.) This procedure has revolutionized the field of cytogenetics and has made possible a series of important observations on human cytogenetics.

The number and type of chromosomes encountered in an individual is known as his or her **karyotype.** Study of karyotypes has revealed chromosomal alterations associated with several types of diseases, including a form of leukemia.

Nucleolus

The nucleolus is a rounded structure, generally acidophilic, and rich in RNA and basic proteins. The nucleus may contain one or more nucleoli of variable dimensions. When the nuclear chromatin is very condensed, as in lymphocytes, it becomes difficult to visualize the nucleoli within the nucleus. A dense portion of chromatin found attached to the nucleolus is known as **nucleolus-associated**

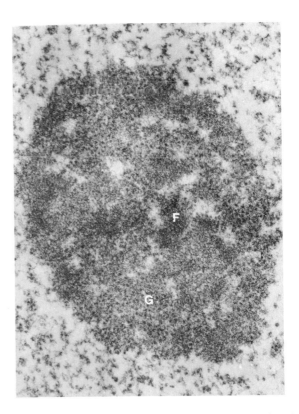

Figure 3 –34. Nucleolus of a newt showing its fibrillar (F) and granular (G) portions. × 40,000.

chromatin. The nucleolus disperses during cell division but reappears in the telophase stage of mitosis.

In the electron microscope, nucleoli usually consist of 3 distinct regions. The **pars granulosa** and the **pars fibrosa** both contain mainly ribonucleoprotein in the form of granules or very fine filaments considered to be precursors of future ribosomes (Fig 3–34). The third region—the chromosomal portion—consists of dispersed filaments of DNA that permeate the other 2 regions.

outer margin

inner core →

It is in this third portion of nucleolus that ribosomal RNA is synthesized. It is then transformed and deposited first in the pars fibrosa and then in the granulosa, before being transferred to the cytoplasm. Larger nucleoli are encountered in young cells during intense proliferative activity, in cells that are actively synthesizing proteins, and in the majority of rapidly growing malignant tumors.

Nucleoplasm

Nucleoplasm is an amorphous substance that fills the space between the chromatin and the nucleoli in the nucleus. It is composed mainly of proteins (some of which have enzymatic activity), metabolites, and ions.

CELL DIVISION

Cell division can be observed with the light microscope. During this process, known as **mitosis,** the mother cell divides and each of the daughter cells receives a chromosomal karyotype identical to that of the mother cell. Essentially, a longitudinal duplication of the chromosomes takes place, and they are distributed to the daughter cells. The phase during which the cell does not undergo division is called **interphase,** and the nucleus appears as it is normally observed in microscope preparations. The process of mitosis is dynamic and continuous but is subdivided into phases to facilitate its study (Figs 3–35 and 3–36).

The **prophase** is characterized by the gradual coiling up of chromatin of the nucleus, giving rise to several individualized rod-shaped or hairpin-shaped bodies that stain intensely. These are the **chromosomes.** The nuclear envelope remains unaltered, and the chromosomes appear coiled in the nucleus. The centrioles duplicate and separate, and a pair migrates to each pole of the cell. Simultaneously, the microtubules of the mitotic spindle appear between the 2 pairs of centrioles (Figs 3–35 and 3–37).

During **metaphase,** the nuclear envelope and the nucleolus disappear. The chromosomes migrate to the equatorial plane of the cell, where each di-

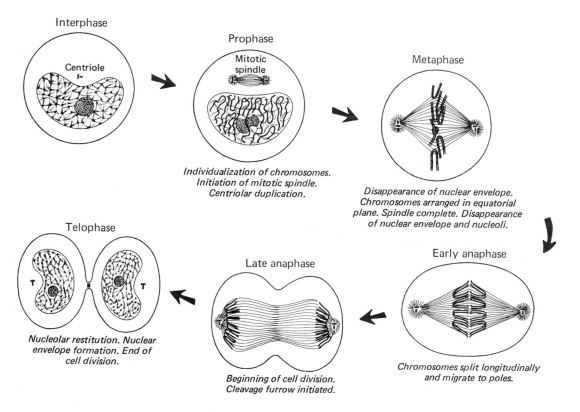

Interphase

Centriole

Prophase

Mitotic spindle

*Individualization of chromosomes.
Initiation of mitotic spindle.
Centriolar duplication.*

Metaphase

*Disappearance of nuclear envelope.
Chromosomes arranged in equatorial
plane. Spindle complete. Disappearance
of nuclear envelope and nucleoli.*

Telophase

*Nucleolar restitution. Nuclear
envelope formation. End of
cell division.*

Late anaphase

*Beginning of cell division.
Cleavage furrow initiated.*

Early anaphase

*Chromosomes split longitudinally
and migrate to poles.*

Figure 3 –35. Phases of mitosis.

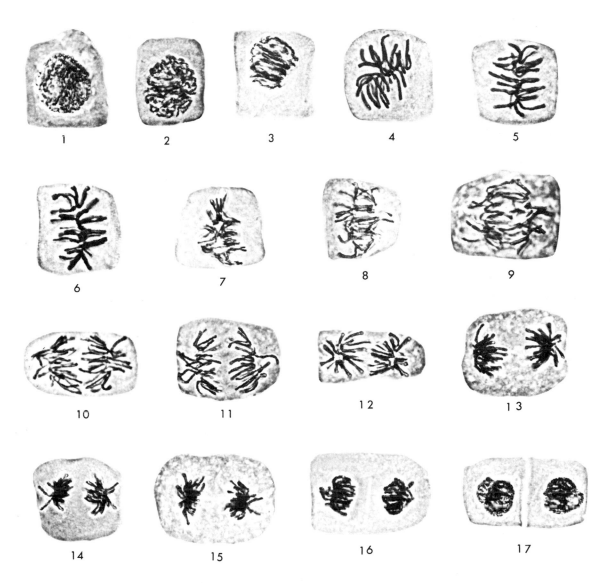

Figure 3–36. Stages of mitosis in the cells of the root of *Allium cepa*. Phase microscopy. 1–3, prophase; 4–7, metaphase; 8–13, anaphase; 17, telophase. (Courtesy of G Gimenez-Martin.)

vides longitudinally to form 2 chromatids. These attach to the microtubules of the mitotic spindle at a special plaquelike, electron-dense region, the **centromere (kinetochore)** (Figs 3–37 and 3–38).

In **anaphase,** the sister chromatids separate from each other and migrate toward the opposite poles of the cell, following the direction of the spindle microtubules. Throughout this process, the centromeres move from the center, pulling along the remainder of the chromosome (Figs 3–35 and 3–36). It has been shown by immunofluorescence that microtubular protein (tubulin), actin, and myosin appear in the spindle region. It is very probable that these proteins participate in the process of chromosome migration to the cell poles.

Telophase is characterized by the reappear-

ance of nuclei in the daughter cells. The chromosomes revert to their semidispersed state and the nucleoli, chromatin, and nuclear envelope reappear. While these nuclear alterations are taking place, a constriction develops at the level of the equatorial plane of the mother cell and progresses until it divides the cytoplasm and its organelles in half (Fig 3–35). An accumulation of microfilaments occurs beneath the cell membrane in the region of mitotic constriction. This and other evidence suggests that the microfilaments participate in the cytoplasmic component of cell division.

Most body tissues undergo a constant turnover because of continuous cell division and continuous death of cells. The nerve tissue and cardiac muscle cells are an exception since they do not regenerate

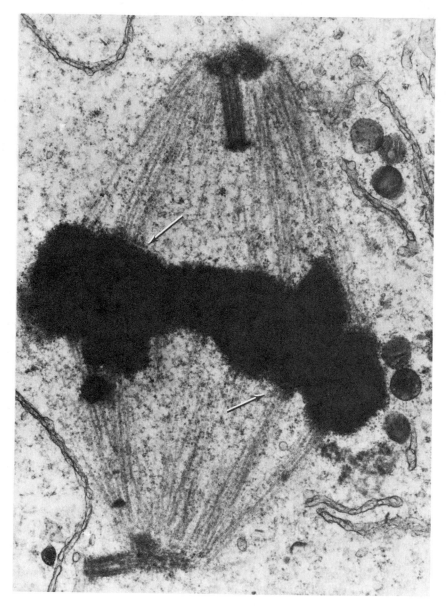

Figure 3 –37. Electron micrograph of a section of a rooster spermatocyte in metaphase. Observe the presence of 2 centrioles in each pole, the mitotic spindle formed by microtubules, and the chromosomes in the equatorial plate. The arrows show the insertion of microtubules in the centromeres. Reduced from × 30,000. (Courtesy of R McIntosh.)

or multiply postnatally. The turnover rate of the cells varies greatly from one tissue to another—rapid in the epithelium of the alimentary canal and the epidermis, slow in the pancreas and thyroid.

THE CELL CYCLE

Mitosis is the visible manifestation of cell division, but there are other processes, not so easily observed with the light microscope, that play a fundamental role in cell multiplication. Principal among these is the phase in which DNA, the main chromosomal component, replicates. This process can be analyzed by the introduction of labeled, radioactive DNA precursors, followed by biochemical and radioautographic methods. DNA duplication has been shown to occur during **interphase,** when no visible phenomena of cell division are observable in the microscope. This alternation between mitosis and interphase in all tissues with cellular turnover is known as the **cell cycle.** A careful study of the cell cycle reveals that it may be divided into 2 stages: mitosis, consisting of the 4

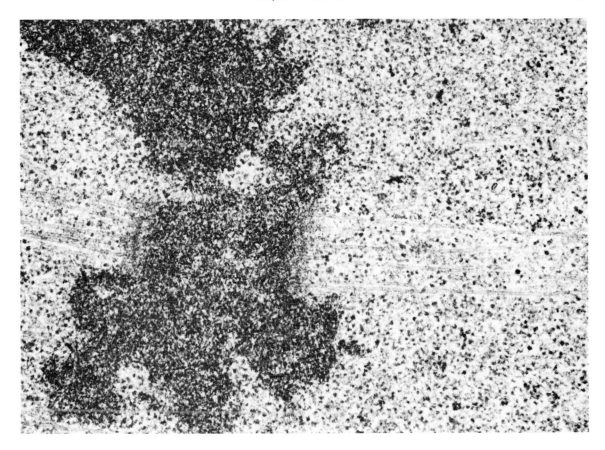

Figure 3–38. Electron micrograph of the metaphase of a human lung cell in tissue culture. Note the insertion of microtubules in the centromeres of the densely stained chromosomes. Reduced from × 50,000. (Courtesy of R McIntosh.)

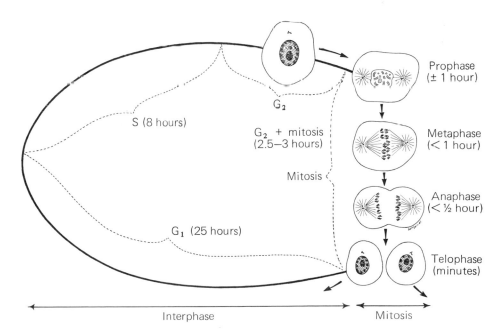

Figure 3–39. Phases of the cell cycle. G_1 (presynthetic) phase is variable and depends on many factors, including the rate of cell division in the tissue. In this particular case of bone tissue, it lasts 25 hours. The S (DNA synthetic) phase lasts about 8 hours. The G_2 plus mitosis phase lasts 2.5–3 hours. The times are from Young RW in J Cell Biol 14:357, 1962.

phases already described (prophase, metaphase, anaphase, and telophase), and interphase.

Interphase is itself divided into 3 phases: G_1 (presynthesis), S (DNA synthesis), and G_2 (post DNA duplication) (Fig 3–39). Synthesis and duplication of DNA take place in the S phase. The sequence of these phases and the time* involved are illustrated in Fig 3–39. The G_1 (for gap) phase is the phase during which RNA and protein synthesis occur and the cell volume, previously reduced to one-half by mitosis, is restored to its normal size. In cells that are not continuously dividing, the cell cycle activities may be temporarily or permanently abated. Cells in such a stage of development are referred to as being in G_0.

Processes that occur during the G_2 phase are the production and accumulation of energy to be utilized during mitosis; reproduction of centrioles; and the assembly of tubulin into microtubules during mitosis.

CELL DYNAMICS

Study of the cell by means of the light or electron microscope gives the false impression that the

*See comment in legend to Fig 3–39.

cell is static. However, cinematography at accelerated rates (5–30 times normal) shows considerable activity in cells. Thus, it has been observed that the nucleus can rotate within the cytoplasm up to 270 degrees per minute. Mitochondria demonstrate active wriggling movements in the cytoplasm. In only a few minutes, they can be seen to become fragmented and fuse together again.

Profound cellular changes are also observed during cell differentiation. Depending upon the function of the cell, some organelles become better developed than others and are major features of the cytoplasm. Cytoplasm in striated muscle cells is composed mainly of contractile fibrils, the myofibrils. Cells of the acinar pancreas that synthesize and secrete protein contain cytoplasm almost completely filled with granular endoplasmic reticulum and zymogen granules. Furthermore, in an already differentiated cell, modification of the organelles can be observed according to the phase of cell activity. This depends on whether the cell is hypoactive or hyperactive. Cells that actively secrete protein have a more highly developed granular endoplasmic reticulum and Golgi apparatus than those that secrete protein in moderate or minimal amounts.

In addition to these morphologic aspects of the cell's continuous activity as reflected in its organelles, it should also be realized that with few exceptions, the cell's chemical components are actively being turned over.

•   •   •

References

Bajer A, Mole-Bajer J: Architecture and function of the mitotic spindle. Adv Mol Biol 1:213, 1971.

Baserga R, Weibel F: The cell cycle of mammalian cells. Int Rev Exp Pathol 7:1, 1969.

Baudhuin P: Liver peroxisomes: Cytology and function. Ann NY Acad Sci 168:214, 1969.

Bertalanffy FD: Tritiated thymidine vs. colchicine technique in the study of cell population cytodynamics. Lab Invest 13:871, 1964.

Bloom W, Fawcett DW: *A Textbook of Histology*, 10th ed. Saunders, 1975.

Brachet J, Mirsky AE (editors): *The Cell.* Academic Press, 1959.

Bradbury EM: La chromatine. La Recherche 9:466, 1978.

Brinkley BR, Porter KR: *International Cell Biology, 1976—1977.* Rockefeller Univ Press, 1977.

Dalton AJ, Haguenau F (editors): *The Nucleus.* Academic Press, 1968.

De Duve C, Wattiaux R: Functions of lysosomes. Annu Rev Physiol 28:435, 1966.

DeRobertis E, Saez FA, DeRobertis EMF: *Cell Biology.* Saunders, 1975.

Dingle JT: *Lysosomes in Biology and Pathology.* 5 vols. Elsevier/North-Holland, 1973–1978.

Favard P: The Golgi apparatus. Page 1131 in: *Handbook of Molecular Biology.* Lima de Faria A (editor). North-Holland Publishing Co, 1969.

Friend DS, Gilula NB: Variation in tight and gap junctions in mammalian tissues. J Cell Biol 53:758, 1972.

Gahan PB: Histochemistry of lysosomes. Int Rev Cytol 21:2, 1967.

Granboulan N, Granboulan P: Cytochimie ultrastructurale de nucléole et le noyau. Exp Cell Res 38:604, 1965.

Grouchy J & others: *Atlas des maladies chromosomiques.* Expansion Scientifique Francaise (Paris), 1977.

Hsu TC: Longitudinal differentiation of chromosomes. Annu Rev Genet 7:153, 1974.

Inoué S, Stephen RE: *Molecules and Cell Movement.* Raven Press, 1975.

Jones AL, Fawcett DW: Hypertrophy of the agranular endoplasmic reticulum in hamster liver induced by phenobarbital. J Histochem Cytochem 14:215, 1966.

Junqueira LCU. Control of cell secretion. In: *Secretory Mechanisms of Salivary Glands.* Schneyer LH, Schneyer CA (editors). Academic Press, 1967.

Lazarides E, Revel J-P: The molecular basis of cell movement. Sci Am 240:88, May 1979.

Mazia D: Mitosis and the physiology of cell division. In: *The Cell.* Vol 3. Brachet J, Mirsky AE (editors). Academic Press, 1961.

Monneron A, Bernhard W: Fine structural organization of the interphase nucleus in some mammalian tissues. J Ultrastruct Res 27:266, 1969.

Neutra M, Leblond CP: The Golgi apparatus. Sci Am 220:100, Feb 1969.

Orrenius S, Ericson JLE, Ernster L: Phenobarbital-induced synthesis of the microsomal drug metabolizing enzyme system and its relationship to the proliferation of endoplasmic membranes: A morphological and biochemical study. J Cell Biol 25:627, 1965.

Paine PL, Feldherr CM: Nucleocytoplasmic exchange of macromolecules. Exp Cell Res 74:81, 1972.

Rabinowitz M, Swift H: Mitochondrial nucleic acids and the problem of biogenesis. Physiol Rev 50:376, 1970.

Rambourg A: Morphological and histochemical aspects of glycoproteins at the surface of animal cells. Int Rev Cytol 31:57, 1971.

Rappaport R: Cytokinesis in animal cells. Int Rev Cytol 31:301, 1972.

Remmer H, Merker HJ: Effect of drugs on the formation of smooth endoplasmic reticulum and drug metabolizing enzymes. Ann NY Acad Sci 123:79, 1965.

Resibois A & others: Lysosome and storage diseases. Int Rev Exp Pathol 9:93, 1970.

Saier MH Jr, Stiles CD: *Molecular Dynamics in Biological Membranes.* Springer-Verlag, 1975.

Schatz G, Mason T-L: The biosynthesis of mitochondrial proteins. Annu Rev Biochem 43:51, 1974.

Singer SJ: The molecular organization of membranes. Annu Rev Biochem 43:805, 1975.

Spooner BS & others: Microfilaments and cell locomotion. J Cell Biol 49:595, 1971.

Staehelin LA, Hull BE: Junctions between living cells. Sci Am 238:41, May 1978.

Tedeschi H: *Cell Physiology: Molecular Dynamics.* Academic Press, 1974.

Vincent WS, Miller OL Jr (editors): *International Symposium on the Nucleolus: Its Structure and Function.* Monograph No. 12. National Cancer Institute, 1967.

Weissman G, Claiborne R: *Cell Membranes: Biochemistry, Cell Biology, and Pathology.* HP Publishing Co (New York), 1975.

Wessels NK & others: Microfilaments in cellular and developmental processes. Science 171:135, 1971.

Zagury D & others: Immunoglobulin synthesis and secretion. 2. Radioautographic study of site of addition of carbohydrate moieties and intracellular transport. J Cell Biol 46:52, 1970.

4 | Epithelial Tissue

Tissues are structures formed by collections of cells that frequently have similar morphologic characteristics and similar functions. Despite its complexity, the human body is composed of only 4 basic types of tissue: epithelial, connective, muscular, and nervous. These tissues do not exist as isolated units but rather in association one with another and in variable proportions, forming different organs and systems of the body.

Connective tissue is characterized by the abundance of intercellular material produced by its cells; muscular tissue is composed of elongated cells that have the specialized function of contraction; and nervous tissue is composed of cells with elongated processes extending from the cell body that have the specialized functions of receiving, generating, and transmitting nervous impulses.

Epithelial tissues, the subject of this chapter, are composed of closely aggregated polyhedral cells with very little intercellular substance. Adhesion between these cells is strong. Thus, cellular sheets are formed that cover the surface of the body and line its cavities.

Epithelial tissues have the following principal functions: (1) covering and lining surfaces (eg, skin); (2) absorption (eg, the intestines); (3) secretion (eg, the epithelial cells of glands); (4) sensory (eg, neuroepithelium); and (5) contractile (eg, myoepithelial cells).

Epithelia are derived from all 3 embryonic germ layers. Most of the epithelium lining the skin, mouth, nose, and anus has an ectodermal origin. The lining of the respiratory system, the digestive tract, and the glands of the digestive tract such as the pancreas and the liver are derived from the endoderm. Other epithelia (eg, the kidney) originate from mesoderm.

GENERAL CHARACTERISTICS OF EPITHELIAL TISSUES

Although the epithelial tissues have varied morphology depending on their function and position in the body, they possess some basic common characteristics.

The Forms of Epithelial Cells

The form and dimensions of epithelial cells are varied, ranging from high columnar to low squamous cells and including all intermediate forms (Fig 4–1). Their common polyhedral form is accounted for by their juxtaposition in cellular layers or masses. A similar aspect might be observed if a large number of inflated rubber balloons were compressed into a limited space. With appropriate stains, the cell nuclei have a distinctive appearance, varying from spherical to elongated or elliptic in

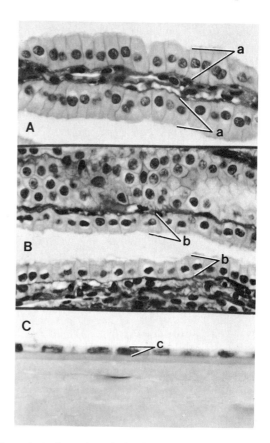

Figure 4 –1. Examples of simple epithelia. *A:* Simple columnar type from the intestine (a). *B:* Simple cuboidal epithelium from the kidney (b). *C:* Simple squamous epithelium from the cornea (c).

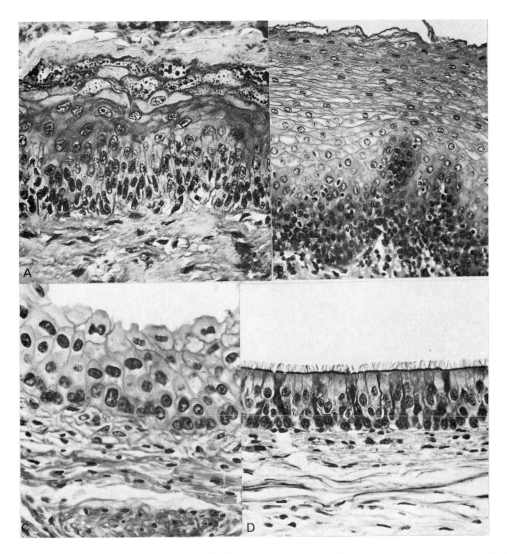

Figure 4 –2. Photomicrographs of several types of epithelial tissue. *A:* Stratified squamous keratinized epithelium. *B:* Stratified nonkeratinized squamous epithelium. *C:* Transitional epithelium. *D:* Pseudostratified columnar ciliated epithelium. H&E stain, × 500.

shape. The nuclear form usually corresponds grossly to the cell shape; thus, cuboidal cells have spherical nuclei whereas squamous cells have horizontal, elliptic nuclei. The long axis of the nucleus is always parallel to the main axis of the cell.

Since the limits between cells are frequently indistinguishable, observation of the form of the cell nucleus is of great importance because it is an indirect clue to the shape of the cell. This is of value not only for itself but also for determining cell disposition—whether or not they are arranged in layers, which is a useful morphologic criterion for classifying epithelia (Fig 4–2).

Presence of a Basal Lamina

All epithelial tissues have on their basal surface, in contact with the underlying connective tissue, a continuous sheetlike extracellular structure called the **basal lamina.** With few exceptions, this structure is visible only with the electron microscope and appears as a thin granular layer in which very fine fibrils comprise a delicate network. It is known to contain the protein collagen and some amorphous protein-polysaccharide complexes.

Until recently, it was not clear whether the basal lamina was of epithelial or connective tissue origin. Recent results obtained with immunofluorescence, combined with the observation that basal laminas are formed in pure epithelial tissue cultures, indicate that epithelial cells are probably the main source of the basal lamina.

Although the thickness of the basal lamina is variable (50–80 nm), it does not present a barrier to the diffusion of most substances. Since epithelial tissues are avascular, basal lamina permeability to substances is a prerequisite for proper nutrition and

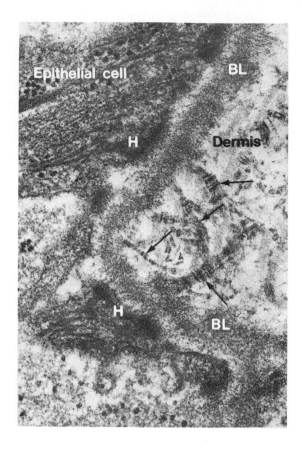

Figure 4 –3 (at left). Section of human skin showing the zone of the epithelial–connective tissue junction. Observe the anchoring fibers (arrows) that apparently insert in the basal lamina (BL). The characteristically irregular spacing of these fibers distinguishes them from common collagen fibers. Note also the hemidesmosomes (H). (See p 65.) × 54,000. (Courtesy of FM Guerra Rodrigo.)

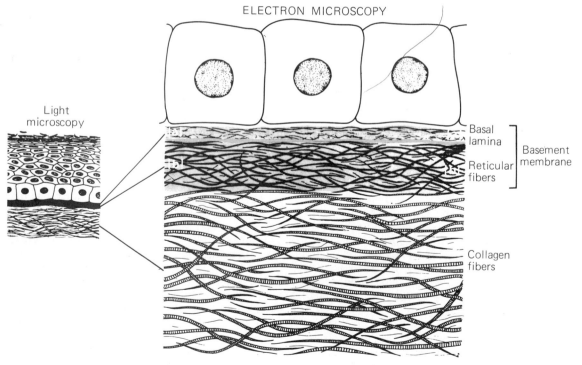

Figure 4 –4. Structure of basement membrane in the skin. *Left:* As seen with the light microscope after staining by PAS or silver impregnation. *Right:* As seen with the electron microscope. Staining by PAS and silver is believed to be due to the high polysaccharide content of the basal lamina and reticular fibers.

function. In some epithelial tissues (eg, the skin) subject to friction, the basal lamina is anchored to the subjacent connective tissue by small fibers of collagen termed **anchoring fibers** (Fig 4–3).

In most epithelia, fibrils of collagen (reticular fibers) complexed with amorphous protein-polysaccharides constitute another layer beneath the basal lamina called the **fibrous** or **reticular lamina.** This considerably thicker structure is clearly visible with the light microscope when stained by 2 methods: the reticular fibers can be impregnated with silver salts, and the amorphous component has a strong PAS reaction. All 3 constituents—basal lamina, ground substance, and reticular fibers—form what is called the **basement membrane** (Fig 4–4). The collagen of the basal lamina is of type IV. That of the subjacent reticular fibers is probably type III collagen. The thick fibers below this layer are known to be formed by collagen type I. (The significance of reticular fibers and types of collagen is explained in Chapter 5.) In this book, the term basement membrane will be reserved for the thicker structures visible with the light microscope. However, it is a somewhat misleading expression, for it has created confusion with the term used to denote those cell membranes from the basal region of the cells. In current usage, the terms basal lamina and basement membrane are frequently used interchangeably; however, this practice is not only incorrect but also has the inconvenience of not distinguishing between these 2 different structures.

Cohesion Among Epithelial Cells

Epithelial cells are extremely cohesive, and relatively strong mechanical forces are necessary to separate them. This quality of intercellular binding is especially marked in those epithelial tissues usually subjected to traction and pressure (eg, the skin). This is due in part to the binding action of the glycoproteins of the plasma membrane. Calcium ions are also important in maintaining this cellular cohesion. Thus, the chelating agent EDTA, which complexes with calcium, is known to decrease cell adhesion and is widely used in cell biology to separate epithelial cells, a necessary step in obtaining a suspension of isolated cells. Intercellular adhesiveness changes with age, as indicated by the cells' different responses to the presence of trypsin or deoxycholate or the removal of calcium.

Probably the most important factors in cell adhesion, however, are special junctional structures the most frequent of which are the **desmosomes,** or **maculae adherentes** (Figs 4–5 and 4–6). These are complex disk-shaped structures that exhibit the juxtaposition of 2 electron-dense regions on the cytoplasmic faces of the cell membranes of 2 neighboring cells. These regions, called **attachment plaques** or **dense cytoplasmic plates,** consist essentially of a granular electron density closely associated with the innermost surface of the cellular

unit membrane. Groups of intermediate filaments are inserted in the intracellular region of the desmosome or make hairpin turns and return into the cytoplasm. Between the membranes of a desmosome region—and therefore in the extracellular space—fibrillar and granular structures are frequently observed that are probably responsible for the intense intercellular adhesion (Fig 4–7).

In the contact zone between an epithelial cell and the basal lamina, **hemidesmosomes** can often be observed. Morphologically, these structures take the shape of half of a desmosome on the epithelial plasmalemma only and probably bind the epithelial cell to the subjacent tissue (Fig 4–3).

The thin intracellular fibrils inserted into the desmosomes are also present at other sites in the epithelial cells. Particularly in the columnar cells of the intestinal epithelium, they may form a horizontal mat of intermediate filaments just below the surface membrane—the **terminal web**—from which the cytoplasmic organelles are excluded (Fig 4–5). These intermediate filaments apparently form a sort of intracellular skeleton (cytoskeleton). The terminal web serves as an anchoring site for the actinlike microfilaments that extend upward into the microvilli.

Desmosomes are distributed in patches along the surface of the cell. Despite the fact that they maintain cell cohesion, they do not occlude the separation of the cell membranes in regions where they are not present. Consequently, fluid material can circulate between epithelial cells, and this phenomenon represents an important pathway in the physiology of epithelial tissues.

The achievement of biologic complexity and specialization depends to a large extent on compartmentalization of the living structure. This occurs on a cellular level with several organelles (see Chapter 3). In the organism, compartmentalization can be established and maintained by the presence of barriers formed by intercellular junctions that bind adjacent epithelial cells together so that they comprise cellular sheets or layers. Specific binding sites or junctions can impede the passage of various substances between adjacent cells. The epithelial lining of the gut and skin are 2 examples where these barriers can be found. In Chapter 12, several other examples of barriers between the blood and other tissues are given.

A structure of importance in maintaining this compartmentalization and adherence is the **junctional complex** (Figs 4–5 and 4–6). Many years ago, the presence of a dense condensation of the cell membrane called the **terminal bar** was discerned by means of the light microscope in the apexes of tall columnar epithelial cells (Figs 4–12C and 4–13C). In horizontal section, they appear as a continuous net around the polygonal perimeter of these cells. Under the electron microscope, it can be seen that this structure corresponds to the 2 upper spe-

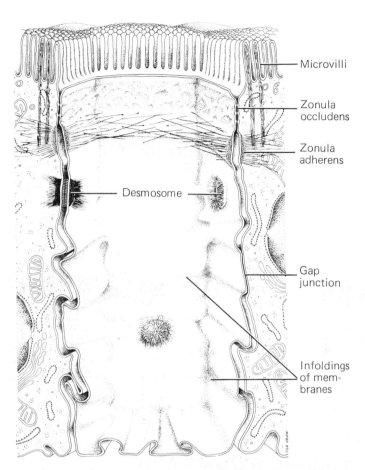

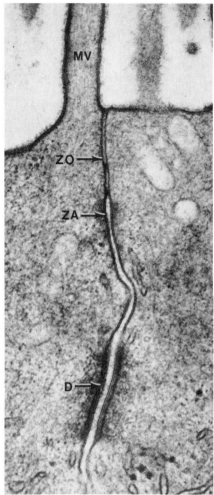

Figure 4 –5. The main structures that participate in cohesion among epithelial cells. The drawing shows 3 cells from the intestinal epithelium. The cell in the middle was emptied of its contents to show the inner surface of its membrane. Observe that the zonulae occludens and adherens form a continuous ribbon around the cell apex, while the desmosomes and gap junctions comprise spotlike plaques. The zonula occludens is formed by multiple ridges where the membranes' outer laminas fuse. (Redrawn and reproduced, with permission, from Krstić RV: *Ultrastructure of the Mammalian Cell.* Springer-Verlag, 1979.)

Figure 4 –6. Electron micrograph of a section of epithelial cells in the large intestine showing a junctional complex with its zonula occludens (ZO), zonula adherens (ZA), and desmosome (D). Also shown is a microvillus (MV). × 80,000.

cialized types of attachment that form a junctional complex.

From the apex of the cell to its base, there is, first, the **zonula occludens** (tight junction), a region in which the outer laminas of 2 adjoining cell membranes converge and fuse into one (Figs 4–5 and 4–6). Studies using the freeze fracture technic show that the zonula occludens is not a localized continuous fusion of 2 adjoining membranes but rather is composed of ridges of IMPs present in the membranes of neighboring cells that fuse at their apexes (Fig 4–8).

The occluding junction is important in the formation of a barrier that prevents the free pas-

sage of substances across an epithelium. The zonula occludens has a **sealing effect** in not permitting the extracellular passage of material from the epithelial surface to the base of the cell. The zonula occludens is indispensable in the formation of an electrical potential between the 2 surfaces of an epithelial membrane and is also important in understanding certain absorptive and secretory processes.

In addition to the zonula occludens, the junctional complex also consists of a **zonula adherens.** This junction consists of electron-dense plaques on each cytoplasmic surface of adjacent membranes. The spacing between the cells ranges from 20 to 90

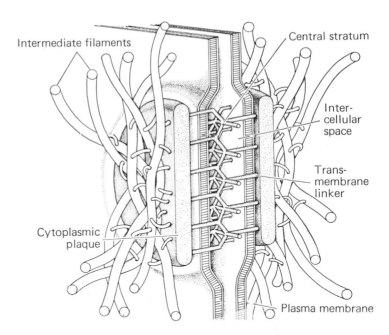

Figure 4 –7 (at right). A model of a desmosome is outlined in this diagram. The intermediate filaments, 10 nm in diameter, form a tensile network that extends throughout the interior of the cell. They are attached to the plaques of the desmosome through poorly defined filamentous structures. Other filaments, called transmembrane linkers, connect the plaques of the spot desmosome across the intercellular space. The junction therefore serves to couple the tonofilament networks of adjacent cells, allowing the dissipation of shearing stresses throughout the tissue. (Reproduced, with permission, from Staehelin LA, Hull BE: Sci Am 238:141, May 1978. Copyright © 1978 by Scientific American, Inc. All rights reserved.)

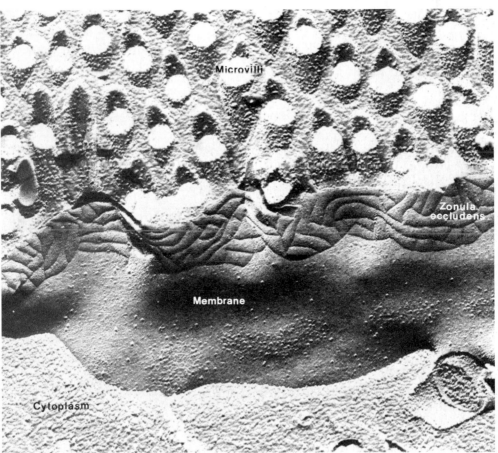

Figure 4 –8. Electron micrograph of a freeze-fractured small intestine epithelial cell. In the upper portion, the microvilli fractured transversely; in the lower portion, the fracture crossed through the cytoplasm of the intestinal epithelial cell. The ridges, which actually lie in the lipid (middle) layer of each plasmalemma, reveal that the membranes of adjoining cells were fused in the zonula occludens. (Courtesy of A Pinto da Silva.)

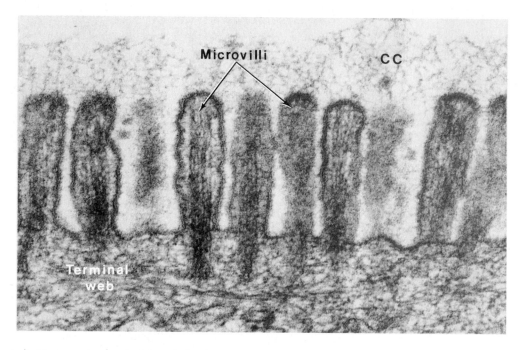

Figure 4 –9. Electron micrograph of the apical region of an intestinal epithelial cell. Observe the terminal web composed of a horizontal network of intermediate filaments, in which are anchored the vertical microfilaments that constitute the core of the microvilli. An extracellular filamentous **cell coat** (CC) is bound to the plasmalemma of the microvilli.

nm (wider than in nonjunction areas). Intermediate filaments, constituting the sheetlike terminal web, insert into the dense plaques that completely encircle the cellular apex. The terminal web serves as a site of insertion for the contractile microfilaments that form the core of the microvilli. The zonula adherens keeps the terminal web taut, so that the microfilaments can use it as an anchoring substrate to aid in contraction of the microvillar border (Figs 4–5 and 4–9).

Adhesion of cells may also be enhanced by membrane interdigitation, often observed between the membranes of the lateral walls of epithelial cells (Fig 4–11). It increases the area of surface contact between the cells and, therefore, their adhesion.

A third type of adhesion is often present in the junctional complex, the gap junction. The structure and function of this junction, which provides ionic coupling between adjacent cells, is fully described in Chapter 3.

SPECIALIZATION OF THE CELL SURFACE

Microvilli

The electron microscopic study of epithelia with absorptive functions (eg, the intestinal epithelium or certain epithelial tissues in the kidney) shows that the surface membrane presents a

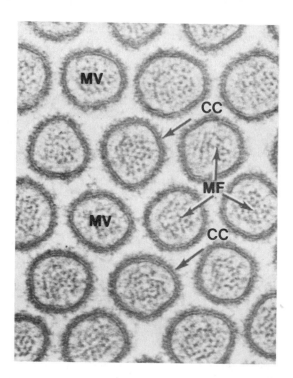

Figure 4 –10. Electron micrograph of a section from the apical region of a cell from the intestinal lining showing cross-sectioned microvilli (MV). In their interiors, note the microfilaments (MF) in cross section. The surrounding unit membrane can be clearly discerned and is covered by a layer of cell coat (CC). × 100,000. (Courtesy of KR Porter.)

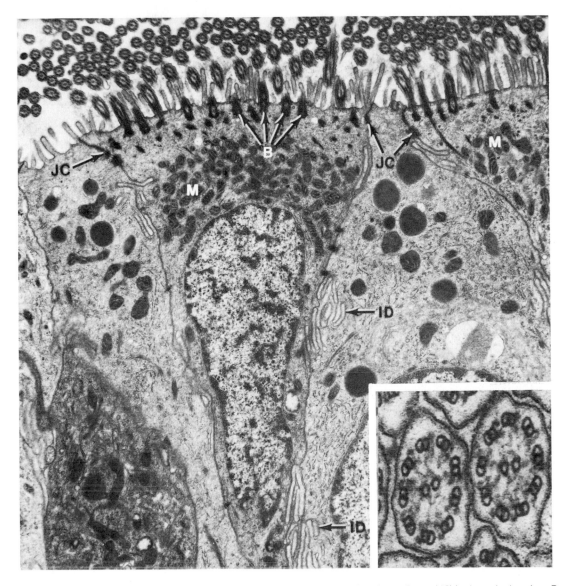

Figure 4 –11. Electron micrograph of a ciliated epithelium. Observe the junctional complexes (JC) in the apical region. Basal bodies (B) are shown at the bases of cilia. Mitochondria (M) are in a supranuclear position. The presence of these organelles is probably related to the provision of energy for the movement of the cilia. Membrane interdigitations (ID) are frequent. The inset shows a transverse section of cilia with a typical microtubular pattern. × 120,000.

multitude of fingerlike evaginations called **microvilli** (Figs 4–9 and 4–10). An extracellular glycoprotein layer, the **cell coat,** frequently covers the apical extremities of the microvilli of absorptive epithelial cells (Fig 4–9). This differential localization of the filamentous cell coat is important for the intense pinocytotic processes occurring here, especially near the base of the microvilli. The microvilli considerably increase the efficiency of absorption and the surface area of the cell, thus enhancing the efficiency of all processes occurring in this region.

Stereocilia

Stereocilia are long, nonmotile processes in the apical region of the cells lining the epididymis. Under the electron microscope, they have the appearance of elongated, flexible microvilli that frequently anastomose. Their name is therefore a misnomer.

Cilia & Flagella

Cilia are numerous elongated, motile structures on the surface of epithelial cells, 5–10 μm long and 0.2 μm in diameter—much longer than and different in structure from the microvilli. Under the electron microscope in cross section, they are observed to be surrounded by the cellular membrane and contain a central pair of microtubules and, at the periphery below the membrane, arranged in a

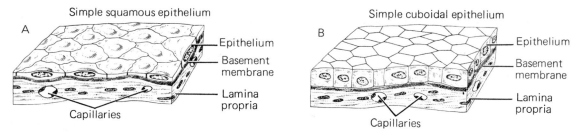

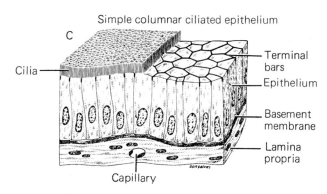

Figure 4–12. Diagrams of epithelial tissue. *A:* Simple squamous epithelium. *B:* Simple cuboidal epithelium. *C:* Simple ciliated columnar epithelium. All are separated from the subjacent connective tissue by a basement membrane. Note in *C* the terminal bars, which correspond in light microscopy to the zonula occludens and zonula adherens of the junctional complex.

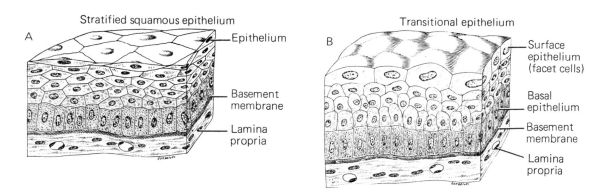

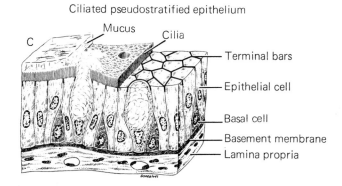

Figure 4–13. Diagrams of epithelial tissue. *A:* Stratified squamous epithelium. *B:* Transitional epithelium. *C:* Ciliated pseudostratified epithelium. The goblet cells secrete mucus that forms a continuous mucous layer over the ciliary layer.

circle, 9 more pairs of microtubules all of which run in the direction of the long axis (Fig 4–11).

The cilia are inserted on the **basal bodies,** which are dense structures present at the apical pole just below the cell membrane. They have an internal structure analogous to that of the centrioles (see Chapter 3).

In living organisms, rapid back-and-forth movement can be observed in cilia. Ciliary movement is frequently coordinated to permit a current of fluid or particulate matter to be propelled in one direction *over* the ciliated epithelium. ATP, which enhances this type of movement, seems to be a source of energy for it.

It is estimated that a ciliated cell of the trachea can have about 250 cilia. Flagella, present in the human body only in the spermatozoa, are similar in structure to cilia but are much longer.

CLASSIFICATION OF EPITHELIAL CELLS

Epithelial cells are customarily classified according to their structure and function into 2 main groups: covering epithelium and glandular epithelium. This is an arbitrary division, for there are covering epithelial tissues in which all cells secrete mucus (eg, the surface epithelium of the stomach) or in which glandular cells are very sparse (eg, mucous cells in the intestine or trachea).

Covering Epithelial Tissue

Covering epithelial tissues are tissues whose cells are organized in membranous layers that cover the external surface or line the cavities of the body. They can be classified morphologically according to

the number of cell layers and the morphology of the cells in the surface layer (Table 4–1). Simple epithelium contains only one layer of cells, and stratified epithelium contains more than one layer (Figs 4–1, 4–12, and 4–13).

Simple epithelium can, according to cell form, be squamous, cuboidal, or columnar. The endothelium lining blood vessels and the mesothelium lining certain body cavities are examples of simple squamous epithelium (Fig 4–12A). Although endothelial and mesothelial cells present the same aspect in the light microscope, they should not be considered as one cell type differently localized. It is known that they differ not only in their embryologic origin and ultrastructural morphology but also in their pathologic responses. Thus, they react differently to several types of aggression and even produce different types of tumors. An example of cuboidal epithelium is the surface lining of the ovary (Fig 4–12B), and an example of columnar epithelium is the intestinal lining (Fig 4–12C).

Stratified epithelium is classified according to the cell form of its superficial layer. These include **squamous, cuboidal, columnar,** and **transitional** epithelium. Pseudostratified epithelium forms a separate group.

Stratified squamous keratinized epithelium is found mainly in the skin. Its cells form many layers; the cells closer to the overlying tissue are usually cuboidal or columnar. In the following layers, however, toward the surface, the cells become irregular in shape and flatten progressively as they get closer to the surface, where they are thin squamous (Fig 4–13A). (For details, see Chapter 19.)

Stratified squamous mucosal or **mucous membranes** are the epithelial membranes that line wet cavities (eg, mouth, bladder, intestines), in contrast to the skin, whose surface is dry. Structurally, the

Table 4–1. Common types of epithelial lining in the human body.

According to the Number of Cell Layers	According to the Form of the Cells	Distribution	Function
Simple (one layer)	Squamous	Lining of vessels (endothelium). Serous lining of cavities: pericardium, pleura, peritoneum (mesothelia).	Facilitates the movement of the viscera (mesothelium), active transport by pinocytosis.
	Cuboidal	Covering the ovary, thyroid.	Covering, secretion.
	Columnar	Lining of intestine, gallbladder.	Protection, lubrication, absorption, secretion.
Pseudostratified (layers of cells with nuclei at different levels; not all cells reach surface but all adhere to basal lamina)		Lining of trachea, bronchi, nasal cavity.	Protection; transport of particles out of the air passages; secretion.
Stratified (2 or more layers)	Squamous keratinized (dry)	Skin	Protection; prevents water loss.
	Squamous nonkeratinized (moist)	Mouth, esophagus, vagina, anal canal.	Protection; prevents water loss; secretion.
	Cuboidal	Sweat glands, developing ovarian follicles.	Protection, secretion.
	Transitional	Bladder, ureters, renal calyces.	Protection.
	Columnar	Conjunctiva	Protection.

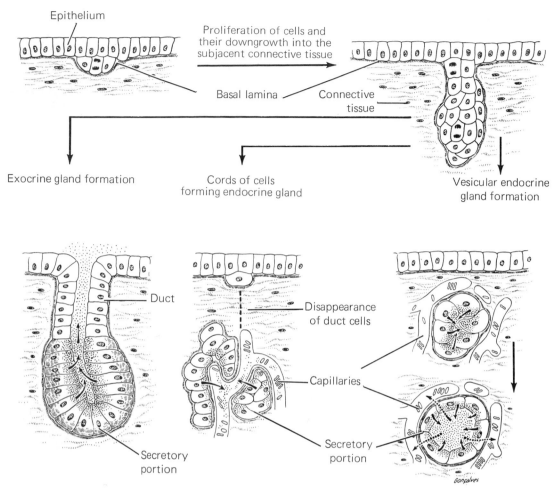

Figure 4 –14. Formation of glands from covering epithelia. Epithelial cells proliferate and penetrate into connective tissue. They may or may not maintain contact with the surface. When contact is maintained, exocrine glands are formed; when contact is not maintained, endocrine glands are formed. The cells of these glands can be arranged in cords or follicles. The lumens of follicles accumulate large quantities of secretion; cells of the cords store only small quantities in their cytoplasm. (Redrawn and reproduced, with permission, from Ham AW: *Histology,* 6th ed. Lippincott, 1969.)

stratified mucosal epithelium is identical to the stratified keratinized epithelium, except that in the latter the surface cells are dead and appear as flattened keratin scales.

Stratified columnar epithelium is rare; it is present on the human body only in small areas such as the ocular conjunctiva and the ducts of large glands.

Transitional epithelium, which lines the urinary bladder, the ureter, and the upper part of the urethra, is characterized by the presence on its surface of globular cells that are neither squamous nor columnar (Fig 4–13B). The form of these cells changes according to the degree of distention of the bladder. This type of epithelium is discussed in detail in Chapter 20.

Pseudostratified epithelium is so called because, although nuclei appear to lie in various layers, all cells are attached to the basal lamina, but

some do not reach the surface. The best-known example of this tissue is the ciliated pseudostratified columnar epithelium present in the respiratory passage (Fig 4–13C).

Two other types of epithelium warrant brief mention. The neuroepithelia are cells of epithelial origin with specialized sensory functions (eg, cells of taste buds). Myoepithelial cells specialize in contraction (eg, in the sweat, mammary, and salivary glands).

Glandular Epithelia

Glandular epithelial tissues are those formed by cells specialized in producing a fluid secretion that differs in composition from blood or intercellular fluid. This process is usually accompanied by the intracellular synthesis of macromolecules. These compounds are generally stored in the cells in small droplets called secretory granules.

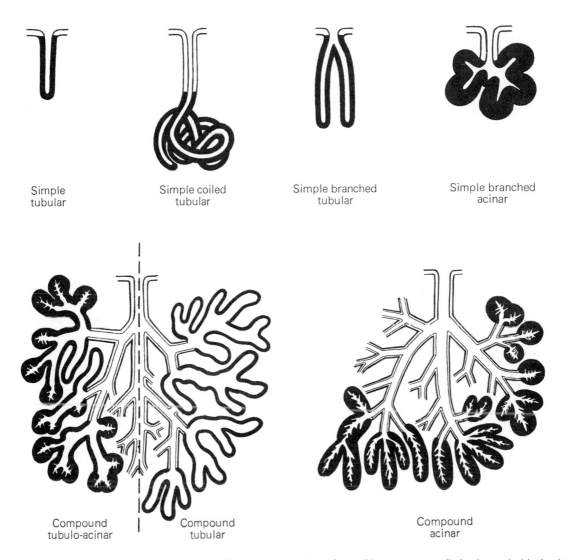

Simple
tubular

Simple coiled
tubular

Simple branched
tubular

Simple branched
acinar

Compound
tubulo-acinar

Compound
tubular

Compound
acinar

Figure 4–15. Principal types of exocrine glands. The part of the gland formed by secretory cells is shown in black; the remainder shows the ducts. The compound glands have ramified ducts.

The nature of these macromolecules is variable; they secrete proteins (eg, pancreas), lipids (eg, adrenal and sebaceous glands), or complexes of carbohydrate and proteins (eg, salivary glands). In the mammary glands, all 3 substances—proteins, lipids, and carbohydrates—are secreted. Less common are the cells of glands which have low synthetic activity (eg, sweat glands) and in which secretion is mostly composed of substances transferred from the blood to the lumen of the gland.

In some cases, a gland may contain active synthesizing cells in association with cells specializing in ion transport. This occurs in most major mammalian salivary glands where secretory acini coexist with ion-transporting structures called **striated ducts** (see Chapter 17).

All gland cells produce and expel to an extracellular compartment products that are not used by the cell itself but are of importance to other parts of the organism.

Types of Glandular Epithelium

The epithelium that forms the glands of the body can be classified according to various criteria, eg, unicellular glands consist of isolated glandular cells and multicellular glands are composed of clusters of cells. An example of a unicellular gland is the goblet cell of the lining of the small intestine or of the respiratory tract. However, most glands are multicellular.

Glands always derive from epithelial covering membranes by means of cell proliferation and invasion of subjacent connective tissue, subsequently followed by further differentiation. Figure 4–14 shows how this occurs. The secretion of **exocrine glands** will, by special structures called ducts, be taken to the epithelial surface from which the glands originate. **Endocrine glands** are ductless, and their secretions are released directly into blood vessels.

Multicellular glands are not merely collections of cells but complete organs with a definite and orderly architecture. They may have a surrounding capsule of connective tissue and septa that divide the gland into lobules. These lobules then subdivide, and in this way the connective tissue separates and binds together the glandular components. Blood vessels and nerves also penetrate and subdivide in the gland.

According to the way the secretory products leave the cell, glands may be classified as **merocrine** or **holocrine.** In merocrine glands (eg, in the pancreas), the secretory granules leave the cell with no loss of cellular material. In holocrine glands (eg, sebaceous glands), the product of secretion is shed with the whole cell—a process which involves destruction of the secretion-filled cells. In an intermediate type—the **apocrine** gland—the secretory product is discharged together with parts of the apical cytoplasm. This type of secretion is observed in certain sweat glands.

Two types of endocrine glands can be differentiated according to cell grouping. In the first type, the agglomerated cells form anastomosing cords interspersed between dilated blood capillaries (eg, adrenal gland, parathyroid, anterior lobe of the pituitary) (Fig 4–14). In the second (**vesicular**) type, the cells line a vesicle or follicle filled with noncellular material (eg, the thyroid gland) (Fig 4–14).

Exocrine glands have a **secretory portion,** which contains the cells responsible for the secretory process; and the **gland ducts,** which transport the secretion to the exterior of the gland (Fig 4–14). In some glands, the excretory ducts also participate in regulating the ionic composition of the secretory fluid (see Salivary Glands in Chapter 17). **Simple glands** have only one unbranched duct. **Compound glands** have ducts that branch repeatedly. The cellular organization within the secretory portion of the gland further classifies the glands. The simple glands can be tubular, coiled tubular, branched tubular, and acinar. The compound glands can be tubular, acinar, or tubuloacinar. Figure 4–15 illustrates these types of glands schematically. Some organs have both endocrine and exocrine functions, and one cell type may function both ways—eg, in the liver, where cells that secrete bile into the duct system also secrete their products into the bloodstream. In other organs, some cells are specialized in exocrine secretion whereas others are concerned exclusively with endocrine secretion, eg, in the pancreas, where the acinar cells secrete digestive enzymes into the intestinal lumen while the islet cells secrete insulin and glucagon into the blood.

GENERAL BIOLOGY
OF EPITHELIAL TISSUES

Covering epithelial tissues are situated on a layer of connective tissue called lamina propria and separated from it by the basal lamina. The lamina propria not only serves to support the epithelium but also binds it to neighboring structures. The contact between epithelium and lamina propria is increased by irregularities in the surface in the form of evaginations called papillae. They occur most frequently in epithelial tissues subject to strain such as the skin and the tongue.

Nutrition & Innervation

Normally, blood vessels do not penetrate to the epithelium, so that there is no direct contact between these cells and blood vessels. Epithelial nutrition depends, therefore, on the diffusion of metabolites through the basal lamina and, frequently, through parts of the lamina propria also. The diffusion process is probably enhanced by the papillae, which increase the area of contact between epithelium and lamina propria, and it probably limits the thickness of the epithelium. Most epithelial tissues receive nerve endings from a rich nervous network.

The Renewal of Epithelial Cells

Epithelial tissues are labile structures whose cells are continuously renewed by means of mitotic activity. This renewal rate is variable. It can be fast in such tissues as the intestinal epithelium, which is changed every 2–5 days; or slow, as in the pancreas, where tissue renewal takes about 50 days. In stratified and pseudostratified epithelial tissues, mitosis occurs within the germinal layer, those cells closest to the basal lamina.

Metaplasia

Under certain physiologic or pathologic conditions, a single type of epithelial tissue may undergo a series of transformations into another epithelial type. This process is called metaplasia. It is reversible, and the following examples illustrate this process: (1) In heavy cigarette smokers, the pseudostratified epithelium lining the bronchi can be transformed into stratified squamous epithelium. (2) In individuals with chronic vitamin A deficiency, epithelial tissues of the type found in the bronchi and urinary bladder are gradually replaced by stratified squamous epithelium. Metaplasia is not restricted to epithelial tissue; it may also occur in connective tissue.

Control of Glandular Activity

The activity of a gland depends on 2 types of mechanisms: The first is genetic and depends on the expression of one or more genes that promote the synthesis and secretion of specific compounds or

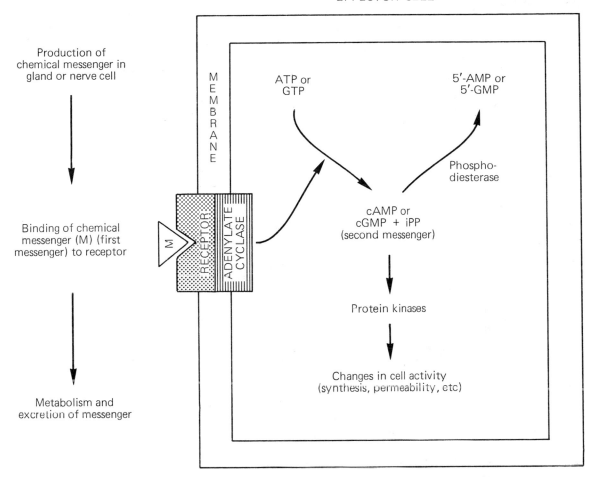

Figure 4 –16. Cyclic AMP or GMP is produced from ATP or GTP owing to the activation of adenylate cyclase by the first messenger. Adenylate cyclase is located in the cell membrane, and a specific first messenger receptor is associated with this enzyme. These second messengers are produced inside the cell, while the first messenger remain outside. The actions of many neurotransmitters and hormones are mediated by cAMP or cGMP. The specificity of the first messengers on different cell types depends on the presence of specific receptors associated with adenylate cyclase. Cyclic GMP is usually found in lower concentrations than cAMP, but it also mediates a variety of cellular activities. In some cells, both cAMP and cGMP are known to interact, one stimulating and the other inhibiting a specific cellular activity. (Based on Sutherland: Studies on the mechanism of hormone action. Science 177:401, 1972. Copyright 1972 by the American Association for the Advancement of Science.)

products. During the differentiation of a glandular cell, a significant developmental event concerns the selection and expression of the genes that control secretion.

The second type of mechanism is related to exogenous or environmental controls. The nervous and endocrine systems are the main participants in its control. Most glands are sensitive to both nervous and endocrine control, but one is frequently more important than the other. Thus, exocrine secretion in the pancreas depends mainly on stimulation by the hormones secretin and pancreozymin. The salivary glands, on the other hand, are essentially under nervous control.

The nervous and endocrine control of glands occurs through the action of chemical substances called **chemical messengers.** Neurotransmitters are those messengers produced by nerve cells, while hormones are the controlling factors produced by the endocrine glands.

Chemical messengers may act by either of 2 mechanisms. In the first case, the messenger enters the cell, reacts with intracellular receptors, and activates one or more genes, initiating the production of specific proteins. Some steroid hormones, which are capable of easily crossing the cell membrane owing to their lipid structure, exhibit this type of action. The antibiotic dactinomycin blocks

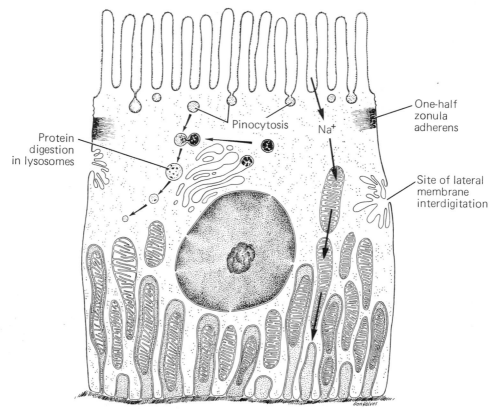

Figure 4 –17. Ultrastructure of a proximal convoluted tubule cell of the kidney. Invagination of the basal cell membrane outlines regions filled with elongated mitochondria. This typical disposition is present in ion-transporting cells. Interdigitations from neighboring cells (stippled structures) interlock with those of this cell. Protein absorbed by pinocytosis and being digested by lysosomes is shown in the upper left portion of the diagram. The arrows at the right indicate the path by which sodium ions presumably cross the cell. Chloride ions probably flow in the cytoplasm between the mitochondria. This is an example of a cell with more than one function, since it transports ions in addition to providing for protein digestion.

the synthesis of messenger RNA and is known to inhibit this type of messenger activity.

A second mechanism is related to the interaction of a chemical messenger with a receptor located in the outer surface of the cell membrane. This chemical substance, referred to as **first messenger,** acts by inducing the synthesis of yet another messenger, called **second messenger,** that initiates a series of events which ultimately promotes a specific cell activity. Figure 4–16 summarizes this concept. Protein or polypeptide hormones and neurotransmitters that do not readily cross the cell membrane are known to act via this second messenger mechanism.

BIOLOGY OF THE MAIN TYPES OF EPITHELIAL CELLS

As cells differentiate, they gradually acquire morphologic and physiologic characteristics related to the various functions they assume. Since these differentiated cells frequently have the same functions in different tissues and organs, descriptions of the main cell types will be given.

Cells That Transport Ions

The observation that certain dyes injected into the bloodstream can be concentrated in the lumens of renal tubules and that this activity depends on the integrity of their energy-yielding metabolism led to the concept of **active transport.** Active transport is an energy-dependent process. Certain metazoan cells utilize this system for ion transport, an important physiologic activity in the maintenance of ionic balance.

The most important ions for ionic balance are sodium and potassium; in the human body, cells have mechanisms to selectively transport these ions through cell membranes. The most conspicuous of these are the columnar or cuboidal cells of the proximal and distal renal tubules and those of the striated ducts of the salivary gland. These cells, which usually have a central nucleus, also exhibit the following characteristics (Fig 4–17): (1) Multiple and deep invaginations of the membrane of the

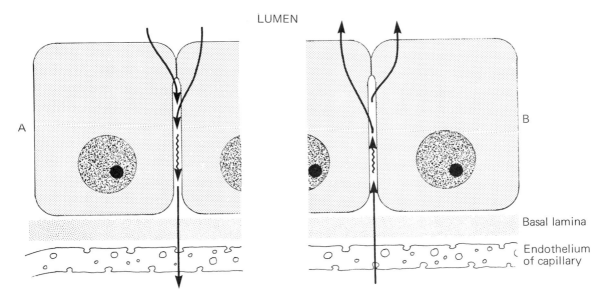

Figure 4–18. Ion and fluid transport can occur in different directions depending on which tissue is involved. *A:* The direction of transport is from the lumen to the blood vessel, as occurs in the gallbladder and intestine. This process is called absorption. *B:* Transport is in the opposite direction, as occurs in the choroid plexus, ciliary body, and sweat gland. This process is called secretion. Note the use of the intercellular space in the transport process.

basal portion of the cell. These invaginations are not followed by the basal lamina, and they divide the basal pole into a series of vertical compartments, thus considerably increasing the basal surface area of the cell. (2) Frequent interdigitations between adjacent lateral cell surfaces. (3) A large number of filamentous mitochondria, with abundant cristae, filling most of the invaginated compartments, near the base of the cell. (4) Extensive ATPase activity in the infolded membrane. (5) As would be expected in cells rich in mitochondria, they exhibit great metabolic activity with high oxygen consumption. The cells exhibit strong histochemical reactions with succinate dehydrogenase and cytochrome oxidase, mitochondrial enzymes necessary for oxidative phosphorylation.

Adding oxidative phosphorylation inhibitors to these cells blocks ionic transport, which suggests that this process is linked to energy metabolism. Although ionic transport may occur in certain cell types that do not have membrane invaginations and mitochondria-filled compartments, these characteristics are always present in cells in which this activity is intense. Studies performed on this material suggest that sodium reabsorbed by the apical pole of the cell passes in part through the mitochondria and that chloride is transported in the cytoplasm (Fig 4–17). The close contact of the mitochondria with cell membrane invagination also suggests that this organelle participates in ion transport. The mechanism of water transport through the cell is obscure. It probably occurs following an osmotic gradient formed by the transport of ions.

Ion transport and the consequent flow of fluid

may occur in opposite directions (ie, apical → basal, basal → apical) in different epithelial tissues. In the intestine, proximal convoluted tubules of the kidney, striated ducts of the salivary glands, gallbladder, etc, the flow is from the apex of the cell to its basal region. Flow is in the opposite direction in other epithelial sheets such as in the choroid plexus and ciliary body (Fig 4–18). In both cases, the tight junctions seal the apical portions of the cells and provide for inner and outer tissue compartments. Fluid transport between the cells probably occurs to a great extent in the extracellular space (see arrows in Fig 4–18). Such a process requires much less energy than if the transported fluid had to cross the entire cell.

Cells That Transport by Pinocytosis

In various cells of the body, pinocytotic vesicles that form abundantly on plasmalemma surfaces permit the transport of macromolecules across the cell membranes. This activity is clearly observed in the simple squamous epithelium lining the blood vessels (endothelia) or the body cavities (mesothelia). These cells have few organelles other than the abundant pinocytotic vesicles found on the cell surfaces and in the cytoplasm (Fig 4–19). These observations, in conjunction with results obtained by injection of electron-dense colloidal particles (eg, ferritin, colloidal gold, thorium) and evidence obtained by electron microscopy, indicate that the vesicles transporting the injected materials flow in both directions through the cells (Fig 4–19).

Calculations based on these studies suggest that a pinocytotic vesicle can cross these cells in 2–3

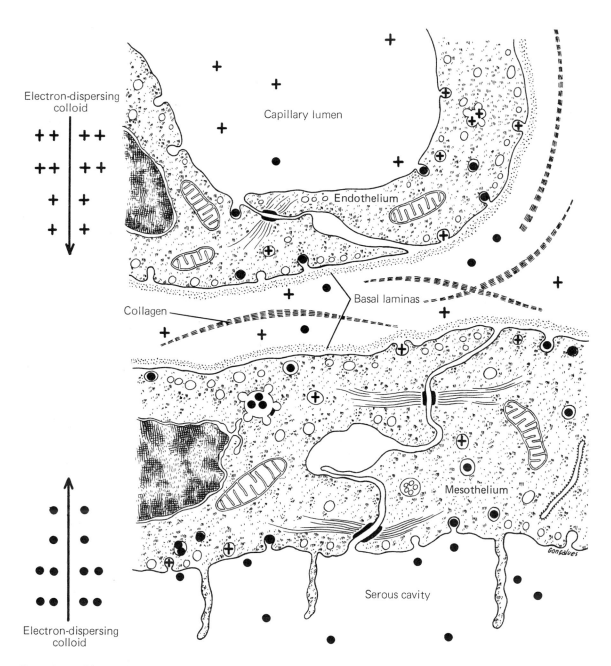

Figure 4 –19. Diagram illustrating how the transport of electron-dense colloids through the mesothelial and endothelial cells was studied. Simultaneous injections of colloids that differ morphologically were made, one intravenously and the other in a serous cavity (eg, the mesentery or pericardial cavity) lined by the cells. After short periods of time (minutes), fragments of the serous membranes were fixed and studied in the electron microscope. It was observed that the transport of colloid occurred in both directions. These particles are engulfed by pinocytosis and are transported across the cells in vesicles. (Redrawn and reproduced, with permission, from Staubesand J: Zur Histophysiologie des Herzbeutels. Z Zellforsch Mikrosk Anat 58:915, 1963.)

minutes. Since the frequency of vesicle formation and vesicle volume can be measured, it has been possible to calculate the quantity of the transferred liquid through the walls of capillaries. In the case of muscle tissue, the amount transported has been estimated to be 2–3 mL/h/kg of tissue.

Chemical Messenger-Producing Cells

The vertebrate body has many cell types whose main function is the production of messenger substances of a varied chemical nature that may influence the activities of other cells. These cells can be classified in 3 groups according to the mode of delivery of the messenger:

(1) **Neurocrine cells** release chemical messages at interfaces where cytoplasmic extensions of the messenger cell approach the surface of the target cells. Neurons are an example of this type of messenger, and the site where its extension makes contact with the effector cell is called a **synapse** (see Chapter 9).

(2) **Paracrine cells** secrete a message that diffuses into the surrounding extracellular fluid and acts upon neighboring target cells. The mast cell, an example of this type of messenger cell, secretes histamine that acts upon nearby capillary endothelial cells (see Chapter 12).

(3) **Endocrine cells** secrete their messenger substances into the blood, which carries them directly to the target cells. Most endocrine cells produce steroid or protein messenger compounds. However, some endocrine cells produce biologically active amines.

Chemical messenger cells are derived from each of the 3 embryologic germ layers and subsequently reside in a variety of tissues within the body. Thus, for example, the neurocrine cells are present in the nervous tissue, and mast cells are present in the connective tissue. However, most chemical messenger cells are constituents of epithelial tissues.

Protein-Synthesizing Cells

All cells continuously synthesize small amounts of protein in order to replace cytoplasmic subunits utilized or lost through the normal turnover of cellular components. Some cells, however, synthesize excessively large amounts of protein as a consequence of their differentiating function. These cells can be divided into 2 classes based on the final distribution of their protein products. In one group, where the protein remains free within the cytoplasm, protein synthesis primarily occurs on free or unbound polyribosomes. Examples of cells within this group include striated skeletal muscle cells and erythroblasts (Fig 14–5).

In the second group, synthesized proteins are segregated from other cytoplasmic components as a result of their encapsulation within membrane-bound vesicles. This group can be further subdivided in regard to whether the synthesized proteins are accumulated within or exported from the cell. Some leukocytes (eg, neutrophils and eosinophils) and macrophages synthesize lytic enzymes stored in membrane-bound granules that are retained within the cytoplasm and subsequently utilized for intracellular digestion (see Chapter 5 and Fig 5–10). However, most protein synthesizers segregate their protein products and eventually release them into the extracellular space in a process called **secretion.** Examples of protein secretors include fibroblasts, plasma cells, and pancreatic acinar cells. Within these cells, proteins are synthesized on membrane-bound polysomes, and the newly synthesized polypeptides are injected directly into the cistern of the rough endoplasmic reticulum.

Some cells **synthesize, segregate,** and **export** proteins without accumulating them within the cytoplasm. In such cells (for example, the **plasma cell** [Fig 5–16]), proteins are transferred from the endoplasmic reticulum to the Golgi apparatus and are then extruded from the cell by a mechanism to be discussed later.

In other cell types, proteins are **synthesized, segregated,** and **accumulated** in the apex of the cell, and then they are **exported.** The acinar cells of the pancreas and parotid glands are typical examples of this cell type. They are polyhedral or pyramidal, with a central, rounded euchromatic nucleus and well-defined polarity. In the basal infranuclear region, these cells exhibit an intense basophilia, which results from local accumulation of granular endoplasmic reticulum in the form of parallel arrays of flattened cisternae and tubular elements (Fig 4–20).

Filamentous mitochondria are frequently interspersed among endoplasmic reticulum cisternae. The position of the nucleus and the presence of an evident basal basophilic region in these cells are characteristic of protein-synthesizing cells and are criteria used to distinguish them from cells secreting acid mucopolysaccharides.

In the apical region just above the nucleus lies a well-developed Golgi apparatus. The rest of the cytoplasm is filled with rounded, protein-rich, membrane-bound **secretory granules.** In cells that produce digestive enzymes (eg, the pancreas), these structures containing inactive enzyme are called **zymogen granules** (Figs 4–20 and 4–21).

Enough evidence has been presented from biochemical and cytologic studies to define the secretory process in these cells as follows:

(1) Amino acids from the bloodstream pass through the capillary walls and their basal lamina, through the secretory cell basal lamina and plasma membrane, and into the cells. The entry of amino acids through the membrane is greatly accelerated by an active transport mechanism.

(2) Within the cell, the amino acids associate with a free ribosome and a strand of messenger (m) RNA in order to initiate the synthesis of a polypep-

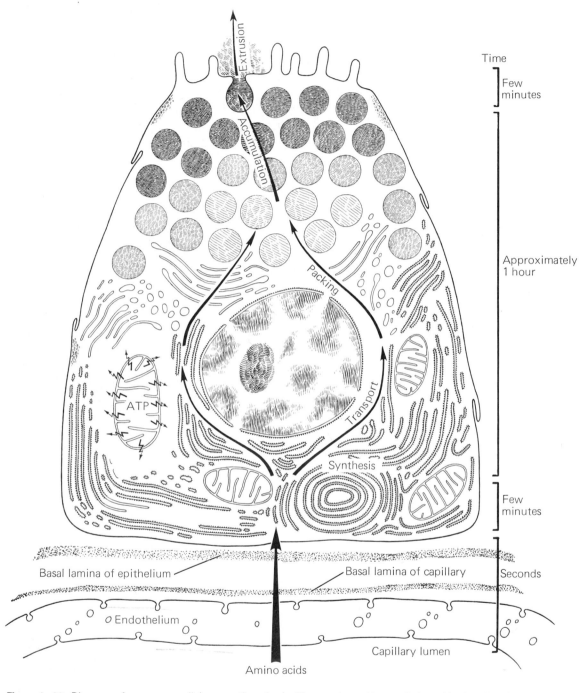

Figure 4 –20. Diagram of a serous cell (pancreatic acinar). Observe its evident polarity with abundant basal granular endoplasmic reticulum (ergastoplasm). The Golgi apparatus and secretory granules are in the supranuclear region. The secretory process is described in the text. To the right is a time scale indicating the approximate time necessary for each step.

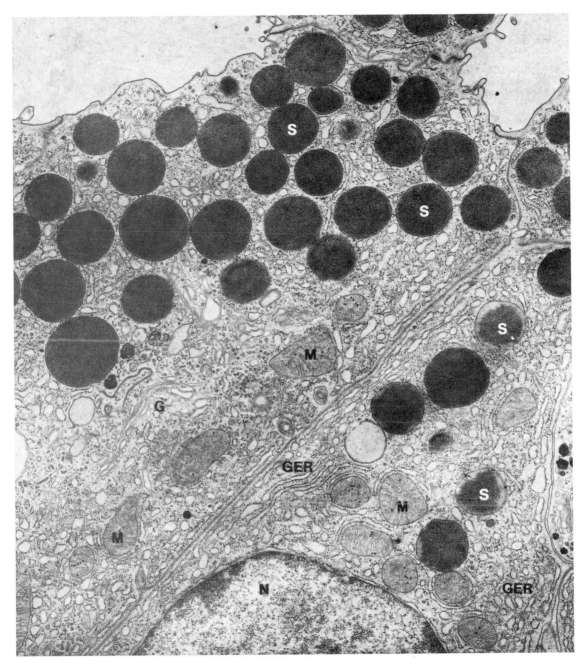

Figure 4–21. Electron micrograph of 2 frog pancreatic cells. Observe the nucleus (N), mitochondria (M), Golgi apparatus (G), secretory granules (S) in various stages of condensation, and granular endoplasmic reticulum (GER). × 13,000. (Courtesy of KR Porter.)

tide chain. The mRNA coding for exported proteins possesses an additional initiation sequence of hydrophobic amino acids called a **signal peptide.** As the newly assembled peptide extends from the central core of the ribosome (Fig 3–10), the hydrophobic signal peptide specifically penetrates the endoplasmic reticulum membrane, which results in binding of the ribosomal complex to the endoplasmic reticulum. As the protein chain is assembled and injected into the endoplasmic reticulum cisterna, additional ribosomes are simultaneously attached to both the mRNA and the endoplasmic reticulum membrane, which results in the formation of a membrane-bound polysome. The hydrophobic signal peptide is enzymatically clipped off after the assembled protein enters the endoplasmic reticulum cisterna. At this stage, the proteins are segregated within an extracytoplasmic space—the interior of the granular endoplasmic reticulum cisternae. This separation is significant in that it avoids direct contact of the secretory product, often digestive enzymes (eg, ribonuclease and protease), with cytoplasmic components.

(3) The proteins thus segregated are transported from the endoplasmic reticulum to the Golgi apparatus. The mechanism by which they reach the interior of the Golgi cisternae is still in question, but evidence shows that in several cell types this occurs by formation of small transfer vesicles containing protein that bud from the endoplasmic reticulum, migrate to, and fuse with the convex surface of Golgi cisternae.

(4) This material is then accumulated in the Golgi cisternae. On the mature (concave) face of the Golgi, bulges form along the surface and lateral margins of the uppermost cisterna. These bulges pinch off to form large membrane-bound **secretory vesicles** or **granules** (Figs 4–20 and 4–21).

(5) The newly formed granules in turn migrate to the cell apex and in doing so become more dense as water is removed from the protein. They have been designated mature granules, in contrast to the less dense, recently formed granules. Granules accumulate until they are mobilized. Accumulation occurs for periods of time that vary with the type of gland and its activity.

(6) When the cells extrude their secretory products, the membranes of the secretory granules fuse to the cell membrane and the granule contents spill out of the cell in a process that roughly resembles (and has been called) **exocytosis.** The energy for these processes is known to be furnished by oxidative phosphorylation at the mitochondrial level.

Polypeptide-Secreting Cells

Recent studies suggest that cells synthesizing low-molecular-weight polypeptides or proteins with hormonal activity have some morphologic and histochemical characteristics in common. They are endocrine cells present in several organs of vertebrates. They have the capacity to concentrate in their cytoplasm either ready-made biogenic amines, such as epinephrine, norepinephrine, or 6-hydroxytryptamine, or precursors from which they synthesize these amines. They also exhibit a high level of amino acid decarboxylase activity—an enzyme related to the synthesis of biogenic amines. These characteristics explain the designation APUD (*a*mine *p*recursor *u*ptake and *d*ecarboxylation) given to these cells. In addition to synthesizing polypeptides with hormonal activity, APUD cells possess an overt or latent capacity to synthesize biogenic amines. If this capacity is overtly expressed, both amines and polypeptides coexist within the cell. If this capacity is latent, the cell will produce amines only if it is overloaded with precursor. APUD cells have low cytoplasmic basophilia, in contrast to the above-described protein-synthesizing cells. Under the electron microscope, their main features are shown to be the presence of unusually small, round secretory granules (100–200 nm) accumulated in the cellular region close to the capillaries, relatively scarce granular endoplasmic reticulum (Fig 4–22), and an undeveloped Golgi apparatus.

In view of their function, which is mainly to

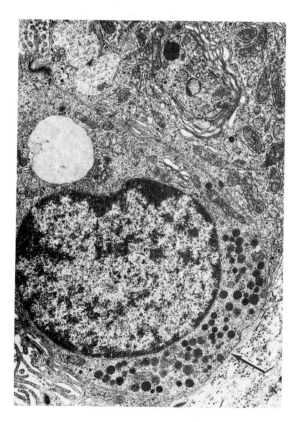

Figure 4–22. Electron micrograph of a somatostatin D cell from human gastrointestinal tract. Observe the accumulation of secretory granules in the cellular basal region. The arrow shows the basal lamina. × 13,500. (Courtesy of AGE Pearse.)

form peptide bonds, it might be expected that these cells would have a well-developed granular endoplasmic reticulum and Golgi apparatus. Radioautographic and physiologic studies suggest, however, that the rate of protein synthesis is low in the polypeptide-secreting cell, which accounts for the cytologic characteristics mentioned above. Thus, it has been calculated that the pancreatic islet beta cells secrete insulin at a rate that is about one-fiftieth the rate of protein synthesis in the exocrine acinar cells.

These cells are believed to be derived from the neural crest, although this view has been contested by some investigators.

Theoretically, APUD cells can react to stimuli by discharging their hormonal content. It is believed that they derive from cells whose original function was to deal with biogenic amines but that they evolved gradually, acquiring the capacity to secrete polypeptides.

APUD cells in humans are diffusely distributed, clustered in groups, or form small glandular structures. Approximately 30 types of cells have been proved to be or are suspected to belong to the APUD series in mammals.

The characterization of polypeptides or low-molecular-weight proteins produced by these cells has been achieved mainly by the immunofluorescence method described in Chapter 2. Using this method, it was possible to identify in humans several APUD cells (Table 4–2). The morphology and histochemistry of these cells vary with the species studied. At present, several polypeptides with biologic activity whose corresponding APUD cells have not thus far been located, as well as several cells with APUD morphology but with undetermined function, are known to exist. It will be necessary to isolate sufficient quantities of polypeptides in order to produce the antibodies required to apply the immunofluorescence method to the study of APUD cells with unknown function.

Several tumors derived from the APUD cells have been described: Tumors of the nonbeta islet cells of the pancreas that produce gastrin are responsible for Zollinger-Ellison syndrome, and the calcitonin-producing tumor of the thyroid. Tumors derived from the APUD cells are called **apudomas** and are one of a group of tumors having their origin in cells of the neuroectoderm.

The close relation between the nervous system and most polypeptide and catecholamine-producing cells has led to a somewhat wider concept of paraneurons that has been proposed to replace the APUD cell concept. It is too early for definite conclusions on this subject, since the field is still being actively studied.

Glycoprotein Cells

The most typical and most thoroughly studied example of glycoprotein cells is the goblet cell of the intestines, which is characterized by the presence

Table 4–2. Some of the better known APUD cells present in the human organism.

Cell Name and Site	Polypeptide Produced
C and M of pituitary	Adrenocorticotropin and melanotropin
A of the Langerhans islet	Glucagon
Non-B of the Langerhans islet	Insulin
D of the Langerhans islet	Somatostatin
AL of the stomach	Glucagon
G of the stomach	Gastrin
EG of the intestine	Glucagon
S of the intestine	Secretin
D of the intestine	Somatostatin
Parafollicular of the thyroid	Calcitonin

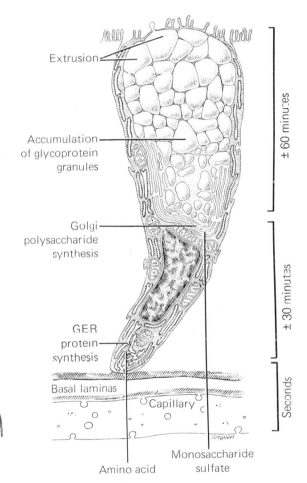

Figure 4–23. Diagram of a mucus-secreting intestinal goblet cell. Its constricted base, where the mitochondria and granular endoplasmic reticulum (GER) are located, is typical. Synthesis of the protein part of the glycoprotein complex occurs in the endoplasmic reticulum. A developed Golgi apparatus is present in the supranuclear region. In cells that secrete sulfated polysaccharides, the process of sulfation occurs in the Golgi complex. (Redrawn after Gordon and reproduced, with permission, from Ham AW: *Histology,* 6th ed. Lippincott, 1969.)

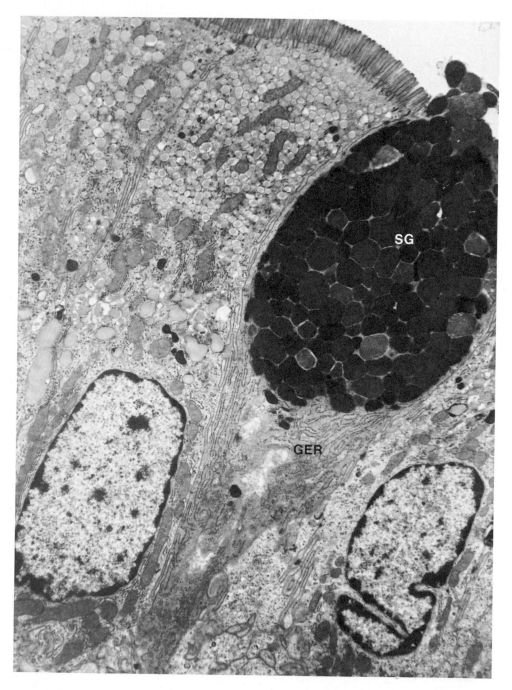

Figure 4 –24. Electron micrograph of a typical goblet cell from the small intestine. The granular endoplasmic reticulum is present mainly in the basal portion of the cell (GER), while the cell apex is filled with dense secretory granules (SG). × 5000. Typical columnar absorptive cells with microvillar borders lie adjacent to the goblet cell. (Courtesy of HI Friedman.)

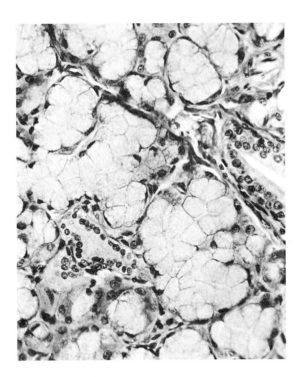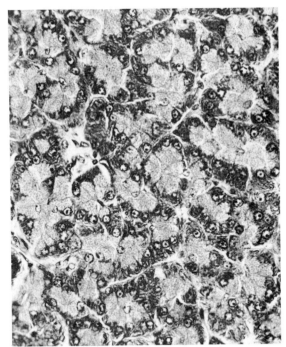

Figure 4 –25. Two photomicrographs illustrating the differences between mucous cells (sublingual gland) at left and serous cells (pancreas) at right.

of abundant, large, lightly staining secretory granules filling its extensive supranuclear apical pole. The nucleus is usually flattened vertically and is localized in the cell base. This region is usually rich in granular endoplasmic reticulum (Figs 4–23 and 4–24). The Golgi apparatus located just above the nucleus is exceptionally well developed, indicative of its important function in this cell. Data obtained by radioautography suggest that in this cell, proteins are synthesized from amino acids at the level of the endoplasmic reticulum present in the cell base. The complex, high-molecular-weight carbohydrates are likely to be synthesized both in the endoplasmic reticulum and Golgi apparatus. In those cells that produce sulfated glycoproteins, the process of sulfation of the polysaccharide moiety occurs in the region of the Golgi apparatus.

The goblet cell of the intestines is only one of several types of cells that synthesize glycoproteins. Other types—discussed later—show great variability in the chemistry of their secretion and present somewhat different morphologic characteristics.

Serous & Mucous Cells

Pancreatic cells and goblet cells are typical examples of cells called serous and mucous cells, respectively, because of the molecular nature and consistency of their products of secretion. Mucous cells are characterized by the presence of large, clear secretory granules that occupy most of the cell and a flattened nucleus containing condensed chromatin at the cell base. Serous cells present a rounded euchromatic nucleus surrounded by granular and endoplasmic reticulum in the basal third of the cell, in addition to clearly visible and easily stained secretory granules at the cell apex (Figs 4–25 and 17–1).

Differences between these 2 types of cells are not always clear, and in mammalian organisms various cell types have been described that produce variable proportions of polysaccharides and proteins. This occurs, for example, in the parotid and submandibular salivary glands. Close analysis of these cell types shows that there is an almost continuous gradient from serous to mucous cells, which consequently makes it impossible to classify certain cell types as either mucous or serous. In doubtful instances, an intermediate classification of **seromucous cells** has been proposed.

Myoepithelial Cells

Several glands (eg, sweat, mammary, and salivary glands) commonly contain a special cell type that surrounds mainly the cells of its secretory portions. This is the star-shaped myoepithelial cell, which has a centrally located nucleus and long cytoplasmic arms bound to the secretory cells by desmosomes. Myoepithelial cells are located between the basal lamina and basal pole of the secretory cells. They embrace gland acini as an octopus would embrace a rounded boulder. The presence of filaments similar to those of smooth muscle, as well as

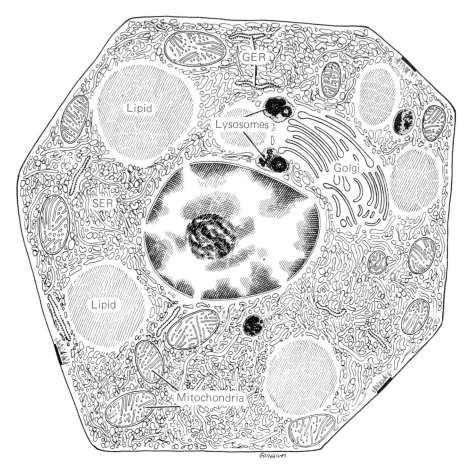

Figure 4 –26. Diagram of the ultrastructure of a hypothetic steroid-secreting cell. Observe the richness of the smooth endoplasmic reticulum (SER), lipid droplets, Golgi apparatus, and lysosomes. The abundant mitochondria have tubular cristae. They not only produce the energy necessary for activity of the cell but are also involved in steroid synthesis. GER, granular (rough) endoplasmic reticulum.

other musclelike characteristics, suggests that these cells are contractile. They are considered to participate actively in secretion by compressing the secretory portion of the glands in which they are present.

Steroid-Secreting Cells

Cells secreting steroids are found in various structures of the body (eg, testicles, ovaries, adrenals). They are endocrine cells specialized for synthesizing and storing steroid substances with hormonal activity. They have the following characteristics (Figs 4–26 and 4–27):

(1) They are polyhedral or rounded acidophilic cells with a central nucleus and a cytoplasm that is usually but not invariably rich in lipid droplets.

(2) The cytoplasm of steroid-secreting cells presents an exceptionally rich smooth endoplasmic reticulum, which takes the form of vesicles and tubules. In properly fixed material, they appear mainly as freely anastomosing tubules. The endoplasmic reticulum contains the necessary enzymes

to synthesize cholesterol from acetate and other substrates and to transform (mainly in the testicles and ovaries) the pregnenolone produced in the mitochondria into androgens, estrogens, and progestogens.

(3) The spherical or elongated mitochondria that are present usually contain tubular rather than lamellar or shelflike cristae, which are common to mitochondria of other epithelial cells. Besides being the main site of energy production for cell function, these organelles have the necessary enzymatic equipment not only to cleave the cholesterol side chain and produce pregnenolone but also to participate in the synthesis of the steroids of the adrenal glands. The process of steroid synthesis results, therefore, from close collaboration between smooth endoplasmic reticulum and mitochondria, a striking example of cooperation between intracellular organelles. It also explains the close proximity observed between these 2 organelles in the steroid-secreting cells.

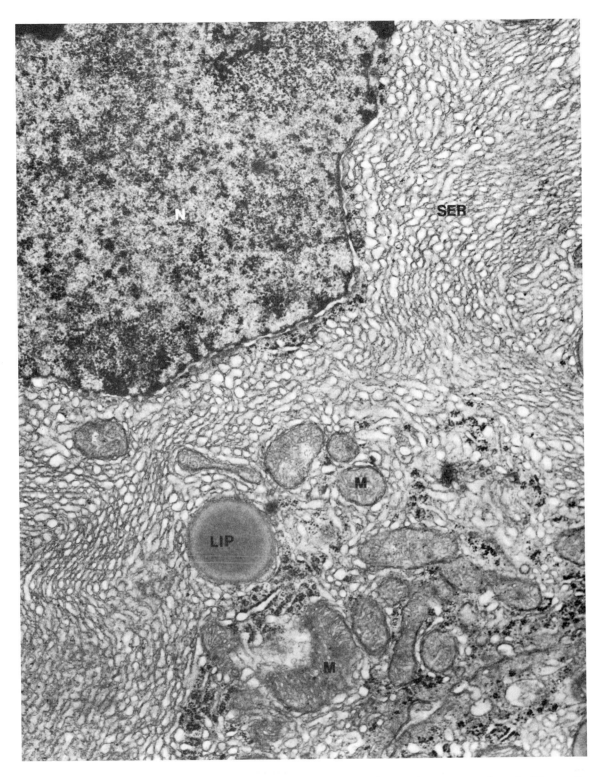

Figure 4 –27. Electron micrograph of a steroid-producing cell from the corpus luteum of a pregnant guinea pig. Observe the nucleus (N), the abundance of smooth endoplasmic reticulum (SER), the lipid droplet (LIP), and the mitochondria (M). Reduced from × 30,000. (Reproduced, with permission, from Christensen & Gillim in: *The Gonads.* McKerns KW [editor]. Appleton-Century-Crofts, 1969.)

•   •   •

References

Amsterdam A, Ohad I, Schramm M: Dynamic changes in the ultrastructure of the acinar cell of the rat parotid gland during the secretory cycle. J Cell Biol 41:753, 1969.

Bennett G, Leblond CP, Haddad A: Migration of glycoproteins from the Golgi apparatus to the surface of various cell types as shown by radioautography after labelled fucose injection into rats. J Cell Biol 60:258, 1974.

Berridge MJ, Oschman JL: *Transporting Epithelia*. Academic Press, 1972.

Blöbel G: Mechanism for the intracellular compartmentalization of newly synthesized proteins. *FEBS Symposium*. Vol 43. Pergamon Press, 1977.

Botelho SY, Brooks FP, Shelley WB: *Symposium on the Exocrine Glands*. Pennsylvania Univ Press, 1969.

Bretscher MS: Some general principles of membrane structure. Page 17 in: *The Cell Surface in Development*. Moscona AA (editor). Wiley, 1974.

Christensen AK, Gillim SW: The correlation of fine structure and function in steroid-secreting cells with emphasis on those of the gonads. In: *The Gonads*. McKerns KW (editor). Appleton-Century-Crofts, 1969.

Farquhar MG, Palade GE: Junctional complexes in various epithelia. J Cell Biol 17:375, 1963.

Freeman JA: Goblet cell fine structure. Anat Rec 154:121, 1966.

Gabe M, Arvy L: Gland cells. Page 1 in: *The Cell*. Vol 5. Brachet J, Mirsky AE (editors). Academic Press, 1961.

Hull BE, Staehelin LA: The terminal web: A reevaluation of its structure and function. J Cell Biol 81:67, 1979.

Jamieson JD, Palade GE: Intracellular transport of secretory protein in the pancreatic exocrine cell. 4. Metabolism requirements. J Cell Biol 39:589, 1968.

Junqueira LCU, Hirch GC: Cell secretion: A study of pancreas and salivary glands. Int Rev Cytol 5:323, 1956.

Kefalides NA: *Biology and Chemistry of Basement Membranes*. Academic Press, 1978.

Kelly DE: Fine structure of desmosomes, hemidesmosomes, and an adepidermal globular layer in developing newt epidermis. J Cell Biol 28:51, 1966.

Kobayashi S, Chiba T: Paraneurons: New concepts on neuroendocrine relatives. Arch Histol Jpn 40 (Suppl), 1977.

Komnick H, Komnick U: Elektronenmikroskopische Untersuchungen zur funktionellen Morphologie des Ionentransportes in der Salzdrüse von *Larus argentatus*. Z Zellforsch Mikrosk Anat 60:163, 1963.

Krstić RV: *Ultrastructure of the Mammalian Cell*. Springer-Verlag, 1979.

Lane N & others: On the site of sulfation in colonic goblet cells. J Cell Biol 21:339, 1964.

Leader DP: Protein synthesis on membrane-bound ribosomes. Trans Int Biol Soc 4:205, 1979.

Leblond CP, Bennett G: Elaboration and turnover of cell coat glycoproteins. Page 29 in: *The Cell Surface in Development*. Moscona AA (editor). Wiley, 1974.

Mukherjee TM, Williams AW: A comparative study of the ultrastructure of microvilli in the epithelium of small and large intestines of mice. J Cell Biol 34:447, 1967.

Neutra M, Leblond CP: Radioautographic comparison of the uptake of galactose-H^3 and glucose ^3H in the Golgi region of various cells secreting glycoproteins or mucopolysaccharides. J Cell Biol 30:137, 1966.

Neutra M, Leblond CP: Synthesis of the carbohydrate of mucus of the Golgi complex, as shown by electron microscope radioautography of goblet cells from rats injected with glucose-H^3. J Cell Biol 30:119, 1966.

Pearse AGE: The cytochemistry and ultrastructure of polypeptide hormone-producing cells of the APUD series and the embryologic, physiologic and pathologic implications of the concept. J Histochem Cytochem 17:303, 1969.

Pearse AGE, Polak JM: Endocrine tumours of neural crest origin: Neurolophomas, apudomas and the APUD concept. Med Biol 52:3, 1974.

Pierce GB & others: Basement membranes. 4. Epithelial origin and immunologic cross reactions. Am J Pathol 45:929, 1964.

Rambourg A, Leblond CP: Electron microscope observations on the carbohydrate-rich cell coat present at the surface of cells in the rat. J Cell Biol 32:27, 1967.

Staehelin LA, Hull B: Junctions between living cells. Sci Am 238:141, May 1978.

Tamarin A: Myoepithelium of the rat submaxillary gland. J Ultrastruct Res 16:320, 1966.

Warshawsky H, Leblond CP, Droz B: Synthesis and migration of proteins in the cells of exocrine pancreas as revealed by specific activity determination from radioautographs. J Cell Biol 16:1, 1963.

Connective Tissue | 5

The connective tissues are responsible for providing and maintaining form in the body. Functioning in a mechanical role, they comprise a matrix that serves to connect and bind the cells and organs and ultimately give support to the body. Unlike the other tissue types (epithelium, muscle, and nerve), connective tissue functions primarily through its extracellular components. In fact, the major constituent of connective tissue is its extracellular **matrix**, composed of protein **fibers**, an amorphous **ground substance**, and **tissue fluid**, the latter consisting primarily of bound water of solvation. Embedded within the extracellular matrix are the connective tissue–specific cell types.

Consequently, in terms of structural composition, connective tissue can be subdivided into 3 classes of components: cells, proteinaceous fibers, and ground substance. The wide variety of connective tissue types in the body represent modulations in the expressions of these 3 components.

Connective tissues have various functions as discussed further in the section on histophysiology (see p 112). The capsules that surround the organs of the body and the internal architecture that supports their cells are composed of connective tissue. This tissue also makes up tendons, ligaments, and the areolar tissue that fills the spaces between organs. Bone and cartilage are types of connective tissue that function to support the soft tissues of the body.

The role of connective tissue in defense of the organism is related to its content of phagocytic and antibody-producing cells. Phagocytic cells engulf inert particles and microorganisms that enter the body. Specific proteins called **antibodies** are produced by plasma cells in the connective tissue. These combine with foreign proteins of bacteria and viruses—or with the toxins produced by bacteria—and combat the biologic activity of these harmful agents. In addition, connective tissue matrix components provide a physical barrier in preventing the dispersion of microorganisms that pass through the epithelial barrier.

The role of connective tissue in nutrition depends upon its close association with blood vessels. The connective tissue matrix serves as the medium through which nutrients and metabolic wastes are exchanged between cells and their nourishing blood supply.

Connective tissue develops from an embryonic tissue, the **mesenchyme,** which is characterized by branched cells embedded in an abundant amorphous intercellular substance. The mesenchymal cells have oval nuclei with well-developed nucleoli and fine chromatin. The mesenchyme that derives from the middle layer of the embryo, the **mesoderm,** spreads throughout the fetus, surrounding the developing organs and penetrating into them. In addition to being the point of origin of all types of connective tissue, the mesenchyme develops into other types of tissue (eg, muscle, blood vessels, epithelium, and some glands).

FIBERS

There are 3 main types of connecting tissue fibers: collagen fibers, elastic fibers, and reticular fibers. These are distributed unequally among the different types of connective tissue. In many cases, the predominant fiber type is responsible for conferring certain specific properties on the tissue. Elastic tissue, with a predominance of elastic fibers, is an obvious example.

Collagen Fibers

Collagen fibers are the most numerous fibers in connective tissue. Fresh collagen fibers are colorless strands, but when present in great numbers they cause the tissues in which they lie to be white—for example, in tendons and aponeuroses.* In the polarizing microscope, collagen fibers are birefringent, which is an indication that they contain long and parallel molecules—an interpretation that has been fully confirmed by electron microscopic and x-ray crystallographic studies. Collagen is completely inelastic and, because of its molecular configuration, has a greater tensile strength than steel. Consequently, collagen imparts a unique combination of flexibility and strength to the tissue in which it lies.

In many parts of the body, collagen fibers are organized in a parallel array, forming **collagen bundles.**

Because of their long and tortuous course, the

*aponeurosis = flat sheet of conn. tiss. serving to attach mus. to bone or other tiss. at their origin.

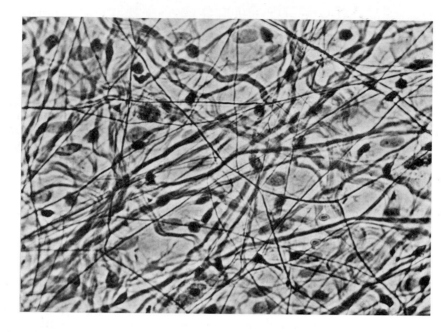

Figure 5–1. Whole mesentery spread on a microscope slide. The preparation was stained by the Weigert method for elastic fibers and photographed under the phase contrast microscope. The thin, taut filaments are elastic fibers that branch and form a woven network. Collagen fibers are the thick and wavy structures. × 200.

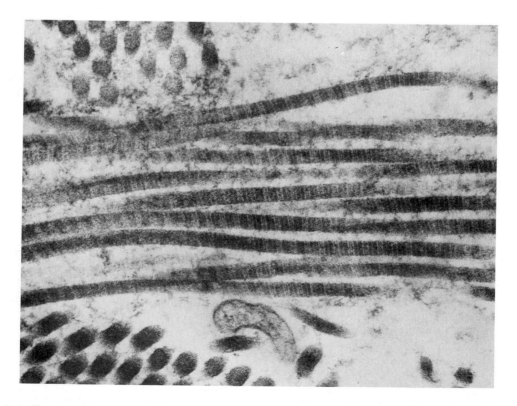

Figure 5–2. Electron micrograph of human collagen fibrils in cross and longitudinal sections. Each fibril consists of regular alternating dark and light bands, which are further divided by cross-striations. Amorphous ground substance completely surrounds the fibrils. × 100,000.

morphologic characteristics of collagen fibers are better studied in spread preparations than in histologic sections. Mesentery is frequently used for this purpose, for when spread on a slide, it is sufficiently thin to be stained and examined under the microscope. Mesentery is composed of a central portion of connective tissue lined on both surfaces by a simple squamous epithelium, the mesothelium. The collagen fibers in a spread preparation appear as elongated and tortuous cylindric structures. Their endings merge with other components of the tissue and cannot be seen. The diameter of collagen fibers varies from 1–20 μm (Fig 5–1). These fibers are longitudinally striated and are composed of **fibrils** with a diameter of 0.2–0.5 μm. The diameter of the fibers depends on the number of fibrils they contain.

The electron microscope also shows that each fibril is made up of finer filaments whose dimensions cannot be resolved by the light microscope. Collagen fibrils present a characteristic cross-banding with a periodicity of 64 nm (Fig 5–2). Each fibril presents a sequence of dark and light bands. The dark bands retain more of the stain used in electron microscopic studies because they have more free chemical radicals than the light bands (Fig 5–3). In addition to the typical 64-nm banding fibrils, collagen fibrils with a periodicity of approximately 250 nm exist in the connective tissue of the eye and in the cartilage of elderly people. These fibrils are called **fibrous long space** collagen.

Seen in the light microscope, collagen fibers are acidophilic; they stain pink with eosin, blue with Mallory's trichrome stain, and green with Masson's trichrome stain.

The principal amino acids composing collagen are glycine (33.5%), proline (12%), and hydroxyproline (10%). The remainder is made up of other amino acids, although it is interesting to note that collagen is very low in sulfated amino acids and in tyrosine. It is the only protein containing an appreciable amount of hydroxyproline. (Elastin is the only other substance that contains hydroxyproline, although in very small quantities.) The amount of collagen in a tissue can therefore be determined by measurement of the hydroxyproline content. Another amino acid unique to collagen is hydroxylysine. Collagen is the most abundant protein of the human body, representing 30% of total body proteins.

The protein subunit that polymerizes to form collagen fibrils is an elongated molecule called **tropocollagen,** which measures 280 nm in length and 1.5 nm in width. Tropocollagen consists of 3 polypeptide chains (Fig 5–4). In type I collagen, 2 of these peptide chains are alike (alpha-1) and differ from the third (alpha-2) in their amino acid sequence. The tropocollagen molecule is asymmetric, ie, each end has a different chemical composition. These molecules are the building blocks from which fibrils are formed. The transverse striation of the collagen fibrils is determined by the overlapping arrangement of the subunit tropocollagen molecules (Fig 5–3).

More detailed studies on the chemical structure of collagen have revealed that the amino acid composition of the alpha-1 chain varies according to its location in the body. The most widespread collagen, known as type I, consists of 2 alpha-1 (type I) chains and one alpha-2 chain. This collagen appears in the dermis of the skin, tendons, bone, teeth, and virtually all other connective tissues. Type II colla-

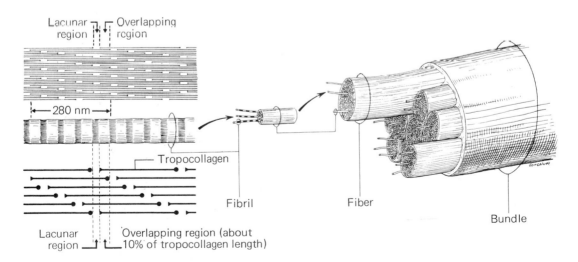

Figure 5–3. Schematic drawing of collagen fibrils, fibers, and bundles. In collagen bundles, the fibers are bound together by a cementing substance. Under the electron microscope, the fibrils show periodicity of dark and light bands. This periodicity is explained by the overlapping arrangement of rodlike tropocollagen subunits, each measuring 280 nm. It is thought that tropocollagen molecules are organized in a step-wise arrangement that produces lacunar and overlapping regions. Lacunar regions contain more stain (uranyl acetate, phosphotungstic acid) and appear dark.

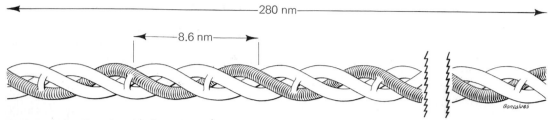

Figure 5-4. In the most abundant form of collagen, known as type I, each molecule (tropocollagen) is composed of 2 alpha-1 and one alpha-2 (shaded area) peptide chains, each with a molecular weight of approximately 100,000, intertwined in a helix and held together by hydrogen bonds. Each complete turn of the helix spans a distance of 8.6 nm.

gen, consisting of 3 alpha-1 (type II) chains, is the principal fibrous constituent of hyaline cartilage. In type III collagen, the tropocollagen subunits are composed of 3 alpha-1 (type III) chains. This form of collagen appears in reticular networks present in blood vessels, dermis, uterus, and other soft connective tissues. During development in a number of differentiating connective tissues, type III collagen is present earlier than—and is subsequently replaced by—type I collagen. Type IV collagen, consisting of 3 alpha-1 (type IV) chains, is present in basal and external laminas and appears to be a product of the cells associated with the laminas and not produced by fibroblasts.

It is possible to extract several collagen fractions with different solubility characteristics from connective tissue that is in an active phase of fibrillogenesis (eg, in growing animals or during wound healing). The first fraction, extracted in neutral solutions, appears to contain tropocollagen molecules not yet polymerized as well as those which, at the beginning of polymerization, form only very fine microfibrils. This is the recently synthesized **neutral-soluble collagen.** For this reason, collagen that is soluble in neutral solutions is the first to become radioactive after the administration of ^{3}H-proline or ^{3}H-glycine, which are radioactive amino acid collagen precursors. If the remaining tissue is treated with sodium citrate solutions at pH 3.0, a second fraction is obtained called **acid-soluble collagen.**

The third fraction, **insoluble collagen,** contains the collagen not extracted by the 2 previous steps. It can only be dissolved by means of very drastic procedures. Because isotope-labeled collagen precursors appear after injection first in the fraction soluble in neutral solution, next in the acid-soluble fraction, and finally in the insoluble fraction, it is believed that these 3 fractions represent successive stages of collagen formation.

The synthesis of collagen proceeds through the following steps (Fig 5-5):

(1) Polypeptide alpha chains known as protocollagen are assembled on polyribosomes bound to endoplasmic reticulum membrane and injected into the cisterna.

(2) Hydroxylation of proline and lysine occurs after these amino acids are incorporated into the polypeptide precursor of collagen, the protocollagen. Free hydroxyproline and hydroxylysine are not incorporated directly into the chains. The hydroxylation begins after the peptide chain has reached a certain minimum length and is still on the ribosomes. The 2 enzymes involved are (a) peptidyl proline hydroxylase and (b) peptidyl lysine hydroxylase.

(3) Glycosylation of hydroxylysine occurs after its hydroxylation; the different collagen types have variable amounts of carbohydrate in the form of galactose or glycosylgalactose linked to hydroxylysine.

(4) Each alpha chain is synthesized with an extra length of peptides on both NH_2- and COOH-terminal ends called **registration peptides** that assist in the proper register of the alpha chains. Electron microscopic measurements show that the newly synthesized molecule is 13 nm longer than tropocollagen. The extra lengths of peptides at the terminal ends play a specific role in that they aid in the assembly or alignment of the 3 alpha chains into the triple helix of the **procollagen** molecule. The alignment peptides probably ensure that the appropriate alpha chains (ie, alpha-1, alpha-2) assemble in the correct proportion. In addition, the extra peptides make the resulting procollagen molecule soluble and prevent premature assembly of the procollagen into precipitable collagen fibrils. Because of the end pieces, the procollagen is readily transported out of the cell and into the extracellular matrix. Outside of the cell, a specific protease called procollagen peptidase cleaves off the extra lengths of peptides. The altered tripeptide is known as tropocollagen, which is insoluble and capable of assembling into the polymeric collagen fibril.

Within the tropocollagen, the alpha chains are covalently bound to one another. The hydroxyproline residues serve an important role in that they not only aid in the helical assembly of the alpha chains but also function in stabilizing the alpha chains through the formation of the interchain covalent links. Hydroxylysine and other specific lysine residues become glycosylated and consequently serve as linking elements in the assembly of tropocollagen into the polymeric collagen fibrils.

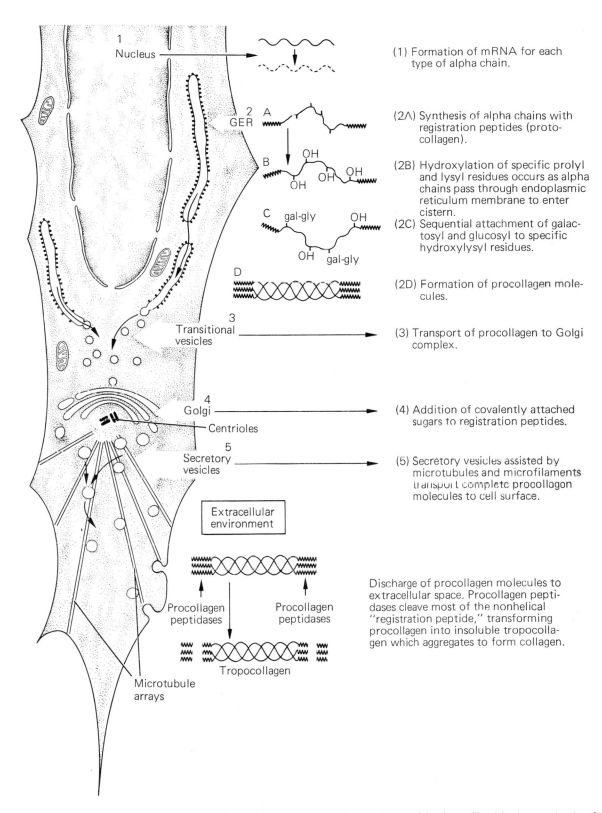

(1) Formation of mRNA for each type of alpha chain.

(2A) Synthesis of alpha chains with registration peptides (proto-collagen).

(2B) Hydroxylation of specific prolyl and lysyl residues occurs as alpha chains pass through endoplasmic reticulum membrane to enter cistern.

(2C) Sequential attachment of galactosyl and glucosyl to specific hydroxylysyl residues.

(2D) Formation of procollagen molecules.

(3) Transport of procollagen to Golgi complex.

(4) Addition of covalently attached sugars to registration peptides.

(5) Secretory vesicles assisted by microtubules and microfilaments transport complete procollagen molecules to cell surface.

Discharge of procollagen molecules to extracellular space. Procollagen peptidases cleave most of the nonhelical "registration peptide," transforming procollagen into insoluble tropocollagen which aggregates to form collagen.

Figure 5–5. Schematic representation of the molecular events and organellar participation utilized in the synthesis of collagen.

Defects in OH-lysine make the fibrils unstable and usually lead to a disassembly of the collagen fibrils when they are under stress.

Polysaccharides are used in linking the lysine and hydroxylysine groups between adjacent tropocollagen subunits. The faint PAS staining of collagen reflects these intramolecular carbohydrate linkages.

Elastic Fibers

Elastic fibers are easily distinguished from the collagen fibers in stretched connective tissue preparations because they are thinner and do not have longitudinal striations (Fig 5–6). They branch and unite with one another, forming an irregular network (Fig 5–1). When they are fresh and present in great quantity, elastic fibers appear characteristically yellow. Elastic fibers predominate in elastic tissue and are known as yellow fibers of connective tissue, while collagen fibers are known as white fibers. Elastic fibers, capable of stretching to one and one-half times their length, yield easily to very small traction forces but return to their original shape when these forces are relaxed. The presence of elastic fibers in blood vessels contributes to the efficiency of blood circulation and has contributed to the successful evolution of vertebrates.

Elastic fibers may stain weakly and irregularly with hematoxylin and eosin, but they usually appear unstained with this method. Selective methods to demonstrate elastic fibers, although they are devoid of histochemical specificity, include resorcin-fuchsin, aldehyde-fuchsin, and orcein, resulting in purple or dark blue staining.

Electron microscopic observations reveal that elastic fibers consist of 2 components: (1) an amorphous central region (elastin) surrounded by (2) a sheath of 10-nm fibrils. During their formation, the fibrils appear first, followed by small droplets of amorphous substance that accumulates in the center of the fibrotubules. The fibrotubules are composed of structural glycoprotein as judged by biochemical, immunochemical, and electron microscopic technics. The proelastin molecules are globular and have a molecular weight of about 76,000. When polymerized, these molecules correspond to the amorphous structure seen in the electron microscope. The amorphous substance becomes more abundant and predominates in the mature fiber.

The principal component of elastic fibers is an amorphous material that is made of a rubberlike scleroprotein called **elastin**, a significantly "younger" protein in terms of evolution than collagen and much more resistant to extracting procedures. It is produced by fibroblasts in skin and tendon and by smooth muscle cells in the large vessels with elastic tissue. Elastin resists boiling, dilute acids, and alkalis and is not digested by trypsin; and all of this, apparently, is due to its tertiary and quaternary structure, stabilized by hydrophobic interactions between the nonpolar peptide chains. This probably also explains the affinity of elastin for lipids. Pepsin at pH 2.0 acts slowly upon elastin, but elastin is easily hydrolyzed by the pancreatic enzyme **elastase**. The amino acid composition of elastin is somewhat similar to that of collagen—it is rich in proline and glycine—but it contains a greater quantity of valine and alanine. It contains the amino acids desmosine and isodes-

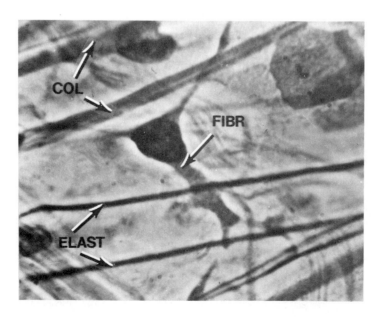

Figure 5–6. Phase contrast photomicrograph of a piece of mesentery spread on a glass slide. Shown are a fibroblast (FIBR), collagen fibers (COL), and elastic fibers (ELAST). H&E stain, × 800.

mosine not found in collagen. Elastin also occurs in a nonfibrillar form as **fenestrated membranes** present in the walls of blood vessels.

Reticular Fibers

Reticular fibers are extremely fine, with a diameter comparable to that of collagen fibrils (Fig 5–7), and are not visible in hematoxylin and eosin preparations. Since they are strongly PAS-positive, however, they can be demonstrated by means of impregnation with silver salts and by the PAS technic. These fibers are called **argyrophilic fibers** because of their affinity for silver salts. When impregnated with silver, they appear black. The argyrophilia and positive PAS reaction of the reticular fibers can be explained on the basis of their high content of hexoses—6–12% as opposed to 1% in collagen—and the configuration of the macromolecular architecture of glycoproteins making end groups available to bind the dyes.

Reticular fibers are composed mainly of the protein collagen. The thin microfibrils present a 64-nm periodicity, which is characteristic of collagen fibers, but reticular fibers have a smaller diameter.

Reticular fibers are particularly abundant in the framework of hematopoietic organs (eg, spleen, lymph nodes, red bone marrow) and constitute a network around the cells of epithelial organs (eg, liver, kidney, and endocrine glands). During embryogenesis, most connective tissues have an abundance of reticular fibers, but these are subsequently replaced by regular collagen fibrils.

CELLS

Cell specialization in connective tissue has given rise to several types of cells, each having its own morphologic and functional characteristics. This population includes fibroblasts, macrophages, mast cells, plasma cells, adipose cells, and leukocytes.

Fibroblasts

The fibroblast is the most common cell found in connective tissue. It is responsible for the synthesis of fibers and amorphous intercellular substance. There are 2 quite different morphologic types of fibroblasts and several with intermediate characteristics. The young cell with intense synthetic activity is morphologically distinct from the quiescent fibroblast that is found scattered within the matrix it has already synthesized. Some histologists reserve the term fibroblast to denote the young cell and call the mature cell a **fibrocyte** (Fig 5–8).

The young fibroblast presents abundant and irregular cytoplasmic processes; its nucleus is ovoid, large, and light, with fine chromatin and an evident nucleolus (Figs 5–8 and 5–9). The cytoplasm is rich in granular endoplasmic reticulum, and the Golgi apparatus is well developed (Figs 5–8 and 5–9).

The fibrocyte is a smaller cell than the fibroblast. It tends to be spindle-shaped and has fewer processes than the young fibroblast. It presents a smaller—and darker—elongated nucleus and an acidophilic cytoplasm (Fig 5–8).

The electron microscope shows that the fibrocyte has a less well developed granular endo-

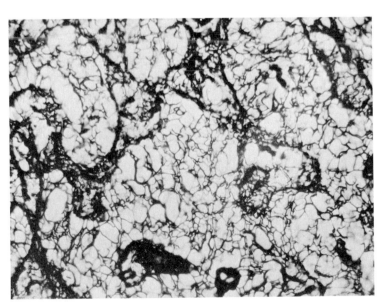

Figure 5–7. Section from a lymph node stained with silver. Note the thin black lines representing the argyrophilic reticular fibers forming an extensive network.

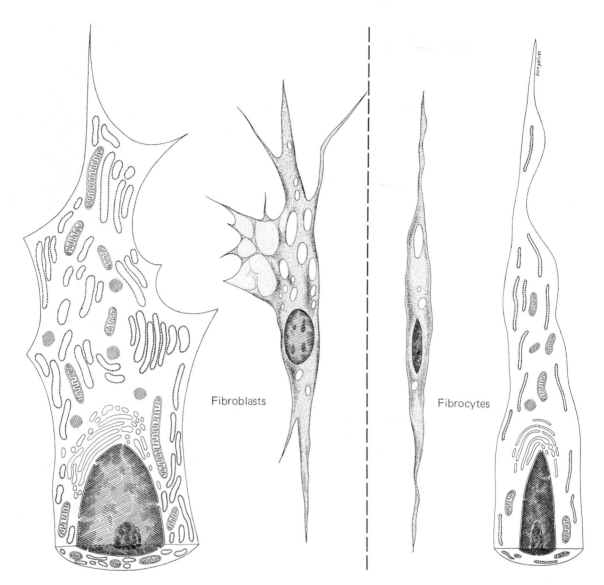

Figure 5–8. Immature *(left)* and mature *(right)* fibroblasts. External morphology and ultrastructure of each cell are shown. Synthetically active immature or young fibroblasts are richer in mitochondria, lipid droplets, Golgi apparatus, and granular endoplasmic reticulum than mature fibroblasts, often called fibrocytes.

plasmic reticulum and Golgi apparatus than the young fibroblast. When it is adequately stimulated, the fibrocyte may again synthesize fibers. This occurs during wound healing, and in such instances the cell resumes the form and appearance of a young fibroblast.

The functions of the fibroblasts have been studied in light and electron microscope radioautographs. These cells synthesize collagen and elastic fibers and the glycosaminoglycans of the amorphous intercellular substance. Proline and glycine labeled with ³H have been used in the study of collagen synthesis.

Radioautographic technics reveal that tropocollagen synthesized by the granular endo-

plasmic reticulum accumulates in the cisternae of this structure. It is subsequently encountered in the Golgi apparatus and is then transported to the outside of the cell. Collagen, therefore, most probably follows the same path as other secreted proteins (see Chapter 4). Evidence has been presented, however, that in some cases part of the synthesized collagen might be secreted by the fibroblast by means of a direct communication between the endoplasmic reticulum and the cell membrane without passing through the Golgi apparatus.

Fibroblasts secrete procollagen molecules into the intercellular matrix, and their polymerization into microfibrils takes place outside the cytoplasm.

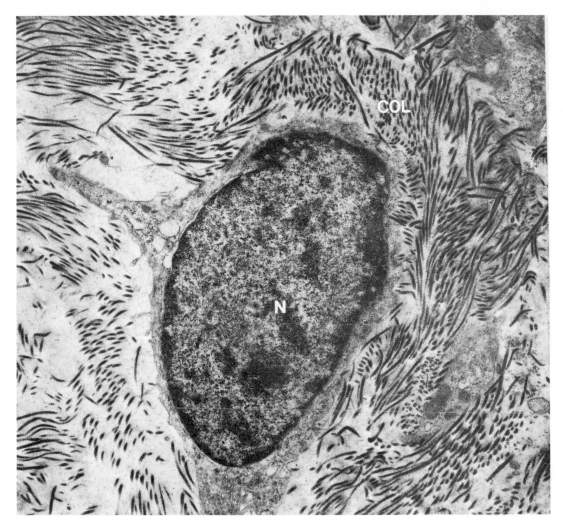

Figure 5–9. Electron micrograph of a fibroblast. There are many collagen fibrils (COL) around the cell. N, nucleus. × 7000.

The synthesis of glycosaminoglycans has been studied mainly by radioautography after the administration of sulfate labeled with ^{35}S since many connective tissue glycosaminoglycans are sulfated. Fibroblasts synthesize collagen and glycosaminoglycans at the same time, although some cell culture experiments indicate that a cell which produces collagen in substantial amounts produces little glycosaminoglycan and vice versa. The rate of secretion of different molecules of connective tissue by the same cell might vary with the age of the individual or in response to hormonal influences.

In adults, fibroblasts in connective tissue rarely undergo division. Mitoses are observed only when the organism requires more fibroblasts, ie, when connective tissue is damaged.

Macrophages

The macrophage is distinguished by its great capacity for pinocytosis and phagocytosis rather than by its morphologic characteristics, which vary according to its functional state and localization. Macrophages are either fixed or wandering. Wandering macrophages migrate by means of ameboid movement.

The phagocytic capacity of the macrophages permits their identification. When a vital dye such as trypan blue, India ink, or lithium carmine is injected into an animal, the macrophages engulf it and accumulate it in their cytoplasm in the form of granules visible under the light microscope. Fixed macrophages are spindle-shaped or star-shaped and have an ovoid nucleus with condensed chromatin. In loose connective tissue, macrophages are morphologically similar to fibroblasts and can be mistaken for them.

The wandering macrophage is more active in phagocytosis than the fixed macrophage. It migrates and phagocytoses by means of short, thick pseudopodia that cause it to have an irregular shape. The nucleus contains condensed chromatin and is usually round.

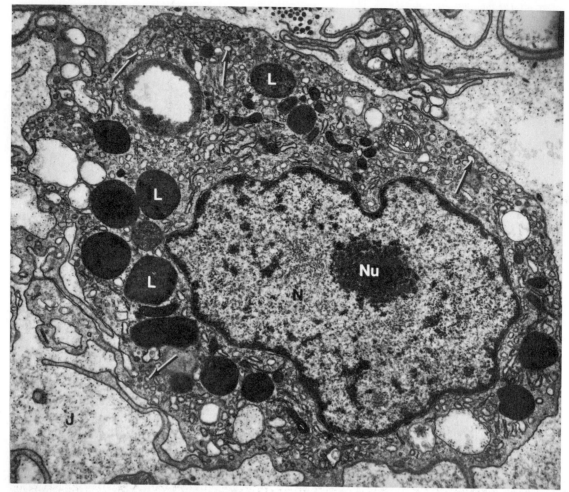

Figure 5–10. Electron micrograph of a macrophage. Note the secondary lysosomes (L), the nucleus (N), and the nucleolus (Nu). The arrows point to pinocytotic vesicles. Reduced from × 15,000.

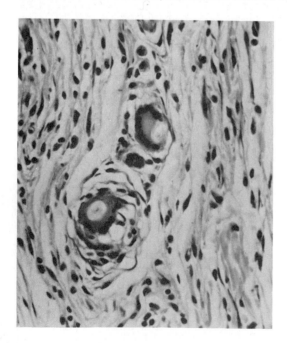

Figure 5–11 (at left). Photomicrograph of 2 foreign body giant cells. Both cells contain, in their cytoplasm, phagocytosed material that appears lightly stained. At the periphery of these cells, many nuclei can be seen. H&E stain, × 320.

The electron microscope reveals that the surface of the macrophage is irregular; its plasma membrane is pleated and contains protrusions and indentations (Fig 5–10). These cells have primary lysosomes that spill their contents into vacuoles containing phagocytosed material, giving rise to secondary lysosomes or phagosomes in which digestion of the engulfed material occurs. The surface charge of the particle to be phagocytosed plays an important role in the initiation of phagocytosis. Materials with positive charge are easily engulfed; those with negative or neutral charge are seldom phagocytosed.

Fixed and wandering macrophages are different phases of the same cell, and one may transform itself into the other.

Because of their capacity for locomotion and phagocytosis, the main function of macrophages is in the defense of the organism. They engulf cellular remains, altered intercellular substances, microorganisms, and inert particles that enter the body. When they encounter large foreign bodies, macrophages fuse together to form large cells with

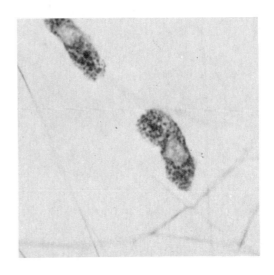

Figure 5–12. Whole mount of spread mesentery Two mast cells appear stained by Gomori's aldehyde-fuchsin. × 400.

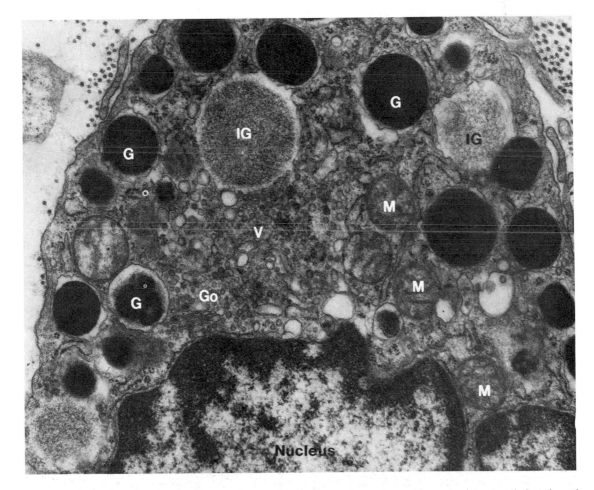

Figure 5–13. Electron micrograph of a mast cell. Mature granules (G) are electron-dense and appear darker than the immature granules (IG). M, mitochondria; Go, Golgi apparatus; V, small and large Golgi vesicles. × 36,000.

100 or more nuclei called **foreign body giant cells** (Fig 5–11). In health, macrophages are the end phase in the life cycle of monocytes, a type of leukocyte originated in bone marrow. After leaving the bone marrow, monocytes stay 8–74 hours in the blood and cross the wall of venules or capillaries to penetrate connective tissue, where they become macrophages.

In the process of monocyte-macrophage transformation, there is an increase in both protein synthesis and cell size. An increase in the size of the Golgi apparatus as well as in the number of lysosomes, microtubules, and microfilaments is also apparent.

Cells of Regeneration

Some believe that in adults there are cells that persist with the same potential as embryonic mesenchymal cells—ie, the ability to give rise to any kind of connective tissue cells. It is also believed that they have the capacity to give rise to smooth muscle cells. This is assumed when an injured blood vessel grows and new muscle cells derived from the multiplication and differentiation of mesenchymal cells appear in its wall. Sometimes these cells are called **adventitial cells** because they are usually found along blood capillaries.

Morphologically, adventitial cells are quite similar to fibroblasts, which makes their identification difficult in some cases. They are usually smaller than fibroblasts and possess elongated nuclei with coarse chromatin.

The opposing view is that new connective tissue arises from existing cells such as fibroblasts, smooth muscle cells, etc, which retain their capacity to divide following certain stimuli.

Mast Cells

A mast cell is large and ovoid. Its cytoplasm is full of intensely staining basophilic granules (Fig 5–12). The nucleus of the mast cell is spherical and centrally situated; it is frequently obscured by cytoplasmic granules.

Mast cells are numerous in several types of connective tissue but are difficult to detect in hematoxylin and eosin preparations. They are easily demonstrated by toluidine blue, which stains their granules reddish purple.

The property that cells and tissues have of changing the color of a dye they are stained with is called **metachromasia.** It is believed to be due to the presence of numerous acidic groups in the structure amenable to metachromatic staining. Mast cell granules, which are surrounded by a unit membrane (Fig 5–13), are metachromatic because of their content of heparin, a sulfated glycosaminoglycan. In addition to heparin, the granules of mast cells contain other pharmacologically active chemical mediators such as histamine and ECF-A (eosinophil chemotactic factor of anaphylaxis). Mast cells also release SRS-A (slow-reacting substance of

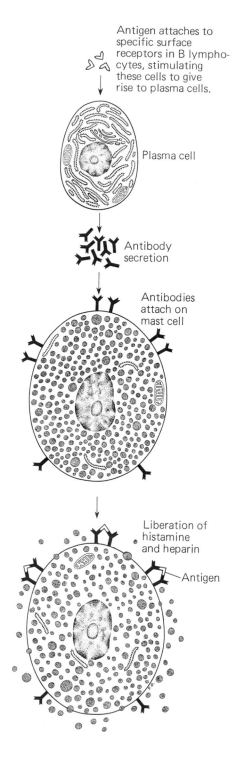

Antigen attaches to specific surface receptors in B lymphocytes, stimulating these cells to give rise to plasma cells.

Plasma cell

Antibody secretion

Antibodies attach on mast cell

Liberation of histamine and heparin

Antigen

Figure 5–14. Schematic drawing showing how antigens act on mast cells. Antibodies synthesized by plasma cells become attached to the surface of mast cells. Another injection of the same antigen promotes the liberation of mast cell granules through the combination of the newly injected antigen with membrane-fixed antibodies. Mast cell granules liberate histamine and heparin in the intercellular space.

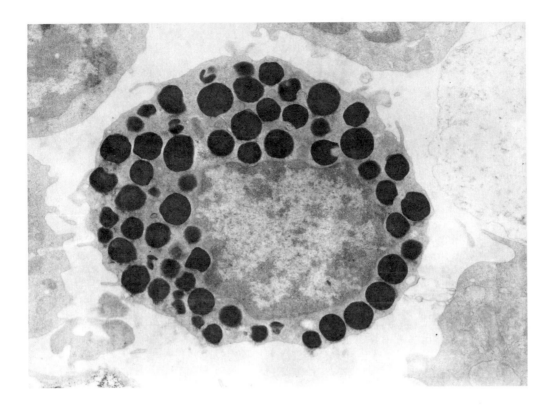

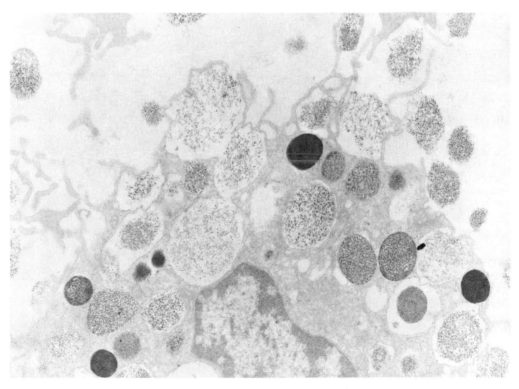

Figure 5–15. This pair of electron micrographs illustrates the liberation of granules by mast cells. *Above:* A resting mast cell with its numerous cytoplasmic granules. *Below:* A similar cell after injection of protamine, which stimulates liberation of the granules. The cell surface is irregular and the granular content is dissolving out. Magnification is the same for both cells: × 20,000. (Courtesy of I Vugman and RM Hofmeister.)

anaphylaxis), but this compound is not preformed in the cell. It is produced and immediately released under certain conditions. In some animals, not including humans, mast cell granules contain serotonin.

The surface of mast cells contains specific receptors for IgE, a type of immunoglobulin produced by plasma cells. Most IgE molecules are fixed on the surface of mast cells and blood basophils, while very few remain in the plasma.

Release of the chemical mediators stored in mast cells promotes the allergic reactions known as "immediate hypersensitivity reactions" because they occur within a few minutes after penetration of antigen into an individual previously sensitized to the same or a very similar antigen. There are many examples of immediate hypersensitivity reaction; a dramatic one is **anaphylactic shock,** a potentially fatal condition. It may occur when a person is injected with tetanus antitoxin months after having had one or several injections of it. The process of anaphylaxis consists of the following sequential events: IgE is formed by plasma cells after the first administration of antitoxin and is absorbed on the surface of mast cells. On the second administration, the antitoxin reacts with the IgE absorbed on the surface of mast cells (Fig 5–14) and triggers the release of mast cell granules, liberating histamine, SRS-A, and ECF-A (Fig 5–15).

Histamine causes contraction of smooth muscle (mainly the bronchioles), dilates blood capillaries, and increases their permeability. SRS-A produces slow contractions in smooth muscle, and ECF-A attracts blood eosinophils. Heparin is a blood anticoagulant, but in humans blood clotting remains normal during anaphylactic shock. Any liberated histamine is inactivated immediately after release.

Mast cells play an important role in all allergic reactions, but other cells also participate.

Extrusion of mast cell granules is an active, energy-consuming process that may be easily observed with the light microscope. Electron microscopic studies show that the membranes of peripheral granules fuse with the cell membrane to discharge their content (Fig 5–15). Simultaneously, peripheral granules fuse with granules located deep inside the mast cell, creating channels that facilitate

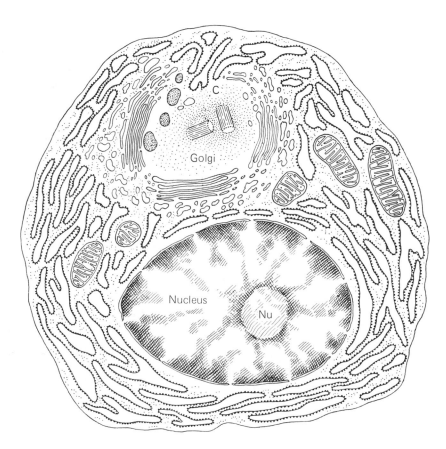

Figure 5–16. Ultrastructure of a plasma cell. The cell contains a well-developed granular endoplasmic reticulum, with dilated cisternae containing gamma globulins (antibodies). In plasma cells, the secreted proteins do not aggregate into secretory granules. Nu, nucleolus; C, centriole. (Redrawn and reproduced, with permission, from Ham AW: *Histology,* 6th ed. Lippincott, 1969.)

a rapid passage of material to the cell exterior. The process of extrusion does not damage the mast cell, since it remains viable and synthesizes new granules. Extrusion is inhibited by cytochalasin, a compound which inhibits the activity of microfilaments, suggesting that microfilaments participate in the release of mast cell granules.

Plasma Cells

Plasma cells are few in number in connective tissue in most areas of the body. They are numerous in sites subject to the penetration of bacteria and foreign proteins (eg, intestinal mucosa) and in areas where there is chronic inflammation.

Plasma cells are large, ovoid cells that have a basophilic cytoplasm due to their richness in granular endoplasmic reticulum. The juxtanuclear Golgi apparatus and the centrioles occupy a region that appears pale in regular histologic preparations (Fig 5–16). The nucleus of the plasma cell is spherical, containing compact, coarse heterochromatin alternating with lighter areas of approximately equal size. The configuration resembles a wheel with spokes, giving the nucleus a clock-face appearance (Fig 5–16).

Plasma cells are responsible for the synthesis of the antibodies found in the bloodstream. Antibodies are specific globulins produced by the organism in response to the penetration of antigens. Each synthesized antibody is specific for the one antigen that gave rise to its production and reacts with it, although it is possible that the antibody could cross-react with antigens possessing a similar molecular configuration. The results of the antibody-antigen reaction are variable. Its capacity to neutralize harmful effects caused by antigens is important. When an antigen is a toxin (eg, tetanus, diphtheria), it may lose its capacity to do harm when it combines with its respective antibody.

By means of immunofluorescence and cytochemical technics, it has been demonstrated that after injection of an antigen, the corresponding antibody appears first in the cytoplasm of the plasma cell. Electron microscopic studies involving injection of a vegetable protein (peroxidase) into animals as an antigen have shown that the first intracellular site in which antibodies appear is the cisternae of the granular endoplasmic reticulum.

Many of the antibodies synthesized by the plasma cells are specific for bacterial antigens and thus protect the body against these mi-

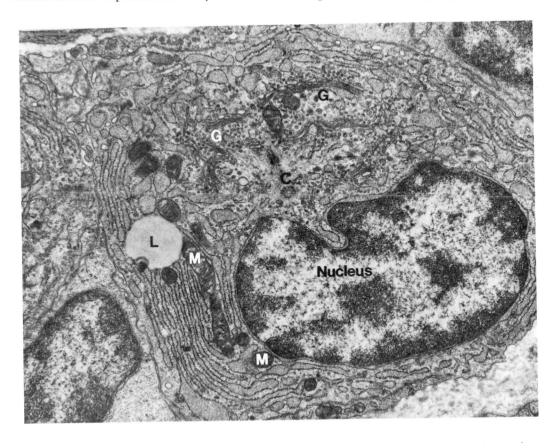

Figure 5–17. A plasma cell seen under the electron microscope. The micrograph shows the abundance of granular endoplasmic reticulum. Observe that many cisternae are dilated. M, mitochondria; G, Golgi apparatus; C, centriole; L, lipid droplet. × 18,000.

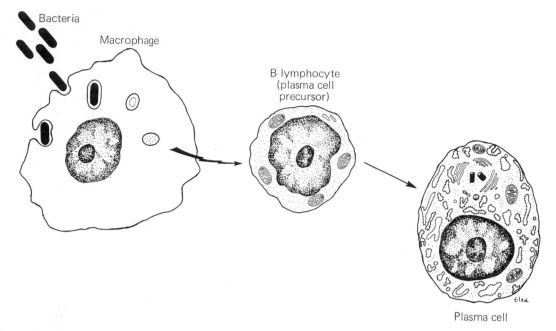

Figure 5–18. Possible relationships between macrophages and plasma cells. It has been shown that some kind of information passes from macrophages to plasma cell precursors.

croorganisms. Since bacteria are never found inside plasma cells but rather are engulfed by the macrophages, it was thought that there was a mechanism by which the plasma cell "learned" about the nature of the antigens present in the bacteria. Although the process by which this information is transmitted has not been completely elucidated, electron microscopic studies have shown that cellular contact occurs between macrophages and presumed precursor plasma cells (see Chapters 14 and 15). This suggests a transfer of information-bearing substances. It has also been demonstrated that extracts of macrophages that have phagocytosed certain antigens are able to induce the appearance of plasma cells which form antibodies against these antigens (Fig 5–18).

Some antigens need contact with macrophages in order to produce antibody-forming plasma cells. Other antigens act directly on plasma cell precursors (B lymphocytes). In such instances, the resulting plasma cells synthesize antibodies without assistance from macrophages.

Adipose Cells

Adipose cells (adipocytes) are cells that have become specialized for storage of neutral fats. They are discussed in Chapter 6.

Leukocytes

Leukocytes or white blood corpuscles are frequently found in connective tissue. In general, they migrate across the capillary and venule walls from the blood. There is a continuous movement of leukocytes from blood to connective tissue, and this process increases greatly during inflammation. Eosinophils, basophils, and lymphocytes are leukocytes frequently encountered in normal connective tissue.

A. Eosinophils: The main morphologic characteristics of eosinophils are the granules in their cytoplasm (lysosomes). Electron microscopic examination shows that they are membrane-bound and, in their interior, possess a flat crystal embedded in a granular substance. The nucleus of these cells usually has 2 lobes (Fig 5–19).

The number of eosinophils increases during the course of allergic and parasitic diseases as well as other types of disease. It is believed that these cells, attracted by histamine liberated by basophils and mast cells, produce prostaglandins that block the release of more histamine, thus decreasing the intensity of the inflammatory reaction.

The injection of antigenic protein causes an increase in the number of eosinophils in the injected area. This attraction is due to the complex formed by the reaction of the injected protein and its antibody. The antigen-antibody complex is promptly phagocytosed by eosinophils, although these cells are not very active in the phagocytosis of bacteria and foreign particles.

The principal experiments that led to this concept were performed by injecting an antigen (bovine albumin) or its antibody into the peritoneal cavities of guinea pigs. The antigen was coupled with a red fluorescent dye; the antibody was coupled with a green fluorescent dye. It was observed that when injected separately, neither the antigens nor the antibodies were phagocytosed by

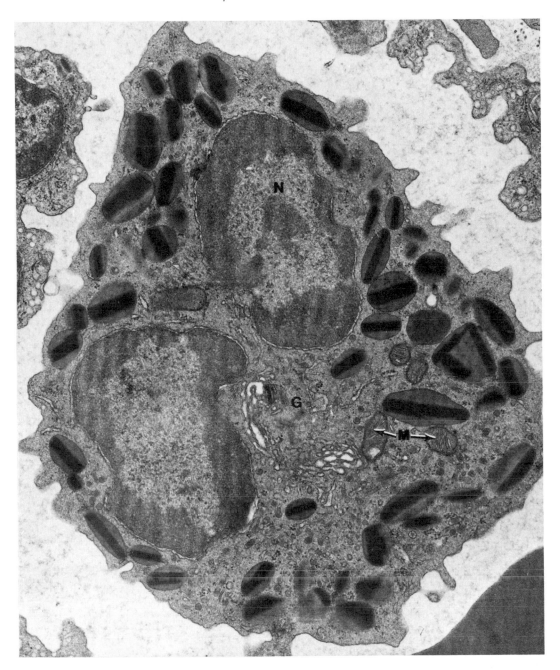

Figure 5–19. Electron micrograph of an eosinophil from rat connective tissue. Typical eosinophilic granules are clearly seen. Each granule has a disk-shaped crystal that is electron-dense and appears surrounded by a matrix which is enveloped by a unit membrane. N, nucleus; G, Golgi apparatus; M, mitochondria. × 20,000. (Courtesy of KR Porter.)

the eosinophils. However, when the fluorescent antigen and antibody were administered together, the eosinophils manifested a yellow fluorescence, which revealed that these cells engulf antigen-antibody complexes.

B. Basophils: Basophils are a form of leukocyte that contains granules similar in composition and function to those of mast cells.

C. Lymphocytes: Connective tissue lym-phocytes have a diameter of 6–8 μm (small lym-phocytes). They have a small amount of slightly basophilic cytoplasm and a large, dark nucleus with condensed chromatin that sometimes shows an in-dentation. The nucleolus is not visible under the light microscope.

The lymphocytes of the connective tissue form a heterogeneous population. Some have a long life span (many months to several years), whereas

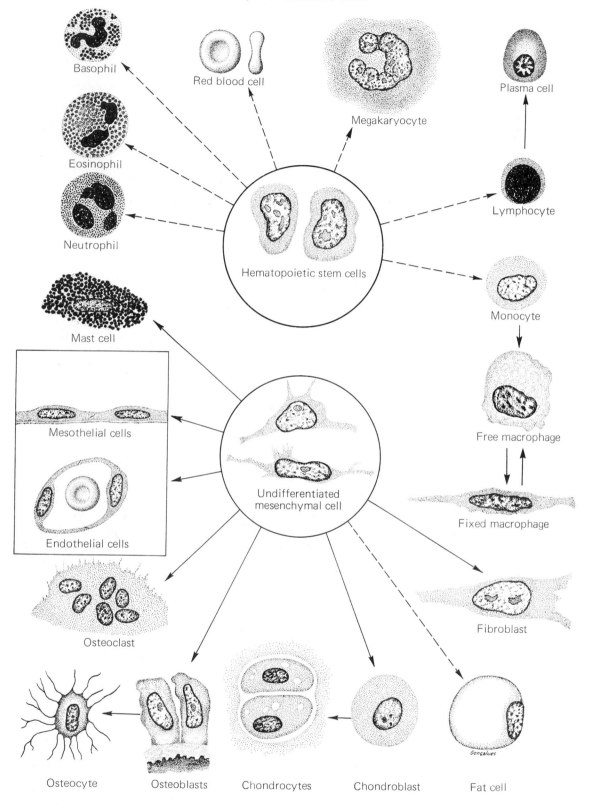

Basophil
Red blood cell
Megakaryocyte
Plasma cell
Eosinophil
Neutrophil
Lymphocyte
Hematopoietic stem cells
Monocyte
Mast cell
Free macrophage
Mesothelial cells
Fixed macrophage
Undifferentiated
mesenchymal cell
Endothelial cells
Fibroblast
Osteoclast
Osteocyte   Osteoblasts   Chondrocytes   Chondroblast   Fat cell

Figure 5–20. Simplified representation of the transformations that take place in connective tissue cells. Dotted arrows indicate that intermediate cell types exist between the pointed ones. The 2 cell types enclosed in the rectangle at left are epithelial morphologically, but they originate from the mesenchyme and retain several mesenchymal properties. These cells are not drawn in proportion to their actual sizes. For example, the fat cell, megakaryocyte, and osteoclast are much larger than shown here.

others live for only a short time (a few days or weeks). At least 2 functional types have been recognized: (1) the **T lymphocytes,** which are responsible for initiating cell-mediated immune responses and have a long life; and (2) the **B lymphocytes,** which, when stimulated by an antigen, divide several times and generate plasma cells which in turn secrete antibodies specific to the antigen. Their function is related to humoral immune responses, and their life span is short.

The lymphocytes in the lamina propria beneath the intestinal epithelium migrate across the epithelium and are destroyed when they enter the lumen of the alimentary canal. This phenomenon also takes place in the tonsils, which accumulate large numbers of lymphocytes beneath the epithelium.

The relationships among cells found in different types of connective tissue are shown in Fig 5–20. For further discussions of lymphocytes, see Chapters 13, 14, and 15.

GROUND SUBSTANCE

The amorphous intercellular ground substance is colorless, transparent, and homogeneous. It is difficult to study it in the fresh state. It fills the space between cells and fibers of connective tissue; it is viscous and acts as a barrier to the penetration of foreign particles into the tissues.

Intercellular substance is poorly preserved by histologic fixatives. In common preparations, it appears as a granular material among the cells and fibers of connective tissue. Histologic preservation of this substance is possible with the freeze-drying technic, which consists of freezing tissue rapidly to the temperature of liquid nitrogen (-200 C) and removing water by means of sublimation performed at high vacuum at a temperature of -30 C. The water, instantaneously solidified during freezing, is removed without passing through the liquid phase during drying. This method does not really fix the tissues, but it dehydrates them so that their morphologic and chemical characteristics are maintained almost unaltered. The tissues can then be fixed by nonpolar substances, and the intercellular substance, stainable by several methods including the PAS technic, appears as a homogeneous component among the structural elements of connective tissue.

The exact chemical nature of amorphous intercellular substance of connective tissue is not completely clear, but it is composed mainly of glycosaminoglycans and complexes of protein with carbohydrates referred to as proteoglycans.

The term **acid mucopolysaccharides** was used originally to designate extracted polysaccharides of connective tissue rich in hexosamine. In the last few years, other terms have been introduced to further classify these substances: **glycosaminoglycans** (polysaccharides that contain amino sugars), **galactosaminoglycans** (polysaccharides that contain galactosamine), **glucosaminoglycuronates** (polysaccharides that contain amino sugars and uronic acids), **glucosaminoglycans** (polysaccharides that contain glucosamine), **deoxyglucosaminoglycans,** etc. The terms proteoglycans, glycoproteins, mucoproteins, etc are often used synonymously with the term acid mucopolysaccharides. In this book, the following terms will be used: (1) **glycosaminoglycans** and (2) **structural proteoglycans.** Glycosaminoglycans have characteristic repeating disaccharide units made of uronic acid and hexosamine.

The most common form of uronic acid is glucuronic acid, and the most common hexosamines are glycosamine and galactosamine. The glycosaminoglycans of connective tissue form large molecules which become even larger by their association with proteins. Polymerization of these glycosaminoglycans is variable and is in direct proportion to the viscosity of the amorphous substance.

The structural proteoglycans are conjugated proteins containing as prosthetic groups one or more saccharides with relatively few sugar residues. These proteoglycans are extracted from connective tissue by a specific procedure and are different from serum glycoproteins. They are synthesized by fibroblasts in the connective tissue—cartilage cells in cartilage and smooth muscle cells in the walls of vessels.

The general type of synthesis for both groups of substances (collectively called glycoconjugates) consists of the formation of a protein core and the subsequent addition of repeating, usually similar glycosaminoglycan units or structural proteoglycans. The polypeptide units of the proteoglycans assembled within the liver cell occur on membrane-bound ribosomes. Initial sugar molecules are added while this core material traverses the lumen of granular or smooth endoplasmic reticulum. Other sugar components on the external surface of the molecule may be added while in the Golgi apparatus. Polymerizing and transfer enzymes have been isolated, the first mainly from smooth and the second from granular endoplasmic reticulum. In different tissues (aorta, cartilage, cornea, heart valves, skin, synovial membranes, and tendons), they yield similar but not identical structural proteoglycans, and they are unrelated to collagen or elastin.

Table 5–1 illustrates the chemical composition of the most common glycosaminoglycans in connective tissue, some of which are sulfated. Hyaluronic acid is the most common nonsulfated glycosaminoglycan in connective tissue. Chondroitin sulfate is the most abundant of the sulfated glycosaminoglycans but not so abundant as hyaluronic acid. Sulfated glycosaminoglycans give a solid consis-

Table 5–1. Main components of connective tissue acid mucopolysaccharides or glycosaminoglycans.

Glycosamino-glycans	Disaccharide Unit	Location
Hyaluronic acid*	D-Glucuronic acid + N-acetyl-D-glucosamine	Skin, umbilical cord, vitreous, synovial fluid, heart valves, cornea; produced also by bacteria
Chondroitin*	D-Glucuronic acid + N-acetyl-D-galactosamine; some sulfate esters	Cornea, embryonic cartilage
Chondroitin 4-sulfate* (sulfate of chondroitin A)	D-Glucuronic acid + N-acetyl-D-galactosamine-4 sulfate	Cartilage, bone, cornea, skin
Chondroitin 6-sulfate* (sulfate of chondroitin C)	D-Glucuronic acid + N-acetyl-D-galactosamine-6-sulfate	Cartilage, tendon, umbilical cord, intervertebral disk, embryonic cartilage
Dermatan sulfate (chondroitin sulfate B)	L-Iduronic acid + N-acetyl-D-galactosamine-6-sulfate	Skin, tendon, ligaments, heart valves
Keratan sulfate	D-Galactose-6-sulfate + N-acetyl-glucosamine-6-sulfate	Cartilage, intervertebral disk, bone, cornea

*Hydrolyzed by testicular hyaluronidase.

tency to tissues where they are present, whereas tissues containing hyaluronic acid are less viscous.

These glycosaminoglycans are covalently bound to proteins. Because they have numerous negative radicals in their molecules, the glycosaminoglycans are polyanions and are able to combine with a great number of cations by electrovalency. In connective tissue, sodium is the most frequent cation bound to glycosaminoglycans.

Glycosaminoglycans play an important role in regulating the amount of water in connective tissue. Each molecule of glycosaminoglycan is extremely hydrophilic and combines with a great number of molecules of water. Almost all water present in the amorphous intercellular substance of connective tissue is in the form of solvation water of glycosaminoglycan molecules. Even so, this water permits the diffusion of numerous water-soluble substances throughout connective tissue without fluid movement. The solvation water forms several layers around the glycosaminoglycan molecules, which become more irregular and unstable as they become more distant from these macromolecules. It is impossible to aspirate liquid from connective tissue with a hypodermic syringe because most of the water in amorphous intercellular substance is conjugated to glycosaminoglycans.

One interesting aspect of the distribution of the different glycosaminoglycans in vertebrate tissue is the variation of their relative proportions with age. Induction of calcification, control of metabolites, ions, and water, and healing of wounds are

important roles of these compounds. They are genetically controlled, and disturbances in their metabolism result in pathologic conditions. In some of these disorders, the degradation of dermatan sulfate or heparan sulfate is blocked at the lysosomal level by biochemically defective fibroblasts. Lack of hydrolase in the lysosomes has been found as the cause of several disorders in humans, including Hurler's syndrome, Hunter's syndrome, Sanfilippo syndrome, and Morquio's syndrome.

Proteoglycan molecules sometimes show significant variations in their side chains in response to changes in environmental conditions. They may influence the processes of development and adaptation, thus functioning as secondary informational macromolecules.

In connective tissue, in addition to the amorphous substance, there is a very small quantity of fluid—called **tissue fluid**—that is similar to blood plasma in its content of ions and diffusible substances. Tissue fluid contains a small percentage of plasma proteins of low molecular weight that pass through the capillary walls as a consequence of the hydrostatic pressure of the blood. Under normal conditions, the quantity of tissue fluid is insignificant.

Edema

Water in the intercellular substance of connective tissue comes from the blood, passing through the capillary walls into the intercellular regions of the tissue. The capillary wall is impermeable to macromolecules but permits the passage of water and small molecules, including low molecular weight proteins.

Blood brings to connective tissue the different nutrients required by the cells and carries metabolic waste products away to the detoxifying and excretory organs (liver, kidney, etc).

There are 2 forces acting on the water contained in the capillaries: (1) the hydrostatic pressure of the blood, a consequence of the pumping action of the heart, which forces water to pass through the capillary walls; and (2) the colloid osmotic pressure of the blood plasma, which draws water back into the capillaries. Osmotic pressure is due mainly to plasma proteins because the ions and crystalloids that pass easily through the capillary walls have approximately the same concentration inside and outside these blood vessels. Therefore, osmotic pressures exerted by these ions and crystalloids are approximately equal on either side of the capillaries and cancel each other. However, the colloid osmotic pressure exerted by the blood protein macromolecules—that are unable to pass through the capillary walls—is not counterbalanced by outside pressure and therefore tends to bring water back into the blood vessel.

Normally, water passes through capillary walls to the surrounding tissues at the arterial end of a capillary. This occurs because the hydrostatic pressure at this level is greater than the colloid osmotic pressure. However, hydrostatic pressure decreases along the length of the capillary toward the venous end. As hydrostatic pressure falls, osmotic pressure rises because of the progressive increase in the concentration of proteins, which is determined by the passage of water from the capillaries. As a result of the increase in protein concentration and the fall in hydrostatic pressure, osmotic pressure becomes greater than hydrostatic pressure at the venous end of the capillary, and water is thus drawn back into the capillary (Fig 5–21).

The quantity of water drawn back is less than that which passes out through the capillaries. The portion of water that remains in the connective tissue returns to the blood by the lymphatic vessels. The smallest lymphatic vessels are the lymphatic capillaries, which originate in connective tissue with blind ends. Terminal lymphatic vessels drain into veins at the base of the neck.

There is, therefore, little free water in the tissue because of the equilibrium that exists between the water entering and the water leaving the intercellular substance of connective tissue.

In several pathologic conditions, the quantity of tissue fluid may increase considerably, causing edema. Histologically, this condition is characterized by enlarged spaces between the components of the connective tissue caused by the increase in liquid. Macroscopically, edema can appear as an increase in volume that yields easily to localized pressure, which results in a depression that slowly disappears ("pitting edema").

Edema may result from venous obstruction or decrease in venous blood flow (eg, congestive heart failure). It may also be caused by starvation because the consequent protein deficiency results in lack of plasma proteins and a fall in colloid osmotic pressure. Water therefore accumulates in the connective tissue and is not drawn back into the capillaries.

Another possible cause of edema is increased permeability of the blood capillary endothelium due to mechanical injury or to some substance produced in the body (eg, histamine).

Edema may be caused also by the obstruction of lymphatic vessels, eg, by plugs of parasites or tumor cells.

TYPES OF CONNECTIVE TISSUE

There are several types of connective tissue that consist of the basic components already described—fibers, cells, and ground substance. The names given to the different types denote either the component that predominates in the tissue or a structural characteristic of the tissue.

The classification shown in Fig 5–22 does not include all possible types of connective tissue.

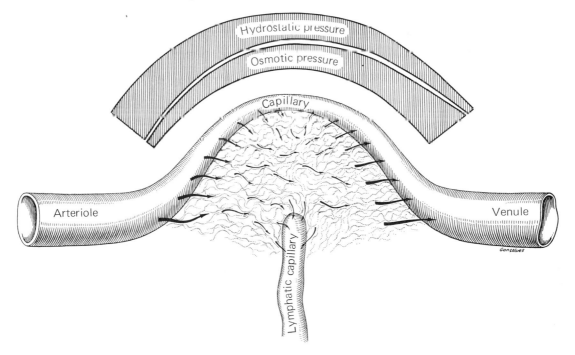

Figure 5–21. Movement of fluid through connective tissue. From the arterial to the venous parts of the blood capillaries there is a decrease in hydrostatic pressure and an increase in osmotic pressure (upper part of drawing). Fluid leaves the capillary through its arterial end and penetrates back into the blood at the venous end of the capillaries. Some fluid is drained by the lymphatic capillaries.

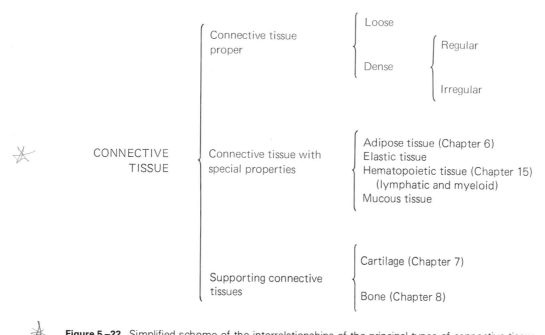

✦

Figure 5–22. Simplified scheme of the interrelationships of the principal types of connective tissue.

Connective Tissue Proper

In connective tissue proper, no single component predominates. There are 2 types: loose and dense.

A. Loose Connective Tissue: This tissue—also called areolar tissue—is the more abundant of the 2 types. It fills spaces between fibers and muscle sheaths, supports epithelial tissue, and forms a layer that encircles the lymphatic and blood vessels. Loose connective tissue is found mainly in the papillary layer of the dermis, in the hypodermis, in the serosal linings of peritoneal and pleural cavities, and in glands and mucous membranes (wet membranes that line the hollow organs) supporting the epithelial cells.

Loose connective tissue is composed of all the main components of connective tissue proper (Fig 5–23). The most numerous cells are the fibroblasts and macrophages, but all of the other types of connective tissue cells are present also. Collagen, elastic, and reticular fibers also appear in this tissue, though the proportion of reticular fibers is small. They tend to accumulate only where connective tissue comes into contact with other structures. A major constituent of loose connective tissue is the amorphous ground substance.

Loose connective tissue has a delicate consistency; it is flexible and not very resistant to stress.

B. Dense Connective Tissue: This type of tissue is composed of the same components found in loose connective tissue, but there is a clear predominance of collagen fibers. Histologic preparations reveal that this tissue has fewer cells than loose connective tissue. The fibroblasts are most common. Dense connective tissue is less flexible

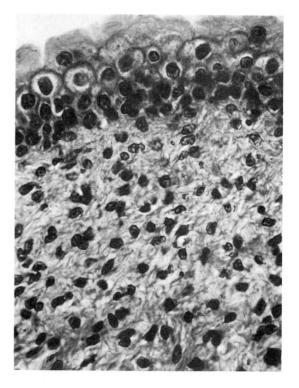

Figure 5–23. Photomicrograph of a section through the wall of the urinary bladder. Under the transitional epithelium there is a layer of loose connective tissue containing numerous cells. H&E stain, × 400.

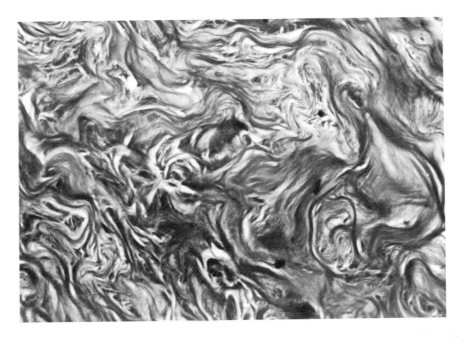

Figure 5–24. Irregular dense connective tissue. This tissue contains many randomly oriented large collagen fibers, sparse ground substance, and few cells. H&E stain, × 320.

and far more resistant to stress. It is known as irregular dense connective tissue when the collagen fibers are arranged in bundles without a definite orientation. The collagen fibers form a 3-dimensional network in this tissue and provide adequate resistance to stress from all directions (Fig 5–24). This type of tissue is encountered in the dermis of the skin, in the submucosa of the digestive tract, and in the connecting tissue capsules around such organs as the spleen, lymph nodes, and ganglia.

The collagen bundles of regular dense connective tissue are arranged according to a definite pattern. The collagen fibers of this tissue are formed in response to prolonged stresses exerted in the same direction and consequently offer great resistance to traction forces.

Tendons are the most common example of regular dense connective tissue. They are elongated, cylindric structures that function to attach striated muscle to bone; they are white and inextensible by virtue of their richness in collagen fibers. They have parallel, closely packed bundles of collagen separated by a small quantity of amorphous intercellular substance. Their fibroblasts contain elongated nuclei parallel to the fibers and a sparse cytoplasm which incompletely envelops the collagen bundles. Their cytoplasm is rarely revealed in hematoxylin and eosin stains—not only because it is sparse but also because it stains the same color as the fibers (Fig 5–25).

The collagen bundles of the tendons (primary bundles) aggregate into larger bundles (secondary bundles) that are enveloped by loose connective

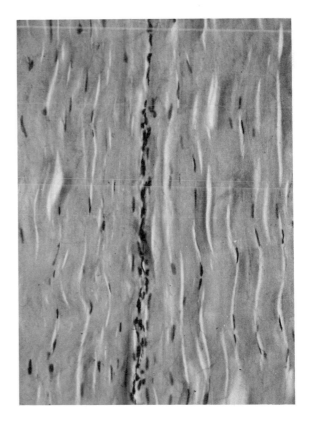

Figure 5–25. Regular dense connective tissue (longitudinal section through a tendon). There are numerous collagen bundles in parallel array. Tendon cell nuclei are seen between the collagen bundles. H&E stain, × 320.

tissue containing blood vessels and nerves. Externally, the tendon is surrounded by a sheath of dense connective tissue. In some tendons, this sheath is made up of 2 layers, both lined by squamous cells of mesenchymal origin. One layer is fixed to the tendon and the other lines the neighboring structures. A cavity containing a viscous fluid (similar to synovial fluid) is formed between the 2 layers. This fluid, which contains water, proteins, glycosaminoglycans, and ions, is a lubricant that permits an easy sliding movement of the tendon.

Elastic Tissue

Elastic tissue is composed of bundles of thick, parallel elastic fibers. Around each bundle there is a small amount of loose connective tissue, and flattened fibroblasts, similar to those of tendons, are found between the elastic fibers. The abundance of elastic fibers in this tissue confers on it a typical yellow color and great elasticity. Elastic tissue occurs infrequently. It is present in the yellow ligaments of the vertebral column and in the suspensory ligament of the penis.

Reticular Tissue

Reticular tissue is composed of reticular cells and the reticular fibers they synthesize. Reticular tissue is encountered in the organs that produce blood cells (hematopoietic organs) and comprises

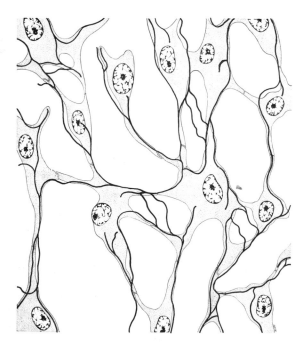

Figure 5–26. Schematic drawing of reticular connective tissue showing only the fixed cells and the fibers. Free cells are not represented. Reticular fibers are enveloped in the cytoplasm of reticular cells; however, the fibers are extracellular, being separated from the cytoplasm by the cell membrane.

the framework which supports the free cells found in these organs (Fig 5–26). Reticular cells have long extensions that are in contact with those of neighboring cells. Their nuclei are large, with fine chromatin and one or more visible nucleoli.

Mucous Tissue

Mucous tissue has an abundance of amorphous ground substance. It is a jellylike tissue containing collagen fibers and a few elastic or reticular fibers. The cells in this tissue are chiefly fibroblasts. Mucous tissue is the chief component of the umbilical cord and is called Wharton's jelly. It is also found in the pulp of young teeth (see Chapter 16).

HISTOPHYSIOLOGY

Connective tissues have the functions of support, packing, storage, transport, defense, and repair. The functions of support and packing are obvious—epithelial, muscular, and nerve tissues are associated with connective tissue that supports and fills the tissue spaces between their cells. The support function is carried out mainly by connective tissue fibers.

Collagen fibers constitute tendons, aponeuroses, capsules of organs, and membranes that envelop the central nervous system (meninges). They also make up the trabeculae and walls inside several organs, forming the most resistant component of the stroma (support tissue) of these organs.

Storage

Lipids, which are important nutritional reserves, are stored in adipose tissue, which is a type of connective tissue (see Chapter 6). In addition, because of its richness in glycosaminoglycans, loose connective tissue stores water and electrolytes. The most abundant electrolyte is sodium. Although only a small percentage of connective tissue consists of plasma proteins, because of its large size it is estimated that as much as one-third of the plasma proteins of the body are stored in the intercellular connective tissue compartment.

Defense

Several defense mechanisms depend upon the cells and intercellular components of connective tissue. This tissue contains phagocytic cells (macrophages) and plasma cells, which synthesize antibodies. In addition, because of its viscosity, the intercellular substance acts as a barrier to the penetration of bacteria and inert particles. Bacteria that produce **hyaluronidase** have great invasive power, for this enzyme hydrolyzes hyaluronic acid and other glycosaminoglycans of the connective tissue, thus reducing the viscosity of the intercellular substance and facilitating their invasion.

The diverse mechanisms that constitute the reaction known as **inflammation** take place principally in connective tissue. Inflammation is a vascular and cellular defensive reaction against foreign bodies. In most cases, it is a reaction against pathogenic bacteria or irritating chemical substances. Blood flow and capillary permeability are increased, partly as a result of the liberation of histamine by the mast cells. Edema is formed in this way, and an increase in the volume of bound water results in a swelling of the inflamed area.

Through their active ameboid movement, leukocytes cross the walls of venules and capillaries, invading the inflamed area. This migration is called **diapedesis.**

During the initial or acute phase of inflammation, the neutrophils predominate; when the inflammation persists and enters the **chronic phase,** the cell population changes. The main types of cells in the chronic phase are lymphocytes and monocytes, which come from the blood, and plasma cells, which originate from B lymphocytes. Macrophages in the area of inflammation represent wandering connective tissue cells which have migrated to that site, or they may differentiate from monocytes which arrive via the circulation.

The cells in the inflamed area engulf the remains of cells and fibers altered by this process and produce antibodies against invading microorganisms. If the bacteria are not destroyed, surrounding connective tissue forms a retaining fibrous wall around the inflammation.

Repair

Connective tissue has great regenerative capacity, and the areas destroyed by inflammation or traumatic injury are easily repaired. The spaces left by injuries to tissues whose cells do not divide (eg, cardiac muscle) are filled by connective tissue, which forms a scar. The healing of surgical incisions depends on the reparative capacity of connective tissue.

Transport

There is a close association between blood capillaries, lymphatic capillaries, and connective tissue. These vessels, except in nerve tissue, are always ensheathed by connective tissue. Consequently, the connective tissue carries nutrients from the blood to various tissues in the body and moves metabolic wastes from the cells to the blood.

Hormonal Effects

Different hormones influence the metabolism of connective tissue. An example is the hormone **cortisol (hydrocortisone),** produced by the cortical layer of the adrenal gland, which inhibits the synthesis of fibers by connective tissue cells. **Adreno-corticotropic hormone (ACTH),** elaborated by the pituitary, which stimulates the production of cortisol, has the same effect. Injection of either cortisol or ACTH has a detrimental effect on wound healing. These hormones also suppress or attenuate the inflammatory process. Their action is also directed against the cells of the connective tissue (lymphocytes, plasma cells, etc).

Hypothyroidism causes an accumulation of glycosaminoglycans in connective tissues. Adult hypothyroidism is called **myxedema (mucous edema)** and is associated with an excess of glycosaminoglycans in the connective tissue.

Nutritional Factors

Vitamin C (ascorbic acid) deficiency leads to **scurvy,** a disease characterized by generalized degeneration of connective tissue. In the absence of this vitamin, the fibroblast synthesizes defective collagen and the defective fibers are not replaced. Ascorbic acid is a cofactor for the enzyme protocollagen proline hydroxylase, which is essential for the normal synthesis of collagen. Recent evidence shows that hydroxylation of prolyl and lysyl residues is necessary for the normal polymerization and stabilization of collagen fibrils. In this step of hydroxylation, iron, molecular oxygen, and α-ketoglutarate are also necessary. Changes in the concentration of these substances within the cell will influence the rate of collagen biosynthesis. The roles of vitamins A, C, and D in connective tissue are also discussed in Chapters 7 and 8.

Renewal of Collagen

Collagen is a stable protein, and its renewal is very slow. Its **turnover rate** is different in different anatomic structures. The collagen of tendons is renewed very slowly or not at all, whereas the collagen of loose connective tissue is renewed more rapidly.

In vitamin C deficiency, once collagen fibers are destroyed they are not replaced. This leads to a generalized degeneration of connective tissue that becomes more pronounced in areas where collagen renewal takes place at a faster rate. The periodontal membrane that holds teeth in their sockets exhibits a relatively high collagen turnover; consequently, this membrane is markedly affected by scurvy and leads to a loss of teeth.

The physiologic destruction of collagen is performed by collagenase, an enzyme produced by the connective tissue cells. This enzyme digests only collagen and not other proteins. It is active at the normal pH of the connective tissue (about 7.0). The existence of collagenase in mammals has recently been confirmed, although the fact of collagen removal has been known for some time. Some bacteria of the genus *Clostridium* that cause gas gangrene produce collagenase, which greatly increases the invasive power of these microorganisms.

•   •   •

References

Allison AC, Davies P, de Petris S: Role of contractile microfilaments in macrophage movement and endocytosis. Nature 232:153, 1971.

Bellamy G, Bornstein P: Evidence for procollagen, a biosynthetic precursor of collagen. Proc Natl Acad Sci USA 68:1138, 1971.

Bouteille M, Pease DC: The tridimensional structure of mature collagenous fibers: Their protein filaments. J Ultrastruct Res 35:314, 1971.

Carneiro J, Leblond CP: Suitability of collagenase treatment for the radioautographic identification of newly formed collagen labeled with ^{3}H-glycine or ^{3}H-proline. J Histochem Cytochem 14:334, 1966.

Chvapil M: Physiology of Connective Tissue. Butterworth, 1967.

Cohn ZA, Fedorko ME, Hirsch JG: The in vitro differentiation of mononuclear phagocytes. 4. The ultrastructure of macrophage differentiation in the peritoneal cavity and in culture. 5. The formation of macrophage lysosomes. J Exp Med 123:747, 757, 1966.

Combs JW: An electron microscope study of mouse mast cells arising in vivo and in vitro. J Cell Biol 48:676, 1971.

Cox JP, Karnovsky ML: The depression of phagocytosis by exogenous cyclic nucleotides, prostaglandins, and theophylline. J Cell Biol 59:480, 1973.

Dehm P & others: A transport form of collagen from embryonic tendon: Electron microscopic demonstration of an NH$_2$-terminal extension and evidence suggesting the presence of cystine in the molecule. Proc Natl Acad Sci USA 69:60, 1972.

De Petris S, Karlsbad G, Pernis B: Localization of antibodies in plasma cells by electron microscopy. J Exp Med 117:849, 1963.

Dische Z: Some biological aspects of structural characteristics of glycoproteins. Page 161 in: The 4th International Conference on Cystic Fibrosis of the Pancreas. Karger (Basel), 1968.

Dougherty TF, Berliner DL: The effects of hormone on connective tissue cells. In: Treatise on Collagen. Vol 2, part A. Gould BS (editor). Academic Press, 1968.

Franzblau C: Elastin. In: Comprehensive Biochemistry. Vol 26, part C. Florkin M, Stoltz EH (editors). Elsevier, 1971.

Fullmer HM: The histochemistry of the connective tissues. Int Rev Connect Tissue Res 3:1, 1965.

Gay S, Miller EJ: Collagen in the Physiology and Pathology of Connective Tissue. Gustav Fischer, 1978.

Grant ME, Prockop DJ: The biosynthesis of collagen. (3 parts.) N Engl J Med 286:194, 242, 291, 1972.

Green H, Goldberg B, Todaro GJ: Differentiated cell types and the regulation of collagen synthesis. Nature 212:631, 1966.

Greenlee TK Jr, Ross R: The development of the rat flexor digital tendon: A fine structure study. J Ultrastruct Res 18:354, 1967.

Greenlee TK Jr, Ross R, Hartman JL: The fine structure of elastic fibers. J Cell Biol 30:59, 1966.

Harkness RD: Mechanical properties of collagenous tissues. In: Treatise on Collagen. Vol 2, part A. Gould BS (editor). Academic Press, 1968.

Hunter JAA, Finlay B: Scanning electron microscopy of connective tissues in health and disease. In: International Review of Connective Tissue Research. Vol 6. Hall DA, Jackson DS (editors). Academic Press, 1973.

Jackson SF: The morphogenesis of collagen. In: Treatise on Collagen. Vol 2, part B. Gould BS (editor). Academic Press, 1968.

Kefalides NA, Winzler RJ: The chemistry of glomerular basement membrane and its relation to collagen. Biochemistry 5:702, 1966.

Kivirikko KI: Biosynthesis of collagen. In: Connective Tissues, Biochemistry and Pathophysiology. Fricke R, Hartmann F (editors). Springer-Verlag, 1974.

Kornfeld-Poullain N, Robert L: Effet de différents solvants organiques sur la dégradation alcaline de l'élastine. Bull Soc Chim Biol 50:759, 1968.

Lagunoff D: Membrane fusion during mast cell secretion. J Cell Biol 57:252, 1973.

Pease DC, Bouteille M: The tridimensional ultrastructure of mature collagenous fibrils: Cytochemical evidence for a carbohydrate matrix. J Ultrastruct Res 35:339, 1971.

Petruska JA, Hodge AJ: A subunit model for the tropocollagen macromolecule. Proc Natl Acad Sci USA 51:871, 1964.

Robert AM, Robert B, Robert L: Chemical and physical properties of structural glycoproteins. Page 237 in: Chemistry and Molecular Biology of the Intercellular Matrix. Vol 1. Balars EA (editor). Academic Press, 1970.

Robert B & others: Studies on the nature of the "microfibrillar" component of elastic fibers. Eur J Biochem 21:507, 1971.

Robert L, Parlebas J: Rapport entre la nature de la trame fibreuse et le taux d'incorporation d'aminoacides marqués dans différentes types de tissu conjonctif. C R Acad Sci [D] (Paris) 261:842, 1965.

Robert L, Robert B: Structural glycoproteins, their metabolism in normal and pathological connective tissue. In: Nutritional Aspects of the Development of Bone and Connective Tissue. Symposium, Cambridge, 1968. Karger (Basel), 1969.

Ross R: The connective tissue fiber forming cell. In: Treatise on Collagen. Vol 2, part A. Gould BS (editor). Academic Press, 1968.

Ross R: The elastic fiber: A review. J Histochem Cytochem 21:199, 1973.

Ross R, Bornstein P: Elastic fibers in the body. Sci Am 224:44, June 1971.

Ross R, Klebanoff SJ: The smooth muscle cell. 1. In vivo synthesis of connective tissue proteins. J Cell Biol 50:159, 1971.

Schoenberg MD & others: Cytoplasmic interaction between macrophages and lymphocytic cells in antibody synthesis. Science 143:964, 1964.

Schubert M, Hamerman D: A Primer on Connective Tissue Biochemistry. Lea & Febiger, 1968.

Simkin JL: Biosynthesis of plasma glycoproteins. Expos Annu Biochim Med 30:19, 1970.

Sutton JS, Weiss LV: Transformation of monocytes in tissue cultures into macrophages, epithelioid cells and multinucleated giant cells: An electron microscope study. J Cell Biol 28:303, 1966.

Szigetti M & others: Distribution of ingested ^{14}C-cholesterol in the macromolecular fractions of rat connective tissue. Connect Tissue Res 1:145, 1972.

Trelstad RL, Coulombre AJ: Morphogenesis of collagen in the chick cornea. J Cell Biol 50:840, 1971.

Velican C: Macromolecular changes in atherosclerosis. In: Handbuch der Histochimie. Vol 8, part 2 (Suppl). Gustav Fischer, 1974.

Adipose Tissue | 6

Adipose tissue is a special type of connective tissue in which adipose cells (adipocytes) predominate. These cells may be found either isolated or in small groups within connective tissue itself, but most are found in the adipose tissue spread throughout the body. Adipose tissue is, in a sense, one of the largest organs in the body. In men of normal weight, adipose tissue represents 15–20% of the body weight; in women of normal weight, 20–25% of body weight.

Adipose tissue is important as a reservoir of energy for mammals because they need energy continuously although they eat intermittently. Fat is a way of storing concentrated chemical energy and occupies much less space per calorie than carbohydrates or proteins. It is in a state of continuous turnover and is sensitive to nervous and hormonal stimuli. Subcutaneous layers of adipose tissue help to shape the surface of the body, while deposits in the form of pads act as shock absorbers, chiefly in the soles and palms. Since fat is a poor heat conductor, it contributes to the thermal insulation of the body. Adipose tissue also fills up spaces between other tissues and helps to keep some organs in position. Animals that hibernate have a special variety of adipose tissue that supplies the heat necessary to permit them to return to activity after hibernation.

The 2 types of adipose tissue are characterized by the structure of their cells, localization, color,

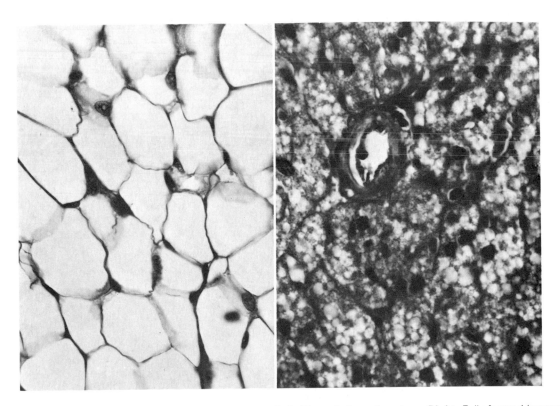

Figure 6–1. Photomicrographs of unilocular adipose tissue. *Left:* Tissue in formative stage. *Right:* Fully formed (mature) tissue. H&E stain, × 320.

vascularization, and functions: **common, yellow,** or **unilocular adipose tissue,** whose cells, when completely developed, contain one large central droplet of fat in their cytoplasm; and **brown** or **multilocular adipose tissue,** composed of cells containing numerous lipid droplets and mitochondria. Both types of adipose tissue have a rich blood supply.

UNILOCULAR ADIPOSE TISSUE

The color of unilocular adipose tissue varies from white to dark yellow, depending on the diet, and is mainly due to the presence of carotenoids dissolved in fat droplets of the cells. Almost all adipose tissue in adults is of this type. It is found throughout the human body except for the eyelids, the penis and scrotum, and the lobule of the auricle. The distribution and density of adipose deposits are determined by age and sex.

In the newborn, unilocular adipose tissue has a uniform thickness throughout the body; with age, it tends to disappear from some parts of the body and increase in others since its arrangement is partly regulated by sex hormones and adrenocortical hormones, which regulate the accumulation of fat and are largely responsible for male or female body contour.

Histologic Structure of Unilocular Tissue

Unilocular adipose cells are spherical when isolated but are polyhedral in adipose tissue, where they are closely packed. Lipid droplets are removed by the alcohol and xylol used in routine histologic technics. In standard microscope preparations, each cell appears as a thin ring of cytoplasm surrounding the vacuole left by the removed lipid droplet, the **signet ring cell** (Fig 6–1). The rim of cytoplasm that remains after removal of the stored triglycerides (neutral fats) frequently ruptures and collapses, distorting the tissue structure.

The thicker portion of cytoplasm surrounding the nucleus of these cells contains a Golgi apparatus, mitochondria of the filamentous and ovoid variety, a paucity of granular endoplasmic reticulum, and free ribosomes. The cytoplasm surrounding the lipid droplet contains vesicles of smooth endoplasmic reticulum, occasional microtubules, and numerous pinocytotic vesicles (Fig 6–2). Electron microscopic studies reveal that each adipose cell usually possesses lipid droplets other than the large one seen with the light microscope. Lipid droplets are not bound by a membrane.

Unilocular adipose tissue is subdivided into incomplete lobules by a partition of connective tissue containing blood vessels and nerves. Reticular fibers form a fine interwoven network that supports individual fat cells and binds them together.

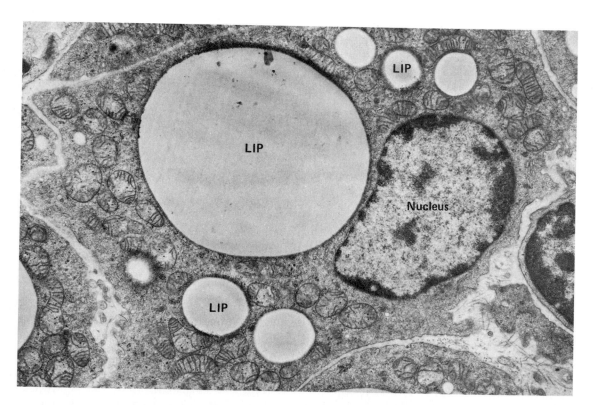

Figure 6–2. Electron micrograph of young fat cells. The cytoplasm is accumulating lipids (LIP), which appear as droplets. × 7500.

Although blood vessels are not always apparent, adipose tissue is richly vascularized. Considering the amount of cytoplasm that exists in fat cells, the ratio of blood volume to volume of cytoplasm is greater in adipose tissue than in striated muscle.

Histophysiology of Unilocular Tissue

The lipids stored in adipose cells are chiefly neutral fats or triglycerides—ie, esters of fatty acids and glycerol. The fatty acids stored by these cells have their origin (1) in digested food that is hydrolyzed and brought to the adipose cells in the form of chylomicrons; (2) in triglycerides synthesized in the liver and transported to the adipose tissue in the form of very low density lipoproteins; (3) in synthesis from glucose in the adipose cells; and (4) in neutral fats formed by the association of free fatty acids and α-glycerol (a product of adipocyte glucose metabolism). The deposition of unaltered fatty acids explains why a mammal fed lipids of another species may have in its adipose tissue neutral fats typical of the species utilized as food.

Chylomicrons are particles up to 3 μm in diameter formed in the intestinal epithelial cells and transported in blood plasma. They are composed of a central core of neutral fats and cholesterol esters surrounded by a stabilizing monolayer consisting of protein-free cholesterol and phospholipids. Chylomicrons and plasma lipoproteins are hydrolyzed in the blood capillaries of the adipose tissue by lipoprotein lipase, an enzyme synthesized in adipocytes and transmitted to the walls of adjacent capillaries. Within pinocytotic vesicles, the hydrolyzed fatty acids pass through the capillary walls to the center of the intercellular space. Free fatty acids (presumably bound to albumin) are transported to the adipocytes, induce pinocytotic vesicle formation, and enter the cell where they

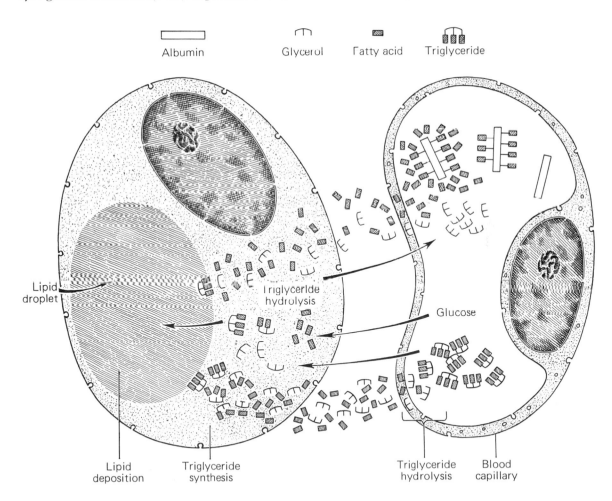

Albumin   Glycerol   Fatty acid   Triglyceride

Lipid droplet

Triglyceride hydrolysis

Glucose

Lipid deposition   Triglyceride synthesis   Triglyceride hydrolysis   Blood capillary

Figure 6–3. Probable pathways of lipid transport from the capillary lumen to the adipocytes and vice versa. The lower half shows the process of lipid deposition, utilizing glucose and triglycerides as precursors; the upper half shows lipid mobilization and its passage to the bloodstream. Triglycerides are hydrolyzed, and the molecules of fatty acid thus formed are carried in vesicles which fuse at the cell membrane. Thus, fatty acids are released into the extracellular space and from there are taken up by endothelial pinocytosis and liberated into the capillary lumen, from which site they are carried away by blood proteins.

combine with an intermediate product of glucose metabolism, α-glycerol phosphate, to form neutral fat molecules. These are then deposited in the fat droplets. Mitochondria and endoplasmic reticulum are organelles that are very active in the process of uptake and storage of lipids. Thus, the fatty acids cross the following layers in passing from the endothelium into the adipose cell: (1) capillary endothelium, (2) basal lamina, (3) connective tissue ground substance, and (4) adipose cell membrane. The movement of fatty acids across the cytoplasm into the lipid droplet is not easily defined.

Adipose cells can synthesize fatty acids from glucose, a process accelerated by insulin. Insulin also stimulates the uptake of glucose into the adipose cells and increases the activity of lipoprotein lipase.

Stored lipids are mobilized by humoral and neurogenic mechanisms, resulting in the liberation of fatty acids and glycerol into the blood. An enzyme known as **hormone-sensitive lipase** (triglyceride lipase) is activated by adenylate cyclase when the tissue is stimulated by norepinephrine. Norepinephrine is liberated at the endings of the postganglionic sympathetic nerves present in adipose tissue. The activated enzyme breaks down triglyceride molecules located mainly at the surface of the lipid droplets. The relatively insoluble fatty acids are transported on albumin to other tissues of the body, while the more soluble glycerol remains free and is taken up by the liver (Fig 6–3).

Growth hormone, glucocorticoids, prolactin, corticotropin, insulin, and thyroid hormone also have roles in different steps in the metabolism of adipose tissue.

Under circumstances of bodily need, mobilization of lipids does not occur in uniform proportion in all parts of the body. Subcutaneous, mesenteric, and retroperitoneal deposits are the first to be mobilized, while adipose tissue in the pads of the hands and feet resists long periods of starvation. After such periods, unilocular adipose tissue loses nearly all of its fat and becomes a tissue containing polyhedral or spindle-shaped cells with very few lipid droplets. These cells remain as such and do not become typical fibroblasts or other types of connective tissue cells.

Both types of adipose tissue are richly innervated by the autonomic nervous system. This innervation plays an important role in the mobilization of fats when the body is subjected to long periods of fasting or severe cold.

Histogenesis of Unilocular Tissue

Most histologists believe that the adipose cells develop from lipoblasts. These cells have the appearance of fibroblasts but are able to accumulate fat in their cytoplasm. The lipid droplets appear initially at one pole of the cell and then at the opposite pole. Lipid accumulations are at first isolated from one another but soon fuse to form the single larger droplet that is characteristic of unilocular tissue cells (Fig 6–4). When lipoblasts or adipose cells contain more than one lipid droplet, they are said to be in the multilocular stage.

Adipose cells were at one time believed not to undergo division. The new lipoblasts develop from undifferentiated mesenchymal cells. The human being is one of the few mammals born with fat stores; they begin to accumulate at the 30th week of gestation. After birth, the development of new adipose cells is common mainly around small blood vessels, where undifferentiated mesenchymal cells are usually found.

It is now possible to estimate the size and number of adipose cells in the body by lipid analysis of a sample of adipose tissue (obtained by needle biopsy) for which a count of adipocytes has also been made. When these data are combined with a mea-

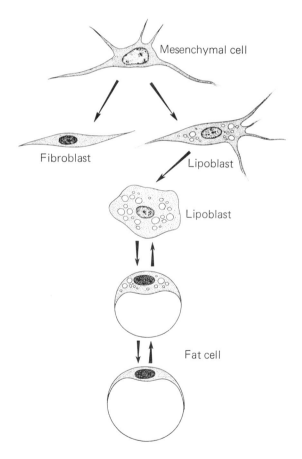

Figure 6–4. Development of unilocular fat cells. Undifferentiated mesenchymal cells are transformed into lipoblasts that accumulate fat and thus give rise to mature fat cells. When a large amount of lipids is mobilized by the body, mature fat cells return to the lipoblast stage. Undifferentiated mesenchymal cells also give rise to other cell types, including fibroblasts. The mature fat cell is in reality larger than shown here when compared with the other cell types of this illustration.

sure of total body fat, it is possible to estimate the total number of fat cells in the body as well as to determine the average lipid content per cell, which is a measure of its size. With these technics, it has been determined that cells of adults of normal weight contain an average of 0.6 μg of lipid and that the average number of cells is 25×10^9. It is believed that during a finite postnatal period, nutritional and other influences can cause an increase in the number of adipocytes, but after that period the cells do not increase in number but only accumulate more lipid under conditions of excess caloric intake. This early increase in the number of adipocytes may predispose an individual to increased adiposity in later life.

MULTILOCULAR ADIPOSE TISSUE

Multilocular adipose tissue is also called **brown adipose tissue** because of its characteristic color, which is due in part to the high content of cytochromes in the mitochondria of its cells. Unlike unilocular tissue, which is present throughout the body, brown adipose tissue has a more limited distribution. It is common in hibernating animals and is improperly called the hibernating gland.

In rats and several other mammals, this tissue is found mainly about the shoulder girdle. In the human embryo and the newborn, multilocular adipose tissue is encountered in several areas and remains restricted to these locations after birth (Fig 6–5). It probably does not persist into adulthood. The function of this tissue in humans appears to be restricted to the first months of postnatal life, when it produces heat and thus protects the newborn against cold.

Histologic Structure of Multilocular Tissue

Multilocular tissue cells are polygonal and smaller than cells of unilocular adipose tissue. Their cytoplasm contains a great number of lipid droplets of different sizes (Fig 6–6) and numerous spherical mitochondria with long cristae occupying their whole width. Granular or smooth endoplasmic reticulum is not abundant.

Brown adipose tissue resembles an endocrine gland, for its cells assume an almost epithelial arrangement of closely packed masses associated with blood capillaries. This tissue is subdivided by partitions of connective tissue into lobules that are better delineated than in unilocular adipose tissue lobules.

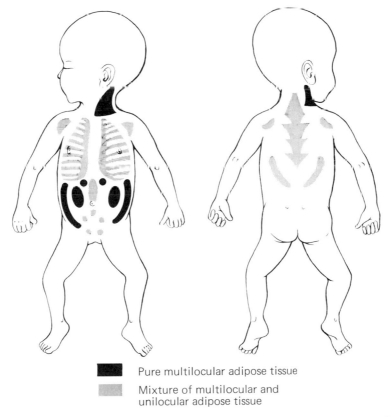

Pure multilocular adipose tissue

Mixture of multilocular and unilocular adipose tissue

Figure 6 –5. Distribution of multilocular adipose tissue in the human fetus. Black areas: multilocular adipose tissue. Shaded areas: mixture of multilocular and unilocular adipose tissue. (Modified, redrawn, and reproduced, with permission, from Merklin RJ: Growth and distribution of human fetal brown fat. Anat Rec 178:637, 1974.)

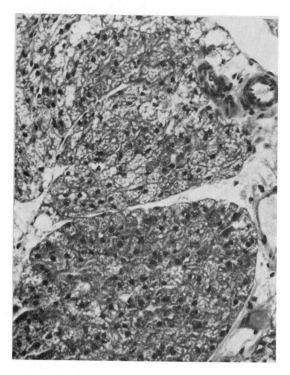

Figure 6–6. Photomicrograph of multilocular adipose tissue (brown fat). The cells exhibit a glandlike arrangement, and their cytoplasm contains numerous small lipid droplets. H&E stain, × 320.

Histophysiology of Multilocular Tissue

The physiology of multilocular tissue is understood best in the study of hibernating species.

In animals ending their hibernation period, nerve impulses liberate norepinephrine into the tissue. This substance activates the hormone-sensitive lipase present in adipose cells, promoting hydrolysis of triglycerides into fatty acids and glycerol. Oxygen consumption and liberation of heat are increased, elevating the temperature of the tissue and warming the blood passing through it. Warmed blood circulates throughout, heating the body and carrying fatty acids not metabolized in the adipose tissue, which will be utilized by other organs.

When a newborn human is submitted to a cold environment, the sympathetic nervous system liberates norepinephrine at the nerve endings to the cells of adipose tissue (brown fat) and promotes a rapid consumption of the stored lipids, with reduction in number and size of lipid droplets. At the same time, the process of oxidative phosphorylation is uncoupled; consequently, no ATP is synthesized, and all the energy derived from electron transport is dissipated as heat.

Mitochondria of multilocular adipose tissue can uncouple and recouple the process of oxidative phosphorylation. The mitochondria can therefore shift, according to the needs of the body, from the production of heat to the accumulation of ATP or vice versa.

Histogenesis of Multilocular Tissue

Multilocular tissue develops differently from unilocular tissue. The mesenchymal cells that constitute the brown tissue resemble epithelium, suggesting an endocrine gland, before they accumulate fat. Apparently there is no formation of brown adipose tissue after birth, nor is one type of adipose tissue transformed into another.

•   •   •

References

Christiansen EN, Pederson JI, Grav HJ: Uncoupling and recoupling of oxidative phosphorylation in brown adipose tissue mitochondria. Nature 222:857, 1969.

Cushman SW: Structure-function relationship in the adipose cell. 1. Ultrastructure of the isolated adipose cell. J Cell Biol 46:326, 1970.

Hales CN & others: Localization of calcium in the smooth endoplasmic reticulum of rat isolated fat cells. J Cell Sci 15:1, 1974.

Imaizumi M: On the fine structure of the surface of lipid droplets in adipose cells. Arch Histol Jpn 30:353, 1969.

Lindberg O & others: Studies of the mitochondrial energy transfer system of brown adipose tissue. J Cell Biol 34:293, 1967.

Merklin RJ: Growth and distribution of human fetal brown fat. Anat Rec 178:637, 1974.

Napolitano L: The differentiation of white adipose cells: An electron microscope study. J Cell Biol 18:663, 1963.

Renold AE, Cahill GF Jr (editors): *Handbook of Physiology*. Section 5: *Adipose Tissue*. American Physiological Society, 1965.

Sheldon H: The fine structure of the fat cell. In: *Fat as a Tissue*. Rodahl K, Issekutz B Jr (editors). McGraw-Hill, 1964.

Slavin BG: The cytophysiology of mammalian adipose cells. Int Rev Cytol 33:297, 1972.

Smith RE, Hock RJ: Brown fat: Thermogenic effector of arousal in hibernators. Science 140:199, 1963.

Stern JS, Greenwood MR: A review of development of adipose cellularity in man and animals. Fed Proc 33:1952, 1974.

Wassermann F, McDonald TF: Electron microscopic study of adipose tissue (fat organs), with special reference to the transport of lipids between blood and fat cells. Z Zellforsch Mikrosk Anat 59:326, 1963.

Williamson JR: Adipose tissue: Morphological changes associated with lipid mobilization. J Cell Biol 20:57, 1964.

Cartilage is a type of connective tissue in which the intercellular material has a rigid consistency, although the tissue is less resistant to pressure than bone. Its surface is usually resilient and smooth. The main functions of cartilage are to support soft tissues and, by virtue of its smooth surface, to provide a sliding area for joints, thus facilitating bone movements. Cartilage is essential for the growth of long bones both before and after birth. As with other differentiated types of connective tissue in general, cartilage contains much intercellular material, known as cartilage matrix, with cavities (lacunas) containing cartilage cells (chondrocytes).

The weight-bearing capacity of cartilage is exceeded only by that of bone, a tissue highly perfected for support and protection.

The physiologic properties of cartilage depend mainly on the physicochemical characteristics of its matrix, which contains either collagen or collagen plus elastin, associated with glycosaminoglycans. Chondrocytes synthesize and maintain the matrix.

Since collagen and elastin are pliable, the hard consistency of most cartilage tissue depends on the glycosaminoglycans, whose molecules appear to combine, by means of electrostatic bonds, with the collagen present in the matrix. Variations in the content and types of collagen and elastic fibers give special properties to cartilage.

In areas subjected to heavy weight-bearing or to strong pulling forces, the content of collagenous fibers is great, and the cartilage in such areas is almost inextensible. Areas of the body where the cartilage is flexible and the demands of weight-bearing and stress are less great contain a matrix with elastic fibers and fewer collagenous fibers, resulting in a more flexible and elastic type of cartilage.

Cartilage, which is devoid of blood vessels, is nourished by diffusion from capillaries in adjacent connective tissue or by means of synovial fluid from joint cavities. In some instances, blood vessels pass through cartilage to nourish other tissues. Cartilage

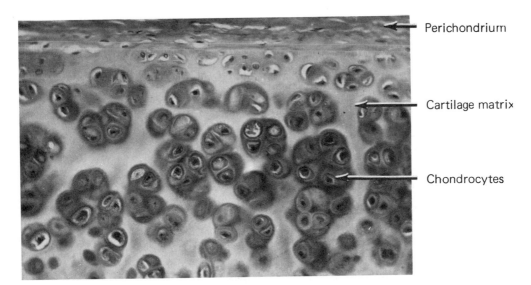

Figure 7–1. Photomicrograph of hyaline cartilage. Most chondrocytes are organized in isogenic groups. An enriched concentration of glycosaminoglycans in the matrix—the capsule—is present around the chondrocytes. The upper part of the figure shows the perichondrium where fibroblasts may differentiate into chondrocytes during cartilage growth. H&E stain, × 300.

has no lymphatic vessels or nerves and has a low metabolic rate.

The 3 types of cartilage are **hyaline** (the most common form), the matrix of which contains a moderate number of collagenous fibers; **elastic**, the matrix of which contains collagenous fibers plus a large number of elastic fibers; and **fibrous (fibrocartilage)**, which contains a dense matrix formed mostly by an interwoven network of coarse collagenous fibers.

The **perichondrium** (Fig 7–1), which forms an interface with the cartilage and its encapsulating connective tissue matrix, is a special capsulelike sheath of connective tissue covering cartilage in most places (see p 125).

HYALINE CARTILAGE

Hyaline cartilage (Fig 7–1) is the most common and best studied of the 3 types. Most experimental data on cartilage have been obtained from studies of hyaline cartilage, but the findings are most likely applicable to the other types as well.

Fresh hyaline cartilage is bluish-white and translucent. In the embryo, it serves as a temporary skeleton until it is replaced gradually by bone. Between the diaphysis and the epiphysis of growing long bones the epiphyseal disk, composed of hyaline cartilage, is responsible for the longitudinal growth of bone (Fig 7–2).

In adults, hyaline cartilage is present mainly in the walls of the respiratory passages (nose through bronchi), on the ventral ends of the ribs, and on bone surfaces within joints (articular cartilages).

Matrix

Forty percent of the dry weight of hyaline cartilage consists of collagen embedded in an amorphous intercellular substance. In routine histologic preparations, the collagen does not stand out from the amorphous substance for 2 reasons: (1) the collagen is mainly in the form of fibrils, the majority of which have submicroscopic dimensions; and (2) the fibers and fibrils have a refractive index very near to that of the amorphous intercellular substance which surrounds them.

Electron micrographs show that isolated collagen fibrils, finer than those in other forms of connective tissue, are the dominant component of the

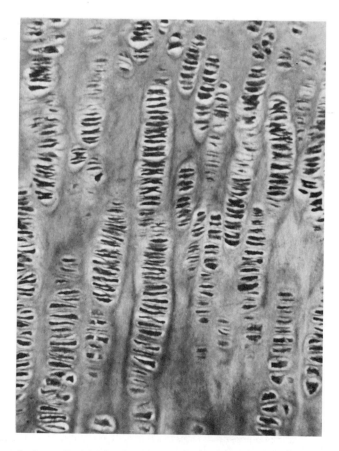

Figure 7–2. Photomicrograph of a portion of the epiphyseal disk cartilage. As illustrated, large numbers of chondrocytes in the proliferative zone of this cartilage are arranged side by side in parallel columns. H&E stain, × 320.

matrix. These fibrils have a 64-nm periodicity similar to that of typical connective tissue collagen (type I). There are also, however, a great number of very fine collagenous fibrils with nearly invisible periodicity and others, even finer, with no periodicity at all. Variations in the assembly and appearance of cartilage collagen reflect its chemical composition. Cartilage matrix primarily contains type II collagen consisting of 3 alpha-1 type II chains ($[\alpha 1(II)]_3$). This type of collagen differs from typical connective tissue collagen in that it possesses high levels of hydroxylysine, an amino acid that provides cross-linking between the tropocollagen subunits of the fibrils and also binds polysaccharides. This and other amino acid substitutions directly influence the assembly and periodicity of the cartilage-

specific collagen fibrils. Coarse collagenous bundles only appear in certain instances, eg, articular cartilage.

Glycosaminoglycans are the main components of the amorphous cartilage matrix. The glycosaminoglycans can be subdivided into 2 major groups: **hyaluronic acid,** an extremely long, unbranched polysaccharide; and a family of **proteoglycans** consisting of a protein core off of which radiate numerous short unbranched sulfated mucopolysaccharides (chondroitin 4-sulfate, chondroitin 6-sulfate, keratan sulfate). Structurally, proteoglycans resemble bottle brushes, the protein core being the backbone and the radiating mucopolysaccharide chains the bristles.

The relative proportions of collagen, hyal-

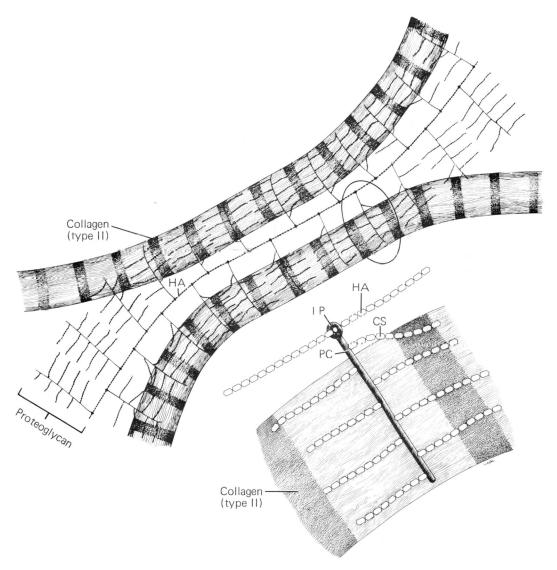

Figure 7 –3. Schematic representation of proposed molecular organization in cartilage matrix. Linking proteins (LP) covalently bind the protein core (PC) of proteoglycans to the linear hyaluronic acid (HA) molecules. The chondroitin sulfate (CS) side chains of the proteoglycan electrostatically bind to the collagen fibrils, forming a cross-linked rigid matrix.

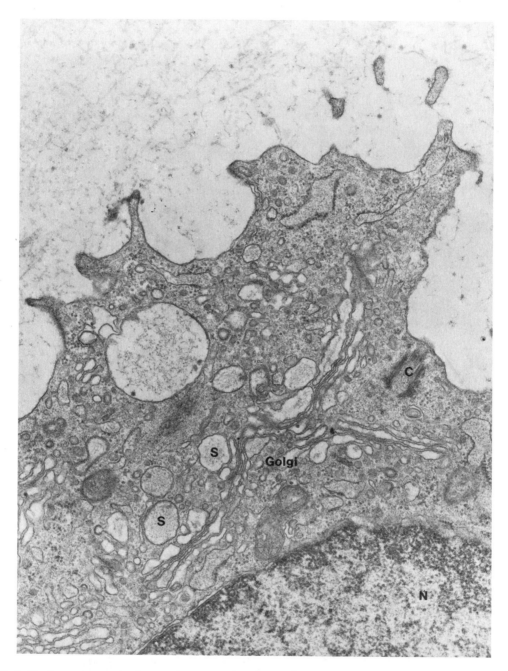

Figure 7–4. Electron micrograph of part of a young chondrocyte from tracheal hyaline cartilage. The surface of the chondrocyte is increased by projections and foldings which facilitate metabolic exchange. There are secretory vacuoles (S) next to the Golgi complex. Observe also a centriole (C) and part of the nucleus (N). Reduced from × 37,000. (Courtesy of M Weinstock.)

uronic acid, and the sulfated proteoglycans in the matrix vary with anatomic site and age. A correlation has been demonstrated between the rigidity of cartilage and the proportion of keratan sulfate to chondroitin sulfates. Structurally, the rigidity of the cartilage matrix is due to the cross-linking between the collagen and glycosaminoglycans. As illustrated in Fig 7–3, the matrix consists of interwoven networks of hyaluronic acid and collagen, firmly cross-linked by the proteoglycans.

Within the cartilage matrix, immediately surrounding each chondrocyte, is a zone of glycosaminoglycan-rich, collagen-poor matrix. This peripheral zone, called the **capsule,** histochemically exhibits an intense basophilia, metachromasia,

and greater PAS positivity than other portions of the matrix (Fig 7–1).

Perichondrium

Except in articular cartilage of joints, all hyaline cartilage is covered by a layer of dense connective tissue, the **perichondrium,** which is essential for the growth and maintenance of cartilage (Figs 7–1 and 7–5). It is rich in collagen (type I) fibers and contains cells that resemble fibroblasts. These extend from the periphery of the perichondrium but are more numerous closer to the cartilage. Morphologically, the cells of the inner layer of the perichondrium (presumptive chondrogenic cells) are similar to the fibroblasts and are consid-

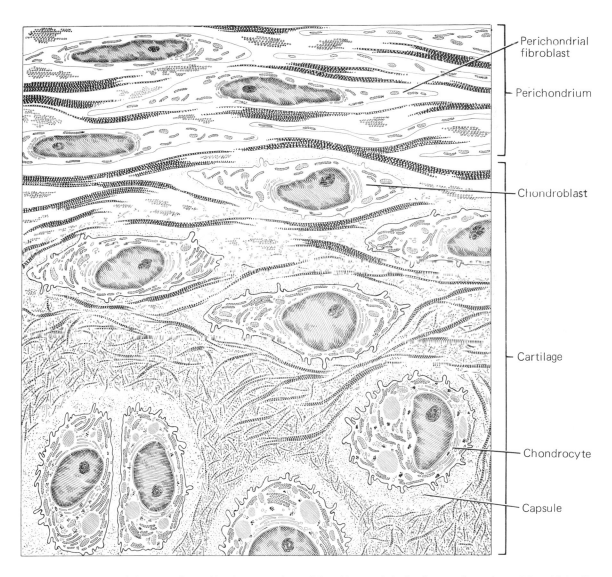

Figure 7–5. Diagram of the area of transition between the perichondrium and the hyaline cartilage. As perichondrial cells differentiate into chondrocytes, they become round, with an irregular surface. Cartilage matrix contains numerous fine collagen fibrils except around the periphery of the chondrocytes, where the matrix primarily consists of glycosaminoglycans; this region is called the capsule.

ered to be so by some authors. Others, however, postulate that they are undifferentiated mesenchymal cells which can be differentiated directly into chondroblasts.

Chondrocytes

At the periphery of hyaline cartilage, the chondrocytes have an elliptic shape, with the long axis parallel to the surface. Farther in, they are round and may appear in groups (Fig 7–1) of up to 8 cells originating from mitotic divisions of a single chondrocyte. These groups are designated isogenous groups. In epiphyseal plate cartilage the proliferating chondrocytes are accumulated in rows (Fig 7–2).

Cartilage cells and the matrix shrink during histologic preparation, causing the irregular shape of the chondrocytes and their retraction from the capsule. In living tissue, the chondrocytes or groups of chondrocytes fill the lacunas completely. Upon examination with the light microscope, their surface appears smooth, but the electron microscope reveals indentations and protrusions, larger and more frequent in young chondrocytes (Fig 7–4). The structural characteristic increases their surface area, permitting easier exchange with the extracellular medium; this has an important function in maintaining nutrition of these cells since they are located at a distance from the bloodstream.

Young chondrocytes are flat, whereas older ones are round and hypertrophied. Cytologically, the cells exhibit organelles typical of protein secretors—primarily an elaborate rough endoplasmic reticulum and well-developed Golgi complex. Characteristic large accumulations of glycogen and lipid vesicles in mature chondrocytes reflect their metabolic activity as influenced by their long distance from the nourishing bloodstream. Recent evidence shows that the chondrocyte is a cell which synthesizes large amounts of glycosaminoglycans and the unique type II collagen $(\alpha 1[\text{II}])_3$. The biosynthesis of proteoglycan appears to be initiated on the granular endoplasmic reticulum where the protein core is formed. Enzymes present in the endoplasmic reticulum but more especially in the Golgi complex add the xylose, galactose, sulfate, and other residues that make up the complete sulfated polysaccharides of the proteoglycan.

Histophysiology

Since cartilage is devoid of blood capillaries, chondrocytes respire under low oxygen tension. Hyaline cartilage cells metabolize glucose mainly by anaerobic glycolysis to produce lactic acid as the end product. Nutrients from the blood diffuse from the perichondrium to the more deeply placed chondrocytes. Because of this, the maximum width of the cartilage is limited. The nutrients diffuse through the solvation water of the matrix. There is almost no free water in cartilage matrix.

By means of radioautography, it has been demonstrated that chondrocytes synthesize all the matrix components of cartilage. In growing cartilage, studies using injection of ^{35}S in the form of sulfate, which is incorporated into the acid-sulfated glycosaminoglycans, revealed that radioactivity appeared first in the cytoplasm of the chondrocytes and afterward in the intercellular substance. Synthesis and sulfation of the glycosaminoglycans take place in the Golgi apparatus. Additionally, the core protein synthesized in the granular endoplasmic reticulum combines here with the repeated units of polysaccharides to form the proteoglycans. Radioautographic studies with the electron microscope after ^3H-proline administration demonstrated that radioactivity appeared first in the granular endoplasmic reticulum, then in the Golgi apparatus, and finally in the intercellular substance.

Chondrocyte function depends on a proper hormonal balance. The synthesis of sulfated glycosaminoglycans is accelerated by growth hormone, thyroxine, and testosterone. It is retarded by cortisone, hydrocortisone, and estradiol.

Histogenesis

Cartilage derives from the mesenchyme (Fig 7–6). The first modification observed is the rounding up of the mesenchymal cells, which retract their protoplasmic extensions, multiply rapidly, and form condensed agglomerations. The cells formed by this direct differentiation of the mesenchymal cells, now called **chondroblasts,** have a ribosome-rich basophilic cytoplasm. Synthesis and accumulation of the matrix then begins to separate the chondroblasts from each other. The differentiation of cartilage takes place from the center outward; therefore, the more central cells have characteristics of chondrocytes while the peripheral cells are typical chondroblasts. The superficial mesenchyme develops into fibroblasts of the perichondrium.

Growth

The growth of cartilage is attributable to 2 processes: **interstitial growth,** due to mitotic division of the preexisting chondrocytes; and **appositional growth,** due to the differentiation of peripheral perichondrial cells. In both cases newly formed chondrocytes synthesize collagen fibrils and amorphous glycosaminoglycans. Real growth is thus much greater than that due to the simple increase in the number of cells. Interstitial growth is the less important of the 2 processes and occurs only during the early phases of cartilage formation when it increases tissue mass by expanding the cartilage matrix from within. As the matrix becomes increasingly more rigid because of cross-linking of matrix components, interstitial growth becomes less pronounced. Cartilage then grows only by apposition. Cells of the perichondrium adjacent to the cartilage multiply and differentiate into chondroblasts, which are then incorporated as chondrocytes into the existing cartilage. During growth, peripheral

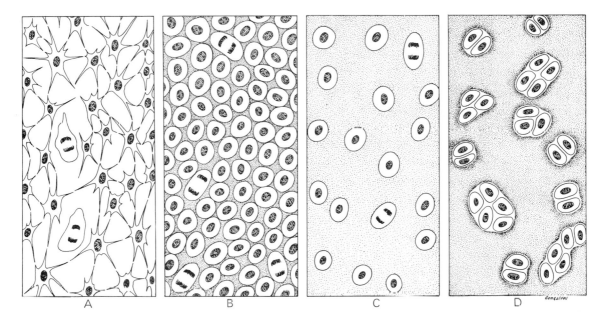

Figure 7 –6. Histogenesis of hyaline cartilage. *A:* The mesenchyme, which is the precursor tissue of all types of cartilage. *B:* Mitotic proliferation of the mesenchymal cell gives rise to a very cellular tissue. *C:* Rounded cells are separated from each other by the formation of a great amount of matrix. *D:* Multiplication of cartilage cells gives rise to isogenic groups which are surrounded by a condensation of the matrix (capsule).

areas of cartilage show chondroblast transitions between chondrocytes and cells resembling the fibroblasts of the perichondrium (Figs 7–1 and 7–5).

Regressive Changes

In contrast to other tissues, hyaline cartilage is frequently subjected to degenerative processes. The most common is calcification of the matrix, and this is preceded by an increase in the size and volume of the cells followed by their death. Although calcification is a regressive alteration, it occurs normally in certain cartilages, providing a model for bone development. (See Endochondral Ossification, Chapter 8.)

Regeneration

Except in young children, damaged cartilage regenerates with difficulty and often incompletely. In adults, regeneration occurs because of the activity of the perichondrium. When cartilage fractures, cells from the perichondrium invade the fractured area and generate new cartilage. In extensively damaged areas (or occasionally in small areas), the perichondrium, instead of forming new cartilage, generates a scar of dense connective tissue.

ELASTIC CARTILAGE

Elastic cartilage is found in the auricle of the ear, in the walls of the external auditory canals, in

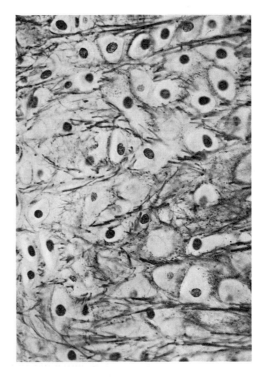

Figure 7 –7. Photomicrograph of elastic cartilage. Weigert staining method for elastic fibers. × 350.

the auditory (eustachian) tubes and epiglottis, and in some of the cartilage in the larynx.

Basically, elastic cartilage is identical to hyaline cartilage except that in addition to collagen fibers, it contains an abundant network of fine elastic fibers. Fresh elastic cartilage has a yellowish color caused by the presence of elastin in the elastic fibers, which may be demonstrated chemically by standard elastin stains (eg, orcein) (Fig 7–7).

Elastic cartilage may be present by itself or in combination with hyaline cartilage. Because the chondrocytes of elastic and hyaline cartilage tissues are very similar, elastic cartilage is frequently found to be gradually continuous with hyaline cartilage. As with hyaline cartilage, elastic cartilage possesses a perichondrium and grows mainly by apposition. It is less susceptible to degenerative processes than hyaline cartilage.

FIBROCARTILAGE

Fibrocartilage is a tissue with characteristics intermediate between those of dense connective tissue and hyaline cartilage. It is found in intervertebral disks, in attachments of certain ligaments to bones, and in the symphysis pubica. Fibrocartilage is always associated with dense connective tissue, and the border areas between these 2 tissues are not clear-cut but show a gradual transition.

Fibrocartilage contains chondrocytes similar to those of hyaline cartilage, either singly or in small isogenous groups. Very often, the chondrocytes are arranged in long columns. Fibrocartilage matrix is

acidophilic because it contains a great number of coarse type I collagen fibers, which are easily seen under the light microscope (Fig 7–8). The matrix is identical to hyaline cartilage except that much of the intercellular hyaline material is displaced by coarse collagen fibers. The woven collagen fibers, which are embedded in the hyaline matrix, so reinforce the cartilage that it can withstand great force yet remain resilient to deformation.

In fibrocartilage, the numerous collagenous fibers either form irregular bundles between the groups of chondrocytes or align in a parallel arrangement along the columns of chondrocytes. This orientation depends upon the stresses acting on fibrocartilage since the collagenous bundles take up a direction parallel to those stresses. There is no perichondrium in fibrocartilage.

Fibrocartilage develops from dense connective tissue by means of differentiation of fibroblasts into chondrocytes.

INTERVERTEBRAL DISKS

Each intervertebral disk is situated between 2 vertebrae and held to them by means of ligaments. The disks have 2 components: the cartilagenous annulus fibrosus and the liquid nucleus pulposus.

The **annulus fibrosus** has an external layer of dense connective tissue, but it is mainly composed of overlapping laminas of fibrocartilage in which collagenous bundles are orthogonally arranged in adjacent laminas. The multiple laminas, with the 90-degree registration of collagen fibers in adjacent

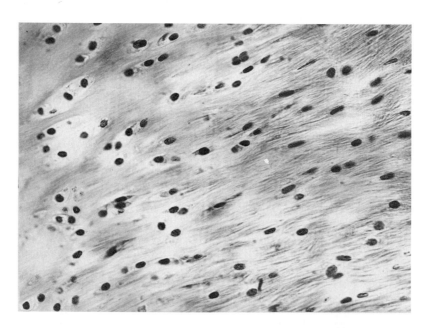

Figure 7 –8. Photomicrograph of fibrocartilage from a human intervertebral disk. H&E stain, × 350.

layers, provide the disk with an unusually strong resilience that enables it to withstand the pressures generated by impinging vertebrae. In tangential section, the disk presents a characteristic herringbone pattern as a result of orthogonal alignment of collagen in alternating lamellas.

The **nucleus pulposus** is situated in the center of the annulus fibrosus. It is derived from the notochord and consists of a few rounded cells embedded in an amorphous syrupy fluid rich in hyaluronic acid. In children, the nucleus pulposus is large, but with age it gradually becomes smaller and is partially replaced by fibrocartilage.

Herniation of the Intervertebral Disk

The intervertebral disk acts as a lubricated cushion that prevents adjacent vertebrae from being eroded by abrasive forces during movement of the spinal column. The liquid nucleus pulposus serves as a shock absorber to cushion the impact between adjacent vertebrae. Rupture of the annulus fibrosus, which most frequently occurs in the posterior region where there are fewer collagenous bundles, results in expulsion of the liquid nucleus pulposus and a concomitant flattening of the disk. As a consequence, the disk frequently dislocates or "slips" from its position between the vertebrae. If it moves toward the spinal cord, it can compress the nerves and result in severe pain and neurologic disturbances. The pain accompanying a slipped disk may be perceived in areas innervated by the compressed nerve fibers—usually the lower lumbar region.

●   ●   ●

References

Anderson DR: The ultrastructure of elastic and hyaline cartilage in the rat. Am J Anat 114:403, 1964.

Campo RD, Dziewiatkowski DD: Turnover of the organic matrix of cartilage and bone as visualized by autoradiography. J Cell Biol 18:19, 1963.

Cooper GW, Prockop DJ: Intracellular accumulation of protocollagen and extrusion of collagen by embryonic cartilage cells. J Cell Biol 38:523, 1968.

Fewer D, Threadgold J, Sheldon H: Studies on cartilage. 5. Electron microscopic observations on the autoradiographic localization of S[35] in cells and matrix. J Ultrastruct Res 11:166, 1964.

Godman GC, Lane N: On the site of sulfation in the chondrocyte. J Cell Biol 21:353, 1964.

Godman GC, Porter KR: Chondrogenesis, studied with the electron microscope. J Biophys Biochem Cytol 8:719, 1960.

Happey F & others: Variations in the diameter of collagen fibrils, bound hexose and associated glycoproteins in the intervertebral disc. In: *Connective Tissues*. Fricke R, Hartmann F (editors). Springer, 1974.

Levitt D, Ho PL, Dorfman A: Differentiation of cartilage. In: *The Cell Surface in Development*. Moscona AA (editor). Wiley, 1974.

Palmoski MJ, Goetinek PF: Synthesis of proteochondroitin sulfate by normal, nanomelic, and 5-bromodeoxyuridine–treated chondrocytes in cell culture. Proc Natl Acad Sci USA 67:3385, 1972.

Revel JP: Role of the Golgi apparatus of cartilage cells in the elaboration of matrix glycosaminoglycans. Page 1485 in: *Chemistry and Molecular Biology of the Intercellular Matrix*. Vol 3. Balazs EA (editor). Academic Press, 1970.

Revel JP, Hay ED: An autoradiographic and electron microscopic study of collagen synthesis in differentiating cartilage. Z Zellforsch Mikrosk Anat 61:110, 1963.

Rosenberg L, Hellmann W, Kleinshmidt AK: Macromolecular models of protein-polysaccharides from bovine nasal cartilage based on electron microscopic studies. J Biol Chem 245:4123, 1970.

Roy S, Meachim G: Chondrocyte ultrastructure in adult human articular cartilage. Ann Rheum Dis 27:544, 1968.

Salpeter MM: ^{3}H-proline incorporation into cartilage: Electron microscope autoradiographic observations. J Morphol 124:387, 1968.

Searls RL: Newer knowledge of chondrogenesis. Clin Orthop 96:327, 1973.

Sheldon H, Kimball FB: Studies on cartilage. 3. The occurrence of collagen within vacuoles of the Golgi apparatus. J Cell Biol 12:599, 1962.

Smith PH: Autoradiographic evidence for the concurrent synthesis of collagen and chondroitin sulfates by chick sternal chondrocytes. Connect Tissue Res 1:181, 1972.

Trelstad RL & others: Isolation of two distinct collagens from chick cartilage. Biochemistry 9:4993, 1970.

Tsiganos CP, Muir H: The natural heterogeneity of proteoglycans of porcine and human cartilage. Page 859 in: *Chemistry and Molecular Biology of the Intercellular Matrix*. Vol 2. Balazs EA (editor). Academic Press, 1970.

8 | Bone

During the process of evolution, a basic structural protein developed that was modified to varying degrees of rigidity, elasticity, and strength depending upon environmental influences and the functional requirements of the animal organism. This protein is **collagen,** and the chief examples among its various modifications are skin, basement membrane, cartilage, and bone.

Bone is one of the hardest tissues of the human body and second only to cartilage in its ability to withstand stress. As the main constituent of the skeleton, it supports fleshy structures, protects vital organs such as those contained in the cranial and thoracic cavities, and contains the bone marrow, where blood cells are formed.

Besides these functions, bones form a system

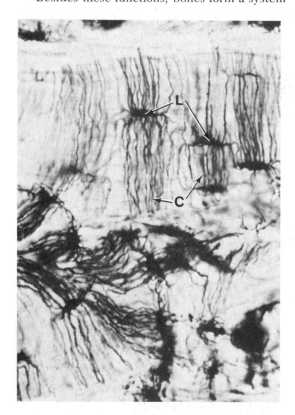

Figure 8–1. Photomicrograph of ground section of bone. Lacunas (L) and canaliculi (C) appear black. × 490.

of levers that multiply the forces generated during skeletal muscle contraction, transforming them into bodily movements.

Bone is composed of intercellular calcified material, the **bone matrix,** and different cell types: **osteocytes,** which are found in cavities (lacunas) within the matrix; **osteoblasts,** which synthesize the organic components of the matrix; and **osteoclasts,** which are multinucleated giant cells involved in the resorption and remodeling of bone tissue.

Since diffusion does not take place through the calcified matrix of bone, the exchanges between osteocytes and blood capillaries depend on cellular communication through the canaliculi, which perforate the matrix. These canaliculi permit the osteocytes to communicate via filopodial processes with their neighbors, with the internal and external surfaces of the bone, and with the blood vessels within the matrix.

Because of its hardness, bone is difficult to section with the microtome; therefore, special technics must be used for its study. One of these consists of grinding slices of bone with abrasives until they are thin enough to be transparent. The preparation thus obtained is referred to as a ground section. This technic does not preserve the cells but does permit detailed study of the matrix, its lacunas, and its canaliculi. Owing to differences in refractive index between lacunas and canaliculi (which are both filled with air in these preparations) and the medium used in mounting, light rays striking the lacunas and canaliculi are deflected and do not penetrate the objective lens of the microscope. Lacunas and canaliculi consequently appear black in ground sections (Fig 8–1).

Another technic that is frequently used because it permits the observation of the cells and organic matrix is based on the decalcification of bone preserved in a standard fixative. The mineral is removed by immersion in a dilute acid solution (eg, 5% nitric acid) or in a solution containing a calcium-chelating substance (eg, ethylenediamine-tetraacetic acid, EDTA). The decalcified tissue is then embedded, sectioned, and stained by routine technics.

All bones are lined on both internal and external surfaces by layers of connective tissue called **endosteum** and **periosteum,** respectively.

BONE CELLS

Osteoblasts

Osteoblasts are responsible for the synthesis of the organic components of bone matrix (collagen and glycoproteins). They are exclusively located at the surfaces of bone tissue, side by side, in a way resembling simple epithelium (Fig 8–2). When they are intensely engaged in matrix synthesis, osteoblasts have a cuboid shape and a basophilic cytoplasm. When their synthesizing activity declines, they flatten, and cytoplasmic basophilia decreases.

Osteoblasts also present cytoplasmic processes which bring them into contact with neighboring osteoblasts. These expansions are more evident when the cell begins to be surrounded by matrix. Once within the newly synthesized matrix, the osteoblast is known as an osteocyte. Lacunas and canaliculi appear because the matrix is formed around a cell and its cytoplasmic processes.

During matrix synthesis, osteoblasts have the ultrastructure of cells synthesizing proteins for export, with well-developed granular endoplasmic reticulum and Golgi apparatus. They are polarized cells; extrusion of the synthesized molecules takes place at the cell surface in contact with bone matrix. The large, round nucleus has a finely dispersed chromatin and is found at the side of the cell away

from the matrix.

The newly synthesized, not yet calcified matrix adjacent to osteoblasts is termed **osteoid** or **prebone.** In active osteoblasts, PAS-positive cytoplasmic granules have been found that are probably precursors of the neutral mucopolysaccharides of the matrix.

The role of osteoblasts in secreting bone collagen has been studied by radioautography in animals injected with ^{3}H-glycine (an amino acid constituting one-third of the residues in collagen). Thirty minutes after ^{3}H-glycine administration, the label was found mainly in osteoblasts; 4 hours later, it was located in osteoid (Fig 8–4A); and after 35 hours, a radioactive band was observed in the calcified matrix. The extracellular label appeared as a radioactive band that was displaced from the proximity of the osteoblasts by the nonradioactive matrix formed after utilization of the injected, labeled glycine. On the seventh (Fig 8–4B) and especially on the 45th day (Fig 8–4C) after the labeling injection, radioactivity was found deep in the matrix. Thus, the unlabeled matrix between the radioactive matrix and the osteoblast layer indicates the amount of bone formed in the interval between the injection of ^{3}H-glycine and the termination of the experiment.

Osteocytes

Osteocytes are mature cells found encapsulated in laminas of the mineralized bone matrix.

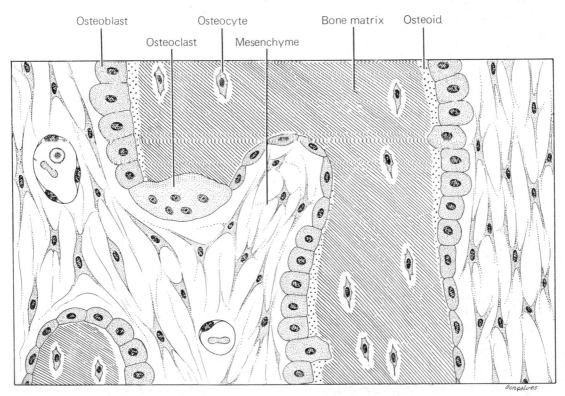

Figure 8–2. Advanced stage of intramembranous ossification. The lower part of the drawing shows an osteoblast being entrapped in the newly formed bone matrix.

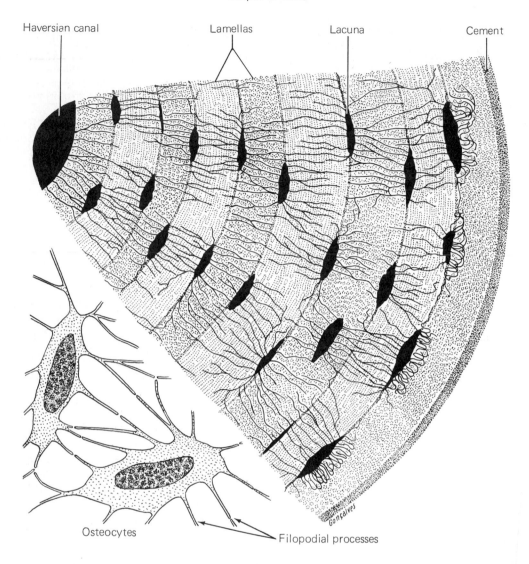

Haversian canal   Lamellas   Lacuna   Cement

Osteocytes   Filopodial processes

Figure 8 –3. Schematic drawings of 2 osteocytes and part of a Haversian system. Collagen fibers of contiguous lamellas are sectioned at different angles. Observe the numerous canaliculi which form intercommunications of the lacunas with each other and with the Haversian canals. Although it is not apparent in this simplified diagram, each indicated lamella actually consists of multiple lamellas in which parallel arrays of collagen fibers are oriented in different directions in adjacent lamellas. The presence of large numbers of lamellas with different fiber orientations provides the bone with great strength despite its light weight. (Redrawn and reproduced, with permission, from Leeson TS, Leeson CR: *Histology,* 2nd ed. Saunders, 1970.)

Within the canaliculi that radiate from the lacunas, osteocyte filopodial processes from adjacent cells are connected via gap junctions. This coupling provides for the intercellular flow of ions and small molecules (eg, hormones controlling bone growth and development). Filopodial contact between encapsulated osteocytes provides a mechanism wherein nutrients and metabolites can be passed between blood vessels and distant osteocytes. This "bucket brigade" phenomenon can provide support for a chain of about 15 cells.

When compared to osteoblasts, the flat, almond-shaped osteocytes exhibit a significantly reduced rough endoplasmic reticulum and Golgi body and more condensed nuclear chromatin. Although these are signs of reduced synthetic activity, these cells are actively involved with the maintenance of the bony matrix. Death of the osteocytes is followed by resorption of this matrix. Histochemical studies show that osteocytes and osteoblasts contain protein- or glycoprotein-bound calcium phosphate. Consequently, bone cells are able to concentrate calcium phosphate within their cytoplasm.

Osteoclasts

Osteoclasts are very large, extensively branched motile cells. Dilated portions of the cell body exhibit from 6 to 50 or more nuclei. The

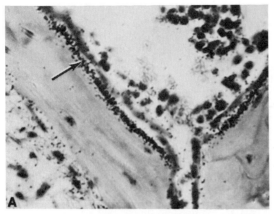

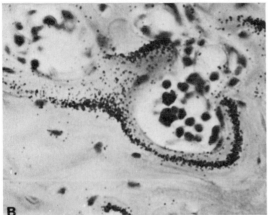

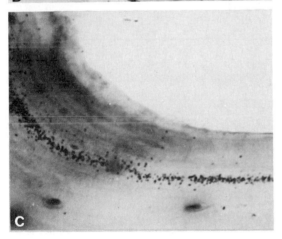

Figure 8–4. Radioautographs of bone tissue from mice injected with ³H-glycine and sacrificed at different intervals after the injection. *A:* From a mouse killed 4 hours after injection. At this time, osteoid is strongly radioactive (arrow). It contains labeled collagen synthesized by the osteoblasts using ³H-glycine. There is some radioactivity remaining in the osteoblasts. Bone marrow cells (upper right) are also radioactive. *B:* From a mouse killed 7 days after injection. The radioactive band is deeper into the calcified matrix because of the subsequent accumulation of the nonradioactive collagen formed after utilization of all labeled glycine. *C:* From a mouse killed 45 days after injection. The radioactive band is more deeply situated in comparison with the sections from previous intervals. H&E stain.

branches of the cell are quite irregular and vary in both thickness and shape. Osteoclasts are generally elevated above the surface of the matrix and sometimes overlap osteoblasts and other osteoclasts. Since sections only reveal a limited aspect of the osteoclast, the true morphology of the cell has only recently been described through the use of the scanning electron microscope. In areas of bone undergoing resorption, portions of the giant osteoclasts are found to lie within enzymatically etched depressions in the matrix known as **Howship's lacunae.** Frequently, some portions of the osteoclast will be actively resorbing bone while other branches of the same cell will appear quiescent.

Until recently, it was thought that osteoclasts were derived from osteoprogenitor cells and that they could revert back to those stem cells by having individual nuclei bud off of the multinucleated osteoclasts and form mononucleated osteoblasts. However, this hypothesis has been in question since recent evidence has revealed that osteoclasts are derived from the fusion of blood-derived mononucleated monocytes. Cytologically, osteoclasts usually present an acidophilic cytoplasm; the cells possess numerous lysosomes and consequently give a positive histochemical reaction for acid phosphatase.

Electron micrographs show that the active osteoclast surface facing bone matrix is folded into irregular, often subdivided projections, forming a ruffled border. Besides establishing a device whereby small particles may be easily trapped and subjected to enzymatic activity, this arrangement considerably increases the active resorptive area. Numerous free polysomes, some rough endoplasmic reticulum, abundant mitochondria, and a well-developed Golgi complex complement the great number of lysosomes that are present within the cell.

Crystals containing calcium have been observed in the spaces between the folds as well as in cytoplasmic vacuoles probably derived from the surface membrane of the osteoclasts. Disintegrating collagenous fibers have also been reported in the extracellular space close to the folds of the osteoclast, but they never occur within the cytoplasm.

The precise role of osteoclasts in bone resorption is not yet clear. They secrete collagenase and other proteolytic enzymes that attack the bone matrix and liberate the calcified ground substance. The cells are actively engaged in elimination of debris formed during bone resorption.

BONE MATRIX

Inorganic matter represents about 50% of the dry weight of bone matrix. Calcium and phosphorus are especially abundant, but bicarbonate, citrate, magnesium, potassium, and sodium are also found. X-ray diffraction studies have shown that calcium and phosphorus form hydroxyapatite crystals with the composition $Ca_{10}(PO_4)_6(OH)_2$. In electron micrographs, hydroxyapatite crystals of bone appear as needles or elongated crystals measuring $40 \times 25 \times 3$ nm. They lie alongside the collagenous fibrils but are surrounded by an amorphous ground substance. The surface ions of hydroxyapatite are hydrated, and a layer of water and ions forms around the crystal. This layer, the **hydration shell,** facilitates the exchange of ions between the crystal and the body fluids.

The organic matter is composed of collagen fibers (95%) and the amorphous ground substance, which contains glycosaminoglycans associated with proteins. One of these proteins, osteomucoid, differs from collagen in the absence of hydroxyproline, the small content of proline and glycine, and the abundance of tyrosine and leucine. Among the glycosaminoglycans of bone are chondroitin 4-sulfate, chondroitin 6-sulfate, and keratan sulfate.

Because of its high collagen content, decalcified bone matrix binds selective stains for collagen fibers. It is also stained by the PAS technic, in which case the color intensity is proportionate to the quantity of galactose, fucose, and other carbohydrates present in glycoproteins.

The association of hydroxyapatite with collagen fibers is responsible for the hardness and resistance that are characteristic of bone. After a bone is decalcified, its shape is preserved, but it becomes as flexible as a tendon. Removal of the organic part of the matrix—which is mainly collagenous in nature—also leaves the bone with its original shape; however, it becomes fragile and breaks easily when handled.

PERIOSTEUM & ENDOSTEUM

Internal and external surfaces of bone are covered by layers of connective tissue named **endosteum** and **periosteum.** Bone surfaces not covered by connective tissue or by osteoblasts are subjected to resorption through the activity of osteoclasts which immediately appear in the area. For this reason, special attention is given to the periosteum and the endosteum in bone surgery.

The **periosteum** is a layer of dense connective tissue that is very fibrous externally but more cellular and vascular near the surface of the bone matrix (Fig 8–5).

Periosteal collagen fibers that penetrate the bone matrix, binding the periosteum to the bone, are called **Sharpey's fibers.**

Periosteal cells with the morphology of fibroblasts are able to proliferate through mitosis and can differentiate into osteoblasts. These cells play a prominent role in bone growth and repair.

The **endosteum** has the same components as the periosteum, and nearly the same structure, but it is considerably thinner and does not exhibit 2 distinct layers, as the periosteum does.

Within the connective tissue of the periosteum and endosteum, blood vessels are found that penetrate within the bone itself through canals called Volkmann's canals. The principal functions of the periosteum and endosteum are nutrition of osseous tissue and provision of a continuous supply of new osteoblast cells for repair or growth of bone.

TYPES OF BONE TISSUE

Gross observation of bone in cross section shows dense areas without cavities—corresponding to **compact bone**—and areas with numerous interconnecting cavities—corresponding to **spongy bone.** Under the microscope, however, both compact bone and the trabecular walls separating the cavities of spongy bone have the same basic histologic structure.

In long bones, the bulbous ends—called **epiphyses**—are composed of spongy bone covered by a thin layer of compact bone. The cylindric part—**diaphysis**—is almost totally composed of compact bone, with a small component of spongy bone in its inner position around the bone marrow cavity (Fig 8–9).

Short bones usually have a core of spongy bone completely surrounded by compact bone.

The flat bones that form the calvaria have 2 layers of compact bone called **plates,** separated by a layer of spongy bone called the **diploë.**

The cavities of spongy bone and the marrow cavity in the diaphyses of long bones contain **bone marrow,** of which there are 2 kinds: **red bone marrow,** in which blood cells are forming; and **yellow bone marrow,** composed mainly of fat cells.

Histologically, there are 2 varieties of bone tissue: **immature, primary,** or **woven bone;** and **mature, secondary,** or **lamellar bone.** Both varieties contain the same structural components, but in immature bone collagen bundles are randomly placed while in mature bone these bundles are organized into **bone lamellas.**

Primary Bone Tissue

In the formation of each bone, as well as in the repair process, the first bone tissue to appear is immature. It is temporary and is replaced in adults by secondary bone tissue except in a very few places in the body, eg, near the sutures of the flat bones of the skull, in tooth sockets, and in the insertions of some tendons.

Besides the irregular array of collagen fibers, other characteristics of primary bone tissue are a smaller content of minerals (it is more easily pene-

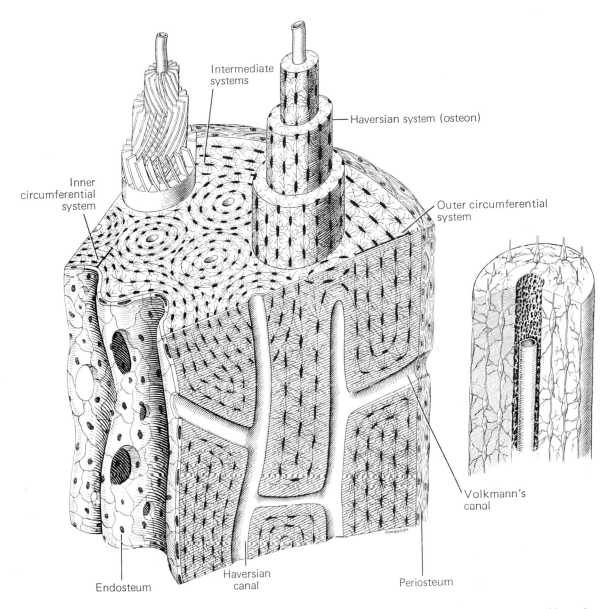

Figure 8–5. Schematic drawing of the wall of a long bone diaphysis. Observe the 4 lamellar arrangements: Haversian system, external and internal circumferential systems, and intermediate system. The Haversian system shows the orientation of collagen fibers in each lamella. At right is a Haversian system showing lamellas, a central blood capillary, and many osteocytes with their processes.

trated by x-rays) and a higher percentage of osteocytes than in the secondary bone tissue.

Secondary Bone Tissue

Secondary bone is the variety usually found in adults. Characteristically, it shows collagen fibers arranged in lamellas of 3–7 μm, that are parallel to each other or concentrically organized around a vascular canal. The whole complex of concentric lamellas surrounding a canal containing blood ves-

sels, nerves, and loose connective tissue is called the **Haversian system** or **osteon** (Fig 8–3). Lacunas with osteocytes are found between and occasionally within the lamellas. In each lamella, collagen fibers are parallel to each other. Surrounding adjacent lamellas or Haversian systems, there is often a deposit of amorphous material called the **cementing substance.**

In the diaphysis, the lamellas exhibit a typical organization consisting of Haversian systems, an

Intermediate or interstitial
lamellas

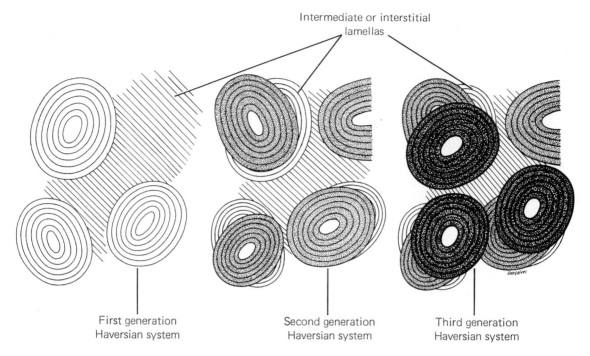

First generation
Haversian system

Second generation
Haversian system

Third generation
Haversian system

Figure 8–6. Schematic view of diaphyseal bone remodeling. Three generations of Haversian systems are shown. At right, the contribution of first and second generation Haversian systems to the formation of intermediate or interstitial systems can be seen.

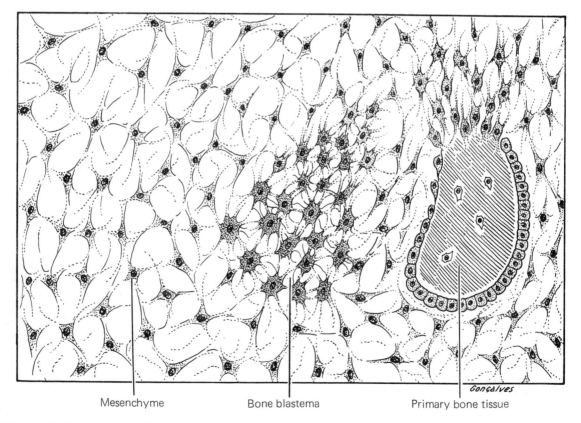

Mesenchyme   Bone blastema   Primary bone tissue

Figure 8–7. The beginning of intramembranous ossification. In the mesenchyme, a blastema from which bone cells are formed.

outer circumferential system, an inner circumferential system, and an intermediate system. The 4 systems are easily identified in cross section (Fig 8–5). Secondary bone tissue that contains Haversian systems is sometimes called **Haversian bone tissue.** It is usually found only in diaphyses, though small Haversian systems may be found in other places.

Each Haversian system is a long, often bifurcated cylinder parallel to the diaphyses. It consists of a central canal (of Havers) surrounded by 4–20 concentric lamellas. Each endosteum-lined canal contains blood vessels, nerves, and loose connective tissue. The Haversian canals communicate with the marrow cavity, with the periosteum, and with each other through transverse or oblique canals called Volkmann's canals (Fig 8–5). Volkmann's canals do not have concentric lamellas. Instead, they seem to perforate the lamellas (Fig 8–5). All vascular canals found in bone tissue come into existence when matrix is laid down around preexisting blood vessels.

Examination of Haversian systems with polarized light shows bright anisotropic layers alternating with dark isotropic layers. When observed under polarized light at right angles to their length, collagen fibers are birefringent (anisotropic). The alternating aspect is due to the distribution of collagen fibers in the lamellas. In each lamella, fibers are parallel to each other and follow a helical course. The pitch of the helix is, however, different for different lamellas, so that at any given point fibers from adjacent lamellas intersect at approximately right angles (Fig 8–5). Cross sections of a Haversian system show transverse sections of collagen fibers from one lamella and oblique, almost longitudinal sections of collagen fibers from the adjacent lamella. The structure of Haversian systems as shown in the light microscope is compatible with this interpretation. In one lamella, the collagen fibers are sectioned transversely and appear granular; in the next, the fibers are sectioned obliquely and have an elongated appearance (Fig 8–3).

There is great variability in the diameter of Haversian canals. Each system is formed by successive deposition of lamellas, starting from the periphery, so that younger systems have larger canals.

During growth—and even in adult bone—there is continuous destruction and rebuilding of Haversian systems, so that one often sees systems with only a few lamellas and a large central canal.

Internal and external circumferential systems are, as their names indicate, located around the marrow cavity and immediately beneath the periosteum. Their lamellas have a circular distribution, with the medullary canal as the center. The external circumferential system has more lamellas than the internal system (Fig 8–5).

Between 2 circumferential systems there are numerous Haversian systems, and among them are triangular or irregularly shaped groups of parallel lamellas called intermediate or interstitial systems. These systems are composed mainly of lamellas left by Haversian systems destroyed during growth and remodeling of bone (Fig 8–6).

HISTOGENESIS

Bone tissue arises either by intramembranous ossification, which occurs within a layer (membrane) of connective tissue, or by endochondral ossification, which takes place within a cartilaginous model. The model is gradually destroyed and replaced by bone formed by incoming cells from adjacent periosteal connective tissues.

In both processes, the bone tissue that appears first is primary or immature. It is a temporary tissue and is soon replaced by the definitive, lamellar variety of bone. During bone growth, areas of primary bone, areas of resorption, and areas of lamellar bone appear side by side. This combination of bone synthesis and removal occurs not only in growing bones but also throughout adult life, though its rate of change then is considerably slower.

Intramembranous Ossification

Intramembranous ossification, the source of most of the flat bones, is so called because it takes place within membranes of connective tissue. The frontal and parietal bones of the skull—as well as parts of the occipital and temporal bones and the mandible and maxilla—are formed by intramembranous ossification. Intramembranous ossification also contributes to the growth of short bones and the thickening of long bones.

In the connective tissue layer, the starting point for ossification is called the **primary ossification center.** The process begins when groups of cells resembling young fibroblasts differentiate into osteoblasts. Osteoid synthesis and calcification follow, resulting in the encapsulation of some osteoblasts which then become osteocytes (Fig 8–7). These islands of developing bone are known as **spicules.** Several such groups arise almost simultaneously at the ossification center, so that the fusion of the spicules gives the bone a spongy structure (Fig 8–8). The connective tissue that remains among the bone spicules is penetrated by growing blood vessels and undifferentiated mesenchymal cells, which give rise to the bone marrow cells.

Cells of the connective tissue membrane divide, giving rise to more osteoblasts, which are responsible for the continued growth of the ossification center. The several ossification centers of a bone grow radially and finally fuse together, replacing the original connective tissue. In newborn infants, the fontanelles are soft areas in the skull that

Bone
spicule   Osteo-   Osteo-
         blast   clast

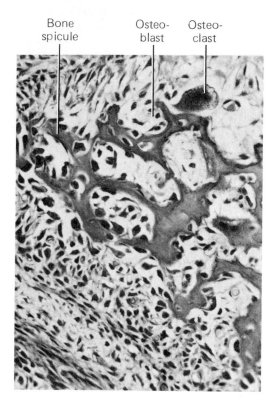

Figure 8–8. Photomicrograph of intramembranous ossification from the head of a young rat. Bone tissue shows osteocytes in lacunas. Around the newly formed bone tissue there are numerous osteoblasts and an osteoclast. Mallory azan stain, × 350.

correspond to parts of the connective tissue not yet ossified.

In cranial flat bones, especially after birth, there is a marked predominance of bone formation over bone resorption at both the internal and the external surfaces. Thus, 2 layers of compact bone (internal and external plates) arise, whereas the central portion (diploë) maintains its spongy nature.

That portion of the connective tissue layer which does not undergo ossification gives rise to the endosteum and the periosteum of the intramembranous bone.

Endochondral Ossification

Endochondral ossification takes place within a piece of hyaline cartilage whose shape resembles a small version of the model of the bone to be formed. This type of ossification is principally responsible for the formation of short and long bones (Fig 8–9).

Basically, endochondral ossification consists of 2 processes. The first process is hypertrophy and destruction of the chondrocytes of the model of the bone, leaving expanded lacunas separated by the septa of a calcified cartilage matrix. In the second process, an **osteogenic bud** consisting of osteogenic

precursors and blood capillaries penetrates into the spaces left by the degenerating chondrocytes. The undifferentiated cells give rise to osteoblasts, which form an osseous matrix on the remnants of the calcified cartilage matrix. In this way, bone tissue appears at the site where there was cartilage, and there is no transformation of the cartilage into bone tissue. The septa of calcified cartilage tissue serve as supports for the beginning of ossification (Fig 8–9).

Long bones are formed from cartilaginous models with dilated extremities (epiphyses) at each end of a cylindric shaft (diaphysis). The first bone tissue to be formed appears by means of intramembranous ossification within the perichondrium surrounding the diaphysis (Fig 8–9). Thus, a hollow bone cylinder, the **bone collar,** is produced in the deep portions of the perichondrium surrounding the cartilage. The perichondrium is then called periosteum because it covers the newly developed bone. Within the forming bone collar, the chondrocytes of the cartilage model begin to degenerate, since the new osseous collar prevents the diffusion of nutrients into the cartilage matrix. As the chondrocytes begin to degenerate, they resorb their surrounding matrix, causing an enlargement of the lacunas—a process known as **hypertrophication.** As the chondrocytes lose their ability to maintain the matrix, calcium deposits form and the cartilage becomes **calcified.**

Blood vessels of the osteogenic bud, coming from the periosteum through holes made by osteoclasts in the bone collar, penetrate the calcified cartilage matrix. Along with the blood vessels, undifferentiated mesenchymal cells also invade the area; they proliferate and give rise to osteoblasts and bone marrow stem cells. These form a continuous layer over the calcified cartilaginous matrix and start to synthesize bone matrix. Thus, primary bone synthesis takes place over the remnants of calcified cartilage (Fig 8–10).

In histologic sections, calcified cartilage can be distinguished as basophilic whereas the bone tissue deposited over it is acidophilic. As the spongy bone matrix develops, calcified cartilage remnants are resorbed by the giant multinucleated **chondroclasts.** These cells are structurally and functionally equivalent to osteoclasts except that they break down cartilage rather than osseous matrix.

The ossification center described above, which appears in the diaphysis, is called the **primary ossification center** (Fig 8–9). Its rapid longitudinal growth ends by occupying the whole diaphysis, which then becomes composed completely of bone tissue. This expansion of the primary ossification center is accompanied by expansion of the periosteal bone collar, which also grows in the direction of the epiphyses. From the beginning of the formation of the ossification center, osteoclasts are active, and resorption of the bone occurs at the center, which results in formation of a hollow marrow cavity that grows toward the epiphyses as ossifi-

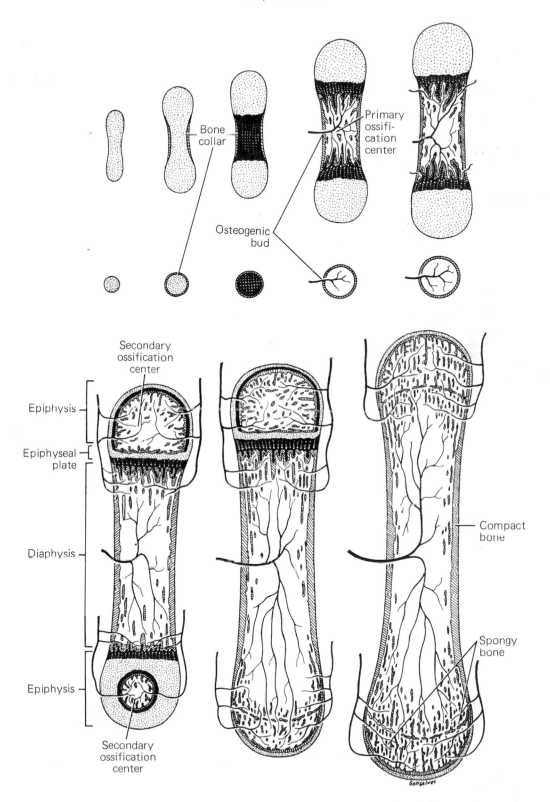

Figure 8 –9. Formation of a long bone on a model made of cartilage. The hyaline cartilage is stippled, the calcified cartilage is black, and bone tissue is indicated by oblique lines. The 5 small drawings in the middle row represent cross sections through the mid regions of the figures shown in the upper row. (For details, see text.) (Redrawn and reproduced, with permission, from Bloom W, Fawcett DW: *A Textbook of Histology,* 9th ed. Saunders, 1968.)

Remnants of cartilage matrix

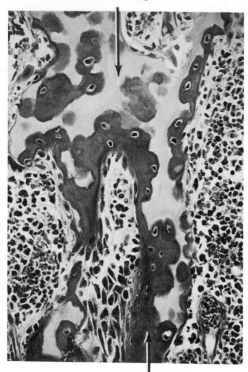

Bone tissue

Figure 8–10. Photomicrograph of endochondral ossification from the finger of a human fetus. Remnants of calcified cartilage matrix appear covered by primary bone tissue. Calcified cartilage matrix has no cells, while bone matrix contains many osteocytes. Mallory trichrome stain, × 238.

cation continues toward the ends of the finally complete bone model.

At later stages in embryonic development, a **secondary ossification center** (Fig 8–9) arises at each epiphysis though, even within one bone, all centers do not develop simultaneously. The function of these centers is similar to that of the primary center, but their growth is radial instead of longitudinal. Furthermore, since the articular cartilage has no perichondrium, the equivalent of a bone collar is not formed here (Fig 8–9).

When bone tissue that originated at the secondary centers occupies the epiphysis, cartilage remains restricted to 2 places: articular cartilage, which persists throughout adult life and does not contribute to bone formation; and epiphyseal cartilage or the epiphyseal plate (Figs 8–11 and 8–12). As the cartilage of the epiphyseal plate grows, it is replaced continuously by expansion of newly formed bone matrix mainly from the diaphyseal center. The epiphyseal plate connects the epiphysis to the diaphysis. No further longitudinal growth of the bone takes place after the growth of the epiphyseal plate ceases.

Epiphyseal cartilage is divided into 5 zones (Fig 8–12), starting from the epiphyseal side of cartilage: (1) The **resting zone** consists of hyaline cartilage without morphologic changes in the cells. (2) In the **proliferative zone,** chondrocytes divide rapidly and form parallel rows of stacked cells along the long axis of the bone. (3) The **hypertrophic cartilage zone** contains large chondrocytes whose cytoplasm has accumulated glycogen. The resorbed matrix is reduced to thin septa between the chondrocytes. (4) Simultaneously with the death of chondrocytes occurring in the **calcified cartilage zone,** the thin septa of cartilage matrix become calcified by the deposition of hydroxyapatite (Figs 8–11 and 8–12). (5) In the **ossification zone,** endochondral bone tissue appears. Blood capillaries and undifferentiated cells formed by mitosis of cells originating from the periosteum invade the cavities left by the chondrocytes. The undifferentiated cells form osteoblasts, which in turn form a discontinuous layer over the septa of calcified cartilage matrix. Over these septa, the osteoblasts lay down bone matrix (Fig 8–10).

The bone matrix calcifies, and some osteoblasts are transformed into osteocytes. In this way, **bone spicules** are formed with a central area of calcified cartilage and a superficial layer of primary bone tissue. The spicules are so called because of their appearance in histologic sections; they are sections of walls which delineate elongated cavities containing capillaries, bone marrow cells, and undifferentiated cells (Fig 8–11).

GROWTH & REMODELING OF BONE

Bone growth is generally associated with partial resorption of preformed tissue and the simultaneous laying down of new bone. This permits the shape of the bone to be maintained while it grows.

Cranial bones grow mainly owing to formation of bone tissue by the periosteum located between the sutures and on the external bone surface. At the same time, resorption takes place on the internal surface. Since bone is an extremely plastic tissue, it responds to the growth of the brain and forms a skull of adequate size. The skull will be small if the brain does not develop completely and larger than normal in a person suffering from hydrocephalus, a disorder characterized by abnormal accumulation of spinal fluid and dilatation of the cerebral ventricles.

The growth of long bones is a complex process. The epiphyses increase in size owing to the radial growth of the cartilage, followed by endochondral ossification. In this way, the spongy part of the epiphysis increases.

The diaphysis (the bone formed between the 2 epiphyseal plates) consists initially of a bone cylinder. Because of the faster growth of the epiphyses,

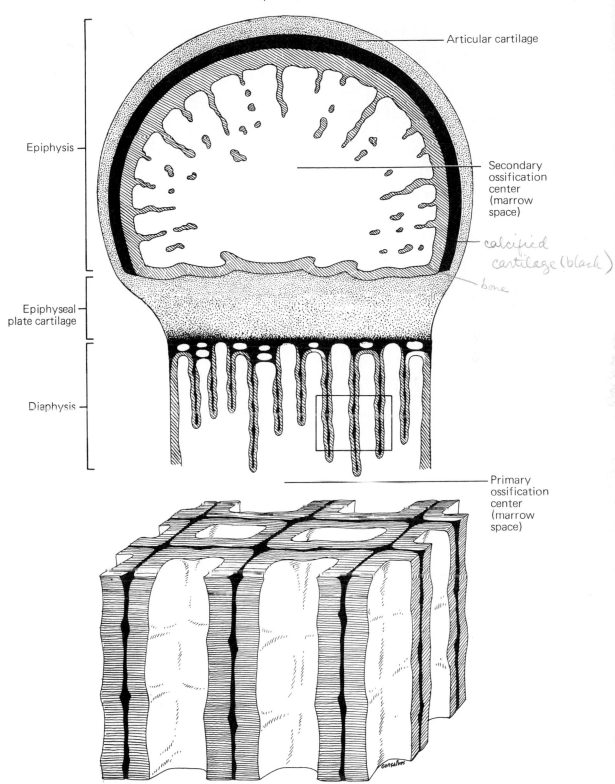

Articular cartilage

Epiphysis

Secondary
ossification
center
(marrow
space)

*calcified
cartilage (black)*

bone

Epiphyseal
plate cartilage

Diaphysis

Primary
ossification
center
(marrow
space)

Figure 8–11. Schematic drawings showing the 3-dimensional shape of bone spicules in the epiphyseal disk area. Hyaline cartilage is stippled, <u>calcified cartilage is black</u>, and bone tissue is indicated by parallel lines. The upper drawing shows the region represented 3-dimensionally in the lower drawing. (Redrawn and reproduced, with permission, from Ham AW: *Histology,* 6th ed. Lippincott, 1969.)

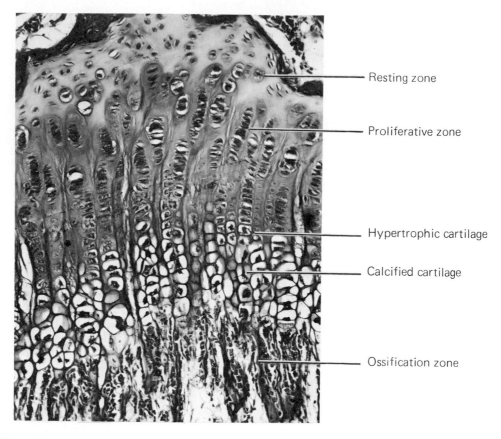

Resting zone

Proliferative zone

Hypertrophic cartilage

Calcified cartilage

Ossification zone

Figure 8–12. Photomicrograph of the epiphyseal plate, showing the changes which take place in the cartilage and the bone spicules formed. H&E stain, × 110.

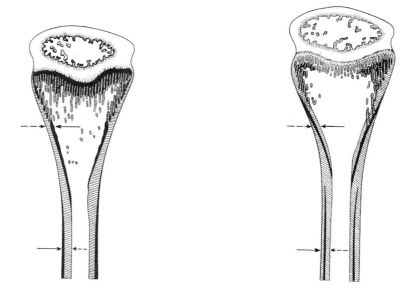

Figure 8–13. Drawings based on radioautographs of animals injected with radioactive phosphate at several time intervals before being killed. Black areas indicate radioactive matrix, solid arrows indicate zones of bone deposition, and broken arrows indicate zones of bone resorption. In diaphyseal funnels, bone deposition occurs mainly at the internal surface. In the diaphysis, bone is laid down mainly on the center surface. (Based on the work of CP Leblond & others. Redrawn and reproduced, with permission, from Greep RO, Weiss L: *Histology,* 3rd ed. McGraw-Hill, 1973.)

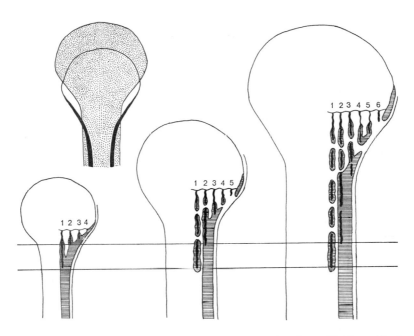

Figure 8–14. *Upper left:* The importance of bone resorption in the external surface of the funnel for bone growth. *Lower drawings:* Bone growth taking place by diaphyseal displacement (Use the 2 parallel lines as reference.) Observe also how epiphyseal bone spicules contribute to the diaphyseal development, eg, spicule 2 is being incorporated into the diaphysis. (Based on the work of CP Leblond & others.)

the extremities of the diaphysis soon become larger, forming 2 **diaphyseal funnels** separated by the **diaphyseal shaft.**

The diaphyseal shaft increases in length mainly as a result of the osteogenic activity of the epiphyseal plate; it increases in width as a result of the formation of bone by the periosteum on the external surface of the bone collar. At the same time, bone is removed from the internal surface, and in this way the bone marrow cavity increases in diameter.

In both diaphyseal funnels, owing to the osteogenic activity of the endosteum, deposition of bone occurs on its internal surface (Fig 8–13). At the same time, bone is resorbed from opposite areas on the external surface. The narrow parts of the diaphyseal funnels therefore become gradually cylindric, and this is due mainly to the osteogenic activity of the epiphyseal plate (Fig 8–14). As a result of this process, the cylindric diaphyseal shaft increases in length, and the 2 diaphyseal funnels grow farther apart as the bone lengthens. Gradually, osteogenic activity in the endosteum of the cylindric portion of the diaphyseal funnel ceases, permitting the bone marrow cavity to maintain or to increase its diameter slowly by resorption. As the central bone spicules become eroded to make room for the bone marrow cavity, the epiphyseal cartilage remains firmly attached to the diaphyseal funnel by means of the peripheral spicules (Figs 8–13 and 8–14).

In brief, it can be said that long bones become longer as a result of the activity of the epiphyseal plates and wider as a result of the apposition of bone

formed by the periosteum. When the cartilage of the epiphyseal plate stops growing, it is replaced by bone tissue through the process of ossification. This occurs around age 20. Afterward, longitudinal growth of bones becomes impossible, although widening may still occur.

FRACTURE REPAIR

When a bone is fractured, the damage suffered by the blood vessels produces a localized hemorrhage with the formation of a blood clot. Destruction of bone matrix and death of bone cells adjoining the fracture also occur.

During repair, the blood clot, the remaining cells, and the damaged bone matrix are removed. The periosteum and the endosteum around the fracture respond with intense proliferation of their fibroblasts, which form a cellular tissue surrounding the fracture and penetrate between the extremities of the fractured bone (Fig 8–15A and B).

Immature bone is then formed by endochondral ossification of small fragments of cartilage appearing in the connective tissue that develops first in the fracture. It is also formed by means of intramembranous ossification. Therefore, areas of cartilage, intramembranous ossification, and endochondral ossification are encountered simultaneously when repair occurs. Repair progresses in

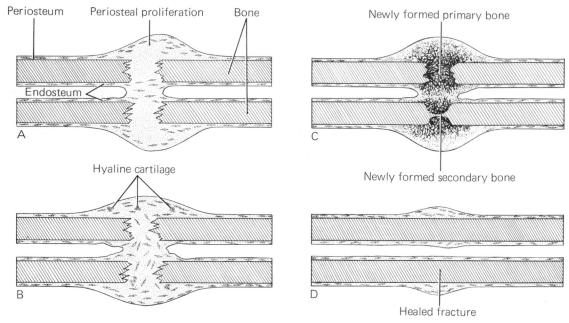

Figure 8–15. Repair of a fractured bone by formation of new bone tissue through proliferation of periosteal and endosteal cells.

such a way that irregularly formed trabeculae of immature bone temporarily unite the extremities of the fractured bone, forming a **bone callus** (Figs 8–15C and 8–16).

Normal stress imposed on the bone during repair and during the patient's gradual return to activity serves to remodel the bone callus. Since these strains are identical to those that occurred during the growth of the bone, thus conditioning its structure, remodeling of the callus reconstitutes the bone as it was prior to fracture. The primary bone tissue of the callus is therefore gradually reabsorbed and replaced by lamellar bone, resulting in restoration of the original bone structure (Fig 8–15D).

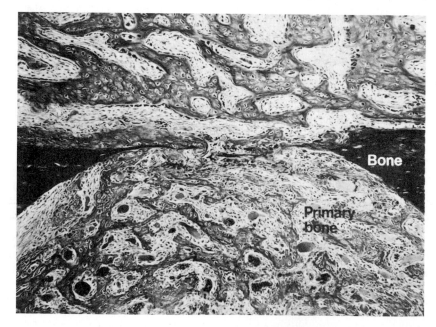

Figure 8–16. Photomicrograph of a mouse bone callus 7 days after fracture. The early callus contains mainly primary bone tissue made by cells originating in the periosteum. This is a micrograph corresponding to an area in Fig 8–15C. Mallory stain, × 118.

HISTOPHYSIOLOGY

Support & Protection

Bones form the skeleton, the function of which is to bear the weight of the body. Voluntary (skeletal) muscles are inserted onto the bones via intercalation of the tendons with the connective tissue of the periosteum. Long bones constitute a system of levers that increase the forces produced by muscular contractions. Bones protect the central nervous system (which is enclosed in the skull and the spinal canal) and the bone marrow.

Plasticity

In spite of its hardness, bone is capable of remodeling its internal structure according to the different stresses to which it is subjected. Thus, for example, the positions of the teeth in the jawbone may be modified by lateral pressures produced by orthodontic appliances. Bone formation takes place on the side where traction is applied and is reabsorbed where pressure is exerted (on the opposite side). In this way, teeth move within the jawbone while the alveolar bone is being remodeled. This capacity for reconstruction is a characteristic of all bones.

Calcium Reserve

The skeleton contains 99% of the total calcium of the body and acts as a calcium reservoir. The concentration of calcium in the blood and in tissues is quite stable. Calcium is important for the activity of several enzymatic systems, including those responsible for muscular contraction and transmission of nerve impulses. Calcium in the extracellular compartment is essential to several functions such as coagulation of the blood and cell adhesion.

There is a continuous interchange between blood calcium and bone calcium. The calcium absorbed from a meal, which would otherwise increase the blood calcium level, is rapidly deposited in bones or excreted in the feces or urine. Calcium in bones is mobilized when the concentration in blood decreases.

Bone calcium is mobilized by 2 mechanisms, one rapid and the other slow. The first is the simple transference of ions from hydroxyapatite crystals to interstitial fluid—from which, in turn, calcium passes into the blood. This purely physical mechanism is aided by the large surface area of the hydroxyapatite crystals. The younger, slightly calcified lamellas that exist even in adult bone because of continuous remodeling receive and lose calcium more readily. These lamellas are more important for the maintenance of calcium concentration in the blood than the older, greatly calcified lamellas, whose role is mainly that of support and protection.

The second mechanism for mobilizing calcium depends on the action of hormones on bone. **Parathyroid hormone** activates and increases the number of cells promoting resorption (osteoclasts) of the bone matrix, with the consequent liberation of calcium.

Another hormone, **calcitonin,** which is synthesized by the clear (C) cells of the thyroid gland, is believed to inhibit matrix resorption by increasing matrix formation and calcium deposition. Its effect on bone, therefore, is opposite to that of parathyroid hormone.

Since the concentration of calcium in tissues and blood must be kept constant, nutritional deficiency of calcium results in decalcification of bones; they then are more liable to fracture and are more permeable to x-rays. Decalcification of bone may also be caused by excessive production of parathyroid hormone (hyperparathyroidism), which results in intense resorption of bone, elevation of blood calcium, and abnormal deposits of calcium in several organs, mainly the kidneys and arterial walls.

Nutrition

Especially during growth, bone is sensitive to several nutritional factors. Insufficient dietary protein causes a deficiency of amino acids and vitamin C necessary for the synthesis of collagen by osteoblasts. Deficiency of calcium leads to incomplete calcification of the organic bone matrix; it may be due either to the lack of calcium in the diet or to the lack of vitamin D, which is important for the absorption of calcium by the small intestine.

Calcium deficiency in children causes rickets, a disease in which the bone matrix does not calcify normally and the bone spicules formed by the epiphyseal plate become distorted when subjected to the normal strains of body weight and muscular activity. Consequently, ossification processes at this level are hindered and the bones not only grow more slowly but also become deformed.

Calcium deficiency in adults gives rise to **osteomalacia,** characterized by deficient calcification of recently formed bone and partial decalcification of already calcified matrix. However, since adults have no epiphyseal cartilage, the deformation of long bones and some retardation of growth that is characteristic of rickets in children does not occur, and of course growth is not affected. Osteomalacia may be aggravated during pregnancy since the developing fetus requires a great deal of calcium.

Osteomalacia should not be confused with **osteoporosis,** a condition not related to nutrition. In the former, there is a decrease in the amount of calcium per unit of bone matrix. Osteoporosis, frequently expressed in immobilized patients and postmenopausal women, is a decrease in bone mass caused by either decreased bone formation or increased bone resorption or both. In osteoporosis, the ratio of mineral to matrix is normal.

Besides the aforementioned effect on intestinal absorption, vitamin D has a direct effect on ossification, as has been demonstrated with in vitro experiments. Bone tissue cultivated in a medium rich in calcium but deficient in vitamin D does not calcify properly. Excessive amounts of vitamin D are toxic and give rise to bone resorption.

Vitamin A, also related to the distribution and activity of the osteoblasts and osteoclasts, affects the balance between production and resorption of bone. This vitamin is essential to normal growth in response to mechanical factors acting on bones, an effect that becomes evident when, as a result of vitamin A deficiency, the bones of the skull do not develop fast enough to respond to the pressure exerted by the growing brain, resulting in damage to the central nervous system. This does not occur in laboratory control animals receiving adequate doses of vitamin A, for the skull then grows to the exact size necessary to contain the brain.

In vitamin A deficiency, the osteoblasts do not synthesize the bone matrix normally and the individual therefore does not reach normal stature. Vitamin A excess accelerates ossification of the epiphyseal plates without a concomitant effect on the growth of cartilage in these plates. Consequently, epiphyseal cartilage is rapidly replaced by bone, and body growth ceases. For these reasons, either vitamin A deficiency or administration of toxic doses of vitamin A may cause small stature.

Another vitamin that acts directly on bone is vitamin C (ascorbic acid), which is essential for collagen synthesis by both osteoblasts and osteocytes. Vitamin C deficiency interferes with bone growth and hinders repair of fractures by altering collagen deposition.

Hormonal Factors

In addition to parathyroid hormone and calcitonin, several other hormones act on bone.

The anterior lobe of the pituitary synthesizes growth hormone, which stimulates overall growth but especially that of epiphyseal cartilage. Consequently, lack of growth hormone during the growing years causes pituitary dwarfism, and growth hormone excess causes gigantism because of excessive growth of long bones. Adult bones cannot increase in length when stimulated by an excess of growth hormone because of the lack of epiphyseal cartilage, but they do increase in width by periosteal growth. In adults, an increase in growth hormone causes **acromegaly**, a disease in which the bones—mainly the long ones—become very thick.

The sex hormones, both male (androgen) and female (estrogens), have a complex effect on bones and are, in a general way, stimulators of bone formation. They influence the time of appearance and the development of ossification centers. Thus, precocious sexual maturity due to sex hormone–producing tumors or to the administration of sex hormones retards bodily growth since the epiphyseal cartilage is quickly replaced by bone. In hormone deficiencies due to abnormal development of the gonads or

castration, epiphyseal cartilage remains functional for a longer period of time, resulting in tall stature.

Interrelationships Between the Cells of Bone

Radioautographic studies performed after the administration of ^{3}H-thymidine to young animals—whose bone cells proliferate rapidly—reveal that these cells represent different aspects of an osteoprogenitor showing modulations between the 3 types of bone cells (Fig 8–17). The osteoblasts and osteocytes do not divide after having been formed from the osteoprogenitor cell, which is a slightly differentiated mesenchymal cell. In the epiphyseal disk, the osteoprogenitor cell has a "generation time" of about 36 hours; this means that during this interval its number doubles. Some of the new cells thus formed are modified, giving rise to osteoblasts.

A. Fate of the Osteoblasts: Most of the osteoblasts give rise to osteocytes; others remain as osteoblasts for long periods of time; and some return to the state of the osteoprogenitor cell.

B. Fate of the Osteocytes: When destruction of the matrix occurs during the process of remodeling, it appears that some of the osteocytes die, but most probably return to the state of the osteoprogenitor cell. As a result of the intensive remodeling of bone that takes place in the epiphyseal disk, many of the osteocytes remain as osteocytes for a short period (minimum of 50 hours). In other sites (eg, in the Haversian system), the cells may persist as osteocytes for a long time.

JOINTS

Bones are joined to one another to form the skeleton by means of connective tissue structures called joints. Joints may be classified as **diarthroses**, which permit free bone movement, and **synarthroses**, in which very limited or no movement occurs. There are 3 types of synarthrosis: synostosis, synchondrosis, and syndesmosis.

Synostosis

In joints of this type, bones are united by bone tissue. No movement takes place. In elderly people, this type of synarthrosis unites the skull bones. In children and young adults, these bones are united by dense connective tissue.

Synchondrosis

Synchondroses are articulations in which the bones are joined by hyaline cartilage. Limited movement may take place. The ribs are attached to the sternum in this way.

Syndesmosis

As is the case with synchondroses, a syndes-

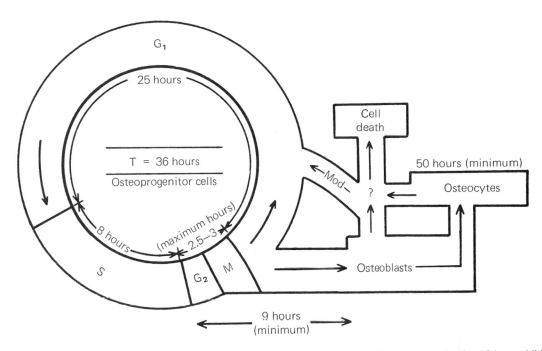

Figure 8–17. Osteoblasts originating from osteoprogenitor cells. Generation time (T) is estimated to be 36 hours (tibia of young rats). The period of DNA synthesis (S) is 8 hours; G₁ consumes 25 hours of the cycle, whereas G₂ and mitosis (M) take 2.5–3 hours. The minimum time for an osteoprogenitor cell to be transformed into an osteoblast is 9 hours. Once formed, osteocytes remain as such for at least 50 hours or, very often, longer. Osteoblasts can modulate (Mod) back to an osteoprogenitor cell; it is not certain whether osteocytes can do so. It has been demonstrated that osteoclasts are derived primarily from blood monocytes. However, it is still possible that some osteoprogenitor cells may fuse and form the multinucleated osteoclasts. (Slightly modified and reproduced, with permission, from Young RW: J Cell Biol 14:357, 1962.)

mosis permits a certain amount of movement. The bones are joined by connective tissue (eg, the inferior tibiofibular articulation).

Diarthrosis

Diarthroses are joints that generally unite long bones and have great mobility. In a diarthrosis, a capsule joins the extremities of the bones and encloses a sealed cavity—the **articular cavity**—which contains a colorless, transparent, viscous fluid, rich in hyaluronic acid, called **synovial fluid.** The sliding of articular surfaces covered by hyaline cartilage and having no perichondrium is facilitated by the lubricating synovial fluid (Figs 8–18 and 8–19).

The capsules of diarthroses (Fig 8–18) vary in structure according to the joint. Generally, however, this capsule is composed of 2 layers, one external (**fibrous layer**) and one internal (**synovial layer**).

The fluid encountered in the articular cavity is formed by the synovial layer, which is arranged in folds that occasionally penetrate deep into the interior of the articular cavity. The internal surface of the synovial membrane is usually lined by a layer of squamous or cuboidal cells. Underneath these cells is a layer of loose or dense connective tissue with areas of adipose tissue. The lining cells of the synovial membrane originate in the mesenchyme. They

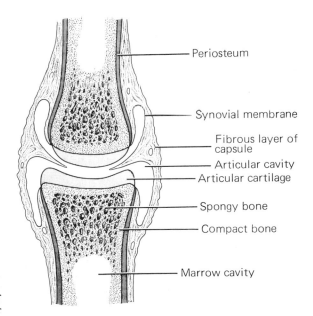

Figure 8–18. Schematic drawing of a diarthrosis. The capsule is formed by 2 parts, not clearly delimited: the external **fibrous layer** and the **synovial layer** (synovial membrane) that lines the articular cavity except the cartilaginous areas.

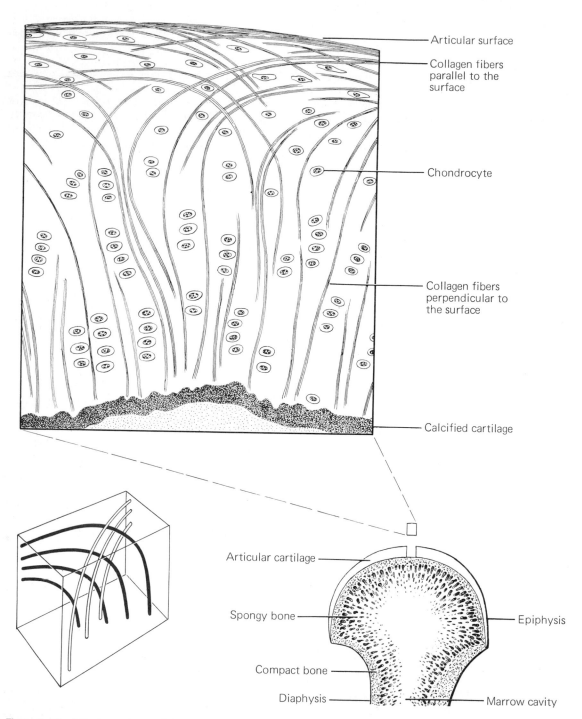

Figure 8–19. Articular surfaces of diarthroses are covered by hyaline cartilage devoid of perichondrium. The upper figure shows that in this cartilage collagen fibers are first perpendicular and then parallel to the cartilage surface. Deeply located chondrocytes are globular and are arranged in elongated rows. Superficially placed chondrocytes are slender and are not organized in groups. The lower left drawing shows the organization of collagen fibers in articular cartilage in 3 dimensions.

are separated from each other by a small amount of connective tissue ground substance (Figs 8–20 and 8–21).

Observations made with the electron microscope have shown 2 cell types lining the synovial membrane (Fig 8–21). Some of these cells resemble macrophages and are called M cells. They have a large Golgi apparatus and many lysosomes but only a small amount of granular endoplasmic reticulum. The other cell type has structural features of a fibroblast and is called an F cell. Cells of this type have a well-developed granular endoplasmic reticulum and are more electron-dense than M cells.

M cells and F cells probably represent different functional stages of the same cell type.

Radioautographs analyzed under the light microscope show that the cells covering synovial membrane synthesize hyaluronic acid and proteins, which are secreted into the synovial fluid. Both M cells and F cells are phagocytic, but M cells are more active in this respect.

The fibrous layer is made of dense connective tissue that is better developed in parts subject to great strain. This layer envelops the ligaments of the joint and some of the tendons inserted into the bone near the joint.

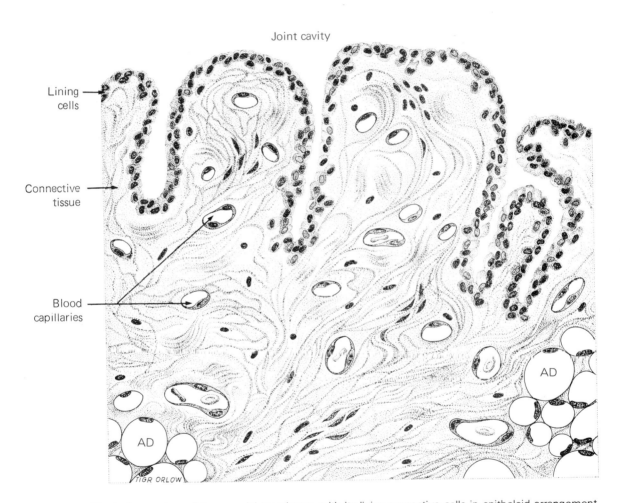

Joint cavity

Lining cells

Connective tissue

Blood capillaries

AD

AD

TIGR ORLOW

Figure 8 –20. Histologic structure of the synovial membrane, with its lining connective cells in epitheloid arrangement. There is no basal lamina between the lining cells and the underlying connective tissue. This tissue is rich in blood capillaries and contains a variable amount of adipose cells (AD). (Reproduced, with permission, from Cossermelli W: *Reumatologia Básica.* Sarvier, 1971.)

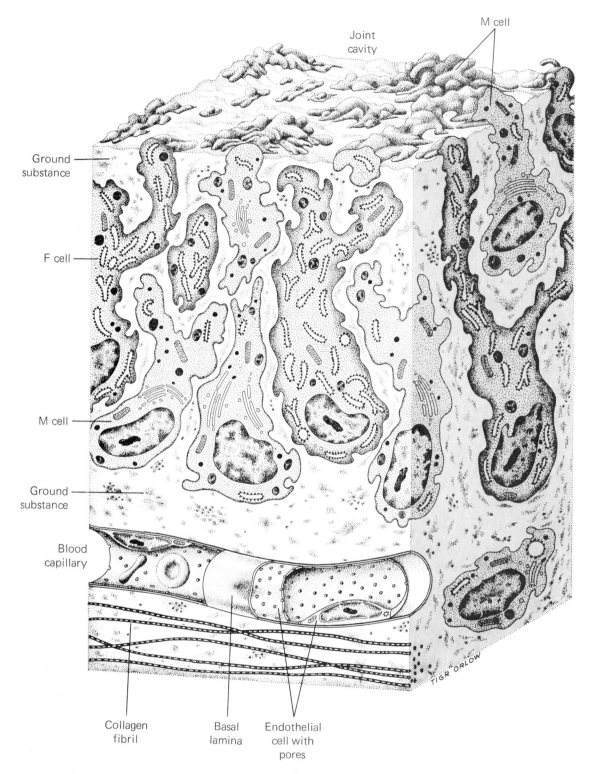

Figure 8 –21. Schematic representation of the ultrastructure of a synovial membrane. F and M cell types are separated by a small amount of connective tissue amorphous ground substance. No basal lamina is seen separating the lining cells from the connective tissue. Blood capillaries are of the fenestrated type, which facilitates exchange of substances between the blood and the synovial fluid. (Redrawn and reproduced, with permission, from Cossermelli W: *Reumatologia Básica.* Sarvier, 1972. Based on a drawing in Barland PA & others: J Cell Biol 14:207, 1962.)

• • •

References

Barland P, Novikoff AB, Hamerman D: Electron microscopy of the human synovial membrane. J Cell Biol 14:207, 1962.

Barland P, Smith C, Hamerman D: Localization of hyaluronic acid in synovial cells by radioautography. J Cell Biol 37:13, 1968.

Blau S & others: Cellular origin of hyaluronate protein in the human synovial membrane. Science 150:353, 1965.

Bourne GH (editor): *The Biochemistry and Physiology of Bone*. Vol 1. *Structure*. Academic Press, 1972.

Cameron DA: The fine structure of osteoblasts in the metaphysis of the tibia of the young rat. J Biophys Biochem Cytol 9:583, 1961.

Carneiro J, Leblond CP: Role of osteoblasts and odontoblasts in secreting the collagen of bone and dentin, as shown by radioautography in mice given tritium-labelled glycine. Exp Cell Res 18:291, 1959.

Carneiro J, Leblond CP: Suitability of collagenase treatment for the radioautographic identification of newly-formed collagen labeled with ³H-glycine or ³H-proline. J Histochem Cytochem 14:334, 1966.

Cherubino P, Kataoka K: Scanning electron microscope observations of the synovial membrane of rabbit knee joints after experimentally induced hemarthrosis. Arch Histol Jpn 35:417, 1973.

Gaillard PJ: The cellular basis of hormone response. Pathol Biol (Paris) 9:619, 1961.

Glimcher MJ, Krane SM: The organization and structure of bone, and the mechanism of calcification. In: *Treatise on Collagen*. Vol 2, part B. Gould BS (editor). Academic Press, 1968.

Ham AW, Harris WR: Repair and transplantation of bone. In: *The Biochemistry and Physiology of Bone*, 2nd ed. Vol 3. Bourne GH (editor). Academic Press, 1976.

Holtrop ME: The ultrastructure of bone. Ann Clin Lab Sci 5:264, 1975.

Horn V, Dvořák MY: Ultrastructure of functional bone components in scanning and transmission electron microscopy. Z Mikrosk Anat Forsch 88:836, 1974.

Jones SJ, Boyde A: Some morphologic observations on osteoclasts. Cell Tissue Res 185:387, 1977.

Jones SJ, Boyde A: The migration of osteoblasts. Cell Tissue Res 184:179, 1977.

Jotereau FV, LeDouarin NM: The developmental relationship between osteocytes and osteoclasts: A study using the quail-chick nuclear marker in endochondral ossification. Dev Biol 63:253, 1978.

Jowsey J: Studies of Haversian systems in man and some animals. J Anat 100:857, 1966.

Kashiwa HA: Localization of phosphate in bone cells of fresh calvaria by means of a dilute silver acetate solution. Anat Rec 162:177, 1968.

Kaufman EJ & others: Collagenolytic activity during active bone resorption in tissue culture. Proc Soc Exp Biol Med 120:623, 1965.

Nichol G Jr (editor): *Workshop Conference on Cell Mechanisms for Calcium Transfer and Homeostasis*. Academic Press, 1971.

Owen M: Cell population kinetics of an osteogenic tissue. (Part 1.) J Cell Biol 19:19, 1963.

Owen M: The origin of bone cells. Int Rev Cytol 28:213, 1970.

Owen M, MacPherson S: Cell population kinetics of an osteogenic tissue. (Part 2.) J Cell Biol 19:33, 1963.

Ramagen W: The bone cell system: Form and function (review). Beitr Pathol 150:1, 1973.

Roberts ED & others: Electron microscopy of porcine synovial cell layer. J Comp Pathol 79:41, 1969.

Taylor AN, Wasserman RH: Immunofluorescent localization of vitamin D–dependent calcium-binding protein. J Histochem Cytochem 18:107, 1970.

Urist MR: Biochemistry of calcification. In: *The Biochemistry and Physiology of Bone*, 2nd ed. Vol 4. Bourne GH (editor). Academic Press, 1976.

Vaughan JM: *The Physiology of Bone*. Clarendon Press, 1970.

Walker DG: Control of bone resorption by hematopoietic tissue: The induction and reversal of congenital osteopetrosis in mice through use of bone marrow and splenic transplants. J Exp Med 142:651, 1975.

Wright V, Dowson D, Kerr J: The structure of joints. In: *International Review of Connective Tissue Research*. Vol 6. Hall DA, Jackson DS (editors). Academic Press, 1973.

9 | Nerve Tissue

The human nervous system contains at least 10 billion neurons. These basic building blocks of the nervous system have evolved from primitive neuro-effector cells that respond to various stimuli by contracting. In higher animals, contraction became the specialized function of muscle cells, while transmission of nerve impulses became the specialized function of neurons.

Nerve tissue is distributed throughout the body as an integrated communications network. Anatomically, the nervous system is divided into the **central nervous system,** consisting of the brain and the spinal cord; and the **peripheral nervous system,** composed of nerve fibers and small aggregates of nerve cells called **nerve ganglia.**

Structurally, nerve tissue consists of **nerve cells** or **neurons,** which usually show numerous long processes; and several types of **glial cells** or **neuroglia,** which support and protect neurons and participate in neural activity, neural nutrition, and the defense processes of the central nervous system.

In the central nervous system, nerve cell bodies are concentrated in groups located at different areas from their processes. The brain and spinal cord are composed of **gray matter** and **white matter.** The former (gray when fresh) contains mainly nerve cell bodies and neuroglia but also a complicated network of nerve cell processes. White matter does not contain nerve cell bodies; it consists of neuronal processes and neuroglia. It takes its name from the presence of a whitish material called **myelin** that envelops most of the neuronal processes. The brain stem exhibits zones containing both nerve cells and myelinated fibers—an area where gray matter is mixed with white matter.

Neurons respond to environmental changes (**stimuli**) by altering electrical potential differences that exist between the inner and the outer surfaces of their membranes. Cells with this property (eg, neurons, muscle cells, some gland cells) are called "excitable." Neurons react promptly to stimuli, and modification of electrical potential may be restricted to the place that received the stimulus or may be spread throughout the neuron by the membrane. This propagation, called the **nerve impulse,** transmits information to other neurons, muscles, and glands.

The 2 fundamental functions of the nervous system are (1) to detect, analyze, utilize, and transmit all information generated by sensory stimuli (such as heat and light) and by mechanical and chemical changes that take place in the internal and external milieu; and (2) to organize and coordinate, directly or indirectly, most functions of the body, especially the motor, visceral, endocrine, and mental activities.

NEURONS

The nerve cells or neurons are independent anatomic and functional units with complex morphologic characteristics. Most neurons consist of 3 parts: the **dendrites,** which are multiple elongated processes specialized in receiving stimuli from the environment, from sensory epithelial cells, or from other neurons; the **cell body** or **perikaryon,** which represents the trophic center for the whole nerve cell and is also receptive to stimuli; and the **axon,** which is a single process specialized in generating or conducting nerve impulses to other cells (nerve, muscle, and gland cells). The distal portion of the axon is usually branched and constitutes the **terminal arborization.** Each branch of this arborization terminates on the next cell in dilatations called **end bulbs,** which facilitate the transmission of information to the next cell in the chain (Fig 9–1).

Neurons usually receive information through dendrites and cell bodies and transmit them via the axons. This sequence, termed **dynamic polarization** by Cajal, constitutes a general mechanism in neuronal function, although several exceptions exist.

Neurons and their processes are extremely variable in size and shape (Fig 9–2). Perikaryons can be spherical, ovoid, or angular in contour; some are very large, measuring up to 150 μm in diameter—large enough to be visible to the naked eye. Other nerve cells are among the smallest cells in the body; for example, the perikaryons of granular cells of the cerebellum are only 4–5 μm in diameter.

According to the size and shape of their processes, most neurons can be placed in one of the

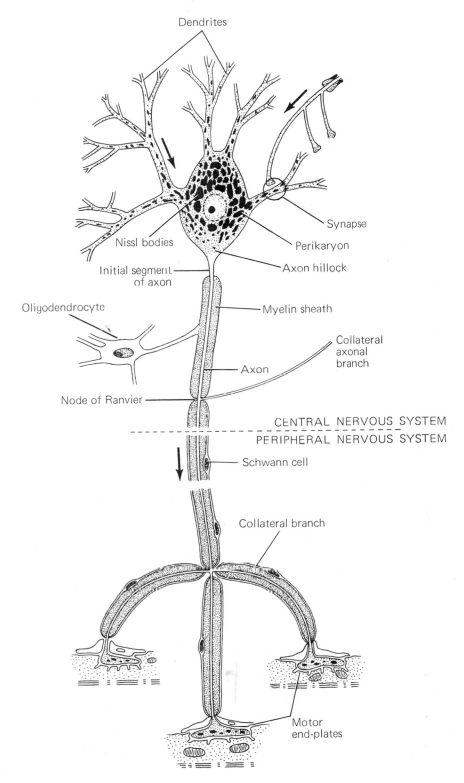

Dendrites

Synapse

Nissl bodies

Perikaryon

Initial segment of axon

Axon hillock

Oligodendrocyte

Myelin sheath

Collateral axonal branch

Axon

Node of Ranvier

CENTRAL NERVOUS SYSTEM
PERIPHERAL NERVOUS SYSTEM

Schwann cell

Collateral branch

Motor end-plates

Figure 9–1. Schematic drawing of a Nissl-stained motor neuron. The myelin sheath is produced by oligodendrocytes in the central nervous system and by Schwann cells in the peripheral nervous system. The neuronal cell body has an unusually large, euchromatic nucleus with a well-developed nucleolus. The perikaryon contains Nissl bodies, which are also found in large dendrites. An axon from another neuron is shown at upper right. It has 3 end bulbs, one of which synapses with the neuron. Note also 3 motor end-plates, which transmit the nerve impulse to striated skeletal muscle fibers. Arrows show the direction of the nerve impulse.

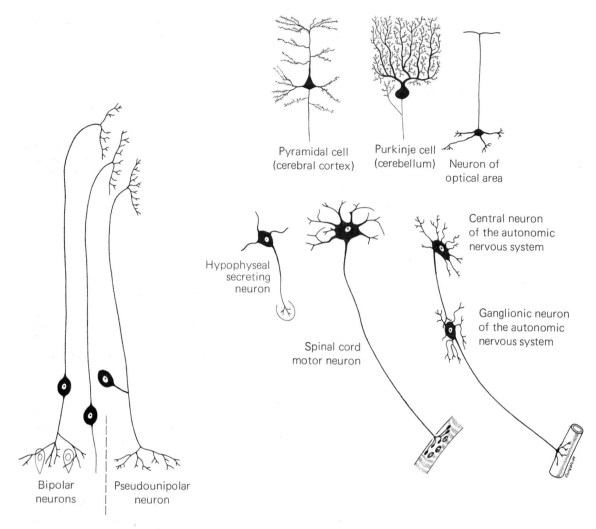

Pyramidal cell
(cerebral cortex)

Purkinje cell
(cerebellum)

Neuron of
optical area

Central neuron
of the autonomic
nervous system

Hypophyseal
secreting
neuron

Ganglionic neuron
of the autonomic
nervous system

Spinal cord
motor neuron

Bipolar
neurons

Pseudounipolar
neuron

Figure 9–2. Diagrams of several types of neurons. Neurons have a very complex morphology. Except for the bipolar and pseudounipolar neurons, which are not very numerous in nerve tissue, all others shown here are of the common multipolar variety.

following categories: **multipolar neurons,** which have more than 2 cell processes, one being the axon and the rest dendrites; **bipolar neurons,** with one dendrite and one axon; and **pseudounipolar neurons,** which show a single process close to the perikaryon but which divides into 2 branches, forming a T shape, one branch extending to a peripheral ending and the other toward the central nervous system (Fig 9–2).

In the embryo, a pseudounipolar neuron starts as a bipolar cell with a dendrite and an axon, each arising from opposite ends of the perikaryon. During later development, the 2 processes come together on one side of the cell and fuse for a certain distance close to the perikaryon. Certain cells, like the amacrine cells of the retina, do not have axons in the ordinary sense, and their processes appear to be both axonic and dendritic. In typical pseudounipolar neurons, both branches are axons on

both structural and electrophysiologic grounds. In pseudounipolar neurons, the arborizations of the peripheral branches receive stimuli and are functional dendrites. The significance of this type of neuron is that stimuli picked up by the dendrites travel directly to the axon terminal without passing through the perikaryon.

Most neurons of the body are multipolar. Bipolar neurons are found in the cochlear and vestibular ganglia as well as in the retina and the olfactory mucosa. Pseudounipolar neurons are found in the spinal ganglia, which are sensory ganglia located at the dorsal roots of the spinal nerves, and they are also found in most cranial ganglia.

Neurons can also be classified according to their functional roles. **Motor neurons** control effector organs (eg, exocrine and endocrine glands) and muscle fibers. **Sensory neurons** are involved in the reception of sensory stimuli from the environment and from within the body. **Interneurons** establish interrelationships among other neurons, forming complex functional chains or circuits.

During mammalian evolution there was a great increase in the number and complexity of interneurons. Highly developed functions of the nervous system cannot be ascribed to simple neuron circuits; rather, they depend on complex interactions established by the integrated processes of many neurons.

In the central nervous system, nerve cell bodies are present only in the gray matter. White matter contains neuronal processes but no perikaryons. In the peripheral nervous system, perikaryons are found in ganglia and in some sensory regions (eg, retina, olfactory mucosa).

PERIKARYON OR SOMA

The perikaryon is the part of the neuron that contains the nucleus and surrounding cytoplasm exclusive of the cell processes. It is primarily a trophic center, but it also has a receptive function.

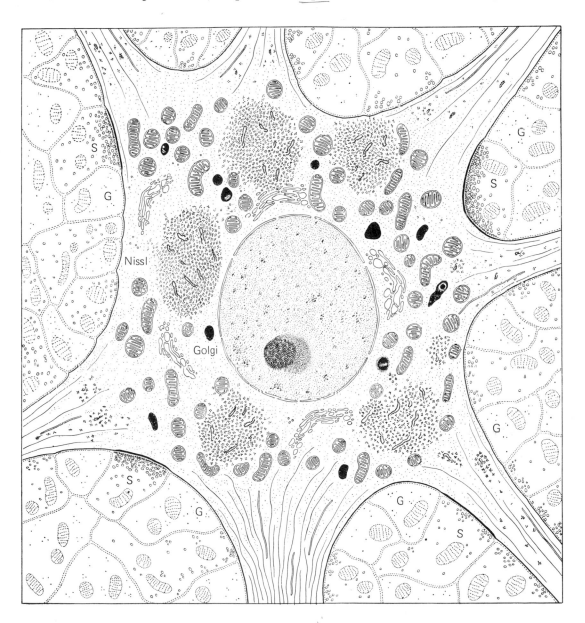

Figure 9–3. Ultrastructure of a neuron. The neuronal surface is completely covered either by synaptic end processes of other neurons (S) or by processes of glial cells (G). At synapses, the neuronal membrane is thicker and is called the postsynaptic membrane. The neuronal process devoid of ribosomes (lower part of figure) is the axon.

The perikaryon of most neurons receives a great number of nerve endings that convey excitatory or inhibitory stimuli generated in other nerve cells (Fig 9–3).

Nucleus

Most nerve cells show a spherical, unusually large, euchromatic (palely staining) nucleus with a prominent nucleolus. The nucleus is most often located in the center of the cell body except in the nerve cells of Clarke's column of the spinal column, where it is situated eccentrically, as in some sympathetic ganglia. Binuclear nerve cells are seen in sympathetic and sensory ganglia. The chromatin is finely dispersed, reflecting the intense synthetic activity of these cells. In females, between the large nucleolus and the nuclear membrane, a special chromatin clump is found in neurons. This is the sex chromatin, first discovered in nerve cells from female cats and later located in other cells of the body of females. This chromatin represents the inactivated X chromosome that remains condensed during interphase.

Granular (Rough) Endoplasmic Reticulum

Perikaryons contain a highly developed granular endoplasmic reticulum organized into aggregates of parallel cisternae. In the cytoplasm between the cisternae, there are great numbers of free ribosomes, which usually form rosettes; these cells synthesize both structural proteins and proteins for transport. When appropriate stains are used, granular endoplasmic reticulum and free ribosomes appear under the light microscope as basophilic granular areas called **Nissl bodies** (Figs 9–1 and 9–4).

The number of Nissl bodies varies according to neuronal type and functional state. They are particularly abundant in large nerve cells such as the motor neurons (Fig 9–4).

Injury to axons or neuron exhaustion resulting from strong or prolonged stimuli causes a reduction in the number of Nissl bodies. This alteration is called **chromatolysis** and occurs simultaneously with nuclear migration to the periphery of the perikaryon. However, moderate stimuli may increase the amount of RNA in the perikaryon.

Golgi Apparatus

The Golgi apparatus is located only in the perikaryon, around the nucleus. The neuronal Golgi apparatus usually consists of multiple parallel arrays of smooth cisternae and lies around the periphery of the nucleus. There are also a number of smaller, spherical vesicles that likely represent both transfer and secretory vesicles (Fig 9–3). With the use of osmic acid or silver impregnation technics, the Golgi apparatus takes on the appearance of a network of irregular filaments. Some profiles of smooth endoplasmic reticulum are seen near the Golgi area.

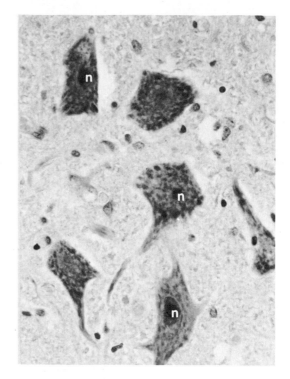

Figure 9–4. Photomicrograph of motor neurons from the human spinal cord. The cytoplasm contains a great number of Nissl bodies, making it difficult to see the cell nucleus; the large nucleoli (n) are more easily seen. Although their cellular boundaries are not evident, nuclei of numerous glial and endothelial cells are present around the neurons. H&E stain, × 360.

Mitochondria

Mitochondria are found in neurons and are especially abundant in the axon terminals. In the perikaryon, they are small and scattered throughout the cytoplasm.

Neurofilaments & Microtubules

Intermediate filaments with a diameter of 10 nm, called neurofilaments, are abundant in perikaryons and cell processes. There is evidence that neurofilaments can agglutinate as a result of the action of fixatives. When impregnated with silver, they form neurofibrils that are visible with the light microscope. Thus, neurofibrils are probably stained artifacts produced by reagents that cause neurofilaments to clump together. In tissue cultures under certain conditions, it is possible to see neurofibrils in living neurons. The neurofilaments can probably be seen because they are often parallel and very close to each other, though they are actually below the limit of resolution of the light microscope. Crisscrossing arrays of neurofilaments cut through the agglomerations of rough endoplasmic reticulum and free polysomes and, as a consequence, carve up this basophilic material into the discrete clusters recognized, after appropriate staining, as Nissl bodies. The perikaryon also contains microtubules with a diameter of 24 nm identical to those found in many other cells (Fig 9–5).

Inclusions

In certain areas of the central nervous system, the perikaryons contain dark brown or black granules. Areas where this pigmentation is seen are the dorsal motor nucleus of the vagus nerve, the spinal and sympathetic ganglia, the substantia nigra of the midbrain, and the locus ceruleus in the floor of the fourth ventricle. The functional role of this melanin pigment in nerve cells is obscure. Another pigment sometimes found in nerve cell bodies is **lipofuscin.** This is a light brown lipid-containing pigment that accumulates in increasing amounts with age. It probably represents a residue of material undigested by lysosomes. Lipid droplets occur quite frequently in nerve cell bodies.

DENDRITES

Most nerve cells have numerous dendrites, which increase considerably the receptive area of the cell. Dendrite arborization makes it possible for one neuron to receive and integrate a great number of axon terminals from other nerve cells. It has been estimated that up to 200,000 axonal terminations establish functional contact with the dendrites of the Purkinje nerve cell found in the cerebellum (Fig 9–2). In other nerve cells, that number may be even higher. Neurons with only one dendrite (bipolar neurons) are uncommon and are found only in special sites. In contrast to axons (nerve fibers), which maintain a constant diameter from one end to the other, dendrites become thinner as they subdivide into branches.

Structurally, dendrites are very similar to perikaryons; however, they are devoid of Golgi apparatus. Nissl bodies and mitochondria are present except in very thin dendrites. Neurofilaments (10 nm) and microtubules (about 24 nm), also found in axons, are more numerous in dendrites. Dendrites are usually short and divide like the branches of a tree. In some instances, however, they assume other forms—for example, the characteristic dendrites of the cerebellar Purkinje cells branch in one plane only, assuming the shape of a fan (Fig 9–2) and increasing the surface area of each Purkinje cell from 250 μm^2 in early development to 27,000 μm^2 in the mature cell. Dendrites are usually covered by a large number of thorny spines or gemmules, which are small dendritic projections representing sites of synaptic contact. However, not all species exhibit axonal synapses, and the spines without synapses may serve in modifying or determining dendritic membrane potentials.

AXONS

Each neuron has only one axon; it is a cylindric process that varies in length and diameter according to the type of neuron. Some neurons have a short axon, but the axons are usually very long processes For example, axons of the motor cells of the spinal cord that innervate the foot muscles may have a length of up to 100 cm (about 40 inches). Since dendrites of a nerve cell are more numerous, their total volume is usually greater than that of the axons.

All axons start from the perikaryon or, in a few cases, from the stem of a major dendrite through a short pyramid-shaped region called the **axon hillock** (Fig 9–5) that can be differentiated from dendrites by distinctive histologic features: (1) The granular endoplasmic reticulum and ribosomes found in perikaryons and dendrites do not extend into the axon hillock. (2) In the axon hillock, the microtubules are arranged in fascicles or bundles. The plasma membrane of the axon is called the **axolemma** and its contents **axoplasm.**

In neurons that give rise to a myelinated axon, the portion of the axon between the axon hillock and the point at which myelination begins is named the **initial segment.** This part of the axon is characterized by a thin layer of electron-dense material underneath the plasma membrane called **dense undercoating.** Microtubules continue in fascicles from the axon hillock into the initial segment.

In contrast to dendrites, axons have a constant diameter and do not branch profusely. Occasionally, the axon, shortly after its departure from the cell body, gives rise to a branch that returns to the area of the nerve cell body. In the central nervous system, the axons give rise to branches at right angles to their main direction. These branches are known as **collaterals** (Fig 9–1).

Axonal cytoplasm (axoplasm) is poor in organelles and primarily possesses few mitochondria, microtubules, and neurofilaments. New cytoplasm and other constituents are formed in the cell body and are transported out into the axon.

SYNAPSES

When axons are artificially stimulated, they conduct the nerve impulse in both directions from the stimulation point. The impulse directed to the cell body, however, does not excite other neurons, and only the impulse reaching the final arborization of the axon, the axon terminal, can excite the next neuron in the chain.

This dynamic polarization and the transmission of the nerve impulse depends on highly specialized structures called **synapses,** which are classically de-

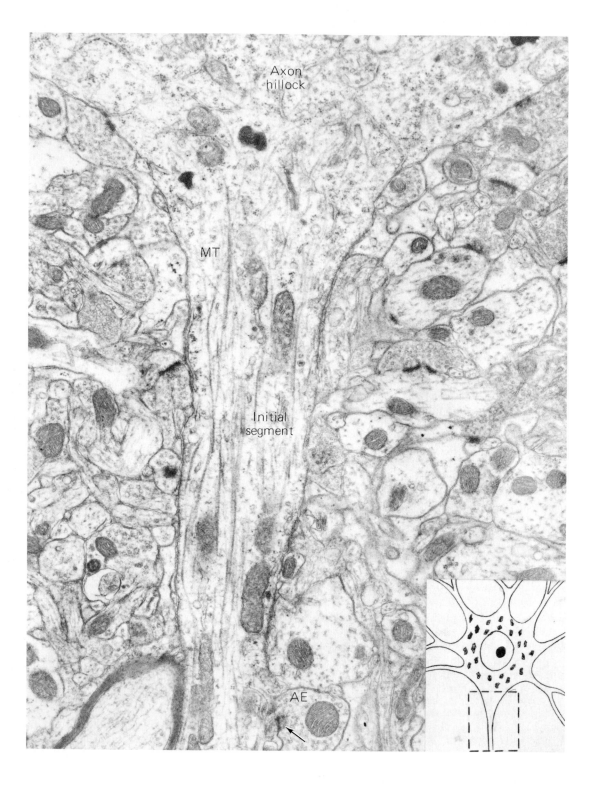

Figure 9 –5. Electron micrograph of the axon hillock and the axon's first segment. (Position in relation to the neuron is indicated in the inset.) The axon hillock is poor in ribosomes and endoplasmic reticulum. The arrangement of the microtubules (MT) in bundles is initiated in the axon hillock and becomes more pronounced in the initial segment of the axon. An axon ending (AE—arrow) synapses with the initial segment in the lower portion of the micrograph. Note that there is virtually no intercellular material in the nerve tissue. (See also Fig 9 –3.) × 26,000. (Courtesy of A Peters.)

fined as the contact of one axon with the dendrites or perikaryon and, very rarely, with the axon of another neuron. Most synapses are between an axon and a dendrite (axodendritic) or between an axon and a cell body (axosomatic). But there are also synapses between dendrites (dendrodendritic) and between axons (axoaxonic). The recent trend is to consider the nerve endings on effector cells, such as gland or muscle cells, as synapses also. Synapses function by altering the membrane potential of neurons. The influence of a particular synapse on a neuron is related to its distance from the axon. Consequently, the influence of incoming information on neuronal activity is intimately related to the distribution and location, as well as number, of synapses on the dendritic tree and cell soma.

Morphologically, several types of synapses can be identified. The axon terminal may form bulbous expansions, basketlike structures, or club-shaped terminations (Fig 9–6). These synaptic end bulbs are often called **boutons terminaux.** More often the axon branch establishes several synapses along its course. In this case, there are varicosities along the axon, called **boutons en passage.** The analysis of a synapse under the electron microscope shows that it is actually a specialized, localized region of a contact between 2 cells (Fig 9–6). It is composed of a terminal membrane (presynaptic membrane), a region of extracellular space (the **synaptic gap**), and a postsynaptic membrane belonging to a dendrite, perikaryon, or axon of another cell. At a synapse, the plasma membranes of the 2 neurons are usually separated by a distance of 20 nm (the synaptic gap). These membranes are firmly bound together at the synaptic region, and in some instances dense filaments form bridges between them. The plasma membranes of the 2 neurons are thicker at the presynaptic and postsynaptic areas of the synapse than elsewhere and show a condensation of the cytoplasm near the synaptic membranes. Cytoplasmic filaments resembling those found in desmosomes are anchored to the inside of each of these membranes.

The cytoplasm in the endings of the terminal typically contains numerous **synaptic vesicles** with a diameter of 20–65 nm, although some vesicles as large as 160 nm have been observed. Neurofilaments are infrequent, but mitochondria are numerous. The synaptic vesicles contain substances called **neurotransmitters** that are responsible for the transmission of the nerve impulse across the synapse. These mediators are liberated at the presynaptic membrane and act on the postsynaptic membrane to promote the transmission of nerve impulses across the synaptic cleft.

Besides the chemical synapses described above, in which a chemical substance mediates the transmission of the nerve impulse, there are also the electrical synapses. Here the nerve cells are linked through a gap junction (see Chapter 3), which permits the passage of ions from one cell to

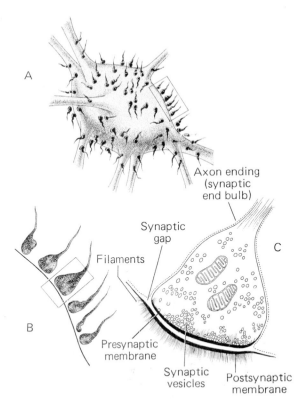

Figure 9 –6. *A:* External morphology of a neuron and some of its processes. Axon endings from other neurons are shown in black. The area outlined by a rectangle appears enlarged at *B. B:* At synaptic junctions, the 2 cell membranes are separated by a slender space—the synaptic gap. *C:* Ultrastructure of the synapse outlined in *B.* Presynaptic and postsynaptic membranes are thicker than the neuronal cell membrane elsewhere. The axon ending shows 2 mitochondria as well as numerous synaptic vesicles that contain neurotransmitters. Liberation of the mediator substance transmits the nerve impulse from the presynaptic to the postsynaptic membrane. (Redrawn and reproduced, with permission, from De Robertis, Novinsky, & Saez: *Biologia Celular,* 8th ed. El Ateneo [Buenos Aires], 1970.)

the other, thus providing for their electrical coupling. Electrical synapses are less numerous than chemical synapses, but they are being observed with increasing frequency owing to technical improvements in electron microscopy.

NEUROGLIA

Several cell types found in the central nervous system in association with the neurons are classified as **neuroglia** or **glial cells.** The several types of neuroglia show morphologic and functional differences.

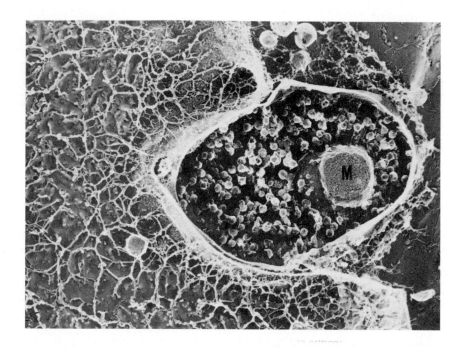

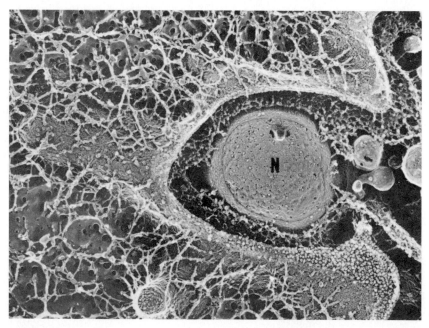

Figure 9 –7. *A:* View of a rotary-replicated freeze-etched synapse. M, mitochondrion. × 25,000. *B:* Another freeze-etched and rotary-replicated synapse that was fractured more obliquely than the specimen in A. The nerve (N) was not broken open, and instead the lacelike basal lamina in the cleft around the nerve was exposed. Also, the filaments that support the postsynaptic membrane were revealed more clearly. × 40,000. (Reproduced, with permission, from Heuser JE, Salpeter SR: Organization of acetylcholine receptors in quick-frozen, deep-etched, and rotary-replicated Torpedo postsynaptic membrane. J Cell Biol 82:150, 1979.)

Routine hematoxylin and eosin preparations are not adequate to study neuroglia, since with this staining technic only their nuclei can be seen among the larger nuclei of nerve cells (Fig 9–4). The cytoplasm and processes of the neuroglia are not visible, for it is impossible to distinguish them from the processes of the neurons. The neuroglia play an important role in the normal function of the nervous system. For the study of the morphology of neuroglia, special procedures involving silver or gold impregnation technics are used.

It has been estimated that in the central nervous system there are 10 neuroglia for each neuron. However, since neuroglia are much smaller, they occupy only about one-half of the total volume of the nerve tissue.

Neuroglia include several varieties: astrocytes, oligodendrocytes, microglia, and ependymal cells. Astrocytes and oligodendrocytes are referred to as the **macroglia.**

Neuroglial cells are thought not to generate action potentials, and they do not form synapses with other cells. They form the myelin sheaths of the axons and are probably necessary for the maintenance and viability of neurons. This latter possibility is supported by the fact that glial cells are necessary for tissue culturing of normal neurons, which cannot be grown unless neuroglia are present in the culture.

1. ASTROCYTES

Astrocytes are the largest of the neuroglia, possessing numerous long processes. They have spherical, centrally located nuclei which stain lightly (Fig 9–8). Many of their processes have expanded pedicles at their ends which attach to the walls of blood capillaries. These pedicles, called the "vascular feet" of the neuroglia, completely surround and ensheath all vessels of the nourishing vascular network. Processes of the astrocytes are also present at the periphery of the brain and spinal cord, forming a layer under the pia mater. This layer, which also contains processes of other neuroglia, separates the connective tissue of the pia mater from the nerve cells. There are usually 2 types of astrocytes: protoplasmic, which are found in the gray matter of the brain and spinal cord; and fibrous, which are found chiefly in the white matter. In tissue culture, astrocytes exhibit constant movement.

Protoplasmic Astrocytes

Protoplasmic astrocytes have abundant granular cytoplasm. Their processes have many branches, are shorter than those of fibrous astrocytes, and are relatively thick (Fig 9–8). Their processes envelop the surface of nerve cells, the synaptic areas, and blood vessels.

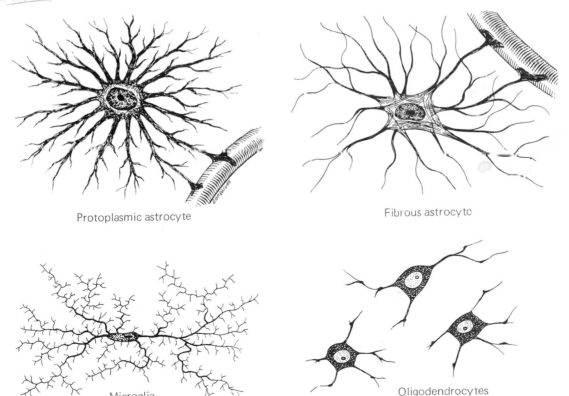

Protoplasmic astrocyte

Fibrous astrocyte

Microglia

Oligodendrocytes

Figure 9–8. Drawings of neuroglial cells as seen in slides specially stained by metallic impregnation. Observe that only astrocytes exhibit vascular end-feet. These processes terminate on the walls of blood capillaries.

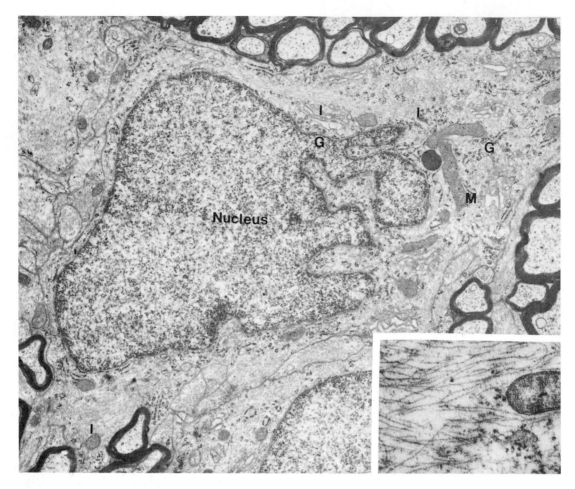

Figure 9–9. Electron micrograph of a fibrous astrocyte. G, Golgi apparatus; M, mitochondrion; I, intermediate (10 nm) filaments. × 12,000. In the inset, the magnification is × 42,000 and shows the abundant filaments in the cytoplasm. (Courtesy of A Peters.)

Fibrous Astrocytes

Fibrous astrocytes have long, slender, smooth processes that branch infrequently. In special silver-stained preparations, their cytoplasm shows fibrillar material that is probably formed by the precipitation of very thin filaments abundant in the cell bodies and processes of fibrous astrocytes (Fig 9–9).

2. OLIGODENDROCYTES

Oligodendrocytes are much smaller than astrocytes, and their processes are less numerous and shorter than those present in other neuroglia (Fig 9–8). Oligodendrocytes are found both in gray and in white matter. In gray matter, they are mainly localized close to perikaryons.

The number of oligodendrocytes increases with increasing complexity of the nervous system in different species. Human nerve tissue has the highest number of oligodendrocytes per nerve cell.

In white matter, oligodendrocytes appear in rows among the myelinated nerve fibers. Under the electron microscope, fetal nerve tissue shows that the myelin sheath of central nervous system tissue is produced by the processes of oligodendrocytes. In this aspect of their function, the oligodendrocytes are analogous to the Schwann cells of peripheral nerves.

The cytoplasm of oligodendrocytes is electron-dense and consists mainly of mitochondria, ribosomes, and microtubles, and these characteristics permit their identification in electron micrographs. Their nuclei are round and small and exhibit condensed chromatin.

On examination in tissue culture, oligodendrocytes show intense movements that seem to possess a specific periodicity.

3. MICROGLIA

The cell bodies of microglia are small, dense, and elongated. Their nuclei show condensed chromatin and an elongated shape along the axis of the cell body. The shape of the nuclei of microglia permits their identification in hematoxylin and eosin preparations, for other neuroglia have spherical nuclei. Microglia have short processes covered by numerous small expansions, giving them a thorny appearance (Fig 9–8). Microglia are not numerous, but they are found in both white and gray matter.

Although many microglia might be evident using special silver-stained light microscope preparations, very few microglial cells are observed in electron microscopic studies. It appears that many of the so-called microglial cells seen in the light microscope actually represent oligodendroglia or immature **glioblasts**. However, there are some macrophagic microglial cells that apparently arise from blood-borne monocytes and are not of neural origin. Following an injury, many invasive macrophages are present; however, under normal circumstances, astroglial cells will function as macrophages in removing cell debris.

4. EPENDYMAL CELLS

Ependymal cells derive from the internal lining of the neural tube and retain their epithelial arrangement, whereas the other cells from the neural tube develop processes and give rise to neurons or to neuroglia. Ependymal cells line the cavities of the brain and spinal cord and are bathed by the cerebrospinal fluid, which fills these cavities. In embryonic life the ependymal cells have cilia, which sometimes are observed in adult organisms in some parts of the lining of the ventricles. In certain parts of the central nervous system, ependymal cells are continuous with and homologous to the cuboidal cells of choroid plexuses.

Although the apical ends of ependymal cells line the cavities, their bases are not uniform but actually consist of long processes that extend from the center of the brain to the peripheral connective tissue. Consequently, ependymal cell processes extend between neural elements and constitute a supporting matrix similar to other glial cells. Because of the organization of the columnar ependymal cells lining the lumen of brain cavities and central canal of the spinal cord, the central nervous system is organized as an unusually thick, stratified columnar epithelium.

The nervous system is in fact a complex epithelium derived from the simple columnar epithelium of the neural plate. Following formation of the neural tube, the cells undergo rapid proliferation and form a stratified epithelium. The constituent cells exhibit abundant filopodial projections interwoven into a complex matrix. In addition to the typical junctions present in other epithelia, the neuroepithelium possesses specialized communicating junctions known as synapses.

In view of its epithelial organization, it is not surprising that the nervous system exhibits an unusual nerve-blood barrier. As described in Chapter 4, epithelia do not have a connective tissue extracellular matrix or a vascular supply. In order to provide nutrition to cells deep within the thick neuroepithelium, blood vessels penetrate the nerve tissue through a maze of tortuous channels. Basal cells of the neuroepithelium lining these channels are primarily the astroglia. Consequently, in order for nutrients to reach the nerve cells, they must pass through the astroglial cells.

HISTOPHYSIOLOGY OF NEUROGLIA

In the central nervous system, connective tissue layers form the enveloping protective and vascular coats (meninges) of the organ. A very small amount of connective tissue, which penetrates into the nerve tissue, is restricted to sheaths that are present around the larger blood vessels.

In spite of its size, the central nervous system is poor in connective tissue content, and its nerve cells and their processes are supported by neuroglia. Because of their number and their long processes, astrocytes seem to be the most important supporting elements.

The vascular feet and the presence of pinocytotic vesicles in astrocytes suggest that they play a role in the transport of substances from blood capillaries to neurons and vice versa. There is evidence that astrocytes transport ions through an energy-dependent mechanism (ion pump) and are responsible for the equilibrium of electrolytes within the central nervous system. It is known that the "scars" formed in the central nervous system after lesions of these tissues result from hyperplasia and hypertrophy of astrocytes.

Perineural oligodendrocytes seem to live symbiotically with the neurons. Cytochemical studies performed on neurons and satellite cells isolated by microsurgery have shown a metabolic dependency between them. Any stimulus that alters the chemical composition of the nerve cell also is reflected in the satellite cell. In tissue cultures, neurons do not survive unless they are kept with their satellite cells.

NERVE FIBERS

Nerve fibers consist of axons enveloped by special sheaths. The axon sheaths are of ectodermal origin. Groups of nerve fibers constitute the tracts of the brain, spinal cord, and peripheral nerves. Nerve fibers exhibit differences in their enveloping sheaths related to whether the fibers are part of the central or peripheral nervous system.

Most axons in adult nerve tissue are ensheathed by single or multiple folds of a sheath cell. In peripheral nerve fibers, the sheath cell is the Schwann cell, or neurolemma sheath, and in central nerve fibers it is the oligodendrocyte. Axons of small diameter are usually **unmyelinated nerve fibers** (Figs 9–10 and 9–15). Progressively thicker axons are generally ensheathed by increasingly numerous concentric wrappings of the enveloping cell. When enveloped by **myelin sheaths,** the fibers are known as myelinated nerves (Fig 9–11). Axonal conduction of the impulse is progressively faster in axons with larger diameters and thicker myelin sheaths. Fresh myelinated fibers appear as homogeneous, glistening tubes.

Myelinated Fibers

In these fibers, the cytoplasm of the covering Schwann cell winds around the axon. In this process, the layers of membranes of the sheath cell unite and form a lipoprotein complex called **myelin,** which can be partly removed (the lipid component) by standard histologic procedures. Its presence can be demonstrated by osmium tetroxide, which preserves myelin and stains it black (Fig 9–13).

The myelin sheath shows gaps along its path called the **nodes of Ranvier,** which represent the spaces between adjacent Schwann cells along the length of the axon. In the node of Ranvier, the membrane of the axon (axolemma) shows an inner layer of electron-dense material forming a dense undercoat. The distance between 2 nodes is called an **internode** of myelin and consists of one Schwann cell (Figs 9–1 and 9–14). The thickness of the myelin sheath varies according to the axonal diameter, but it is constant along the extent of a particular axon. The length of the internodes varies from 0.08–1 mm. Under the light microscope, the myelin sheath shows cone-shaped clefts called **clefts** or **incisures of Schmidt-Lanterman** that are actually helical tunnels from the outside of the

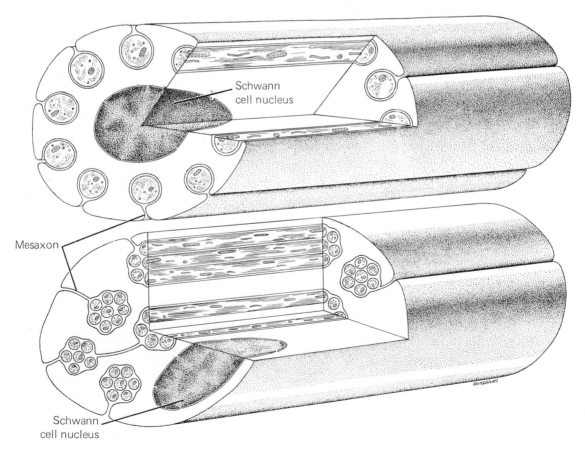

Figure 9–10. *Above:* The most frequent type of unmyelinated nerve fiber, in which each axon has its own mesaxon. *Below:* Many very thin axons are sometimes found together surrounded by the Schwann cell. In such cases there is one mesaxon for several axons.

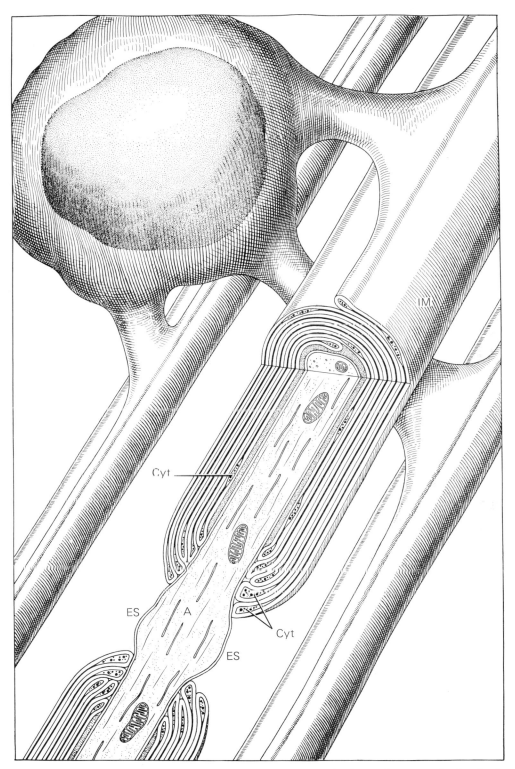

Figure 9–11. Myelin sheath of the central nervous system. The same oligodendrocyte forms myelin sheaths for several nerve fibers (3–50). In the central nervous system, the nodes of Ranvier are covered sometimes by processes of other cells or there is at that point considerable extracellular space (ES). The axolemma shows a thickening where the cell membrane of the oligodendrocyte comes into contact with it, thus limiting the periaxonal space as in the peripheral nervous system (not represented in this drawing). At upper left is a surface view of the cell body of an oligodendrocyte. IM, inner mesaxon; Cyt, cytoplasm of glial cell; A, axon. (Redrawn and reproduced, with permission, from Bunge & others: J Biophys Biochem Cytol 10:67, 1961.)

sheath to the inside. They represent distentions within the myelin cell layers due to the localized presence of Schwann cell cytoplasm. This cytoplasm and, consequently, the clefts move up and down the sheath. Their apexes do not always point in the same direction (Fig 9–14).

Myelin is composed of bimolecular lipid layers alternating with layers of protein molecules parallel to the axon. Thus, myelin actually consists of many layers of modified cell membranes. Embryo studies have shown that the first step in myelin formation is axon penetration into an existing groove of the Schwann cell cytoplasm. The edges of the groove come together to form a mesaxon, so that the plasma membranes of the 2 edges fuse together on their outer surface. Next, through a process not yet fully understood, the mesaxon wraps itself around the axon several times, the number of turns determining the thickness of the myelin layer. After this process, an internal and an external mesaxon can be seen (Figs 9–12 and 9–13). The clefts of Schmidt-Lanterman are areas in which the cytoplasm of the Schwann cells is present within the myelin layer. These cytoplasmic areas were left behind during the winding process of the cytoplasm around the axon (Figs 9–14 and 9–15).

Schwann cells have elongated nuclei that lie parallel to the axon. With the myelin sheath, they assume a cylindric form. The nodes of Ranvier, which are indentations in the myelin sheath, are covered by interdigitating processes of adjacent Schwann cells (Figs 9–14 and 9–15). When involved with myelin formation, Schwann cells are only associated with one axon segment.

There are no Schwann cells in the central nervous system; the myelin sheath is formed by the processes of the oligodendrocytes. Oligodendrocytes differ from Schwann cells in that different branches of one cell can envelop segments of several axons (Fig 9–11). The nodes of Ranvier may be uncovered in the central nervous system; Schmidt-Lanterman clefts are absent.

Unmyelinated Fibers

In both the central and peripheral nervous systems, not all axons are ensheathed in myelin. In the peripheral system, all **unmyelinated axons** are enveloped within simple clefts of the Schwann cells (Fig 9–10). Unlike their associations with individual myelinated axons, each Schwann cell can ensheath many unmyelinated axons. Unmyelinated nerve fibers do not have nodes of Ranvier, since abutting

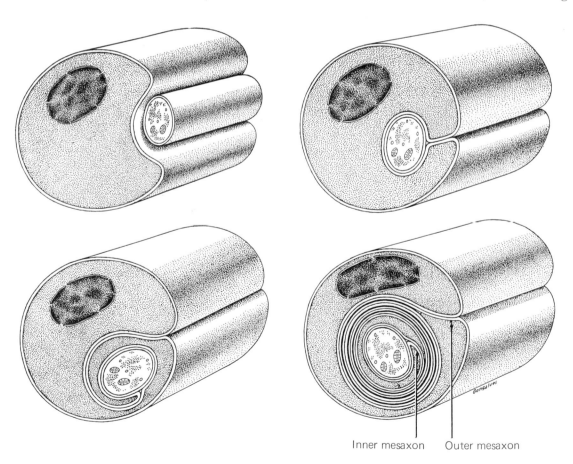

Inner mesaxon   Outer mesaxon

Figure 9–12. Four consecutive phases of myelin formation in peripheral nerve fibers.

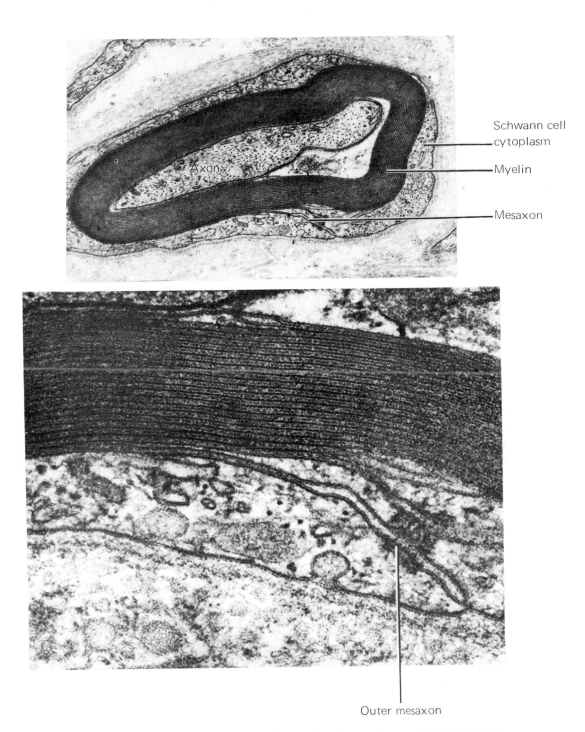

Figure 9–13. Electron micrographs of a myelinated nerve fiber. × 20,000; × 80,000.

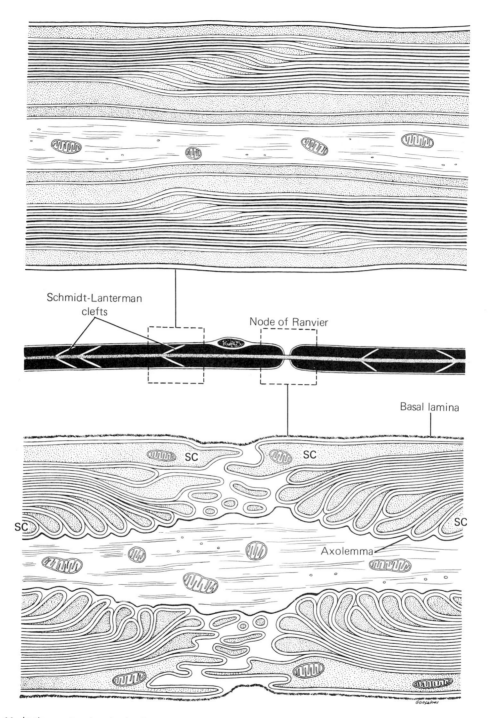

Schmidt-Lanterman clefts

Node of Ranvier

Basal lamina

SC   SC

SC   SC

Axolemma

Figure 9–14. In the center drawing is shown a myelinated peripheral nerve fiber as seen under the light microscope. The stippled process is the axon enveloped by the myelin sheath (in black) and by the cytoplasm of Schwann cells or neurolemma. A Schwann cell nucleus is seen, as well as the Schmidt-Lanterman clefts and a node of Ranvier. The upper drawing shows the ultrastructure of the Schmidt-Lanterman cleft. This cleft is formed by portions of the Schwann cell cytoplasm, separated by the myelin layers during its formation. The lower drawing shows the ultrastructure of a node of Ranvier. Note the appearance of loose interdigitating processes of the outer leaf of the cytoplasm of the Schwann cells (SC) and that a close contact of the inner leaf of the cytoplasm with the axolemma exists, thus acting as a sort of barrier to the movement of materials in and out of the space between the axolemma and the membrane of the Schwann cell. This space is called periaxonal space. The basal lamina around the Schwann cell is continuous. Covering the nerve fiber is a connective tissue layer—mainly reticular fiber—which forms the outer sheath of the peripheral nerve fibers and is known as the sheath of Key and Retzius.

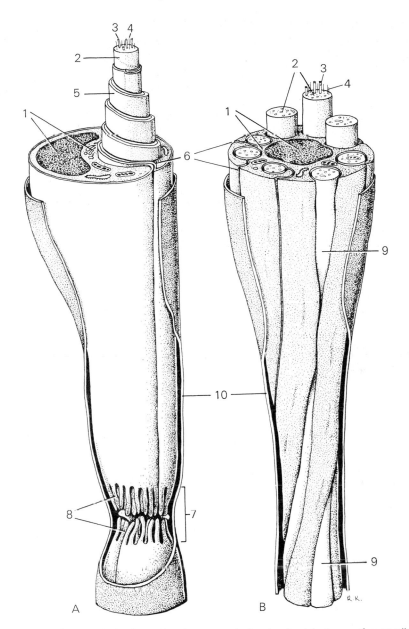

Figure 9 –15. Schematic tridimensional drawings showing several ultrastructural features of a myelinated *(A)* and an unmyelinated *(B)* nerve fiber. 1, nucleus and cytoplasm of Schwann cell; 2, axon; 3, microtubule; 4, neurofilament; 5, myelin sheath; 6, mesaxon; 7, node of Ranvier; 8, interdigitating processes of Schwann cells at the node of Ranvier; 9, side view of an unmyelinated axon; 10, basal lamina. (Slightly modified and reproduced, with permission, from Krstić RV: *Ultrastructure of the Mammalian Cell.* Springer-Verlag, 1979.)

Schwann cells are laterally united to form a continuous sheath.

The central nervous system is rich in unmyelinated axons, but these axons, unlike those in the peripheral system, are not ensheathed. In the brain and spinal cord, unmyelinated axonal processes run free among the other neuronal and glial processes.

NERVES

In the peripheral nervous system, the nerve fibers are grouped in bundles to form the nerves. Except for a few very thin nerves made up of unmyelinated fibers, nerves have a whitish appearance because of their myelin content.

The stroma of the nerves consists of an external fibrous coat of dense connective tissue called

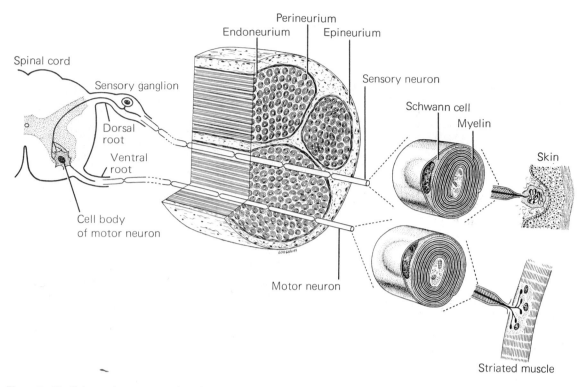

Figure 9 –16. Schematic representation of a nerve and also of the simplest reflex arc. In this example, the sensory stimulus starts in the skin and the motor fiber innervates a striated skeletal muscle. (Redrawn and reproduced, with permission, from Ham AW: *Histology,* 6th ed. Lippincott, 1969.)

epineurium, which also fills the space between the bundles of nerve fibers. Each bundle is surrounded by the **perineurium,** a sleeve formed by layers of epithelium-like fibroblasts. The fibroblasts of each perineurial sleeve are joined at their edges by tight junctions, an arrangement that makes the perineurium a barrier to the passage of most macromolecules. Within the perineurial sheath run the Schwann cell–ensheathed axons and their enveloping connective tissue, called the **endoneurium,** which consists of a very thin layer of loose connective tissue in close contact with the individual nerve fibers (Figs 9–16 and 9–17). Very delicate reticular fibers of the endoneurium form an incomplete envelope—called the connective tissue sheath of Key and Retzius—around each nerve fiber. While the other axonal sheaths (Schwann cells, myelin) originate from the neural ectoderm, the sheath of Key and Retzius derives from the mesenchyme.

The nerves establish communication between the nerve centers and the sense organs and effectors (muscles, glands, etc). They possess afferent and efferent fibers in relation to the central nervous system. The afferent fibers carry the information obtained from the interior of the body and the environment to the nerve centers. The efferent fibers carry impulses from the central nervous system to the effector organs commanded by these centers. Nerves possessing only sensory fibers (afferent) are called **sensory nerves;** those composed only of fibers carrying impulses to the effectors are called **motor nerves.** Most nerves have both sensory and motor fibers and are called **mixed nerves** (Fig 9–16); these nerves have both myelinated and unmyelinated axons (Fig 9–17).

AUTONOMIC NERVOUS SYSTEM

The autonomic nervous system is related to the control of smooth muscle, the secretion of some glands, and the modulation of cardiac rhythm. Its function is to make adjustments in certain activities of the body in order to maintain a constant internal environment (homeostasis). Although the autonomic nervous system is by definition a motor system, fibers that receive sensation originating in the interior of the organism accompany the motor fibers of the autonomic system.

Although the term autonomic implies that this part of the nervous system functions independently, this is not the case; its functions are constantly subject to the influences of conscious activity.

The concept of the autonomic nervous system is mainly functional. Anatomically, it is composed of

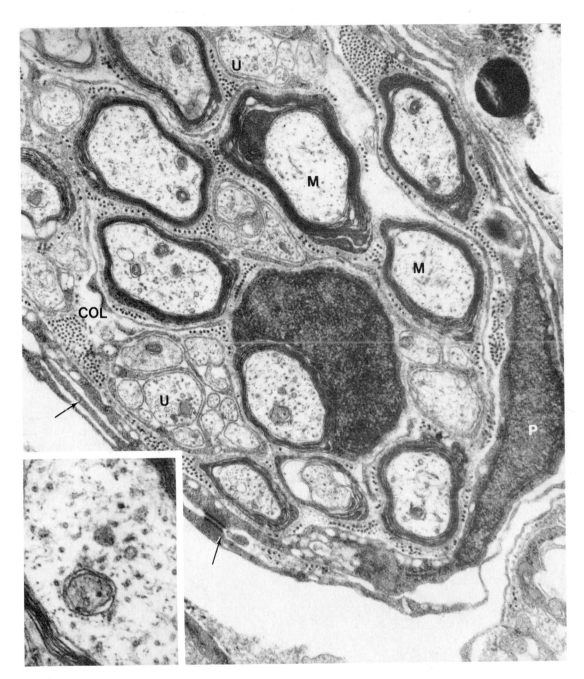

Figure 9–17. Electron micrograph of a peripheral nerve containing both myelinated (M) and unmyelinated (U) nerve fibers. The collagen fibers (COL) seen in cross section belong to the endoneurium. Near the center of the figure there is a Schwann cell nucleus. The perineurial cells (P and arrows) form a cellular sheath that provides an enclosed conduit for the axonal processes. × 30,000. The inset shows part of an axon, where numerous neurofilaments and microtubules are seen. × 60,000.

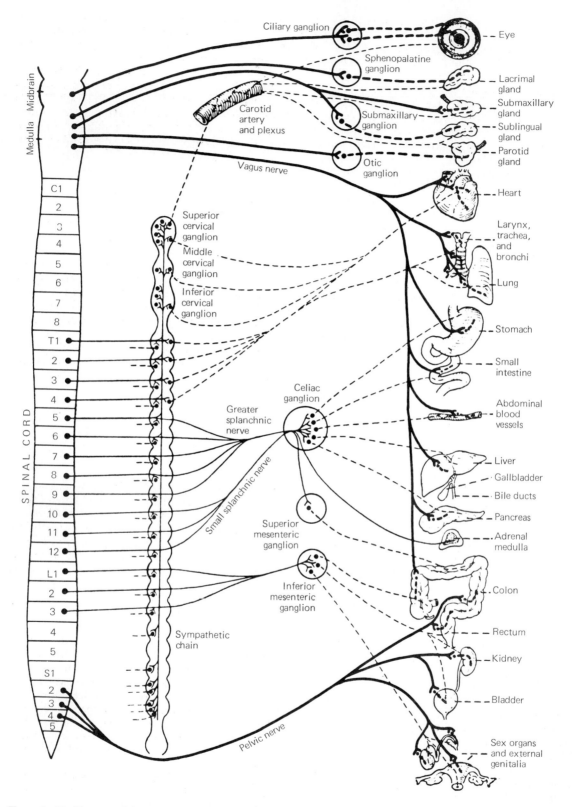

Figure 9–18. Diagram of the efferent autonomic pathways. Preganglionic neurons are shown as solid lines, postganglionic neurons as dotted lines. The heavy lines are parasympathetic fibers; the light lines are sympathetic. (Reproduced, with permission, from Youmans W: *Fundamentals of Human Physiology,* 2nd ed. Year Book, 1962.)

collections of nerve cells located in the central nervous system; of fibers which leave the central nervous system through cranial or spinal nerves; and of nerve ganglia situated in the paths of these fibers. The term "autonomic" covers all the neural elements concerned with visceral function.

The first neuron of the autonomic chain is located in the central nervous system. Its axon forms a synapse with the second multipolar neuron in the chain, located in a ganglion of the peripheral autonomic system. The nerve fibers (axons) of the first neuron to the second are called preganglionic fibers; the axons of the second neuron to the effectors—muscle or gland—are called postganglionic fibers. The chemical mediator present in the synaptic vesicles of all preganglionic endings and at anatomically parasympathetic postganglionic endings is acetylcholine. It is released from the terminals by nerve impulses.

The adrenal medulla is the only organ that receives preganglionic fibers because the majority of the cells, after migration into the gland, do not differentiate into ganglion cells but into secretory cells. Consequently, its innervation is still preganglionic.

The autonomic nervous system is composed of 2 parts that differ both anatomically and functionally: the sympathetic system and the parasympathetic system (Fig 9–18).

Sympathetic System

The nuclei (nerve cell bodies) of the sympathetic system are located in the thoracic and lumbar segments of the spinal cord. The axons of these neurons—preganglionic fibers—leave the central nervous system by the ventral roots and white communicating rami of the thoracic and lumbar nerves. The sympathetic system is also called the thoracolumbar division of the autonomic nervous system. The ganglia of the sympathetic system form the latero-vertebral chain and plexuses situated near the viscera. The chemical mediator of the postganglionic fibers of the sympathetic system is norepinephrine, which is also produced by the medulla of the adrenal. The adrenal secretion has an effect similar to that of stimulation of the sympathetic nervous system.

Parasympathetic System

The parasympathetic system has its nuclei in the medulla and midbrain and in the sacral portion of the spinal cord. The preganglionic fibers of these neurons leave through 4 of the cranial nerves (III, VII, IX, and X) and also through the second, third, and fourth sacral spinal nerves. The parasympathetic system is therefore also called the craniosacral division of the autonomic system.

The second neuron of the parasympathetic chain is found in ganglia smaller than those of the sympathetic system; it is always located near or within the effector organs. These neurons are frequently located in the walls of organs (eg, stomach, intestines), in which case the preganglionic fibers penetrate into the organs and synapse there with the second neuron in the chain.

The chemical mediator released by the pre- and postganglionic nerve endings of the parasympathetic system is acetylcholine. Acetylcholine is readily inactivated by acetylcholinesterase—one of the reasons parasympathetic stimulation has both a more discrete and a more localized action than sympathetic stimulation.

Distribution

Most of the organs innervated by the autonomic nervous system receive both sympathetic and parasympathetic fibers (Fig 9–18). Generally, in organs where the sympathetic system is the stimulator, the parasympathetic system has an inhibitory action, and vice versa. For example, stimulation of the sympathetic system accelerates cardiac rhythm, whereas stimulation of parasympathetic fibers slows it down. In some instances, the activity of these 2 components is complementary and not antagonistic. This is true in the case of some salivary glands, whose secretion is greater when stimulated by both systems than when stimulated by either one separately.

HISTOPHYSIOLOGY OF NERVE TISSUE

The integrative function of nerve tissue depends basically on the generation and spreading of nerve impulses and on the production of neurohormones by special nerve cells. (The neurohormones are discussed in Chapter 21.)

Axonal conduction of nerve impulses is one of the basic and better understood functions of nerve tissue. Several cell components were thought to be implicated in the process of impulse conduction, but it is now well established that the key role is played by the cell membrane.

Passage of the impulse is characterized by changes in membrane permeability, resulting in an inward movement of sodium and an outward movement of potassium. Since the increase in permeability is greater for sodium than for potassium, positive ions accumulate on the undersurface of the cell membrane. During the passage of the impulse, therefore, the outer surface of the axon membrane becomes negatively charged relative to the internal surface (Fig 9–19).

In unmyelinated fibers, the impulse is conducted as a spreading wave of modification in membrane permeability. As this wave moves along the fiber, the membrane behind the wave returns to its resting stage (Fig 9–19). This is possible because of the presence of an active ion-transporting mecha-

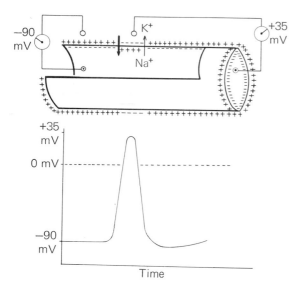

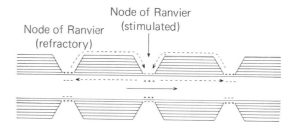

Figure 9–19. Conduction of the nerve impulse through an unmyelinated nerve fiber. In the resting axon there is a difference of −90 mV between the interior of the axon and the outer surface of its membrane (resting potential). During the impulse passage, Na⁺ (thick arrow) passes into the axon interior, while K⁺ (thin arrow) migrates in the opposite direction. The amount of Na⁺ that enters the axon is larger than the amount of K⁺ that leaves it; there is a change in membrane polarity. It becomes relatively positive on its inner surface. The resting potential is thus replaced by an action potential, which in the example given above is equal to +35 mV. In unmyelinated fibers, the nerve impulse is a wave of change in membrane permeability that moves along the axon and promotes the liberation of a chemical mediator when it reaches the axon terminal (telodendron). The above graph shows schematically what is registered by a cathode ray oscilloscope during passage of the nerve impulse through a small segment of the nerve fiber. (Conduction in a myelinated nerve fiber is illustrated in Fig 9–20.) The electrodes were placed as shown in the upper drawing, one inside the axon and the other on the external surface of the axonal membrane.

nism that redistributes the sodium and potassium ions on both sides of the axon membrane in concentrations equal to those present before stimulation. The wave progresses along the axon up to the axon terminal, where it promotes the liberation of neurotransmitters into the synaptic gap.

In myelinated nerve fibers, local changes occur only at the nodes of Ranvier. Along the internodes, the insulating effect of myelin prevents the continuous propagation of the impulse. Therefore, the impulse jumps from one node to the other. This **saltatory conduction** is faster than continuous conduction (Fig 9–20). Because membrane permeability is changed only at the nodes of Ranvier and not along the internodes, there is less ion transport in saltatory conduction than in continuous conduction; consequently, less energy is expended in the process.

The energy used in the conduction of the impulse is restored by an increase in the axonal metabolism, with enhanced oxygen consumption and heat production.

Nerve impulse conduction can be blocked by cold, heat, or pressure on the nerve fiber. More complete blocking is obtained by application of local anesthetics.

According to their conductive properties, nerve fibers may be divided into 3 classes: A, B, and C. Type A fibers are myelinated, have large diameters and long internodes, and conduct impulses with high velocity (15–100 m/s). Type B fibers have smaller diameters, shorter internodes, and medium velocity of conduction (3–14 m/s). Type C fibers are thin and unmyelinated, with slow conduction velocity (0.5–2 m/s).

Nerve impulses are transmitted from one neuron to another or to an effector cell by the neurotransmitters liberated at synapses (Figs 9–21 and 9–22). The transmission substance is stored in synaptic vesicles and liberated by the nerve impulse. It crosses the presynaptic membrane and attaches to specific receptors in the postsynaptic membrane, where it causes a localized increase in the permeability to ions. This change in membrane permeability spreads along the nerve cell and is responsible for the propagation of the impulse.

After performing its function, the excess neurotransmitter, acetylcholine, is removed by the degradative action of the enzyme acetylcholinesterase. The entire process is very rapid and can occur, for brief periods of time, over 100 times a second.

The neurotransmitter in postganglionic endings of the sympathetic system is norepinephrine.

Node of Ranvier (stimulated)

Node of Ranvier (refractory)

Figure 9–20. Conduction of the nerve impulse through a myelinated nerve fiber. In this fiber, the movements of Na⁺ and K⁺ described in unmyelinated fibers (Fig 9–19) take place only at the nodes of Ranvier. The presence of a myelin sheath covering each internode makes a continuous transmission of the impulse impossible, for myelin is a good electrical insulating material. The electrical field generated at each node jumps the internode and excites the next node. This type of conduction is called saltatory and is very fast. After its stimulation, the node of Ranvier remains refractory for a short time. For this reason, even if the electrical field produced at each node spreads in both directions (dotted arrows), physiologic nerve impulses move in one direction only (solid arrow in the center of the fiber).

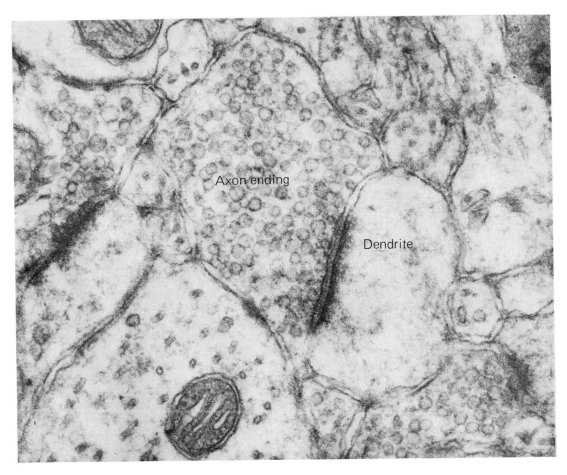

Figure 9–21. Electron micrograph of cerebral cortex. Near the center of the figure there is a cholinergic synapse between one axon ending and a dendrite. At the synapse, both the axonal (presynaptic) membrane and the dendritic (postsynaptic) membrane are thicker. The axon ending contains numerous synaptic vesicles. × 90,000. (Courtesy of A Peters.)

Synaptic vesicles containing norepinephrine are usually larger than those containing acetylcholine, and they usually have an electron-dense core separated from its limiting membrane by a light zone (Fig 9–22).

Other neurotransmitters exist besides acetylcholine and norepinephrine. This function has been demonstrated for gamma-aminobutyric acid (GABA), glutamic acid, dopamine, serotonin (5-hydroxytryptamine, 5-HT), and glycine.

In mammals, gamma-aminobutyric acid is localized exclusively in the central nervous system. There is evidence suggesting that it may function as an inhibitory chemical transmitter. In the nervous system of crustaceans, the role of gamma-aminobutyric acid as an inhibitory transmitter seems well established. Recent investigations have demonstrated the presence of a new class of peptide neurotransmitters that are potent inhibitors of pain receptors. Endorphins and enkephalins are natural brain peptides exhibiting morphinelike analgesic powers that may also regulate behavior. The present concepts of the production, liberation, and inac-

tivation of the 2 best-known chemical mediators are summarized in Fig 9–23.

The abundance of RNA in the perikaryon suggests intense protein synthesis, which has been confirmed by radioautographic studies using ³H-leucine and other labeled amino acids. The actively synthesized and labeled protein molecules migrate down the axons (anterograde transport) at several speeds, but there are 2 main rates: a fast rate in the range of hundreds of millimeters per day and a slow rate in the range of several millimeters per day. In nongrowing animals, these protein molecules are probably used to replace similar molecules broken down in the axon. It has been shown that smaller molecules can also be transported along the axon. Experimental evidence has been presented to show that transport of protein can also occur in a centripetal direction (retrograde transport) from the axon to the perikaryon.

Almost no ribosomes are present in the axon, and these cellular processes depend on their perikaryons for the synthesis of proteins. The observations recently reported of substances that in-

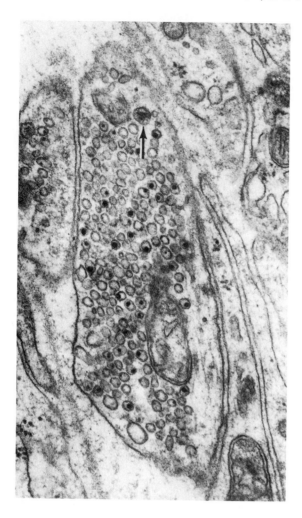

Figure 9–22. Norepinephrine nerve ending of pineal gland. There are many vesicles of 50 nm with a dark, electron-dense core. There are also a few large, pale vesicles, whose function is not known. (Courtesy of A Machado.)

hibit protein synthesis acting on the memory of animals call attention to the importance of Nissl bodies and protein metabolism in the function of the nervous system.

A trophic function has been ascribed to the nervous system of mammals for the structures it innervates. It is known that denervation of organs such as glands and muscles can lead to their atrophy, with functional and morphologic recuperation after reinnervation. Whether this atrophy is solely a consequence of disuse is an open question. In the lower vertebrates, the peripheral nerves have a trophic function that is not dependent on the nerve impulse.

DEGENERATION & REGENERATION

Central or peripheral neurons do not divide; their degeneration represents a permanent loss. Neuronal processes in the central nervous system are, within very narrow limits, replaceable by growth through the synthetic activity of their perikaryons. Peripheral nerve fibers can regenerate if their perikaryons are not destroyed.

Death of a nerve cell is limited to its perikaryon and processes. The neurons functionally connected to the dead neuron do not die, except for those neurons with only one link. In this instance, the isolated neuron undergoes **transneuronal degeneration.**

In contrast to nerve cells, neuroglia of the central nervous system and Schwann cells and ganglionic satellite cells of the peripheral nervous system are able to divide by mitosis. Spaces left in the central nervous system by nerve cells lost by disease or injury are occupied by neuroglia.

Since nerves are widely distributed throughout the body, they are often subjected to injury. When a nerve axon is transected, degenerative changes take place, followed by a reparative phase.

In a wounded nerve fiber, it is important to distinguish the changes occurring in the proximal segment from those in the distal segment. The proximal segment maintains its continuity with the trophic center (perikaryon) and frequently regenerates. The distal segment, separated from the nerve cell body, degenerates totally and is absorbed by the tissue macrophages (Fig 9–24).

Axonal injury causes the following changes in the perikaryon: (1) chromatolysis, ie, dissolution of Nissl substances with a consequent decrease in cytoplasmic basophilia; (2) increase in the volume of the perikaryon; and (3) migration of the nucleus to a peripheral position in the perikaryon. The proximal segment of the axon degenerates close to the wound for a short distance, but growth starts as soon as debris is removed by macrophages.

In the nerve stub distal to the injury, both the axon (now separated from its trophic center) and the myelin sheath degenerate completely, and their remnants, excluding their connective tissue and perineurial sheaths, are removed by macrophages (Fig 9–24B). While these regressive changes take place, the Schwann cells proliferate within the remaining connective tissue sleeve, giving rise to solid cellular columns. These rows of Schwann cells serve as guides to the sprouting axons formed during the reparative phase.

After these regressive changes, the proximal segment of the axon which is connected to the trophic center (perikaryon) grows and branches, forming several filaments that progress in the direction of the columns of Schwann cells (Fig 9–24C). Only those fibers that penetrate these Schwann cell columns will continue to grow and reach an effector

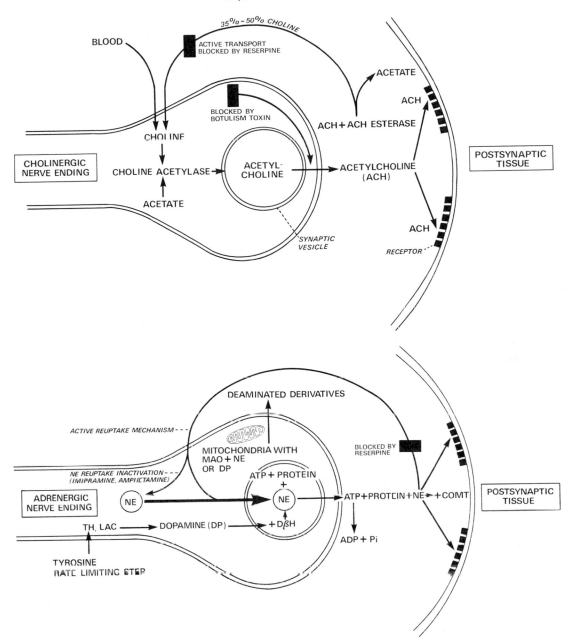

Figure 9–23. Schematic view of the production, liberation, and utilization of acetylcholine and norepinephrine. *Top:* Acetylcholine (ACH) is synthesized at the nerve ending from choline and acetate with the participation of the enzyme choline acetylase. The acetylcholine thus produced is stored in synaptic vesicles. When the nerve impulse reaches the axonal terminal, quanta of acetylcholine are liberated; they activate specific receptors located in the outer part of the cell membrane of perikaryons, dendrites, or effector cells (muscles, glands). Immediately after this activation, acetylcholine is hydrolyzed to acetate and choline by the enzyme acetylcholinesterase. By active transport, choline molecules reenter the axon ending, where they are utilized again. Reserpine inhibits the active transport of choline, thus preventing its reutilization. *Bottom:* Norepinephrine (NE) is synthesized in the nerve ending and probably also in the perikaryon, migrating through the axon to its terminal. It is synthesized from tyrosine through a dopamine step by the action of 3 enzymes: tyrosine hydrolase (TH), aromatic L-amino acid decarboxylase (LAC), and dopamine β-hydroxylase (DβH). Norepinephrine is stored in vesicles which also contain protein and ATP. Norepinephrine is released in quanta, and the ATP and protein are liberated at the same time. Cells sensitive to norepinephrine contain specific receptors in their membranes to which the mediator is attached, thus producing its effects. A portion of norepinephrine is degraded by the enzyme catechol-O-methyltransferase (COMT); however, some norepinephrine is transported back into the nerve endings and is used again. The ATP serves as energy source for this reuptake of norepinephrine. Reentry is blocked by reserpine. Exogenous norepinephrine injected into an animal is also stored in synaptic vesicles. Note that monoamine oxidase (MAO) is intracellular, so that some norepinephrine is being constantly deaminated in adrenergic endings.

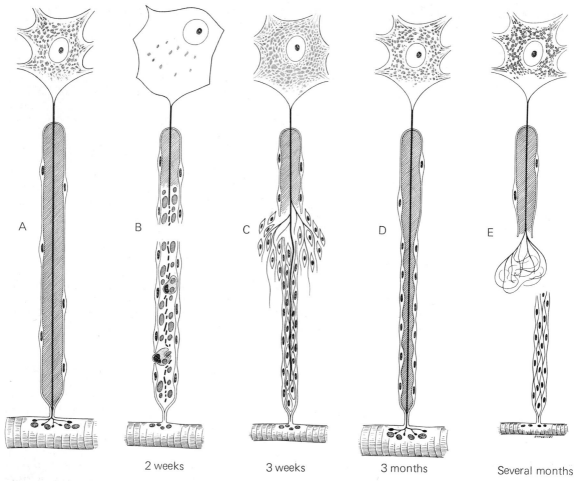

| 2 weeks | 3 weeks | 3 months | Several months |

Figure 9–24. Main changes that take place in an injured nerve fiber. *A:* Normal nerve fiber, with its perikaryon and the effector cell (striated skeletal muscle). Note the position of the neuron nucleus and the amount and distribution of Nissl bodies. *B:* When the fiber is injured, the neuronal nucleus moves to the cell periphery and Nissl bodies become greatly reduced in number. The nerve fiber distal to the injury degenerates along with its myelin sheath. Debris is phagocytosed by macrophages. *C:* The muscle fiber shows a pronounced disuse atrophy. Schwann cells proliferate, forming a compact cord penetrated by the growing axon. The axon grows at a rate of 0.5–3 mm/d. *D:* In this example, the nerve fiber regeneration was successful. Note that the muscle fiber was also regenerated after receiving nerve stimuli. *E:* When the axon does not penetrate the cord of Schwann cells, its growth is not organized. (Redrawn and reproduced, with permission, from Willis RA, Willis AT: *The Principles of Pathology and Bacteriology,* 3rd ed. Butterworth, 1972.)

organ (Fig 9–24D). When there is an extensive gap between the distal and proximal segments, or when the distal segment disappears altogether (as in the case of amputation of a limb), the newly grown nerve fibers may form a painful bulbous mass, improperly called an **amputation neuroma** (Fig 9–24E).

Regeneration is functionally efficient only when the fibers find the columns of Schwann cells directed to the correct place. This possibility is increased for the reason that each regenerating fiber gives origin to several processes and each column of Schwann cells receives processes from several regenerating fibers. In an injured mixed nerve, however, if regenerating sensory fibers grow into columns connected to motor end-plates that were occupied by motor fibers, the function of the muscle will not be reestablished.

GANGLIA

An aggregation of nerve cell bodies outside the central nervous system is called a **nerve ganglion.** Ganglia are usually ovoid structures encapsulated by dense connective tissue and associated with nerves.

Intramural ganglia are very small, consisting of only a few nerve cells, and are located within viscera, especially the walls of the digestive tract.

All intramural ganglia belong to the parasympathetic system.

Two types of nerve ganglia can be distinguished on the basis of differing morphology and function: **craniospinal** or **dorsal root ganglia** (sensory), which occur at the dorsal (posterior) root of the spinal nerves and also in the path of some cranial nerves; and **autonomic ganglia,** which are associated with nerves of the autonomic system.

A capsule of connective tissue surrounding each ganglion is continuous with the connective tissue within it and with the perineurium and epineurium of the pre- and postganglionic nerves.

In ganglia, the body of each ganglion cell is enveloped by a layer of small cuboidal cells called **satellite cells.** A thin fibrous layer of connective tissue envelops each satellite cell-encapsulated perikaryon.

Craniospinal Ganglia

Craniospinal ganglia are located in the dorsal roots of the spinal nerves and in the paths of some cranial nerves. Their function is to carry to the central nervous system impulses generated by various sensory receptors.

Craniospinal ganglia have pseudounipolar neurons whose T-shaped process sends one branch to the periphery and the other to the central nervous system. The 2 branches of the single T-shaped process constitute one axon, and the peripheral branch has a dendritic arborization. In this instance, the dendrites are not expansions of the cell body but of an axon. The nerve impulse goes directly from the periphery to the central nervous system, bypassing the perikaryon. The perikaryons of pseudounipolar neurons therefore do not receive nerve impulses, and their function is exclusively

trophic. The single axonal process of this cell makes several irregular turns around the cell body before its bifurcation, which occurs outside the capsule of satellite cells.

The ganglia from the acoustic nerve are the only cranial ganglia whose cells are bipolar. During the expansion of the craniospinal ganglia, the neurons, which are initially bipolar, fuse the initial segments of their prolongations, giving rise to the T-shaped process.

Craniospinal ganglia contain, side-by-side, small nerve cell bodies 15–30 μm in diameter and large ones about 120 μm in diameter. The cell bodies predominate in the periphery of the ganglion, where they form the cortical zone, which is poor in nerve fibers. The central part of the ganglion shows a great predominance of nerve fibers, forming an axial or medullary zone where only a few perikaryons occur in isolated groups.

In histologic sections, perikaryons of pseudounipolar neurons appear as globular bodies. The site of emergence of the single process is rarely seen. These neurons usually show fine Nissl bodies and droplets with lipofuscin (Fig 9–25).

Autonomic Ganglia

Autonomic ganglia appear as bulbous dilatations in autonomic nerves. Some are located within certain organs, especially in the walls of the digestive tract, where they constitute the intramural ganglia. Intramural ganglia are devoid of connective tissue capsules, and their cells are supported by the stroma of the organ in which they are found.

In autonomic ganglia, the cell bodies do not show the peripheral localization seen in craniospinal ganglia; consequently, a cortical layer is not observed. Autonomic ganglia usually have multipo-

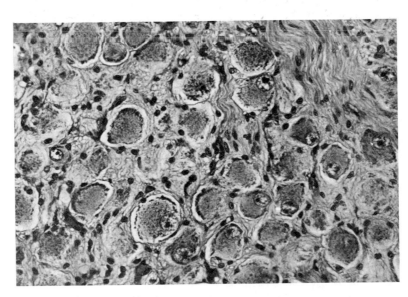

Figure 9–25. Photomicrograph of a spinal ganglion section, showing neurons, satellite cells, and nerve fiber. H&E stain, × 300.

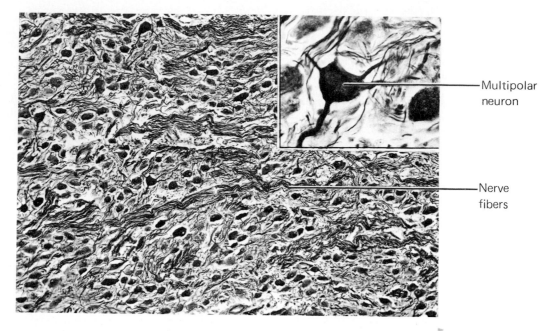

Figure 9–26. Photomicrographs of silver-stained section from an autonomic nerve ganglion. Neurons and nerve fibers appear black. × 80. The inset shows a multipolar ganglion neuron. × 250.

lar neurons, which may appear star-shaped in histologic sections (Fig 9–26). As with craniospinal ganglia, autonomic ganglia show neurons with fine Nissl bodies.

The neurons of autonomic ganglia are frequently enveloped by a layer of satellite cells, which is usually incomplete. In intramural ganglia, only a few satellite cells are seen around each neuron.

GRAY MATTER & WHITE MATTER

The central nervous system is composed of white matter and gray matter. White matter contains myelinated and unmyelinated fibers, oligodendrocytes, fibrous astrocytes, and microglial cells. Gray matter contains perikaryons, unmyelinated and myelinated fibers (mostly the former), protoplasmic astrocytes, oligodendrocytes, and microglial cells. The characteristic color of the white matter is a clue to the large number of myelinated nerve fibers.

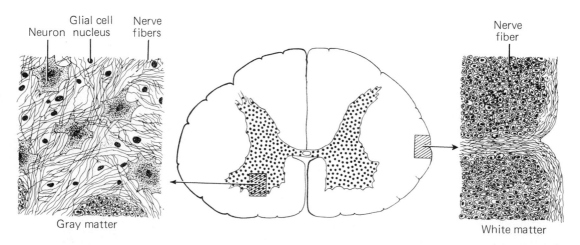

Figure 9–27. *Center:* Cross section through the spinal cord. *Left:* Gray matter. *Right:* White matter.

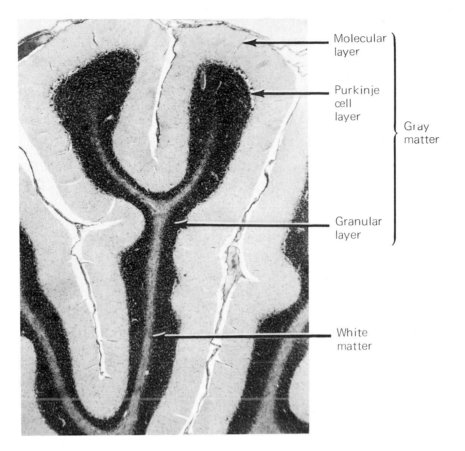

Molecular
layer

Purkinje
cell
layer

Gray
matter

Granular
layer

White
matter

Figure 9−28. Photomicrograph of a portion of cerebellum. Each lobule contains a core of white matter and 3 layers of gray matter: granular, Purkinje, and molecular layers. H&E stain, × 28.

In cross sections of the spinal cord, white matter appears externally around the periphery and gray matter appears centrally, assuming the shape of an H (Fig 9–27). In the horizontal bar of this H is an opening, the central canal, which is a remnant of the embryonic neural tube lumen lined by ependymal cells. The gray matter of the ventral bars of the H forms the anterior horns, which contain

motor neurons that make up the ventral roots of the spinal nerves. It also forms the posterior horns, which receive sensory fibers from neurons in the spinal ganglia (dorsal roots).

Spinal cord neurons are large and multipolar, especially in the anterior horns, where large motor neurons are found (Fig 9–27).

The cerebellum has 2 hemispheres separated

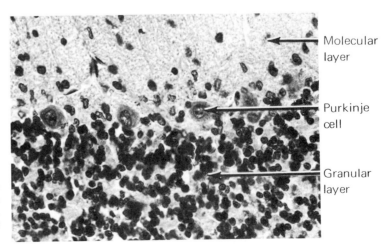

Molecular
layer

Purkinje
cell

Granular
layer

Figure 9−29 (at right). Photomicrograph of cerebellar cortex. This staining procedure does not reveal the unusually large dendritic arborization of the Purkinje cell, which is diagrammatically illustrated in Fig 9–2. H&E stain, × 250.

by the **vermis.** The surface of the cerebellum has
many furrows perpendicular to the vermis. These
furrows divide the organ into lobules, each of which
has a superficial layer of gray matter (cortex) and a
core of white matter (Fig 9–28). In the interior of
the white matter, deep in the cerebellum, isolated
regions of gray matter also appear.

The cerebellar cortex has 3 layers: an inner
molecular layer, a central layer of Purkinje cells,
and an outer granular layer (Fig 9–29). The neurons
of the granular layer are the smallest in the human
body (5 μm in diameter) and have a typical structure. Each granular cell (cerebellar granule) has 3–6
dendrites and, as usual, one axon. The Purkinje
cells are quite large. The dendrites of Purkinje cells
divide repeatedly in one plane, forming a sort of fan
(Fig 9–2). The most superficial layer of the cerebellum (the molecular layer) has few perikaryons and
many unmyelinated nerve fibers.

Like the cerebellum, the cerebrum also has a
cortex of gray matter and a central area of white
matter in which are found the nuclei of gray matter.
The surface of the cerebrum is increased by many
gyri, which are elevations separated by depressions
named sulci. The cytology of the cerebral cortex
varies according to the area. The majority of the
cells of the cortex have perikaryons which are pyramidal, stellate, or spindle-shaped.

MENINGES

The central nervous system is protected by the
skull and the vertebral column. It is also encased in
membranes of connective tissue called the meninges.

Starting with the outermost layer, the meninges are named **dura mater, arachnoid,** and **pia
mater.** Dura mater is also called **pachymeninx.** The
arachnoid and the pia mater are linked together and
are often considered as a single membrane called
the **pia-arachnoid** or **leptomeninx** (Fig 9–30).

Dura Mater

The dura mater is the external meninx, made of
dense connective tissue continuous with the periosteum of the skull bones. The dura mater that envelops the spinal cord is separated from the periosteum of the vertebrae by the epidural space, which
contains thin-walled veins, loose connective tissue,
and fat.

The dura mater is always separated from the
arachnoid by a thin space, the subdural space. The
internal surface of all dura mater, as well as its
external surface in the spinal cord, is covered by
simple squamous epithelium of mesenchymal origin (Fig 9–30).

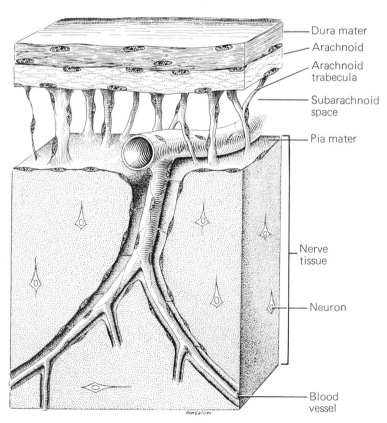

Figure 9–30. Schematic drawing of the meninges. The blood vessel initially located in the subarachnoid space penetrates
the nerve tissue and is partly enveloped by the pia mater.

Arachnoid

The arachnoid has 2 components: a layer in contact with the dura mater and a system of trabeculae connecting that layer with the pia mater. The cavities between the trabeculae form the **subarachnoid space,** which is filled with cerebrospinal fluid and is completely separated from the subdural space.

The arachnoid is composed of connective tissue devoid of blood vessels. Its surfaces are covered by the same type of simple squamous epithelium that covers the dura mater. Since, in the spinal cord, the arachnoid has fewer trabeculae, it can be more clearly distinguished from pia mater.

In some areas, the arachnoid perforates the dura mater, forming protrusions that terminate in venous sinuses in the dura mater. These protrusions, which contain centrally located trabeculae, are called **arachnoid villi.** Their function is to transfer cerebrospinal fluid to the blood of the venous sinuses.

Pia Mater

The pia mater contains many blood vessels and is located quite close to the nerve tissue, but it is not in contact with nerve cells or fibers. Between the pia mater and the neural elements is a thin layer of neuroglial processes, firmly adherent to the pia mater.

The pia mater follows all the irregularities of the surface of the central nervous system and penetrates into it to some extent along with the blood vessels. It is covered by squamous cells of mesenchymal origin.

Blood vessels penetrate the central nervous system through tunnels covered by pia mater and called the **perivascular spaces** (Fig 9–30). The pia mater disappears before the blood vessels are transformed into capillaries. In the central nervous system, the blood capillaries are completely covered by expansions of the neuroglial cell processes.

Blood-Brain Barrier

There is a barrier that prevents the passage of certain substances from the blood to nerve tissue. This functional barrier is termed the **blood-brain barrier.** For example, intravenously injected trypan blue appears in the intercellular spaces of all tissues except the central nervous system.

The blood-brain barrier results from the reduced permeability that is a property of blood capillaries of nerve tissue. Occluding junctions, which provide continuity between the endothelial cells of these capillaries, represent the main structural component of the barrier. The cytoplasm of these endothelial cells does not have the fenestrations found in many other locations. It is also possible that expansions of neuroglial cell processes that envelop the capillaries are partly responsible for their low permeability.

THE CHOROID PLEXUS & THE CEREBROSPINAL FLUID

Choroid Plexus

The choroid plexuses (telae choroideae) are invaginated folds of pia mater that penetrate into the interior of the ventricles. They are found in the roofs of the third and fourth ventricles and in part in the walls of the lateral ventricles.

The choroid plexuses are composed of loose connective tissue of the pia mater, covered by a simple cuboidal or low columnar epithelium of neural tube origin (Fig 9–31). The epithelial cells possess numerous irregular microvilli whose free ends are dilated. Their cytoplasm is rich in mitochondria, and there are junctional complexes near their free ends.

The connective tissue of the choroid plexuses is quite cellular, containing many macrophages. These cells avidly engulf intravenously injected supravital dyes such as trypan blue. The blood-brain barrier does not exist in the choroid plexuses. The endothelium of their fenestrated capillaries exhibits pores closed by thin diaphragms. The endothelial cells are held together by tight junctions. These cells are the site of the so-called "blood-cerebrospinal fluid barrier."

The main function of the choroid plexuses is to secrete cerebrospinal fluid, a thin watery fluid actively secreted by the epithelial cells covering the plexuses. Among the plexuses are a few absorbing cells.

Cerebrospinal Fluid

This liquid, elaborated by the choroid plexuses, contains only a small percentage of solids and completely fills the ventricles, central canal of the spinal cord, subarachnoid space, and perivascular space. It is important for the metabolism of the central nervous system and represents a protective device, forming a liquid layer in the subarachnoid space. This layer cushions the nerve tissue against trauma.

Adult males have about 100 mL of cerebrospinal fluid. The fluid is clear, has a low density (1.004–1.008), and is very low in protein content. It contains relatively high concentrations of sodium, potassium, and chloride, a few desquamated cells, and 2–5 lymphocytes per microliter.

Cerebrospinal fluid is continuously produced, with an outflow (up to 200 mL/d) in cranial lesions that penetrate the arachnoid. Substances entering the cerebrospinal fluid must pass through the cells of the choroid plexus.

Cerebrospinal fluid circulates through the central nervous system and is absorbed by the veins around nerve tissue. Nerve tissue is completely devoid of lymphatic vessels.

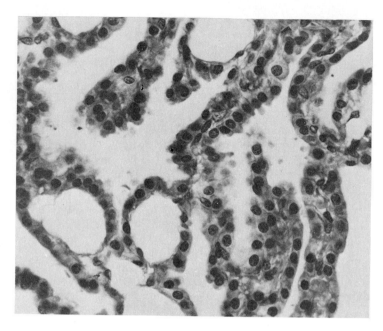

Figure 9 –31. Photomicrograph of the choroid plexus. The numerous folds are covered by simple cuboidal epithelium. H&E stain, × 400.

•   •   •

References

Akert K & others: The fine structure of the perineurial endothelium. Cell Tissue Res 165:281, 1976.

Axelrod J: Neurotransmitters. Sci Am 230:58, June 1974.

Blunt MJ, Wendell-Smith CP, Baldwin F: Glia-nerve fibre relationships in mammalian optic nerve. J Anat 99:1, 1965.

Bourne GH (editor): *The Structure and Function of Nervous Tissue.* Vol 1. Academic Press, 1968.

Brightman MW, Palay SL: The fine structure of ependyma in the brain of the rat. J Cell Biol 19:415, 1963.

Bunge RP: Glial cells and the central myelin sheath. Physiol Rev 48:197, 1968.

Bunge RP, Bunge MB, Cochran M: Some factors influencing the proliferation and differentiation of myelin-forming cells. Neurology 28:59, 1978.

Cajal S: *Histologie du Système Nerveux de l'Homme et des Vertébrés.* Vol 2. Paris: Librairie Maloine, 1911.

Davis R, Koelle GB: Electron microscopic localization of acetylcholinesterase at the neuromuscular junction by the gold-thiocholine and gold-thiolacetic acid methods. J Cell Biol 34:157, 1967.

De Robertis EDP: Ultrastructure and cytochemistry of the synaptic region. Science 156:907, 1967.

Droz B: Protein metabolism in nerve cells. Int Rev Cytol 25:363, 1969.

Friede RL: Enzyme histochemistry of neuroglia. In: *Biology of Neuroglia.* De Robertis EDP, Correa R (editors). Elsevier, 1965.

Friede RL, Samorajski T: The clefts of Schmidt-Lanterman: A quantitative electron microscopic study of their structure in developing and adult sciatic nerves of the rat. Anat Rec 165:89, 1969.

Friede RL, Samorajski T: Myelin formation in the sciatic nerve of the rat: A quantitative electron microscopic, histochemical, and radioautographic study. J Neuropathol Exp Neurol 27:540, 1968.

Hamberger A, Hansson HA, Sjostrand J: Surface structure of isolated neurons: Detachment of nerve terminals during axon regeneration. J Cell Biol 47:319, 1970.

Hydén H: *The Neuron.* Elsevier, 1967.

Jacobson M, Hunt RK: The origins of nerve-cell specificity. Sci Am 228:26, Feb 1973.

Katz B: Elementary components of synaptic transmission. Naturwissenschaften 66:606, 1979.

Kreutzberg GW: Neuronal dynamics and axonal flow. 4. Blockage of intra-axonal enzyme transport by colchicine. Proc Natl Acad Sci USA 62:722, 1969.

Krstić RV: Observations on the nodes of Ranvier of rat sciatic nerve fibers under the scanning and transmission electron microscope. Period Biol 76:105, 1974.

Landon DN (editor): *The Peripheral Nerve.* Chapman & Hall, 1976.

Ling EA & others: Identification of glial cells in the brain of young rats. J Comp Neurol 149:43, 1973.

Morales R, Duncan D: Specialized contacts of astrocytes with astrocytes and other cell types in the spinal cord of the cat. Anat Rec 182:255, 1975.

Palay SL, Chan-Palay V: *Cerebellar Cortex, Cytology and Organization.* Springer-Verlag, 1974.

Pappas GD, Waxman SG: Synaptic fine structure—Morphological correlates of chemical and electronic transmission. In: *Structure and Function of Synapses.* Pappas GD, Purpura DP (editors). Raven Press, 1972.

Peters A, Palay SL, Webster HF: *The Fine Structure of the Nervous System: The Neurons and Supporting Cells.* Saunders, 1976.

Schmitt FO, Samson FE: Neuronal fibrous proteins. Neurosci Res Program Bull 6:117, 1968.

Shepherd GM: Microcircuits in the nervous system. Sci Am 238:93, Feb 1978.

Sotelo C, Palay SL: The fine structure of the lateral vestibular nucleus in the rat. 1. Neurons and neuroglia cells. J Cell Biol 36:151, 1968.

Thomas PK, Olsson Y: Microscopic anatomy and function of the connective tissue components of peripheral nerve. In: *Peripheral Neuropathy.* Dyck PJ, Thomas PK, Lambert EH (editors). Saunders, 1975.

Webster HD: The geometry of peripheral myelin sheaths during their formation and growth in rat sciatic nerves. J Cell Biol 48:348, 1971.

Weiss P: Neuronal dynamics. Neurosci Res Program Bull 5:371, 1967.

Wuerker RB, Kirkpatrick JB: Neuronal microtubules, neurofilaments, and microfilaments. Int Rev Cytol 33:45, 1972.

10 | The Sense Organs

Sensory organs receive information from both external and internal environments of the body and subsequently transmit that information to the central nervous system. In the distal portions of these organs are **receptors,** biologic transducers that convert various forms of physical (touch, light, sound) and chemical (taste, blood gas, pH) stimuli into changes of membrane potential. Following receptor stimulation, the resulting **generating** or **receptor potentials** are transferred to nerve fibers in the form of action potentials, and the information is directly integrated into the central nervous system.

Based on the cells that receive and transduce the incoming stimuli, 3 different types of receptors can be distinguished. The most ubiquitous receptors are dendritic expansions of specific ganglionic neurons. The transducing portions of their dendrites, which may range from simple free endings to complex encapsulations, generally relay information regarding pain, temperature, and tactile stimulation. A second group of receptors, consisting of specialized sensory cells, exhibit synaptic contacts with peripheral nerves. For example, cells in the taste buds or audioreceptors in the organ of Corti can transduce incoming stimuli and pass it on to innervating nerve fibers via chemical synapses. The third type of receptor consists of modified neurons that differentiate from specialized neuroepithelial cells. These receptor cells, which are present in the eye or olfactory region of the nose, for example, possess their own axons that send information directly into the brain.

These receptors create action potentials from various kinds of physical and chemical stimuli, eg, mechanical stimuli (pressure, tactile sensitivity, etc), thermal stimuli (heat and cold), electromagnetic energy (light), and chemical stimuli and concentration (taste, olfaction, blood CO_2 and O_2 concentration).

Most of these generating potentials are probably produced by changes in permeability of the membrane of the receptors, but the exact mechanism is not well understood.

Classification of Receptors

According to their functions, the principal receptors can be provisionally classified as follows:

(1) A system of receptors related to **somatic** and **visceral sensitivity.** These receptors are sensitive to pressure, vibration, temperature, and pain. In this group we include the mechanoreceptors responsible for relaying information on the degree of distention of hollow viscera, the digestive tract, the carotid sinus, etc.

(2) A **proprioceptor system,** which provides information on the position in space of different parts of the body. This system comprises the receptors of the vestibular part of the ear and receptors from the muscles, tendons, and joints.

(3) A **chemoreceptor system,** which participates in the gustatory and olfactory senses, including the receptors sensitive to CO_2 and O_2 present in the walls of blood vessels and those sensitive to food found in the digestive tract.

(4) An **audioreceptor system** responsible for hearing.

(5) A **photoreceptor system** responsible for vision.

RECEPTORS RELATED TO SUPERFICIAL & DEEP SENSATION

These receptors can be divided on morphologic grounds into free and encapsulated nerve terminals according to the absence or presence of a special connective tissue capsule. They consist of dendritic nerve endings and are responsible for the senses discussed below.

Touch

The sense of touch is related to Meissner's corpuscles and to free nerve endings in the epidermis. Meissner's endings are most numerous in hairless (glabrous) skin (eg, tips of fingers and toes, palms, soles, nipples, and lips). They are elongated structures in which wedge-shaped modified Schwann cells interdigitate, creating a multilaminar stack ensheathed in connective tissue. The axon enters at one pole, zigzags upwards through the stacked cells, and terminates at the other pole (Fig 10–1). Meissner's corpuscles generally lie in dermal

Pacinian

Meissner

Free endings

Ruffini

Krause

Muscle spindle

Golgi tendon organ

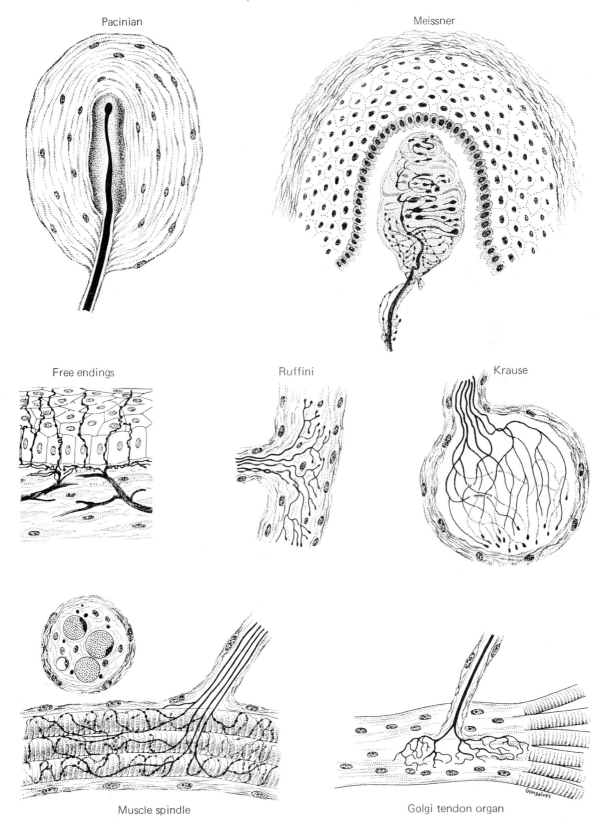

Figure 10–1. Various types of sensory endings of nerves. (Based partially on a drawing in Ham AW: *Histology,* 6th ed. Lippincott, 1969.)

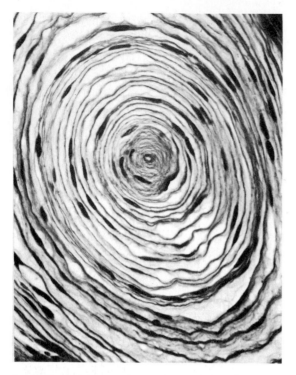

Figure 10–2. Photomicrograph of a transverse section of a human pacinian corpuscle. Observe the concentric layers of connective tissue surrounding the centrally disposed myelinated nerve. H&E stain, × 320.

papillae subjacent to the epidermis.

Dendrites of the free nerve endings lose their Schwann cells as they penetrate the basal layer of the epidermis. These naked nerve endings may reach up to the stratum corneum by passing through deep invaginations of the epidermal cells. When surrounding hair follicles, the naked nerve endings create an encapsulating network of longitudinal and circumferential branches. A number of free endings form associations with specialized tactile epidermal cells found in the basal layer of the epithelium. These cells, which stain differently from other epidermal cells, and their associated nerve endings are known as **Merkel's corpuscles.** Only a small proportion of free nerve endings participate in the reception of tactile stimuli.

Pressure

The main receptors for perception of pressure are the Meissner corpuscles described above and the pacinian corpuscles, which take the form of a nonmyelinated nerve ending surrounded by thin concentric layers of epitheliumlike fibroblasts. In transverse section, this corpuscle resembles a sliced onion. It is found mainly in the deep layer of the dermis, loose connective tissue in general, mesentery and visceral ligaments, and external genitalia of both males and females (Figs 10–1 and 10–2). **Ruffini's corpuscles** are one of the most common pres-

sure mechanoreceptors. They consist of a simple connective tissue capsule surrounding bundles of elongated collagen fibers and fluid. As the myelinated axon penetrates the capsule, the Schwann cell sheath is lost and the free nerve processes arborize and terminate among the collagen bundles. At present, all encapsulated nerve endings (pacinian, Meissner, and Ruffini) are of importance in transducing tactile stimulation.

Cold, Heat, & Pain

Receptors for these stimuli are the unmyelinated, unencapsulated free nerve endings that penetrate the epidermis. Although all free nerve endings are structurally similar, they are physiologically specific, and each will respond to only one cutaneous sensation. Temperature and pain receptors presently are considered to be unencapsulated nerve endings (Fig 10–1).

THE PROPRIOCEPTOR SYSTEM

The proprioceptor system comprises the vestibular receptors of the ear (discussed below) and sensory nerve endings of muscles, tendons, and joints. All human striated muscles contain encapsulated proprioceptors known as **muscle spindles.** The elongated spindles consist of a connective tissue capsule surrounding 2 types of sensory myofibers known as **intrafusal** fibers, which are easily distinguishable from the normal mechanical **extrafusal** muscle fibers. Within each spindle are 1–2 **nuclear bag fibers,** thin striated muscle cells extending through the spindle and exiting at each end. Near the center of the spindle, these fibers exhibit a baglike dilatation in which are clustered numerous myonuclei. Myofibrils are discontinuous in the region of the bag. The other intrafusal fiber found in the spindle is the **nuclear chain fiber,** an extremely thin striated muscle cell in which the nuclei are centrally aligned along the length of the fiber. Myelinated sensory (alpha) nerves penetrate the capsule and lose their Schwann cell sheath when they encounter the intrafusal fibers. **Primary sensory nerves** enwrap the central region of each intrafusal fiber, forming a spirallike sheath. **Secondary sensory nerves** branch and end in clusters called **flower spray endings.** The nerve endings lie within troughlike clefts of the sarcolemma. Each intrafusal fiber is also innervated by motor (gamma) nerves which regulate their contraction.

As muscles contract and relax, the spindle fibers passively follow along. Changes in the length of the intrafusal fibers result in the generation of action potentials in the enveloping sensory nerve fibers. The larger primary nerve endings are more responsive to dynamic stretching, while secondary nerve endings are more responsive to maintained (static) stretch. The gamma motor nerves cause intrafusal fibers to contract and increase the tension on the central (sensory) portion of the fibers, which results in an increased sensitivity of these stretch receptors. During cycles of contraction and relaxation, the spindles relay information to the brain, which deciphers this spatial information. Muscles controlling delicate movements (eg, those of the eye, hand, and neck) have proportionately more spindles than other muscles.

In the tendons, near the insertion sites of the muscle fibers, a connective tissue sheath encapsulates several collagen bundles that insert into adjacent myotendinous junctions. Sensory nerves penetrate the connective tissue capsule, lose their Schwann cell sheath, and arborize into an extensive network that envelops the collagen fibers of the tendon. These structures, known as **Golgi tendon organs,** are sensory receptors activated by the impinging pressure of the tendon collagen fibers as the muscle contracts or stretches.

Within the connective tissue of the joints, sensory receptors include free nerve endings, Ruffini corpuscles, and a few pacinian corpuscles. These receptors sense and relay spatial information to the central nervous system.

The structures mentioned above are sensitive to increases in tension and permit blindfolded persons to know the exact position of their limbs and also to regulate the amount of effort required to perform certain movements that call for variable amounts of muscular force.

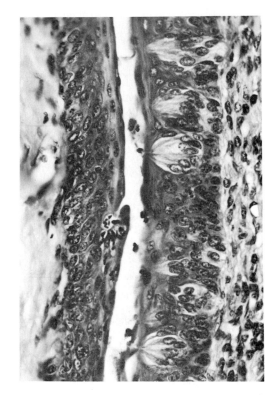

Figure 10 –4. Photomicrograph of a section of a circumvallate papilla of the tongue, showing the taste buds embedded in the epithelial layer. H&E stain, × 400.

THE CHEMORECEPTOR SYSTEM

Taste

Taste is a sensation perceived by the **taste buds,** receptors principally located on the tongue but also present in smaller numbers on the soft palate and laryngeal surface of the epiglottis. Lingual taste buds are found embedded within the stratified epithelium of the circumvallate, foliate,

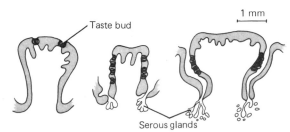

Figure 10 –3. Position of the taste buds on the 3 types of gustatory papillae. (Redrawn and reproduced, with permission, from Schmidt R [editor]: *Fundamentals of Sensory Physiology.* Springer-Verlag, 1978.)

and fungiform papillae. The oval taste buds extend from the basal lamina to a point below the surface, a structural organization that protects the sensory cells from abrasion. Chemicals enter through the **taste pore,** a small aperture providing access to the submerged taste bud.

Taste buds are composed of 3 cell types: basal cells, supporting cells, and sensory cells (Fig 10–5). Radioautographic studies using labeled DNA precursors have shown that the sensory cells have a short life span (about 10–12 days) and consequently a high turnover rate. New sensory cells are derived from the mitotic activity of the basal cells. The supporting cells have been considered to represent intermediate stages in sensory cell differentiation. Both sensory and supporting cells are columnar and exhibit microvilli on their apical surfaces. Chemical stimuli received by sensory cells are transduced into electrical impulses that are passed to innervating nerves through the release of membrane-active neurotransmitters.

Four fundamental taste sensations have been described in humans: acid, bitter, sweet, and salty. Putting small drops of solutions with different tastes on the fungiform papillae shows that some papillae are insensitive to some tastes whereas others are able to transmit more than one taste sensation. No structural differences have been described that

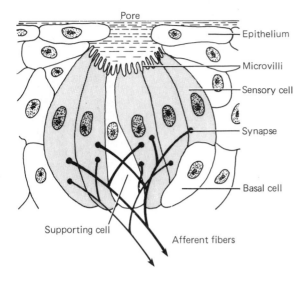

Figure 10 –5. Structure and innervation of a taste bud. The elements of the taste organ, the sensory, supporting, and basal cells, are arranged rather like the leaves in a bud. The whole structure is set below the epithelial surface, so that the microvilli of the sensory cells project into a fluid-filled space above them. Only 2 afferent fibers are shown; actually, about 50 fibers enter and branch within a single taste bud. (Redrawn and reproduced, with permission, from Schmidt R [editor]: *Fundamentals of Sensory Physiology.* Springer-Verlag, 1978.)

might explain the differences in sensitivity of the taste buds to various substances.

The 4 basic taste receptors are not evenly distributed in the tongue, so some regions of this organ are more sensitive to certain tastes than to others. The distribution of taste buds containing papillae on the lingual surface and their innervation are illustrated in Fig 10–6.

Olfaction

The olfactory chemoreceptors are located in a specialized area of the mucous membrane in the roof of the nasal cavity, the **olfactory epithelium.** This is a columnar pseudostratified epithelium composed of 3 types of cells:

The **supporting cells** have broad, cylindric apexes and narrower bases. On their free surface are microvilli which are submerged in the layer of serous fluid that covers the entire epithelial layer. Well-developed junctional complexes bind the supporting cells to the adjacent olfactory cells. The cells have a reddish-brown pigment that is responsible for the dark gray color of the olfactory mucosa (Fig 10–7).

The **basal cells** are small, spherical or cone-shaped, and form a single layer at the base of the epithelium. They have branching processes that extend among the other cells in the epithelium.

Between the basal cells and the supporting cells are the **olfactory cells,** bipolar neurons distinguished from the supporting cells by the posi-

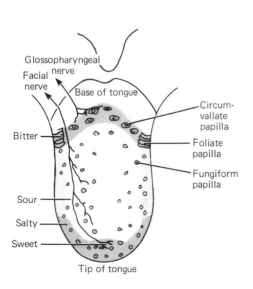

Figure 10 –6. Diagram summarizing the distribution of gustatory papillae, their innervation, and the regions of maximum sensitivity to the different qualities on the human tongue. (Redrawn and reproduced, with permission, from Schmidt R [editor]: *Fundamentals of Sensory Physiology.* Springer-Verlag, 1978.)

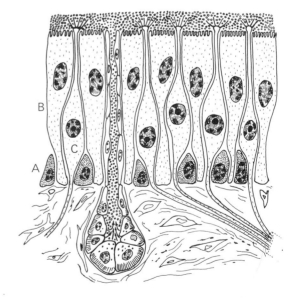

Figure 10 –7. Olfactory mucosa showing the 3 cell types and the gland. *A:* basal cells; *B:* supporting cells; *C:* olfactory cells.

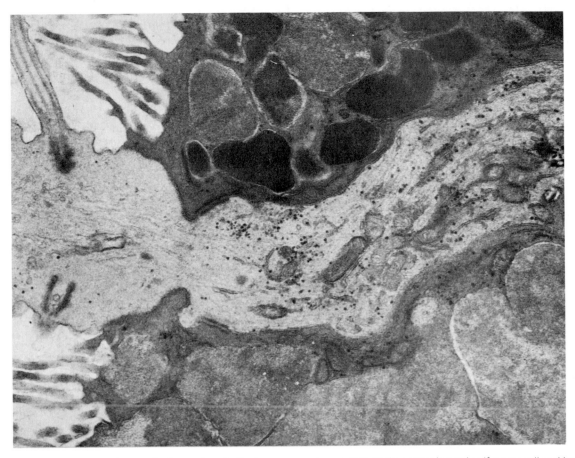

Figure 10 –8. Electron micrograph of a section of olfactory mucosa from a frog. In the center is a pale olfactory cell and its terminal dilatation with 2 basal bodies from which cilia emerge. × 28,000. (Courtesy of KR Porter.)

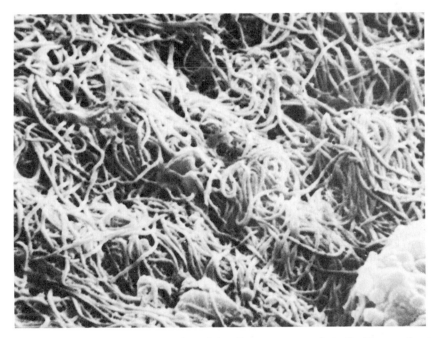

Figure 10 –9. Scanning electron micrograph of the surface of the olfactory mucosa of a turtle. Observe the dense net of cilia covering its surface. × 6600. (Courtesy of PP Graziadei.)

tion of their nuclei, which lie below the nuclei of the supporting cells. Their apexes show dilated areas from which arise 6–8 cilia (Fig 10–8). These cilia are long and nonmotile and are considered to be receptors, ie, the structures that respond to odoriferous substances by generating a receptor potential. Ciliary proximal segments show the usual 9 plus 2 microtubule axonemes. In the outer part of the cilium (70% of its length), all tubular filaments are single instead of the 9 double microtubules found in other cilia. Cilia are sensitive to chemical stimuli, and their mass enlarges considerably the receptor's surface (Fig 10–9). The efferent axons of these neurons unite in small bundles that are directed toward the central nervous system. It has been calculated that a human being has 10^7 receptors distributed in an area of 5 cm^2. In the lamina propria of the olfactory mucosa, in addition to the abundant vessels and nerves, glands of the tubulo-alveolar type are observed that have PAS-positive seromucous cells. The excretory ducts of these glands open onto the epithelial surface, and the continuous flow of their secretion cleans the apical portion of the olfactory cells. In this manner, compounds that stimulate the sense of olfaction are constantly being removed, thus keeping the receptors in a state of readiness to respond to new stimuli.

THE EYE

The eye is a complex and highly developed photosensitive organ that permits a fairly accurate analysis of the form, light intensity, and color reflected from objects. The eyes are located in protective bony structures of the skull—the **orbits**—and are basically made up of a globe, a lens system to focus the image, a layer of photosensitive cells, and a system of cells and nerves whose function it is to collect, process, and transmit visual information to the central nervous system. Each eye is composed of 3 concentric layers: (1) an external layer that consists of the **sclera** and the **cornea**; (2) a middle layer—also called the **vascular layer** or **uveal tract**—consisting of the **choroid, ciliary body,** and **iris;** and (3) an inner layer of nerve tissue, the **retina,** which communicates with the central nervous system through the **optic nerve** (Figs 10–10 and 10–11) and extends forward at the **ora serrata.** Beyond this point, it forms a continuous layer of unpigmented epithelium over the ciliary body and a layer of pigment epithelium over the posterior iris.

The **lens** of the eye is a biconvex transparent structure kept in position by a circular ligament, the **zonule** or **ligament of Zinn,** which extends from the lens into a thickening of the middle layer called the **ciliary body,** and by close apposition to the vitreous on its posterior side (Figs 10–10 and 10–11). Par-

tially covering the anterior surface of the lens is an opaque pigmented expansion of the middle layer called the **iris.** The round hole in the middle of the iris is the **pupil** (Fig 10–10).

The eye is composed of 3 compartments: the **anterior chamber,** which occupies the space between the cornea, the iris, and the lens; the **posterior chamber,** between the posterior iris, the ciliary process, the zonular attachments, and the lens; and the **vitreous space** behind the lens and zonular attachments and surrounded by the retina (Figs 10–10 and 10–11). Both the anterior and the posterior chambers contain a protein-rich fluid called **aqueous humor.** The vitreous space is filled by a viscous, gelatinous substance called **vitreous.**

External Layer or Tunica Fibrosa

The opaque white posterior five-sixths of the external layer of the eye is the **sclera,** forming in the human a segment of a sphere approximately 22 mm in diameter (Figs 10–10 and 10–11). The sclera consists of tough, dense connective tissue made up mainly of flat collagen bundles intersecting in various directions—maintaining a parallel position in relation to the surface of the organ—a moderate amount of ground substance, and a few fibroblasts. The external surface of the sclera—the **episclera**—is connected by a loose system of thin collagen fibers to a dense layer of connective tissue called **Tenon's capsule.** It comes into contact with the loose conjunctival stroma at the junction of the cornea with the sclera, also called the **limbus.** Between Tenon's capsule and the sclera is **Tenon's space.** It is because of this loose space that the eyeball can make rotating movements in all directions. Between the sclera and the choroid is a thin layer of loose connective tissue rich in melanocytes, fibroblasts, and elastic fibers called the **suprachoroidal lamina.** The sclera is relatively avascular.

In contrast to the posterior five-sixths of the eye, the anterior one-sixth—the **cornea**—is colorless and transparent (Figs 10–10 and 10–11). A transverse section of the cornea shows that it consists of 5 regions: epithelium, Bowman's membrane, stroma, Descemet's membrane, and endothelium (Fig 10–12). The corneal epithelium is stratified, squamous, and nonkeratinized and consists of 5 or 6 layers of cells. In the basal regions of these cells there are numerous mitotic figures responsible for the remarkable regenerating capacity of the cornea. The turnover time for these cells is approximately 7 days. The surface corneal cells show microvilli protruding into the space filled by the precorneal tear film, a protective layer of lipid and glycoprotein. The cornea has one of the richest sensory nerve supplies of any eye tissue.

Beneath the corneal epithelium lies a thick homogeneous layer 7–12 μm in diameter. It consists of collagen fibers crossing at random and a condensation of the intercellular substance, but no cells are found (Fig 10–13). This is **Bowman's mem-**

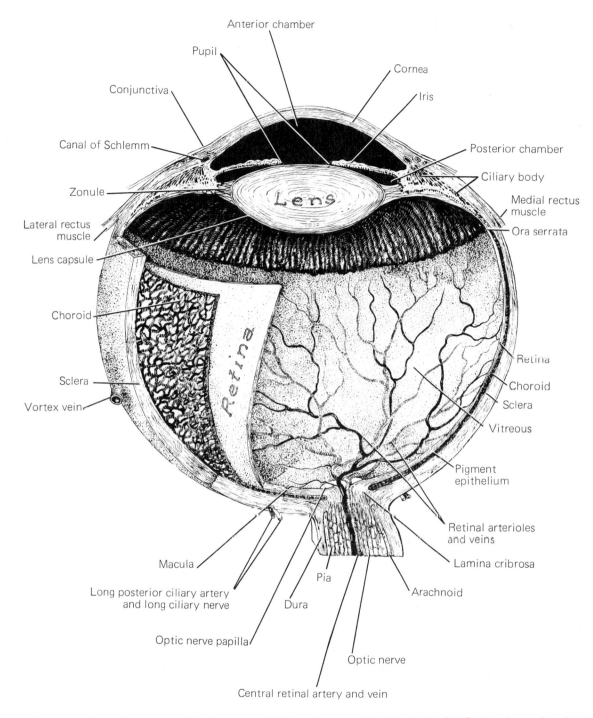

Figure 10 –10. Internal structures of the human eye. (Redrawn from an original drawing by Paul Peck and reproduced, with permission, from *The Anatomy of the Eye.* Courtesy of Lederle Laboratories.)

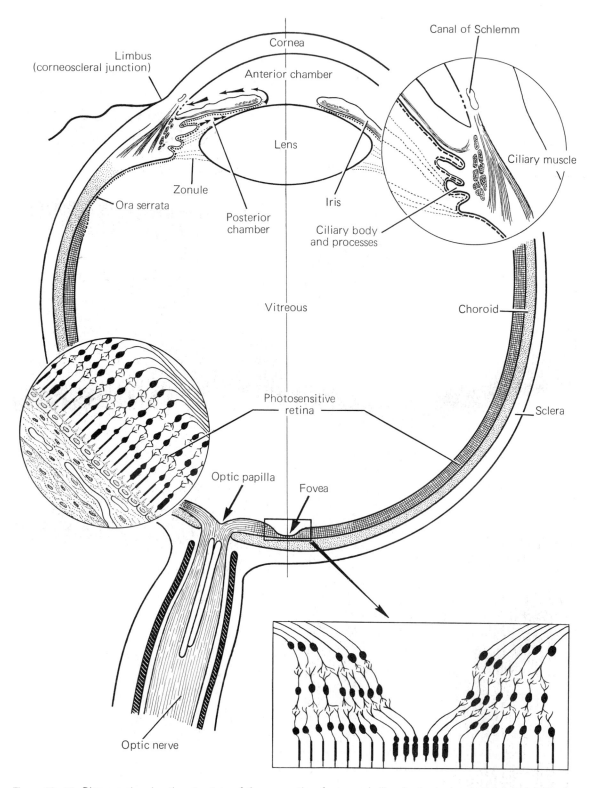

Figure 10–11. Diagram showing the structure of the eye, retina, fovea, and ciliary body. Arrows in the anterior chamber show the direction of flow of aqueous. (Modified and reproduced, with permission, from Ham AW: *Histology,* 6th ed. Lippincott, 1969.)

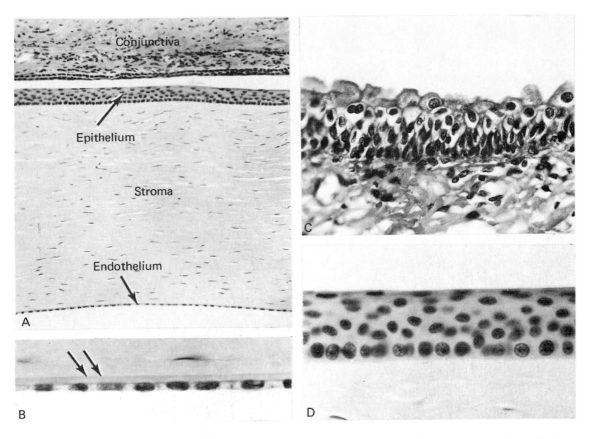

Figure 10–12. Photomicrographs of a transverse section of cornea. *A:* The cornea and conjunctiva seen in small enlargement. × 80. *B:* The posterior corneal epithelium (arrows indicate Descemet's membrane). × 400. *C:* Conjunctival epithelium. × 300. *D:* Anterior corneal epithelium. × 400.

brane, which contributes greatly to the stability and strength of the cornea. Below, the **stroma** is formed by several lamellas of parallel collagenous bundles that cross at an angle to each other. The collagen fibrils within each lamella are parallel to each other and run the full length of the cornea. Between the several layers, the cytoplasmic extensions of the fibroblasts are flattened like the wings of a butterfly. Both cells and fibers of the stroma are immersed in an amorphous metachromatic glycoprotein substance rich in chondroitin sulfate. Although the stroma is avascular, migrating lymphoid cells are normally present in the cornea.

Descemet's membrane is a thick (5–10 μm in diameter) homogeneous structure composed of fine collagenous filaments organized in a 3-dimensional network.

The **endothelium** of the cornea is typical simple squamous epithelium. These cells possess organelles characteristic of cells engaged in active transport and protein synthesis for secretion, which may relate to the synthesis and maintenance of Descemet's membrane.

The **corneoscleral junction** or **limbus** is an area of transition from the transparent collagenous bun-

dles of the cornea to the white opaque fibers of the sclera. It is highly vascularized, and its blood vessels assume an important role in corneal inflammatory processes. The cornea—an avascular structure—receives its metabolites by diffusion from adjacent vessels and from the fluid of the anterior chamber of the eye. In the region of the limbus in the stromal layer, an irregular endothelium-lined channel and other collecting channels merge to form the **canal of Schlemm** (Figs 10–10 and 10–11), which drains fluid from the anterior chamber of the eye. The fluid passes through the trabecular meshwork into the canal of Schlemm, which communicates externally with the venous system.

Middle or Vascular Layer

The middle (vascular) layer of the eye consists of 3 parts: choroid, ciliary body, and iris (Fig 10–10).

A. Choroid: The choroid is a highly vascularized coat. Between its blood vessels is found loose connective tissue rich in fibroblasts, macrophages, lymphocytes, mast cells, plasma cells, collagen fibers, and elastic fibers. Melanocytes are

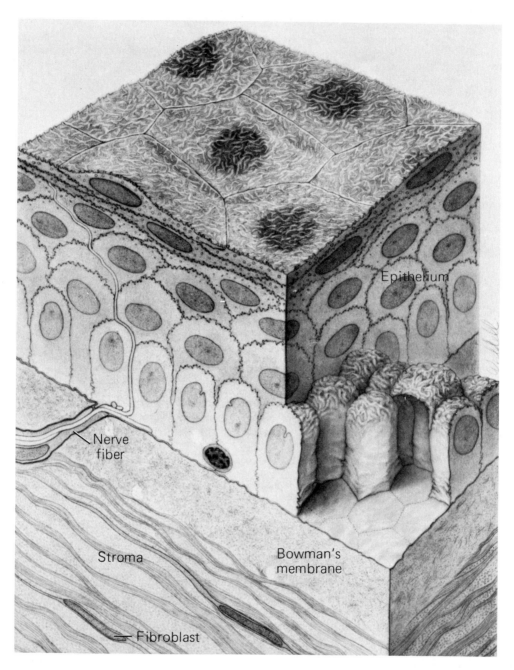

Figure 10 –13. Tridimensional drawing of the cornea. (Reproduced, with permission, from Hogan MJ, Alvarado JA, Weddell JE: *Histology of the Human Eye.* Saunders, 1971.)

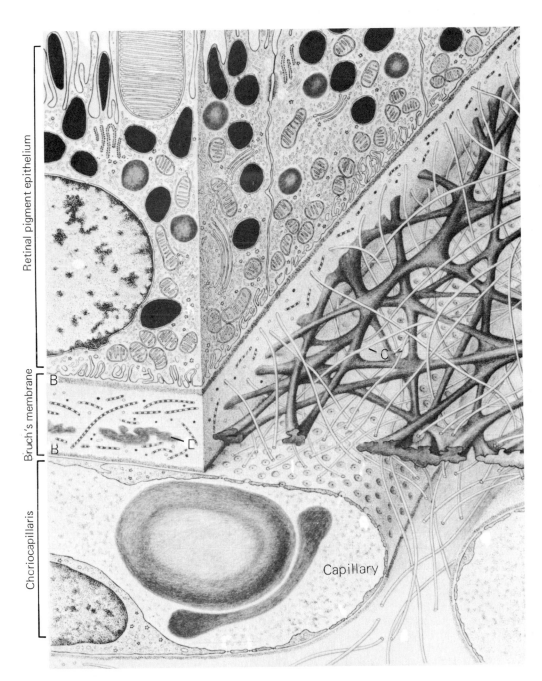

Figure 10 –14. Tridimensional drawing showing the constitution of Bruch's membrane and its relation to the pigment cell layer and choriocapillary layer. B, basal lamina; E, elastic fibers; C, collagen fibers. (Slightly modified and reproduced, with permission, from Hogan MJ, Alvarado JA, Weddell JE: *Histology of the Human Eye.* Saunders, 1971.)

abundant in this layer and give it its characteristic black color. The inner layer of the choroid is richer in small vessels than the outer layer and is called the **choriocapillary layer.** It has an important function in nutrition of the retina, and damage of this tissue causes serious damage to the retina. A thin (3–4 μm), amorphous hyaline membrane separates the choriocapillary layer from the retina. This is known as **Bruch's membrane** and extends from the **optic disk** to the ora serrata. It is PAS-positive. The optic disk, also called **optic papilla,** is the region where the optic nerve enters the eyeball (Fig 10–11).

Bruch's membrane is formed of 5 different layers. The central layer is made of a network of elastic fibers. This network is lined on its 2 surfaces by layers of collagen fibers that are covered by the basal lamina of the capillaries of the choriocapillary layer on one side and basal lamina of the pigment epithelium on the other side (Fig 10–14). (See p 200 for a description of the pigment epithelium.) The choroid is bound to the sclera by means of a loose layer of connective tissue rich in melanocytes called the **suprachoroidal lamina.**

B. Ciliary Body: The ciliary body is an anterior dilatation of the choroid at the level of the lens (Figs 10–10 and 10–11). It constitutes a continuous thickened ring which lines the inner surface of the anterior portion of the sclera. In transverse section, it forms a triangle. One of its faces is in contact with the vitreous, one with the sclera, and the third with the lens and the posterior chamber of the eye. This last face has an irregular surface and presents outgrowths called **ciliary processes** (Figs 10–10 and 10–11). The histologic structure of the ciliary body is basically loose connective tissue (rich in elastic fibers, vessels, and melanocytes) surrounding the **ciliary muscle** (Fig 10–11). This structure is composed of 3 bundles of smooth muscle fibers that insert on the sclera on one side and on different regions of the ciliary body on the other. One of these bundles has the function of stretching the choroid; another bundle, when contracted, relaxes the tension on the lens. These muscular movements are important in visual accommodation, as will be seen later in discussing the lens. The 2 surfaces of the ciliary body which face the vitreous, posterior chamber, and lens are covered by the anterior extension of the retina (Fig 10–11). In this region, the retina consists of only 2 cell layers. The layer directly adherent to the ciliary body consists of simple columnar cells rich in melanin. It corresponds to the forward projection of the pigment layer of the retina. The second layer, which covers the first, is derived from the sensory layer of the retina and consists of simple nonpigmented columnar epithelium (Fig 10–15A).

C. Ciliary Processes: The ciliary processes are ridgelike extensions of the ciliary body that have a loose connective tissue core and are covered by the 2 simple epithelial layers described above (Fig 10–15B). From the ciliary processes emerge their fibers

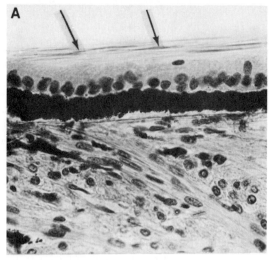

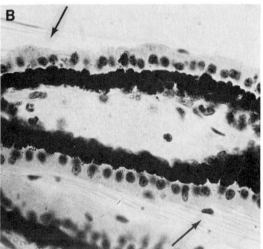

Figure 10–15. Photomicrographs of a ciliary body. *A:* Note the double layer, of which one consists of pigmented cells. *B:* The ciliary process is covered by epithelium on both sides. Arrows indicate zonular fibers. H&E stain, × 400.

(zonule fibers), which adhere to the lens and anchor it to the ciliary body (Fig 10–16). The outer nonpigmented layer in the ciliary processes is called the **ciliary epithelium,** and its cells, when observed in the electron microscope, have basal membrane infoldings characteristic of ion- and water-transporting cells (see Chapter 4). These cells secrete **aqueous humor.** This fluid, produced at the ciliary processes, flows toward the lens and passes between it and the iris, reaching the anterior chamber of the eye (see arrows in Fig 10–11). Once in the anterior chamber, it reverses direction and proceeds to the angle formed by the cornea with the basal part of the iris. It penetrates the tissue of the limbus in a series of labyrinthine spaces (trabecular meshwork) and finally reaches the irregular canal of Schlemm, lined by endothelial cells (Figs 10–10 and 10–11). This structure communicates with

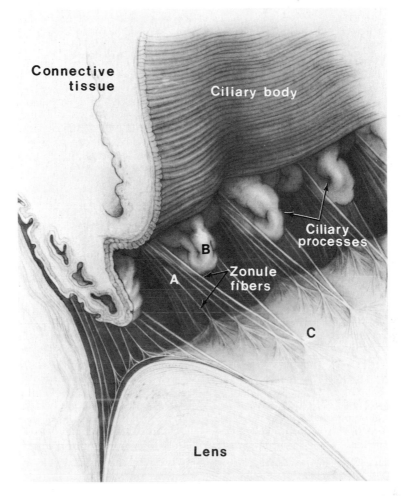

Figure 10 –16. Anterior view of the ciliary processes showing the zonules attaching to the lens. Zonules form columns (A) on either side of the ciliary processes (B), which meet on a single site (C) as they attach to the lens. (Reproduced, with permission, from Hogan MJ, Alvarado JA, Weddell JE: *Histology of the Human Eye.* Saunders, 1971.)

small veins of the sclera through which the aqueous humor escapes. Any impediment to the drainage of aqueous humor caused by an obstruction in the outflow channels results in an increase in intraocular pressure, causing **glaucoma**.

D. Iris: The iris is a membranous extension of the choroid that partially covers the lens, leaving a round opening in the center called the **pupil** (Fig 10–10). The anterior surface of the iris is irregular and rough, with grooves and ridges; the posterior surface is smooth. The anterior surface is formed by a discontinuous layer of pigment cells and fibroblasts. Beneath this layer is a poorly vascularized connective tissue with few fibers and many fibroblasts and melanocytes. The next layer is rich in blood vessels embedded in loose connective tissue. The posterior surface of the iris is covered by 2 layers of epithelium that also cover the ciliary body and its processes. The outer epithelium, in contact with the posterior chamber, is heavily pigmented with melanin granules. The inner epithelial cells undergo a transformation presenting tonguelike extensions of their basal region directed radially and filled with myofilaments that overlap, creating the **dilator muscle** of the iris. The heavy pigmentation prevents the passage of light into the interior of the eye except through the pupil.

The function of the abundant melanocytes or melanin-containing pigment cells in several regions of the eye is to keep stray light rays from interfering with image formation. In so doing, they resemble a camera. The melanocytes of the stroma of the iris are responsible for the so-called color of the eyes, ie, the color of the iris. Thus, if the layer of pigment in the interior region of the iris consists of only a few cells, the light reflected from the black pigment epithelium present in the posterior surface of the iris will be blue. As the amount of pigment increases, the iris assumes various shades of greenish-blue, gray, and finally brown. Albinos have almost no pigment, and the pink color of their irides is due to the reflection of light incident from the blood vessels of the iris.

The interior of the iris contains smooth muscle bundles disposed in circles concentric to the pupillary margin, forming the **sphincter muscle** of the iris. The dilator and sphincter muscles have parasympathetic and sympathetic innervation, respectively.

Lens

This biconvex structure is characterized by great elasticity, a feature that it loses with age as the lens hardens. The lens has 3 principal components:

A. Lens Capsule: The lens is enveloped by a thin (10–20 μm), homogeneous, refractile, carbohydrate-rich capsule coating the outer surface of the epithelial cells. It is elastic and consists mainly of thin lamellas of collagen fibers and amorphous glycoprotein.

B. Subcapsular Epithelium: This consists of a single layer of cuboidal epithelial cells present only on the anterior surface of the lens. Lens fibers originate from cells in the anterior epithelium. The lens increases in size and grows throughout life as new lens fibers develop from cells located at the equator of the lens. The cells of this epithelium exhibit many interdigitations with the lens fibers. Their cytoplasm has few organelles and stains lightly. They are bound together occasionally by gap junctions.

C. Lens Fibers: These are elongated and appear as thin hexagonal prismatic elements. They are highly differentiated cells derived from cells of the embryonic lens. They eventually lose their nuclei and become greatly elongated, attaining dimensions of 7–10 mm in length, 8–10 μm in width, and 2 μm in thickness. They usually follow the direction of the lens surface.

The lens is held in position by a radially oriented layer of fibers, the **zonule,** which inserts on one side on the lens capsule and on the other on the ciliary body (Fig 10–16). This system is important in the process known as **accommodation,** which permits focusing on near and far objects by changing the curvature of the lens. Thus, when the eye is at rest or gazing at distant objects, the lens is kept stretched by the zonule in a plane vertical to the optical axis. To focus on a near object, part of the ciliary muscle contracts, resulting in forward displacement of the choroid and ciliary body. Consequently, the tension exerted by the zonule is relieved and the lens becomes thicker, thus keeping the object in focus.

Vitreous

The vitreous occupies the region of the eye behind the lens. It is a transparent gel that consists of water (about 99%), highly hydrophilic glycosaminoglycans whose principal component is hyaluronic acid, and collagen fibrils.

Retina

The retina, the inner layer of the eyeball, consists of 2 portions. The posterior portion is photosensitive; the anterior part is not photosensitive and constitutes the inner lining of the ciliary body and the posterior part of the iris (Figs 10–11 and 10–17). The retina derives from an evagination of the anterior cephalic vesicle or prosencephalon. This so-called **optic vesicle,** upon coming into contact with the ectoderm, gradually invaginates in its central region, forming a double-walled calyx or cup. In the adult, the outer wall gives rise to a thin membrane called the **pigment epithelium;** from the inner layer is derived the optical or functioning part of the retina.

The pigment epithelium consists of columnar cells with a basal nucleus. The basal regions of the cells adhere firmly to Bruch's membrane, and the cell membranes have numerous invaginations (Fig 10–22). Mitochondria are more abundant in the region of the cytoplasm near these invaginations.

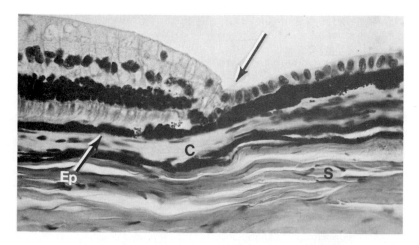

Figure 10–17. Photomicrograph of a section of retina in the transition (arrow) between the photosensitive *(left)* and blind *(right)* parts. Note the pigment epithelium (Ep), the choroid (C), and the sclera (S). H&E stain, × 200.

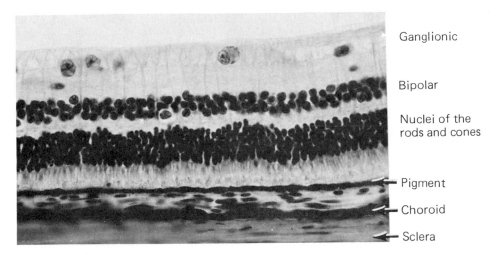

Ganglionic

Bipolar

Nuclei of the
rods and cones

← Pigment

← Choroid

← Sclera

Figure 10–18. Photomicrograph of a section of the photosensitive part of a retina, showing its layers. H&E stain, × 200.

These 2 characteristics suggest an ion-transporting activity for this region.

The lateral cell membranes show cell junctions with conspicuous zonulae occludentes and zonulae adherentes at their apexes as well as desmosomes and gap junctions. These morphologic details show that the apical and basal regions of this epithelial sheet are sealed off and that intercellular communication exists. The existence of an electrical potential difference resulting from ion transport between the 2 surfaces of this epithelium can be accounted for by these junctional specializations.

The cell apex has abundant extensions of 2 types: slender microvilli and cylindric sheaths that invest the tips of the photoreceptors. Neither type of extension is anatomically joined to the photoreceptors, so that these regions can become separated, as occurs in a **detachment of the retina,** a common and serious disorder in humans. The cytoplasm of the pigmented epithelial cells has abundant smooth endoplasmic reticulum, believed to be a probable site of vitamin A esterification and transport to the photoreceptors. Melanin granules are numerous in the apical cytoplasm and microvillous extensions. Melanin is synthesized in these cells by a mechanism similar to that described for the melanocytes in the skin (see Chapter 19). This dark pigment has the function of absorbing light after the photoreceptors have been stimulated, thus creating a dark chamber effect in the eye.

The cell apex has numerous dark bodies of variable shape that represent various stages in the phagocytosis and digestion of the tips of the rod cells' outer segments. The structure of these cells and the peeling of their tips are discussed below (Fig 10–22).

The optical part of the retina—the posterior or photosensitive part—is a more complex structure and consists of the following layers: (1) a deep layer of photosensitive cells, the **rods** and **cones** (Figs 10–11, 10–18, and 10–19); (2) an intermediate layer of **bipolar neurons,** which binds the rods and cones to the ganglion cells; and (3) a surface layer of **ganglion cells,** which establishes contact with the bipolar cells through its dendrites and sends axons to the central nervous system. These axons converge, forming the **optic nerve.**

Between the layer of rods and cones and that of the bipolar cells, a region called the **external plexiform** or **synaptic layer** exists where synapses between these 2 types of cells occur. The region where the synapses between the bipolar and ganglion cells are established is called the **internal plexiform layer** (Fig 10–19). The retina has an inverted structure, for the light will first cross the ganglion layer and then the bipolar layer to reach the rods and cones.

A needle inserted through the posterior part of the eyeball would pass through the sclera, the choroid, the pigment epithelium of the retina, the rods and cones, the bipolar layer, and the ganglion layer to enter the vitreous.

The structure of the retina will now be examined in greater detail. The rods and cones are bipolar cells; at one pole is a single photosensitive dendrite and at the other are synapses with cells of the bipolar layer (Figs 10–19 and 10–20). These photosensitive dendrites assume the form of a rod or cone, giving these cells their names. Both rod cells and cone cells penetrate a thin layer called the **external limiting membrane.** The nuclei of the cones are generally disposed near the limiting membrane, while rod nuclei lie near the center of the inner segment. The external limiting membrane is not a membrane in the customary sense but consists of zonulae adherentes that usually join the inner segments of rods and cones to the terminal extensions of the Müller cells; infrequently, Müller cell extensions are bound among themselves; and, rarely, photoreceptors are bound to photoreceptors.

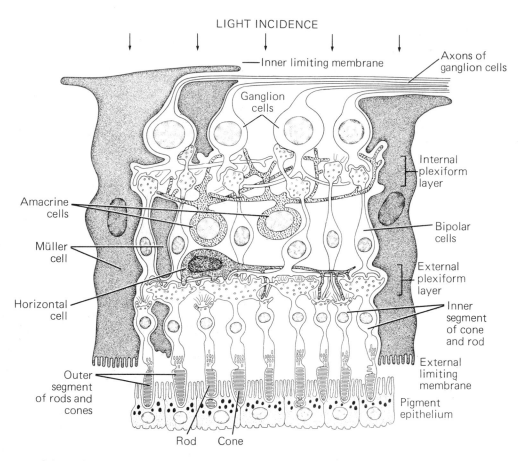

LIGHT INCIDENCE

Inner limiting membrane

Axons of ganglion cells

Ganglion cells

Internal plexiform layer

Amacrine cells

Bipolar cells

Müller cell

External plexiform layer

Horizontal cell

Inner segment of cone and rod

External limiting membrane

Outer segment of rods and cones

Pigment epithelium

Rod   Cone

Figure 10–19. Schematic drawing of the 3 layers of retinal neurons. The arrows represent the direction of the light path. The stimulation generated by the incident light on the rods and cones proceeds in opposite directions. (Redrawn and reproduced, with permission, from Boycott & Dowling: Proc R Soc Lond [Biol] 166:80, 1966.)

The **rod cells** are thin, elongated cells (50 × 3 μm) composed of 2 portions as shown in Figs 10–19 and 10–20. The external photosensitive rod-shaped dendrite is composed mainly of numerous (600–1000) flattened membranous vesicles piled up like a stack of coins. The **outer segment** is separated from the **inner segment** by a constriction. Just below this constriction there is a basal corpuscle from which a cilium arises and passes to the outer segment. The inner segment is rich in glycogen and has a remarkable aggregation of mitochondria, most lying near the constriction (Figs 10–20 and 10–22). This local accumulation of mitochondria is related to the production of energy necessary for the visual process. Polysomes are present in large numbers below the mitochondrial region of the inner segment and are involved in protein synthesis. Some of these proteins migrate to the outer segment of the rod cells, where they are incorporated into membranous vesicles.

The flattened vesicles of the rod cells contain the pigment called **visual purple** or **rhodopsin**, which is bleached by light and initiates the visual stimulus. This substance is globular in form and is located in the outer surface of the lipid bilayer of the flattened membranous vesicles. It has been estimated that the human retina has approximately 120 million rods. They are extremely sensitive to light and are considered to be the receptors used when low levels of light are present, such as during the period of dusk or at night. The outer segment is considered to be the site of photosensitivity, whereas the inner segment contains the metabolic machinery necessary for the biosynthetic and energy-producing processes of these cells.

Radioautographic studies show that proteins of the vesicles of the rods are synthesized in the inner segment of these cells, which is rich in polysomes. From there, they migrate to the outer segment and aggregate at its basal region, where they are assembled into membranes formed by a double layer of phospholipids producing flattened disks (Figs 10–20 and 10–23). These structures gradually migrate to the cell apex, where they peel off and are phagocytosed and digested by the cells of the pigment epithelium. This phenomenon is notable for the large amount of new protein synthesized by these photoreceptors (Fig 10–24). It has been calcu-

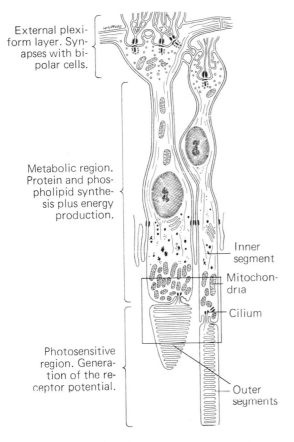

External plexi- form layer. Syn- apses with bi- polar cells.

Metabolic region. Protein and phos- pholipid synthe- sis plus energy production.

Inner segment

Mitochon- dria

Cilium

Photosensitive region. Genera- tion of the re- ceptor potential.

Outer segments

Figure 10 –20. The ultrastructure of the rods *(right)* and cones *(left).* The enclosed region is illustrated in the electron micrograph in Fig 10–23. (Redrawn and reproduced, with permission, from Chevremont M: *Notions de Cytologie et Histologie.* S.A. Desoer Editions [Liège], 1966.)

lated that in the monkey approximately 90 vesicles per cell are produced daily. The whole process of migration, from assembly at the basal cell region to its apical peeling off, takes 9–13 days. In **hereditary retinal dystrophy** in the rat, the vesicles peeled off from the rods are not phagocytosed, probably as a result of a dysfunction of the pigment epithelium, and are instead deposited at the surface of the pigment layer.

The **cone cells** are also elongated (60 × 1.5 μm). They have a structure similar to that of the rods, with internal and external segments, basal body with cilium, and an accumulation of mitochondria and polysomes (Fig 10–20). The cones differ from the rods in their conical form and the structure of their external segments. This region is also composed of stacked flattened vesicles, but they are not independent of the outer enveloping membrane, arising as invaginations of this structure (Fig 10–20). In the cones, the synthesized protein is not concentrated in recently assembled disks (as it is in rods) but is distributed uniformly

throughout the external segment. The cones contain the visual pigment **iodopsin,** which is most sensitive to red light; and the human retina has approximately 6 million cones. While the cones are only sensitive to light of a higher intensity than the rods, they are believed to permit better visual acuity than the rods.

The layer of bipolar cells consists of 2 types of cells (Fig 10–19): (1) **diffuse bipolar cells,** which have synapses with 2 or more photoreceptors; and (2) **monosynaptic bipolar cells,** which establish contact with the axon of only one cone photoreceptor and only one ganglion cell. There are, therefore, a certain number of cones which transmit their impulses directly to the central nervous system.

The cells of the ganglion layer, besides establishing contact with the bipolar cells, project their axons to a specific region of the retina where they come together to form the **optic nerve** (Fig 10–19). This region is deprived of receptors and is therefore called the **blind spot** of the retina, the **papilla of the optic nerve,** or the **optic nerve head** (Fig 10–11). The ganglion cells are typical nerve cells with a large euchromatic nucleus, basophilic Nissl substance, etc. These cells, like the bipolar cells, are also classified as diffuse or monosynaptic types in their connections with other cells.

Besides these 3 main types of cells (photoreceptors, bipolar cells, and ganglion cells), other types of cells are distributed more diffusely in the layers of the retina:

(1) The **horizontal cells** (Fig 10–19) establish contact between different photoreceptors. Their exact function is not known, but it is possible that they act to integrate stimuli.

(2) The **amacrine cells** are various types of neurons that establish contact between the ganglion cells. Their function is also obscure.

(3) The **supporting cells** are neuroglia which possess, in addition to the astrocyte and microglial cell types, some large, extensively ramified cells called **Müller cells.** These cells extend from the inner to the outer limiting membranes of the retina (Fig 10–19). They contain abundant microfilaments and glycogen in their cytoplasm and are known to have a high metabolic rate. These characteristics suggest that the cells have supporting and probably nutrient functions. Observe that both the so-called inner and outer limiting membranes are really thin layers of the retina formed by terminal expansions of Müller cells. They are believed to be functionally analogous to neuroglia in that they serve to support and insulate the retinal neurons and fibers (Fig 10–24).

Retinal Histophysiology

Light passes through the layers of the retina to the rods and cones, where it is absorbed, thus initiating a series of reactions that result in what we call vision. This is an extraordinarily sensitive process, for there is experimental evidence to suggest that

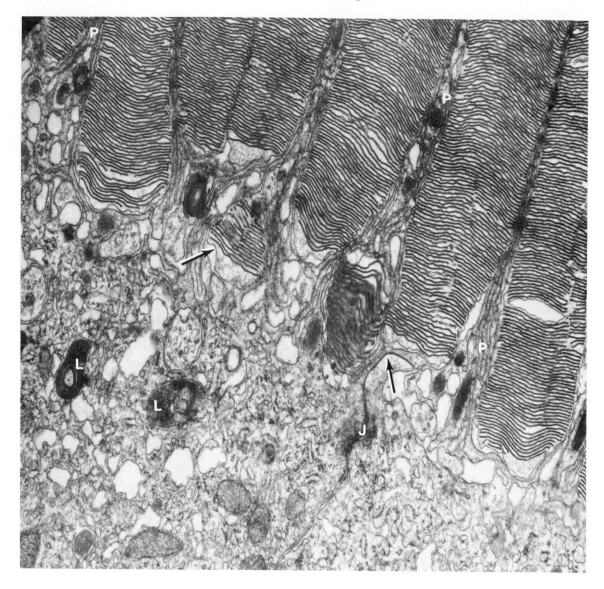

Figure 10 –21. Electron micrograph of the interface between the photosensitive and pigmented layer in a rat retina. Below are portions of 2 pigment epithelial cells revealing junctional specializations between their opposing plasmalemmas (J). Above the pigment cells are the tips of 7 photosensitive portions of rod cells that interdigitate with apical processes of the pigment epithelium (P). The large vesicles containing flattened membranes (arrows) have peeled off from the tips of the rods. Lysosomal vesicles are indicated by an L.

one photon is enough to trigger the production of a receptor potential in a rod. Light acts to bleach the visual pigments, and this photochemical process is amplified by mechanisms that cause the local production of responses which will be transmitted to the central nervous system.

The bleaching of the visual pigment incorporated in the flat membrane vesicles increases the calcium conductance of the vesicular membranes and promotes a diffusion of calcium to the intracellular space of the outer segment of the photoreceptor. This calcium acts on the cell membrane, reducing its permeability to sodium ions and promoting cell hyperpolarization.

In a second step, the visual pigment is reassembled and the calcium ions transported back into the vesicles by an energy-consuming process. The energy requirement would account for the abundance of mitochondria near the photosensitive site of rods and cones. Contrary to what happens in other receptors where action potentials are generated through cell depolarization, the rods and cones are hyperpolarized by light. This signal is transmitted to the bipolar cells, and only the ganglion cells generate action potentials along their axons that serve to relay information to the central nervous system.

The visual pigment of rods, called **rhodopsin,**

THE 4 FUNCTIONS OF A RETINAL PIGMENT CELL

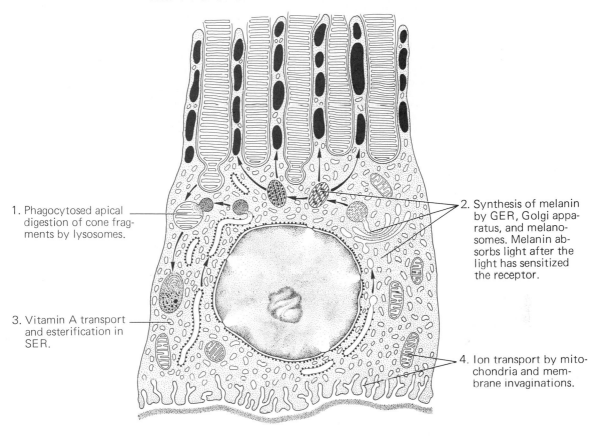

1. Phagocytosed apical digestion of cone fragments by lysosomes.

2. Synthesis of melanin by GER, Golgi apparatus, and melanosomes. Melanin absorbs light after the light has sensitized the receptor.

3. Vitamin A transport and esterification in SER.

4. Ion transport by mitochondria and membrane invaginations.

Figure 10–22. Drawing of a pigment epithelial cell. Observe that the apical portion presents abundant cell processes that fill the spaces between the outer segments of the sensitive cells. The membrane of the basal region has invaginations into the cytoplasm. This is a cell type with several functions. One of them is the synthesis of melanin granules (by a process described in Chapter 19) that absorb stray light in the eye chamber. This is depicted on the right side of the figure, which shows the organelles that participate in melanin synthesis. On the left side of the figure, lysosomes synthesized in the granular endoplasmic reticulum coalesce to the phagocytosed peeled apical parts of the cones, digesting them. Besides these activities, these cells are probably active in ion transport since they maintain a potential between the 2 surfaces of the epithelial membrane. The relatively well developed smooth endoplasmic reticulum probably participates in the processes of vitamin A esterification and transport. SER, smooth endoplasmic reticulum; GER, granular endoplasmic reticulum.

is composed of an aldehyde of vitamin A_1 (called retinene$_1$) bound to specific proteins. Cones contain 3 (not yet completely identified) different pigments in humans, thus providing a chemical basis for the classic tricolor theory of color vision.

The retina is a poorly vascularized structure presenting few capillaries practically restricted to the ganglion and bipolar cell layers. In the photosensitive cell layer, capillaries are almost nonexistent. This poor vascularization accounts for the high glycolytic activity of this tissue. The clinical observation that the retina is damaged when it becomes detached suggests that the photosensitive cells derive their metabolites from the choriocapillary layer. The superficial localization of the vessels of the retina provides for their easy observation with an ophthalmoscope. This examination is of great

value in the diagnosis and evaluation of disorders that affect blood vessels such as diabetes and hypertension.

At the posterior pole of the optical axis lies the **fovea,** a shallow depression in whose center the retina is very thin. This is because the bipolar and ganglion cells accumulate in the periphery of this depression, so that its center consists only of cone cells (Fig 10–11). In this area, blood vessels do not cross over the photosensitive cells. Light falls directly on the cones in the central part of the fovea—a peculiarity related to the extremely precise visual acuity of this region.

Light not absorbed by the photoreceptors is absorbed by the pigment cells of the retinal pigment layer and the choroid.

The structure of the retina varies according to

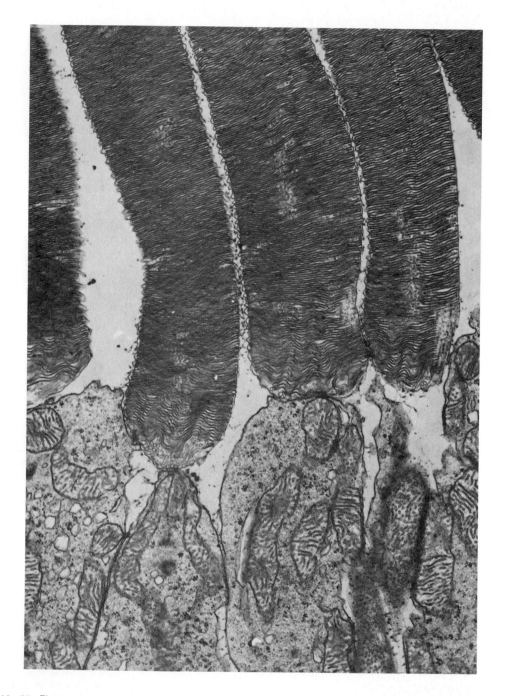

Figure 10 –23. Electron micrograph of a section of the retina of a mouse. In the lower part of the picture are the outer segments. The photosensitive region consists of parallel membranous flat vesicles. Mitochondrial accumulation occurs in the inner portion. × 10,000. (Courtesy of KR Porter.)

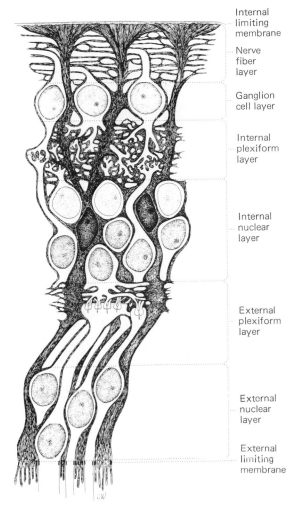

Internal limiting membrane

Nerve fiber layer

Ganglion cell layer

Internal plexiform layer

Internal nuclear layer

External plexiform layer

External nuclear layer

External limiting membrane

Figure 10–24. An illustration revealing the close association of Müller cells with neural elements in the sensory retina. Müller cells (dark fibrous cells) appear to be structurally and functionally equivalent to astrocytes of the central nervous system in that they envelop and support the neurons and nerve processes of the retina. (Reproduced, with permission, from Hogan MJ, Alvarado JA, Weddell JE: *Histology of the Human Eye.* Saunders, 1971.)

the region studied. The fovea has only cones, and the blind spot or papilla has no receptors (Fig 10–11). Other structural variations of physiologic significance are also observed in the retina. The number of ganglion cells per unit area is such an example. In the periphery of the retina, these cells are relatively few in number—hundreds of cells per square millimeter—which is in sharp contrast to the periphery of the fovea, where the cells are counted in hundreds of thousands per square millimeter. Thus, vision at the peripheral part of the retina is much less sharp than at or near the fovea.

Although the retina has approximately 126 million receptors, not all the information gathered by receptors is relayed to the central nervous system. This is because the optic nerve does not have more than 1 million axons. Much of the information collected by the photoreceptors is selected and processed during its flow through the bipolar and ganglion cells. These cells integrate and code the information obtained, sending to the central nervous system a summary of the data. The retina in humans is mainly a **receptor-integrating structure,** which is not surprising since, embryologically, the retina is an outgrowth of the central nervous system.

The retina is an extremely complex organ. In the primate retina at least 15 different types of neurons are present, and these cells form at least 38 distinct kinds of synapses with one another.

ACCESSORY STRUCTURES OF THE EYE

Conjunctiva

The conjunctiva is a thin, transparent mucous membrane that covers the anterior portion of the eye up to the cornea and the internal surface of the eyelids. It has a stratified columnar epithelium, and its lamina propria is composed of loose connective tissue.

Eyelids (Fig 10–25)

Eyelids are movable folds of tissue that serve to protect the eye. The skin of the lids is loose and elastic, permitting extreme swelling and subsequent return to normal shape and size. The **tarsal plates** consist of dense fibrous and elastic tissue. They are lined posteriorly by conjunctiva and fuse medially and laterally to form the **medial** and **lateral palpebral tendons (ligaments),** which attach to the orbital bones. The **orbital septum** is the fascia lying posterior to the orbicularis oculi muscle and is the barrier between the lid and the orbit.

The **orbicularis oculi** muscle, supplied by the seventh cranial nerve, is roughly circular. Its function is to close the lids. The **levator palpebrae** muscle, supplied by the third nerve, inserts into the tarsal plate and the skin and serves to elevate the lid. The superior tarsal muscle (of Müller), supplied by sympathetic nerves, originates in the levator muscle and inserts at the superior edge of the tarsus, coursing deep to the levator aponeurosis.

Three types of glands in the lid are the meibomian glands and the glands of Moll and Zeis. The meibomian glands are long sebaceous glands in the tarsal plate. They do not communicate with the hair follicles. There are about 25 in the upper lid and 20 in the lower lid, appearing as yellow vertical streaks deep to the conjunctiva. The meibomian glands produce a sebaceous substance that creates an oily layer on the surface of the tear film. This helps to prevent rapid evaporation of the normal tear layer.

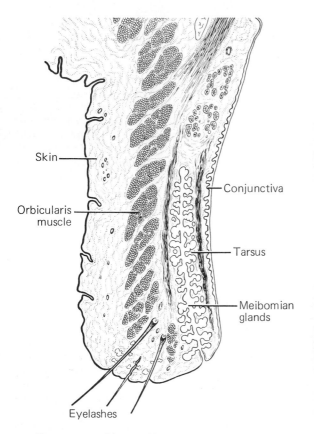

Figure 10–25. Diagram illustrating the lid structure.

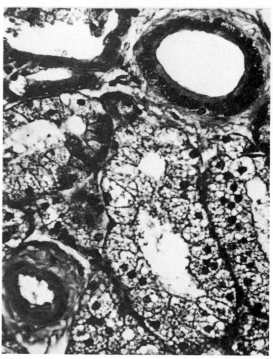

Figure 10–26. Photomicrograph of a section of a human lacrimal gland. A duct is shown in the upper right region. In the center is the secretory portion. H&E stain, × 350.

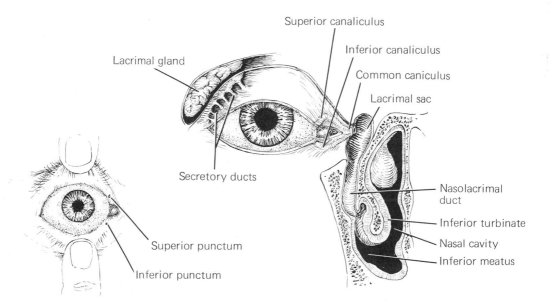

Figure 10–27. The lacrimal drainage system. (Redrawn with modifications and reproduced, with permission, from Thompson: Radiography of the nasolacrimal passageways. Med Radiogr Photogr 25:66, 1949.)

The glands of Zeis are smaller, modified sebaceous glands connected with the follicles of the eyelashes. The sweat glands of Moll are unbranched sinuous tubules that begin in a simple spiral and not in a glomerulus as do ordinary sweat glands.

There is a **gray line** (mucocutaneous border) on the margins of both the upper and the lower eyelids. If an incision is made along this line, the lid can be cleanly split into a posterior portion, containing the tarsal plate and conjunctiva, and an anterior portion, containing the orbicularis oculi muscle, skin, and hair follicles.

The blood supply to the lids is derived mainly from ophthalmic and lacrimal arteries. The lymphatics drain into the preauricular, parotid, and submaxillary lymph glands.

Lacrimal Apparatus

The lacrimal apparatus (Figs 10–26 and 10–27) consists of the lacrimal gland, accessory glands, canaliculi, tear sac, and nasolacrimal duct. The lacrimal gland is a tear-secreting gland located in the anterior superior temporal portion of the orbit. It consists of several separate glandular lobes with 6–12 excretory ducts that connect the gland to the superior conjunctival fornix. (Fornices are the conjunctiva-lined recesses between the lids and the eyeball.) It is a tubulo-alveolar gland that usually has distended lumens. It is composed of columnar-shaped cells of the serous type resembling the parotid acinar cells. They show lightly stained secretory granules, and a basal lamina separates them from the surrounding connective tissue. Well-developed myoepithelial cells surround the secretory portions of this gland. The secretion of the gland passes down over the cornea and the bulbar and palpebral conjunctiva, moistening the surfaces of these structures. They drain into the lacrimal canaliculi through the lacrimal puncta, round apertures about 0.5 mm in diameter on the medial aspect of both the upper and lower lid margins. The canaliculi are about 1 mm in diameter and 8 mm long and join to form a common canaliculus just before opening into the lacrimal sac. Diverticuli of the common canaliculus may be a part of the normal structure and are frequently susceptible to fungal infection.

The lacrimal sac is the dilated portion of the lacrimal drainage system that lies in the bony lacrimal fossa.

The nasolacrimal duct is the downward continuation of the lacrimal sac. It opens into the inferior meatus lateral to the inferior turbinate.

All of the passages of the lacrimal drainage system are lined with epithelium. The tears pass into the puncta by capillary attraction. The combined forces of the capillary attraction in the canaliculi, gravity, and the pumping action of the orbicularis oculi muscle on the lacrimal sac cause the flow of tears down the nasolacrimal duct into the nose and nasopharynx. The lacrimal glands secrete the enzyme lysozyme, whose main activity is to hydrolyze the cell walls of certain species of bacteria.

THE EAR OR VESTIBULOCOCHLEAR APPARATUS

The functions of the vestibulocochlear apparatus (Fig 10–28) are related to equilibrium and hearing (stato-acoustic). It consists of 3 parts: (1) the **external ear,** which receives the sound waves; (2) the **middle ear,** where these waves are transmitted from air to bone and by bone to the internal ear; and (3) the **internal ear,** where these vibrations are transduced to specific nerve impulses that pass via the acoustic nerve to the central nervous system. The internal ear also contains the vestibular organ, which functions to maintain equilibrium.

External Ear

The external ear has an irregular form and consists mainly of a plate of elastic cartilage covered by a layer of skin on both sides. Sebaceous glands and a few sweat glands are present in its dermis.

The **external auditory meatus** extends from the external ear to the tympanic membrane. It appears as a somewhat flattened canal with rigid walls. The external third of the meatus is supported by an elastic cartilage continued from the external ear. The remainder is formed by the temporal bone. The meatus is lined by skin with numerous hairs, sebaceous glands, and a type of modified sweat gland—the **ceruminous glands**—coiled tubular apocrine glands that produce a brownish, semisolid fatty substance called **cerumen** (earwax). Hairs and cerumen probably have a protective function.

Across the deep end of the external auditory meatus lies an oval membrane, the **tympanic membrane.** It is covered by a thin outer layer of epidermis and, on its inner surface, by simple cuboidal epithelium. Between these 2 epithelial coverings is a tough connective tissue layer composed of collagen and elastic fibers and fibroblasts. In the anterior upper quadrant of the tympanic membrane, it is flaccid and devoid of fibers, forming **Shrapnell's membrane.** The tympanic membrane is the structure that transmits impinging sound vibrations to the ossicles of the middle ear (Fig 10–28).

Middle Ear

The middle ear, in the interior of the temporal bone, is an irregular cavity that separates the tympanic membrane (and external ear) from the bony surface of the internal ear. It communicates anteriorly with the pharynx by the **auditory tube (eustachian tube)** and posteriorly with the air-filled cavities of the mastoid process of the temporal bone. The middle ear is lined by simple squamous

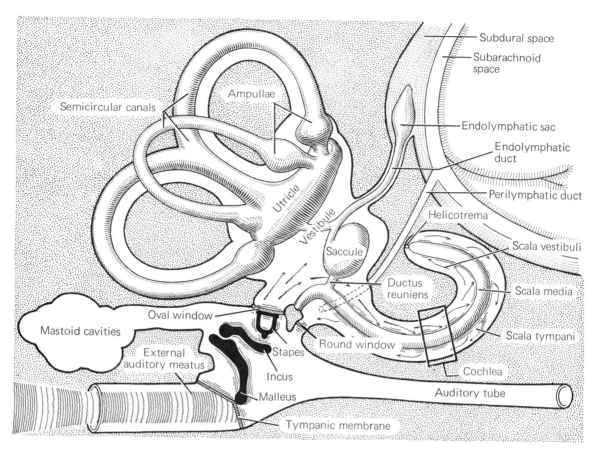

Figure 10–28. Schematic drawing illustrating the vestibulocochlear organ and the path of sound waves in the external, middle, and internal ear. (Redrawn and reproduced, with permission, from Best CH, Taylor NB: *The Physiological Basis of Medical Practice,* 8th ed. Williams & Wilkins, 1966.)

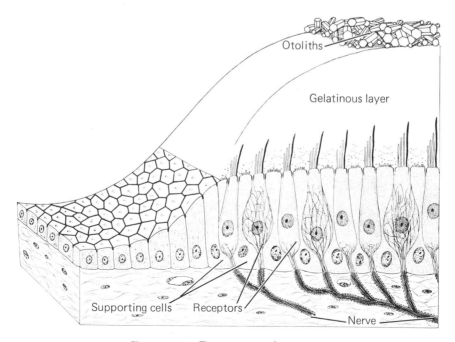

Figure 10–29. The structure of maculae.

epithelium resting on the thin lamina propria strongly adherent to the subjacent periosteum. Near the auditory tube and in its interior, the simple epithelium that lines the middle ear is gradually transformed into pseudostratified columnar ciliated epithelium. The walls of the tube are usually collapsed, but they separate during the process of swallowing, thus balancing the pressure of the air in the middle ear with the atmospheric pressure. In the medial bony wall of the middle ear are 2 oblong regions devoid of bone and covered by membranes; these are the **oval** and **round windows** (Fig 10–28), which will be described later.

The tympanic membrane is connected to the oval window by 3 small bones—the **auditory ossicles: malleus, incus,** and **stapes** (Fig 10–28)—that transmit the mechanical vibration generated in the tympanic membrane to the inner ear. The malleus inserts itself in the tympanic membrane and the stapes in the membrane of the oval window. These bones are articulated by synovial joints, and like all structures of this cavity they are covered by simple squamous epithelium. In the middle ear, 2 small muscles are present that insert themselves in the malleus and stapes. They have a function in sound conduction, as will be seen later.

Internal Ear

The internal ear—also called the **labyrinth**—is a complex structure that consists of a series of fluid-filled membranous sacs and canals lodged in cavities corresponding in form to the petrous part of the temporal bone. The membranous sacs and canals form the **membranous labyrinth**, whereas the corresponding osseous portion is the **osseous labyrinth** (Fig 10–28). The membranous structures sometimes impinge upon and adhere to the osseous labyrinth. Usually, there is a fluid-filled space between both labyrinths. This **perilymphatic fluid** contrasts with the **endolymphatic fluid** in the interior of the membranous labyrinth. The space filled with perilymph—the **perilymphatic space**—is a continuation of the subarachnoid space of the meninges, contains stellate cells, and has, therefore, the same composition as cerebrospinal fluid (Fig 10–28). The membranous labyrinth is bound to the periosteum by thin vascularized strands of connective tissue. The membranous labyrinth consists mainly of a lining of simple squamous epithelium surrounded by a thin connective tissue layer. The epithelium—despite being deeply situated in the temporal bone—is of ectodermal origin. It derives from the **auditory vesicle** developed from the ectoderm of the lateral part of the embryo's head. During embryonic development, this vesicle invaginates into the subjacent connective tissue, loses contact with the cephalic ectoderm, and moves deeply into the rudiments of the future temporal bone. During this process, it undergoes a complex series of changes in form, giving rise to the compartments of the membranous labyrinth. In certain regions, its epithelial lining becomes differentiated to form special receptor organs known as the **maculae,** the **cristae,** and the **organ of Corti.**

The osseous labyrinth consists of a central irregular cavity, the **vestibule,** with **semicircular canals** on one side and the **cochlea** on the other (Fig 10–28). The arrangement of the membranous labyrinth in the osseous labyrinth is illustrated in Fig 10–28. Note that the vestibule houses 2 distinct elongated structures: the **saccule** and the **utricle.** The semicircular canals open into the utricle. Each of these canals has a dilatation—the **ampulla**—in one of its extremities. The saccule—also in the vestibule—communicates with the utricle and cochlea by short ducts. The duct which connects the utricle to the saccule assumes the form of a Y whose stalk ends as a blind sac in a special structure, the **endolymphatic sac** (Fig 10–28).

Histology of the Membranous Labyrinth

A. Saccule and Utricle: These structures are composed of a thin sheath of connective tissue lined by simple squamous epithelium. The membranous labyrinth is bound to the periosteum of the osseous labyrinth by thin strands of connective tissue. In the wall of the saccule and utricle, one can observe small regions, called **maculae,** of differentiated neuroepithelial cells innervated by branches of the vestibular nerve. The maculae of the saccule and of the utricle are perpendicular to one another and have a similar histologic structure (Fig 10–29). They consist basically of 2 cell types: **receptors** and **supporting cells.** In the **receptor cells** one can distinguish 2 forms. Both, however, are characterized by the presence of long extensions, resembling stereocilia, of its surface membrane and of one typical cilium with its accompanying basal body (Figs 10–29 and 10–30). These cells are classically referred to as **hair cells.** The abundance of mitochondria present in these cells is probably related to their sensory activity. One of these cells has the form of a goblet and is surrounded by a net of afferent nerve endings; the other is columnar and presents afferent and efferent nerve endings (Fig 10–29).

The **supporting cells** disposed between the receptors are columnar and prismatic, with their nuclei at the base of the cell and microvilli on its apical surface (Fig 10–29). Covering this neuroepithelium is a thick, gelatinous glycoprotein layer, probably secreted by the supporting cells, with surface deposits of crystal bodies composed mainly of calcium carbonate and called **otoliths (otoconia)** (Figs 10–29 and 10–31).

B. Semicircular Canals: These structures have the same general form as the osseous labyrinth. The receptor areas present in their ampullae (Fig 10–28) have an elongated ridgelike form and are called **cristae ampullares.** They have a structure similar to that of the maculae, but their glycoprotein layer is thicker, has a conical form called a **cupula,** and is not

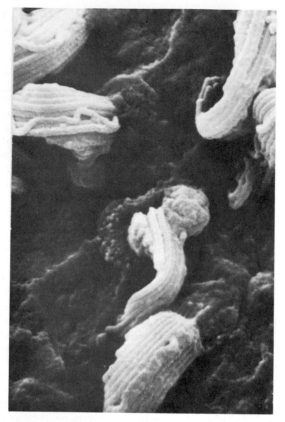

Figure 10–30. Scanning electron micrograph of the surface of the macula of a guinea pig's saccule. Observe the stereocilia grouped in bundles, in which a motile cilium—usually with a wavy aspect—can often be observed. × 7000. (Courtesy of Lim DJ, Lane WC: Arch Otolaryngol 90:283, 1969.)

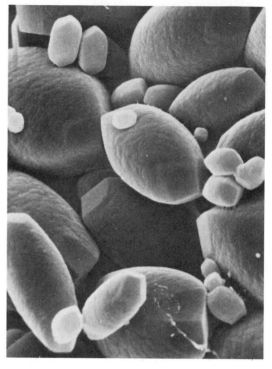

Figure 10–31. Scanning electron micrograph of the surface of a pigeon's macula showing the statoconia or otoliths. (Courtesy of DJ Lim.)

covered by otoliths. The cupula extends across the ampullae, establishing contact with its opposite wall (Fig 10–32).

C. Endolymphatic Duct and Sac: The endolymphatic duct initially has a simple squamous epithelial lining. As it nears the endolymphatic sac, it gradually changes into tall columnar epithelium composed of 2 cell types, one of which has microvilli on its apical surface and abundant pinocytotic vesicles and vacuoles. It has been suggested that these cells are responsible for the absorption of endolymph and the digestion of foreign material and cellular remnants.

Cochlea

This structure—a diverticulum of the saccule—is highly specialized as a sound receptor. It is a spiral osseous canal 35 mm long. The spiral cochlea is coiled around a cone-shaped structure composed of spongiform bone, the **modiolus,** in which there are channels for nerve fibers and vessels. This structure also contains the **spiral ganglion** (Figs 10–33 and 10–34). Lateral to the modiolus is a thin

osseous ridge called the **osseous spiral lamina** (Figs 10–33 and 10–34). The modiolus and spiral lamina form a cone-shaped screw with the spiral lamina analogous to the thread.

Transverse section of the coils of the cochlea shows that its membranous portion is triangular in shape with its smallest angle pointed to the modiolus and resting on the osseous spiral lamina (Fig 10–33). The base of this triangle, in contact with the lateral bony walls of the osseous labyrinth, exhibits differentiated cells of stratified epithelium called the **stria vascularis** (Fig 10–33). Another side of the triangle forms the **vestibular (or Reissner's) membrane** (Fig 10–33).

A complex structure, the **organ of Corti,** can be seen over the spiral lamina; it contains receptor cells responsible for hearing. The membranous triangle divides the space limited by the osseous cochlea into 3 different portions: an upper portion, the **scala vestibuli;** a middle portion, the **scala media;** and a lower portion, the **scala tympani.** The scala vestibuli opens into the vestibule (Fig 10–28), whereas the scala tympani communicates through

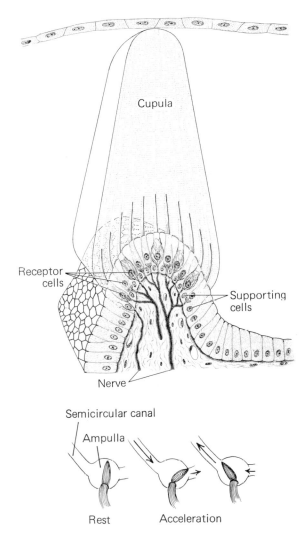

Figure 10–32. *Above:* Schematic drawing of the structure of the crista ampullaris. *Below:* Movements of cupula in ampullary crista during rotational acceleration. Arrows indicate direction of fluid movement. (Redrawn and reproduced, with permission, from Wersäll J: Studies on the structure and innervation of the sensory epithelium of the cristae ampullares in the guinea pig. Acta Otolaryngol [Stockh] Suppl 126:1, 1956.)

the round window with the tympanic cavity or middle ear (Fig 10–28). The vestibular and tympanic cavities are filled with perilymph and communicate in their extremities through a small hole (the **helicotrema**). At its point of origin, the scala media communicates through a duct with the saccule and ends as a blind sac (Fig 10–28).

The cochlea has the following histologic structure: The **vestibular membrane** consists of a very thin layer of connective tissue covered by simple squamous epithelium (Fig 10–33). The **stria vascularis** is lined by stratified epithelium containing 2 main cell types. One is rich in mitochondria and has deep and abundant infoldings of the membrane in

its basal portion—characteristics of an ion- and water-transporting cell. The epithelium of the stria vascularis is one of the few examples of an epithelium that contains blood vessels. This region may be involved in the secretion and maintenance of the unusual ionic composition of the endolymph. This fluid is rich in potassium and contains little sodium—a composition characteristic of cytoplasm. This contrasts with extracellular fluids, including perilymph, that have just the opposite ionic composition, ie, they are rich in sodium and poor in potassium.

Spiral Organ of Corti

This organ is in contact with the osseous and membranous spiral lamina. It consists of a series of complex structures sensitive to the vibrations induced by sound waves. The membranous lamina presents a thickened region composed of a layer of organized collagenlike fibers—the **basilar membrane**—which supports the organ of Corti. The membranous lamina begins medially in the osseous spiral lamina and ends laterally on an eminence of the periosteum called the **spiral crest** (Fig 10–33). Examining Fig 10–33 from right to left, one observes, first, a region composed of loose connective tissue covered by epithelium—called **spiral limbus**—from which derives a glycoprotein-rich amorphous structure, the **tectorial membrane.** This is oriented in a lateral and horizontal direction, establishing contact with the sensory cells of Corti's organ. It creates a channel known as the **internal spiral tunnel** (Fig 10–33). The lateral wall of this tunnel is composed of 3 groups of cells: the **inner sensory** or **hair cells;** the **pillar cells** on the side of the inner tunnel (Fig 10–33); and 3 rows of **outer sensory hair cells.** The cochlear sensory cells, when examined under the electron microscope, show 2 types of cells similar to those in the macula.

The **inner sensory** (or **hair**) **cells** are gobletlike and have modified stereocilia at their free surface and an accumulation of mitochondria in the base of the cell. Afferent and efferent nerve endings can be seen on these cells. The **outer sensory cells** are elongated and also have local accumulations of mitochondria and modified stereocilia. Neither type has cilia, as does the macula. The outer sensory cells are innervated by the cochlear nerve.

Histophysiology of the Vestibule & Cochlea

A. Vestibular Function: Increase or decrease in the velocity of circular movement—also called angular acceleration and deceleration—stimulates a flow of liquid in the semicircular canals as a consequence of the inertia of the endolymph. This flow induces lateral movement of the conic cap (cupula) that covers the crista ampullaris. This movement exerts bending and tensile forces on the sensory cells of the crest. Measurement of electrical impulses along the vestibular nerve fibers indicates that movement of the cupula in one direction pro-

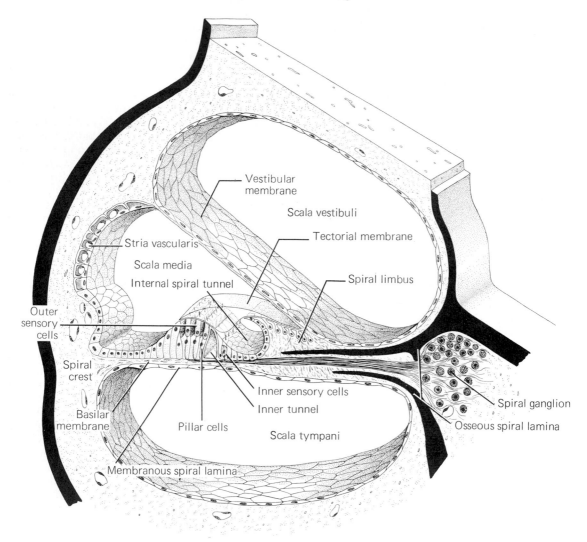

Figure 10–33. The structure of the cochlea. (Redrawn and reproduced, with permission, from Bloom W, Fawcett DW: *A Textbook of Histology,* 9th ed. Saunders, 1968.)

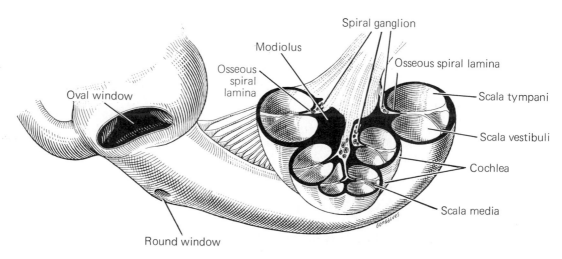

Figure 10–34. Schematic drawing of the disposition of the spiral ganglion and scalas of the cochlea.

vokes excitation of the receptors, with production of potentials in the vestibular nerves; movement in the opposite direction inhibits neuronal reactivity. When uniform movement returns, acceleration ceases, the cupula returns to its normal position, and excitation or inhibition of the receptors no longer occurs (Fig 10–32).

The mechanism of transformation of mechanical into electrical energy is still unknown. The semicircular canals serve to facilitate the reception of information about fluid displacement and therefore body position following circular acceleration; in lower mammals the macula of the saccule and of the utricle also responds to linear acceleration. By virtue of their greater density, the otoliths are displaced when there is an increase or decrease of linear velocity, causing tension in the gelatin layer and deforming the sensory cells. This leads to an excitation of the receptors, with production of action potentials transmitted to the central nervous system by the vestibular nerves. The macula is also sensitive to the action of gravity on the otoliths. Their stimulation is important for the conscious perception of movement and orientation in space and for the maintenance of equilibrium.

B. Cochlear Function: In the cochlea, mechanical stimuli (vibrations) induced by sound waves stimulate the production of a generating potential conveyed to the central nervous system by the cochlear nerve. The sound sets up vibrations in the tympanic membrane that are transmitted across an assembly of small bones to the oval window. The eardrum vibrates when exposed to sound waves but ceases to vibrate when the stimulus is withdrawn. The result is that it functions like a resonator softener. The small bones of the ear function as a series of levers which convert the vibrations of the tympanic membrane into mechanical displacement that is conveyed to the oval window and then to the perilymph of the vestibular scala (Fig 10–28). Contraction of the tensor muscles of the malleus and incus results in consecutive traction on the small bones with a decrease in the transmission of sound. An excessively loud sound produces contraction of these muscles, and this has a protective effect on the sensitive neurons of the spiral ganglia, which can be damaged irreversibly by prolonged or repetitive exposure to loud sounds. Vibrations that reach the perilymph of the vestibular scala are then transmitted to the tympanic scala and dissipate in the round window (Fig 10–28).

Contrary to former opinion, the membranous spiral lamina situated under the organ of Corti is not a dense structure, so the whole membranous cochlea vibrates when a sound passes from the vestibular scala to the tympanic. Vibration of the organ of Corti results in displacement of the tectorial membrane, resulting in pressure on the sensory cells and causing deformation of the stereocilia. This process could generate the action potential in the auditory nerve by an unknown mechanism. In the cochlea, sensitivity to sound varies in accordance with the region. High sounds generate waves that reach maximal vibration in the base of the cochlea, whereas low sounds vibrate maximally in the apex of the cochlea.

•　　•　　•

References

Cutaneous & Other Sensory Mechanisms

Beidler LM (editor): Olfaction. In *Handbook of Sensory Physiology*. Vol 4. Springer, 1971.

Beidler LM (editor): Taste. In: *Handbook of Sensory Physiology*. Vol 4. Springer, 1971.

Chouchkov CV: Cutaneous receptors. In: *Advances in Anatomy, Embryology and Cell Biology*. Vol 54. Springer-Verlag, 1978.

Frisch D: Ultrastructure of the mouse olfactory mucosa. Am J Anat 121:87, 1967.

Iggo WE: Cutaneous and subcutaneous sense organs. Br Med Bull 33:97, 1977.

Jaenicke L (editor): *Biochemistry of Sensory Functions*. Springer-Verlag, 1974.

Kornhuber HH, Aschoff JC (editors): *Somato-sensory System*. Thieme (Stuttgart), 1976.

Lowenstein WR (editor): Principles of receptor physiology. In: *Handbook of Sensory Physiology*. Vol 1. Springer, 1971.

Murray RG: The ultrastructure of taste buds. In: *The Ultrastructure of Sense Organs*. Friedman J (editor). North Holland Publishing Co, 1973.

Nishi K, Oura C, Pallie W: Fine structure of Pacinian corpuscles in the mesentery of the cat. J Cell Biol 43:539, 1969.

Okano M, Weber AF, Frommes SP: Electron microscopic studies of the distal border of canine olfactory epithelium. J Ultrastruct Res 17:487, 1967.

Ovalle WK Jr: Fine structure of rat intrafusal muscle fibers. The equatorial region. J Cell Biol 52:382, 1972.

Schmidt RF (editor): *Fundamentals of Sensory Physiology*. Springer-Verlag, 1978.

Straile WE: Encapsulated nerve end-organs in the rabbit, mouse, sheep and man. J Comp Neurol 136:317, 1969.

Zotterman Y (editor): *Sensory Function of the Skin in Primates*. Pergamon Press, 1976.

The Eye

Bok D, Hall MO: The role of the retinal pigment epithelium in the etiology of inherited retinal dystrophy in the rat. J Cell Biol 49:664, 1971.

Botelho SY: Tears and the lacrimal gland. Sci Am 211:78, Oct 1964.

Breipohl W & others: Scanning electron microscopy of the retinal pigment epithelium in chick embryos and chicks. Z Zellforsch Mikrosk Anat 146:543, 1973.

Dowling JE: Organization of vertebrate retinas. Invest Ophthalmol 9:665, 1970.

Duke-Elder S, Wybar KC: *System of Ophthalmology: The Anatomy of the Visual System*. Mosby, 1961.

Farnsworth PN & others: Ultrastructure of rat eye lens fibers. Invest Ophthalmol 13:274, 1974.

Hogan MJ & others: *Histology of the Human Eye*. Saunders, 1971.

Orzalesi N, Riva A, Testa F: Fine structure of the human lacrimal gland. J Submicrosc Cytol 3:283, 1971.

Raviola E: Intercellular junctions in the outer plexiform layer of the retina. Invest Ophthalmol 15:881, 1976.

Rodieck RW: *The Vertebrate Retina*. Freeman, 1974.

Smelser GK (editor): *The Structure of the Eye: A Symposium*. Academic Press, 1961.

Stell WK: The morphological organization of the vertebrate retina. In: *Physiology of Photoreceptor Organs*. Vol 7. Fuortes MGF (editor). Springer, 1972.

Young RW: Visual cells and the concept of renewal. Invest Ophthalmol 15:700, 1976.

The Ear

Anson BJ, Donaldson JA: *Surgical Anatomy of the Temporal Bone and Ear*. Saunders, 1973.

Hinojosa R, Rodriguez-Echandia EL: The fine structure of the stria vascularis of the cat inner ear. Am J Anat 118:631, 1966.

Hunter-Duvar IM: Hearing and hair cells. Can J Otolaryngol 4:152, 1975.

Kimura RS: The ultrastructure of the organ of Corti. Rev Cytol 42:173, 1975.

Lim DJ: Ultrastructure of the otolithic membrane and cupula. Adv Otorhinolaryngol 19:35, 1973.

Rosenhall U, Engström B: Surface structures of the human vestibular sensory regions. Acta Otolaryngol (Stockh) 319:3, 1974.

Soudijn ER: Scanning electron microscopy of the organ of Corti. Ann Otol Rhinol Laryngol 86:16, 1976.

Wersäll J, Flock A, Lundquist P-G: Structural basis for directional sensitivity in cochlear and vestibular sensory receptors. In: *Sensory Receptors*. Vol 30. Cold Spring Harbor Symp Quant Biol, 1965.

Muscle tissue is responsible for body movements. It consists of elongated muscle cells that are characterized by the presence of great numbers of contractile cytoplasmic filaments. The muscle cells are of mesodermal origin, and their differentiation occurs mainly by a gradual process of lengthening, with simultaneous synthesis of the protein of the filaments.

Three types of muscle tissue may be distinguished in mammals on the basis of morphologic and functional characteristics (Fig 11–1). **Smooth muscle** consists of collections of fusiform cells which, in the light microscope, do not show striations. Their contraction process is slow and not subject to voluntary control. **Striated skeletal muscle** is composed of bundles of very long cylindric multinucleated cells that present cross-striations. Their contraction is quick, forceful, and usually under voluntary control. **Striated cardiac muscle** also presents cross-striations and is composed of

elongated or branched individual cells that run parallel to each other. At sites of end-to-end contact are the **intercalated disks,** structures found only in cardiac muscle. Cardiac muscle contraction is involuntary, vigorous, and rhythmic.

We shall see in this chapter that each type of muscle tissue has a structure adapted to its physiologic role.

Muscle cells are highly differentiated, and their components are named according to their structural characteristics. Thus, the cytoplasm of muscle cells (excluding the myofibrils) is called **sarcoplasm;** the smooth endoplasmic reticulum is called **sarcoplasmic reticulum;** and their mitochondria are called **sarcosomes.** The **sarcolemma** is the cell membrane. These cells are surrounded by a distinct collagenous external (basal) lamina and a fine net of reticular fibers. In current usage, the sarcolemma is often called simply the **cell membrane** or **plasmalemma.**

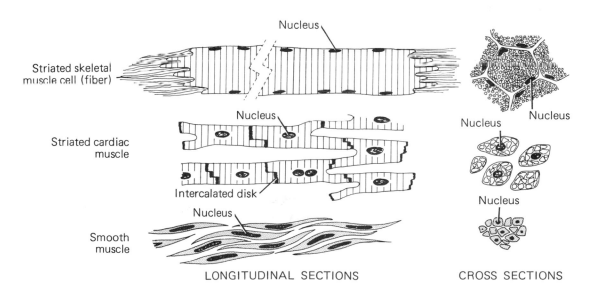

Figure 11–1. Diagram of the structure of the 3 muscle types. *Above:* Striated skeletal muscle. *Center:* Cardiac muscle. *Below:* Smooth muscle. The drawings at right show these muscles in cross section. Skeletal muscle is composed of large, elongated, multinucleated units (fibers). Cardiac muscle is composed of irregular branched cells bound longitudinally. Smooth muscle is an agglomerate of fusiform cells. The packing between cells may be more or less dense depending on the amount of extracellular connective tissue.

STRIATED SKELETAL MUSCLE

Striated skeletal muscle consists of bundles of very long (up to 4 cm) cylindric multinucleated cells with a diameter of 10–100 μm called **muscle fibers**. Multinucleation results from the fusion of embryonic mononucleated myoblasts (muscle stem cells). The oval nuclei are usually found at the periphery of the cell under the cell membrane. This characteristic nuclear location is helpful in distinguishing skeletal muscle from cardiac muscle, which has centrally located nuclei.

Organization of Striated Skeletal Muscle

The masses of fibers that make up the different types of muscle are not grouped in random fashion but are arranged in regular bundles surrounded by an external sheath of dense connective tissue sur-

rounding the entire muscle called the **epimysium** (Fig 11–2). From the epimysium, thin septa of connective tissue extend inward, surrounding bundles of fibers within a muscle. These septa are called **perimysia**. Bundles of perimysial-bound fibers are known as **fascicles**. Each muscle fiber is surrounded by a delicate layer of connective tissue composed mainly of an external (basal) lamina and reticular fibers, the **endomysium** (Figs 11–2 and 11–11). The epimysium, perimysium, and endomysium are all true connective tissue structures, complete with collagen, elastic fibers, fibroblasts, and blood vessels.

The connective tissue not only binds the muscle fibers together and permits some freedom of movement among them but also binds the muscle tissue to the structures (tendon, periosteum, skin, aponeurosis, etc) with which it comes in contact.

One of the most important roles of connective tissue is as a mechanical transducer for the forces

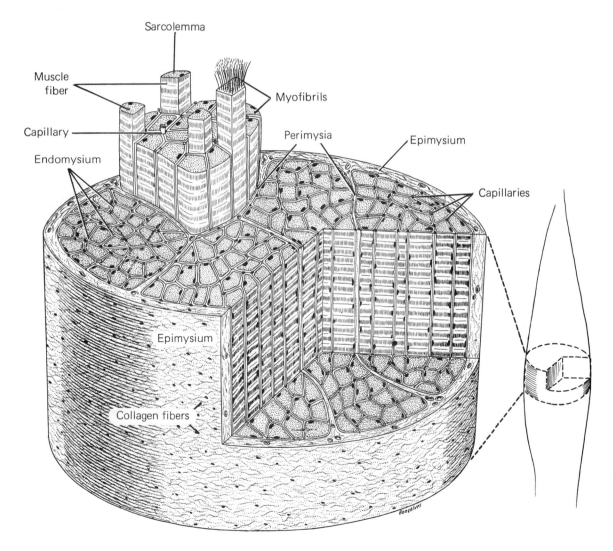

Figure 11–2. Structure of striated skeletal muscle. To the right is a drawing showing where the enlarged segment was taken from a muscle.

generated by contracting muscle cells. In most instances, individual muscle cells do not extend from one end of a muscle to the other. The force of contraction generated by these cells is therefore mediated by the ensheathing connective tissue.

The blood vessels penetrate into the muscle inside the connective tissue septa and form a rich capillary network that runs between and parallel to the muscle fibers. The capillaries are of the continuous type. Lymphatics are found in the connective tissue area.

The muscles taper off at their extremities, where a myotendinous junction is formed. Analysis of this transitional region with the aid of the electron microscope reveals that collagen fibers of the tendon insert themselves into complex infoldings of the plasmalemma of the muscle fibers present at this zone. Normally, each individual muscle fiber has on its surface a motor nerve ending, the so-called **motor end-plate,** whose structure is shown in Fig 11–10 and will be described in detail later in this chapter.

As observed with the light microscope, longitudinally sectioned muscle cells or muscle fibers, when stained with hematoxylin and eosin, show cross-striations composed of alternating light and dark bands (Fig 11–3). The darker bands are called **A bands** (**anisotropic,** ie, birefringent in polarized light); the lighter bands are called **I bands** (**isotropic,** ie, does not alter polarized light). Each I band is bisected by a dark tranverse line, the **Z line.**

The smallest repetitive subunit of the contractile apparatus, the **sarcomere,** extends from Z line to Z line (Figs 11–4 and 11–5).

The sarcoplasm of each muscle fiber is filled with long cylindric filamentous bundles called **myofibrils.** The myofibrils, which have a diameter of 1–2 μm and run parallel to the long axis of the muscle fiber, are composed of an end-to-end chain-like arrangement of sarcomeres (Figs 11–4 and 11–5). As a consequence of the registration of sarcomeres in adjacent myofibrils, the entire muscle fiber exhibits a characteristic pattern of transverse striations.

Electron microscopic studies reveal that the sarcomere pattern described above is due mainly to the presence of 2 types of filaments—thick and thin filaments—disposed parallel to the long axis of the myofibrils in a symmetric pattern.

The thick filaments occupy the A band, the central portion of the sarcomere. The thin filaments run between and parallel to the thick ones and have one end attached to the Z line (Figs 11–4 and 11–5). As a result of this arrangement, the I bands consist of the portions of the thin filaments that are not overlapping the thick filaments. The A bands are mainly composed of thick filaments in addition to portions of overlapping thin filaments. Closer observation of the A band shows the presence of a lighter zone in its center, the **H band** (Figs 11–4 and 11–5). The H band is that portion of the A band that consists of only thick filaments.

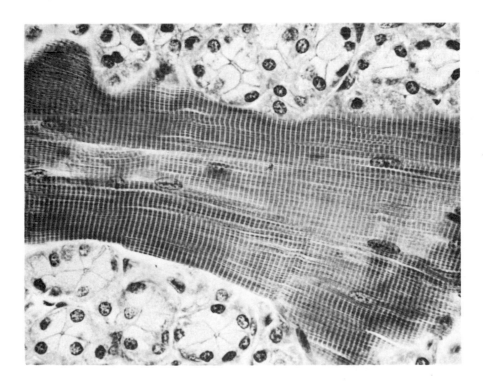

Figure 11 –3. Photomicrograph of a section of the tongue of a rat, showing the transverse (cross) striations of the skeletal muscle fibers cut longitudinally. × 700.

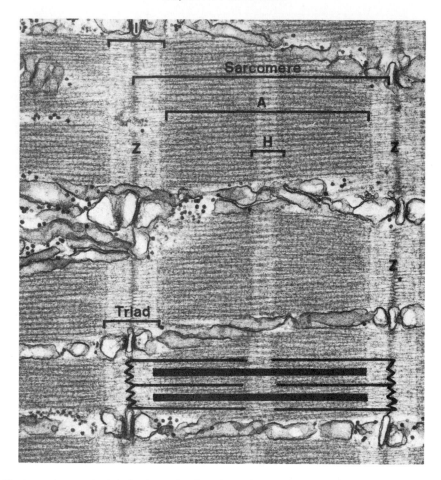

Figure 11–4. Electron micrograph of skeletal muscle of a tadpole. Observe the sarcomere, with its A, I, and H bands and Z line. The position of the thick and thin filaments in the sarcomere is shown in the lower part. Reduced from × 42,000. (Courtesy of KR Porter.)

Thin and thick filaments overlap for some distance within the A band. As a consequence, a cross section in the region of filament overlap shows each thick filament surrounded by 6 thin filaments in the form of a hexagon (Fig 11–5I).

The striated muscle filaments contain at least 4 main proteins: actin, tropomyosin, troponin, and myosin. Thin filaments are composed of the first 3 proteins, while thick filaments consist primarily of myosin.

Myosin and actin together represent 55% of the total protein of striated muscle. Other contractile proteins such as actinin and β-actinin are present in smaller amounts, and their functions are not well understood.

Actin is present as long filamentous (F-actin) structures consisting of 2 strands composed of spherical or globular (G-actin) monomers 5.6 nm in diameter twisted around each other in a double helical formation (Figs 11–5J and 11–5K). A notable characteristic of all G-actin molecules is their structural asymmetry. When G-actin molecules polymerize to form the F-actin, they bind back to front, producing

a filament with distinguishable polarity (Fig 11–6). Each G-actin monomer contains a binding site for myosin (Fig 11–7). Actin filaments, which anchor perpendicularly on the Z line, exhibit opposite polarity on each side of the Z line (Fig 11–5).

Tropomyosin is a long, thin polar molecule about 40 nm in length containing 2 polypeptide chains in the form of an α-helix. These polypeptide chains are coiled one on the other. Tropomyosin molecules are bound head to tail, forming filaments that run over the actin subunits alongside the outer edges of the groove between the 2 twisted actin strands (Fig 11–6).

Troponin is a complex of 3 subunits: **TnT**, which strongly attaches to tropomyosin; **TnC**, which binds calcium ions; and **TnI**, which inhibits the actin-myosin interaction. A troponin complex is attached at one specific site on each tropomyosin molecule (Fig 11–6).

In thin filaments, the tropomyosin molecule covers 7 G-actin molecules and has one troponin complex bound to its surface (Fig 11–6).

Myosin is a much larger molecule, with a

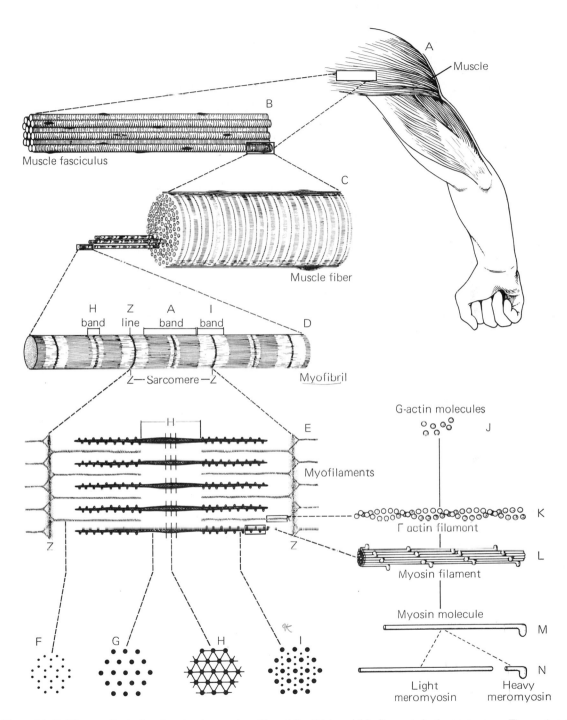

Figure 11–5. Diagram illustrating the structure and position of the thick and thin filaments in the sarcomere. The molecular structure of these components is shown at right. (Drawing by Sylvia Colard Keene. Reproduced, with permission, from Bloom W, Fawcett DW: *A Textbook of Histology,* 9th ed. Saunders, 1968.)

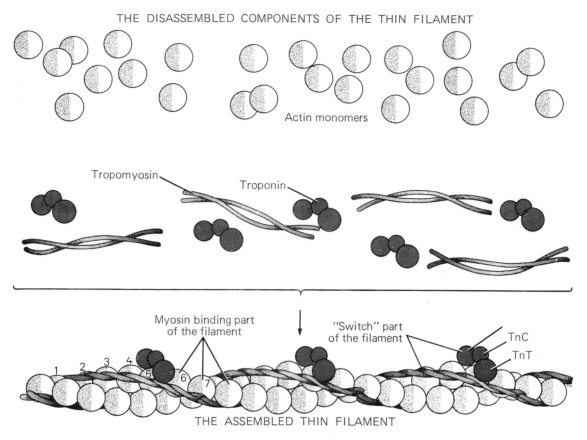

Figure 11–6. Schematic representation of the thin filament, showing the spatial configuration of the 3 major protein components—actin, tropomyosin, and troponin. The individual components in the top half of the drawing are shown in polymerized form in the bottom half. The globular actin molecules are polarized (dark and light areas) and polymerize in one direction. Observe that each tropomyosin molecule extends over 7 actin molecules. TnI, TnC, TnT, see text.

molecular weight of about 500,000. It is a thin rodlike molecule (200 nm long and 2–3 nm in diameter) made up of 2 peptide helices twisted together and running from one end of the rod to the other. A small globular projection or **head,** which extends at one end, possesses a specific ATP binding site. This head is the part of the myosin molecule where all biochemical reactions involved in the hydrolysis of ATP take place. It is also the region where the binding site to actin is located. When subjected to brief proteolysis, myosin can be cleaved into 2 fragments, **light** and **heavy meromyosin.** The light fragment represents the greater part of the rodlike portion of the molecule; heavy meromyosin represents its globular projection plus a small part of the rod (Fig 11–5N). The myosin molecules are arranged within the thick filaments with their rodlike portions overlapping and their globular heads directed toward either end. A bare zone in the middle, which corresponds to the H band, represents a region of myosin overlap consisting of only the rodlike part of the molecule (Fig 11–5E).

Analysis of thin sections of striated muscle shows the presence of crossbridges between thin and thick filaments. These bridges are known to be formed by the head of the myosin molecule plus a short part of its rodlike portion. The ATPase heads are considered to be directly involved in the transduction of chemical into mechanical energy (Fig 11–7).

Contraction Mechanism

Resting sarcomeres consist of partially overlapping thick and thin filaments. During a contraction cycle, both the thick and thin filaments retain their original length. Since contraction is not due to a shortening of individual filaments, it must be due to an increase in the amount of overlap between the filaments. The **sliding filament** hypothesis of muscle contraction proposed by Huxley has received the most widespread acceptance.

Contraction is initiated in the A band, where thick and thin filaments overlap. The following is a brief scheme of how actin and myosin interact during a contraction cycle: At rest, ATP binds to the ATPase site on the myosin heads. Myosin requires

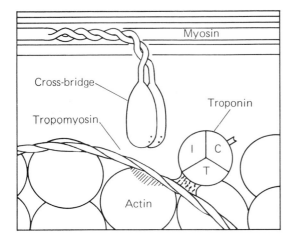

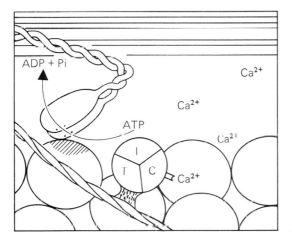

Figure 11 –7. Initiation of muscle contraction occurs by the binding of Ca²⁺ to the TnC unit of troponin, which exposes the actin binding site (cross-hatched area) to myosin. In a second step, the myosin head binds to actin and the ATP breaks down into ADP and energy, which produces a movement of the myosin head. As a consequence of this change in myosin, the bound thin filaments slide over the thick filaments. This process, which repeats itself many times during a single contraction, leads to a complete overlap of the actin and myosin and, concomitantly, a shortening of the whole myofiber. (Reproduced, with permission, from Ganong WF: *Review of Medical Physiology,* 9th ed. Lange, 1979.)

actin as a cofactor in order to break down the ATP and release energy. In a resting muscle, myosin cannot associate with actin because of repression of the binding site by the troponin-tropomyosin complex on the F-actin filament. However, when Ca²⁺ ions are available, they bind to the TnC unit of troponin. The spatial configuration of the 3 troponin subunits changes and drives the tropomyosin molecule deeper into the groove of the actin helix (Fig 11–7). This exposes the active binding site of the actin globular components, so that actin is free

to interact with the head of the myosin molecule. The binding of calcium ions to the TnC unit corresponds to the stage at which myosin-ATP is converted into the active complex. As a result of bridging between the myosin head and the G-actin subunit of the thin filament, the ATP is split into ADP, Pi, and energy. This activity leads to a deformation or bending of the head and a part of the rodlike portion of the myosin (Fig 11–7). Since the actin is bound to the myosin, movement of the myosin head pulls the actin over the myosin filament. Although a large number of myosin heads extend from the thick filament, at any one time during the contraction only a small number of heads align with available actin binding sites. However, as the bound myosin heads move the actin, they provide for alignment of new actin-myosin bridges. The old actin-myosin bridges only detach after the myosin binds a new ATP molecule; this action also resets the myosin head and prepares it for another contraction cycle. If no ATP is available, the actin-myosin complex becomes stable; this accounts for the extreme muscular rigidity (**rigor mortis**) that occurs after death. A single muscle contraction is the result of hundreds of bridge-forming and bridge-breaking cycles. The contraction activity that leads to a complete overlap between thin and thick filaments continues until Ca²⁺ ions are removed and the troponin-tropomyosin complex again covers the myosin binding site.

During contraction, the I band decreases in size as actin filaments penetrate into the A band. Concomitantly, the H band—the part of the A band with only thick filaments—diminishes as the thin filaments completely overlap the thick filaments. A net result is that each sarcomere, and consequently the whole cell (fiber), is greatly shortened.

Sarcoplasmic Reticulum

As described above, muscle contraction depends on the availability of Ca²⁺ ions, while muscle relaxation is related to an absence of Ca²⁺. The sarcoplasmic reticulum (SR) specifically regulates calcium ion flow, which is necessary for rapid contraction and relaxation cycles. Cytologically, the sarcoplasmic reticulum system consists of a branching network of smooth endoplasmic reticulum cisternae that surrounds the myofilaments and carves them up into discrete cylindric myofibril bundles (Fig 11–11). Following a neurally mediated depolarization of the sarcoplasmic reticulum membrane, Ca²⁺ ions concentrated within the sarcoplasmic reticulum cisternae are passively released into the vicinity of the overlapping thick and thin filaments, whereupon they bind to troponin and allow bridging between the actin and myosin. When the neural depolarization ends, the sarcoplasmic reticulum acts as a calcium sink and actively transports the Ca²⁺ back into the cisternae, which results in cessation of contractile activity.

Using cell homogenization and differential centrifugation, it has been possible to isolate the sarco-plasmic reticulum. In vitro, isolated sarcoplasmic reticulum acts as a **relaxation factor** that inhibits muscle contraction. This inhibition, related to the removal of available Ca^{2+} by the vesicular portions of the sarcoplasmic reticulum, demonstrates the existence of an active calcium transport mechanism in the sarcoplasmic reticulum membrane.

Transverse Tubule System

The depolarization of the sarcoplasmic reticulum membrane, which results in the release of Ca^{2+} ions, is initiated at a specialized myoneural junction on the surface of the muscle cell (structure described below). Surface-initiated depolarization signals would have to diffuse throughout the cell to effect Ca^{2+} release from internal sarcoplasmic reticulum cisternae. In larger muscle cells, the diffusion of the depolarization signal would lead to a wave of contraction, wherein peripheral myofibrils would contract prior to more centrally positioned myofibrils. To provide for a uniform contraction, skeletal muscle possesses a system of **transverse (T) tubules.** These sarcolemma-derived, fingerlike invaginations form a complex anastomosing network of tubules that encircle both A-I junctions of each sarcomere in every myofibril (Figs 11–8, 11–9, and 11–11).

Bound to opposite sides of each T tubule process are expanded **terminal cisternae** of the sarcoplasmic reticulum. This specialized complex, consisting of SR-T tubule-SR components, is known as the **triad** (Figs 11–4, 11–9, and 11–11). At the triad, depolarization of the sarcolemma-derived T tubules is transmitted via protein bridges to the sarcoplasmic reticulum.

Neural Innervation

In order to contract, each skeletal muscle fiber normally requires innervation by a motor nerve branch. Myelinated motor nerves branch out within the perimysial connective tissue, where each nerve gives rise to several terminal twigs. At the site of innervation, the nerve loses its myelin sheath and forms a dilated termination that sits within a trough on the muscle cell surface (Fig 11–10). This structure is called the **motor end-plate** or **myoneural junction.** At this site the axon is covered by a thin cytoplasmic layer of Schwann cells. Within the axon terminal are numerous mitochondria and synaptic vesicles, the latter containing the neurotransmitter **acetylcholine** (described in Chapter 9). Between

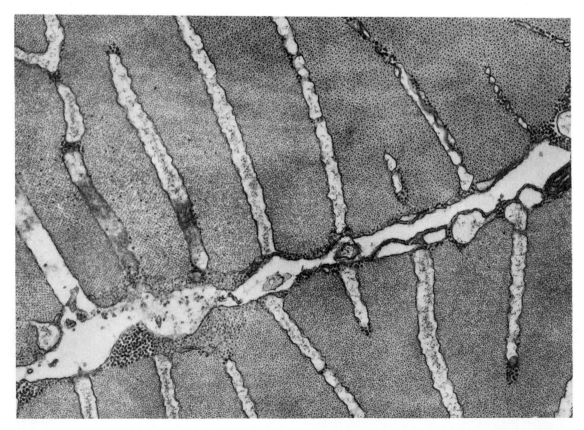

Figure 11–8. Electron micrograph of a transverse section of fish muscle, showing the surface of 2 cells limiting an intercellular space. Observe the invagination present in the sarcolemma, forming the tubules of the T system. The dark, coarse granules in the cytoplasm *(lower left)* are glycogen particles. × 60,000. (Courtesy of KR Porter.)

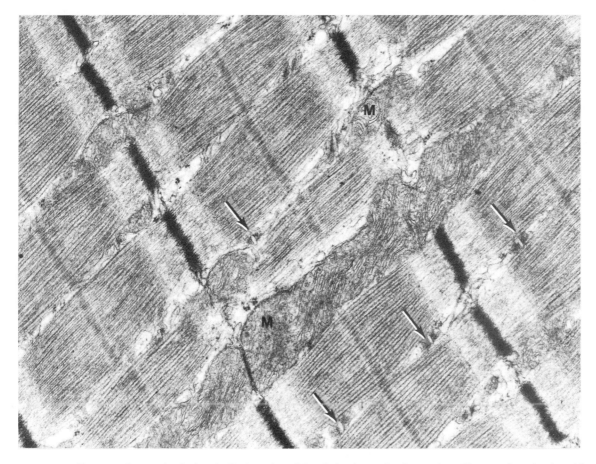

Figure 11 –9. Electron micrograph of a longitudinal section of the skeletal muscle of a monkey. Observe the mitochondria (M) between the myofibrils and the various bands of the sarcomere. The arrows show triads—2 for each sarcomere in this muscle. × 30,000.

the axon and the muscle is a space, the **synaptic cleft,** in which lies an amorphous basal lamina matrix. At the junction, the sarcolemma is thrown into numerous deep **junctional folds.** In the sarcoplasm below the folds lie several myonuclei, numerous mitochondria, ribosomes, and glycogen granules.

When the motor nerve fires, acetylcholine is liberated from the axon terminal, diffuses through the cleft, and binds to acetylcholine receptors in the sarcolemma of the junctional folds. Binding of the transmitter makes the sarcolemma more permeable to sodium, which results in **membrane depolarization.** Excess acetylcholine is hydrolyzed by cholinesterase enzymes situated within the collagenous matrix of the synaptic cleft. Acetylcholine breakdown is necessary to avoid prolonged contact of the transmitter with receptors present in the sarcolemma.

The depolarization initiated at the motor endplate is propagated along the surface of the muscle cell and deep into the fibers via the transverse tubule system. At each triad, the depolarization signal is passed to the sarcoplasmic reticulum and

results in the release of Ca^{2+}, which initiates the contraction cycle. When depolarization ceases, the Ca^{2+} is actively transported back into the sarcoplasmic reticulum cisternae and the muscle relaxes.

Evidence has firmly established that the myoneural disorder **myasthenia gravis,** characterized by a progressive muscular weakness, is an autoimmune disease. In myasthenics, circulating antibodies bind to acetylcholine receptors in the junctional folds and inhibit normal muscle-nerve communication.

A single nerve fiber may innervate one muscle cell or may branch and be responsible for innervating up to 160 or more muscle cells. In the case of multiple innervation, a single nerve fiber and all the muscle cells it innervates is called a **motor unit.** Striated muscle cells do not show degrees of contraction—they either contract all the way or not at all. In order to vary the force of contraction, not all the cells within a muscle bundle should contract at the same time. Since muscles are broken up into motor units, the firing of a single nerve will elicit a

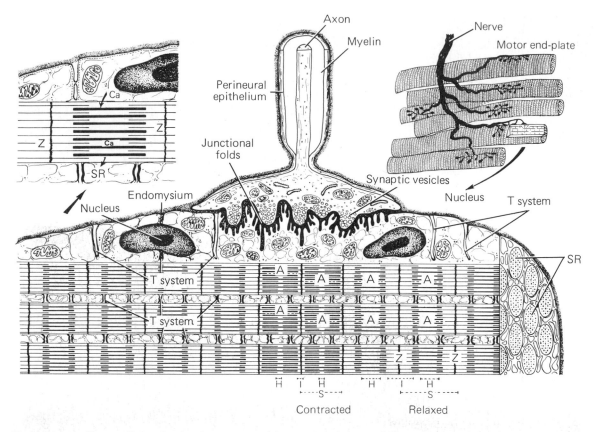

Figure 11 –10. Diagram illustrating the ultrastructure of the motor end-plate and the mechanism of muscle contraction. The upper right drawing shows branching of a small nerve with a motor end-plate for each muscle fiber. The aspect of one of the bulbs of an end-plate is highly enlarged in the central drawing. Observe that the axon terminal bud presents synaptic vesicles. The region of the muscle cell membrane covered by the terminal bud presents clefts and cristae called **junctional folds.** The axon loses its myelin sheath and dilates, establishing close, irregular contact with the muscle fiber. Muscle contraction begins with the release of acetylcholine from the synaptic vesicles of the end-plate. This substance promotes a local increase in the permeability of the sarcolemma. This process is propagated to the rest of the sarcolemma, including its invaginations, all of which constitute the T system, and is transferred to the sarcoplasmic reticulum (SR). The increase of permeability in this organelle liberates calcium ions that trigger the sliding mechanism of muscle contraction. Thin filaments slide between the thick filaments and reduce the distance between the Z lines. This promotes a reduction in the size of all bands except the A band.

contraction that is proportionate to the number of cells innervated by that "motor unit." Thus, the number of motor units and the variable size of each unit can control the intensity of a muscle contraction. The size of motor units within a given muscle is dependent upon the delicacy of movement required by that muscle. For example, because of the fine control required by eye muscles, each of their fibers is innervated by a different nerve. However, in larger muscles exhibiting coarser movements, like those of the limb, many single nerves provide for motor units that consist of over 100 individual muscle cells.

System of Energy Production

Striated skeletal muscle cells are highly adapted for discontinuous production of mechanical work through chemical energy and must have de-

pots of energy to cope with bursts of activity. The most readily available energy is stored in the form of ATP and phosphocreatine, both of which are energy-rich compounds. Chemical energy is also available in glycogen depots, which constitute about 0.5–1% of muscle weight. A small part of the energy from glycogen is made available during glycolysis. The major portion of energy used by the muscle is produced in mitochondria through oxidative phosphorylation of blood metabolites. This process uses oxygen from the bloodstream or from myoglobin, an oxygen-binding protein in muscle.

In mammals, the main sources of energy for skeletal muscle are the circulating fatty acids and acetoacetate. When these muscles are very active, they rapidly metabolize glucose, which becomes the main source of energy.

From the morphologic, histochemical, and

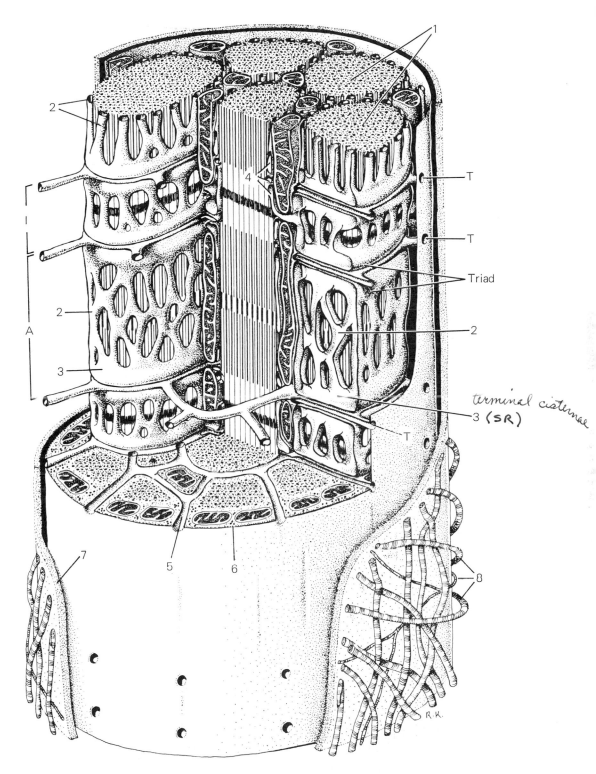

terminal cisternae

3 (SR)

Figure 11 –11. Diagram of a segment of mammalian skeletal muscle. The sarcolemma and muscle fibrils are partially cut, showing the following components: The invaginations of the T system (T and 5) occur at the level of transition between the A and I bands twice in every sarcomere. They associate with terminal cisternae of the sarcoplasmic reticulum (3), forming **triads.** Abundant mitochondria (4) lie between the myofibrils. The cut surface of the myofibrils (1) shows the thin and thick filaments. Surrounding the sarcolemma are a basal lamina (7) and reticular fibers (8). (Reproduced, with permission, from Krstić RV: *Ultrastructure of the Mammalian Cell.* Springer-Verlag, 1979.)

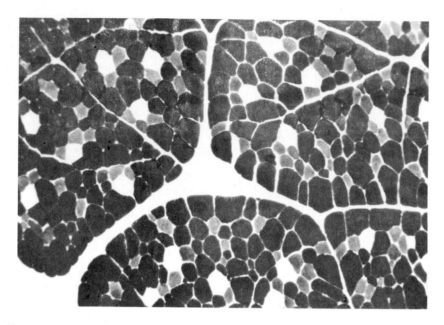

Figure 11 –12. Transverse section of a striated muscle (rectus lateralis), stained by the histochemical technic for myosin ATPase, showing 3 types of fibers in the muscle. This method shows the red fibers in black (high ATPase activity), the white fibers in light gray (low ATPase activity), and the intermediate fibers in various shades of gray and illustrates the histochemical differences between these types of muscle fibers. (Reproduced, with permission, from Khan MA & others: Stain Technol 47:277, 1971.)

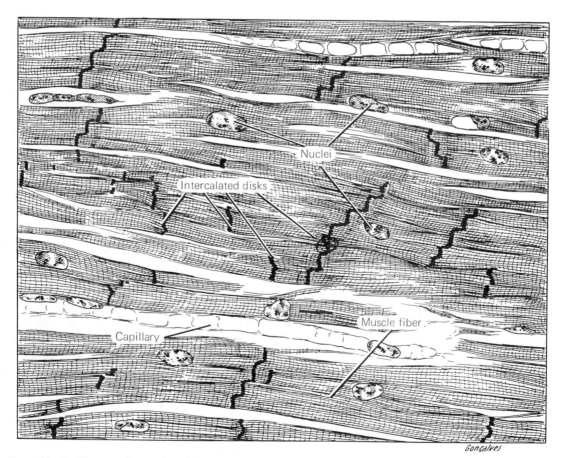

Figure 11 –13. Diagram of a section of heart muscle. Observe the presence of central nuclei and intercalated disks.

functional point of view, we may classify skeletal muscle fibers into 3 types: red, white, and intermediate. **Red fibers** have a high content of myoglobin and cytochrome, which are responsible for the dark red color. They contract at a slower rate than white fibers but are capable of continuous and vigorous activity. Their energy derives mainly from oxidative phosphorylation, and these fibers thus contain great numbers of mitochondria. These are the fibers in the breast muscle of migrating birds and mammalian limbs. The long muscles of the human back, adapted for long slow posture-maintaining contractions, are also an example of red muscle. **White fibers** have a low content of myoglobin and cytochrome and fewer mitochondria. The breast muscles of chickens and turkeys as well as the extraocular muscles of the human eye consist of these fibers. They contract rapidly but do not support continuous heavy work. The energy for their activity is derived mainly from anaerobic glycolysis. **Intermediate fibers** have characteristics between the 2 extremes described above. In humans, the skeletal muscles are frequently composed of mixtures of these 3 types of fibers, as shown in Fig 11–12.

The differentiation of muscle into red, white, and intermediate fiber types is controlled by its innervation. In experiments where the nerves to red and white fibers are cut, crossed, and allowed to regenerate, the myofibers change their morphology and physiology in order to conform to the innervating nerve. Simple denervation of muscle will lead to fiber atrophy and paralysis.

Other Components of the Sarcoplasm

Glycogen is found in abundance in the sarcoplasm in the form of coarse granules (Fig 11–8). It serves as a depot of energy that is mobilized during muscle contraction.

Another component of the sarcoplasm is **myoglobin,** a pigment similar to hemoglobin that is principally responsible for the dark red color of some muscles. Myoglobin acts as an oxygen depot and is present in great amounts in the muscle of deep-diving ocean mammals (eg, seals and whales). Muscles that must maintain activity for prolonged periods usually are red and have a high content of myoglobin.

Mature muscle cells have negligible amounts of granular endoplasmic reticulum and ribosomes,

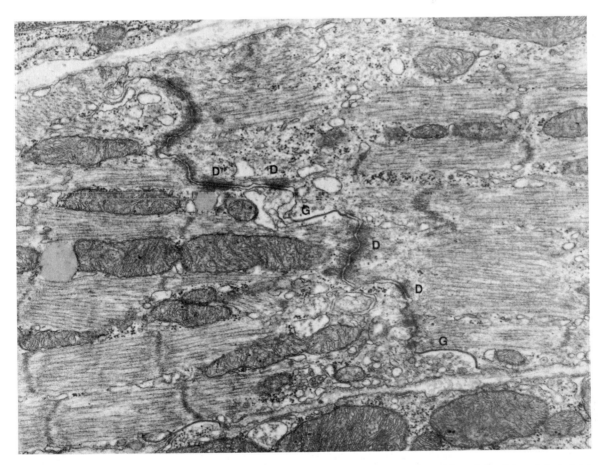

Figure 11–14. Longitudinal section of heart muscle. Observe the typical steplike disposition of the intercalated disks, presenting gap junctions (G) and desmosomes (D). × 23,000. (Courtesy of OP Almeida.)

an observation that is consistent with the low level of protein synthesis occurring in this tissue.

CARDIAC MUSCLE

During development, the splanchnic mesoderm cells of the primitive heart tube align into chainlike arrays. Rather than fusing into syncytial cells like skeletal muscle, the cardiac cells form complex junctions between their extended processes. Cells within a chain often bifurcate or branch and bind to cells in adjacent chains. Consequently, the heart consists of tightly knit bundles of cells, interwoven in such fashion as to provide for

a characteristic wave of contraction that leads to a "wringing out" of the heart ventricles.

Mature cardiac muscle cells exhibit a cross-striated banding pattern identical to that of skeletal muscle. However, unlike multinucleated skeletal muscle, each cell possesses only one or 2 centrally located euchromatic nuclei. Surrounding the columns of muscle cells is a delicate sheath of endomysial connective tissue in which lies a rich capillary network.

A unique and distinguishing characteristic of cardiac muscle is the presence of darkly staining transverse lines that cross the chains of cardiac cells at irregular intervals (Fig 11–13). These intercalated disks represent junctional complexes found at the interface between adjacent cardiac myocytes (Figs 11–14 and 11–15). These junctions may ap-

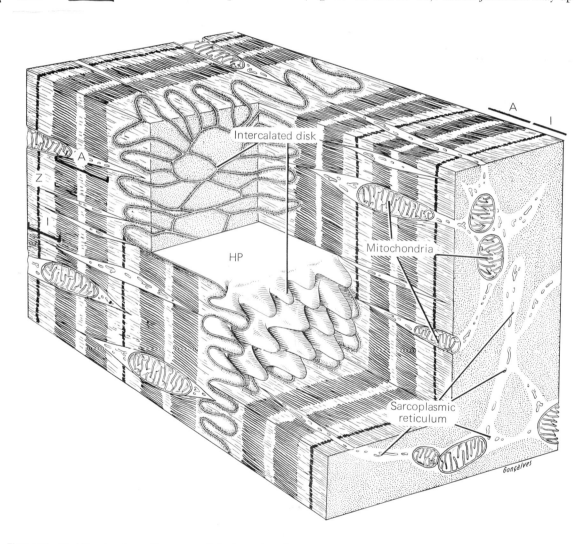

Figure 11–15. Ultrastructure of heart muscle in the region of an intercalated disk. Contact between cells is accomplished by interdigitation in the vertical region and is smooth in the horizontal plane (HP). (Redrawn and reproduced, with permission, from Marshall JM: The heart. In: *Medical Physiology,* 13th ed. Vol 2. Mountcastle VB [editor]. Mosby, 1974. Based on the results of Fawcett DW, McNutt NS: J Cell Biol 42:1, 1969; modified from Poche R, Lindner E: Z Zellforsch Mikrosk Anat 43:104, 1955.)

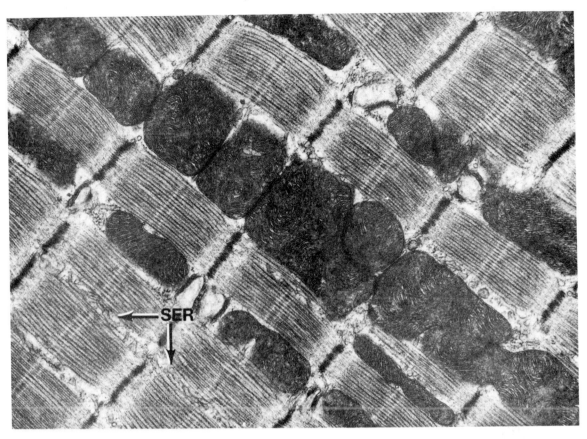

Figure 11 –16. Electron micrograph from a longitudinal section of heart muscle. Observe the striation pattern and the alternation of myofilaments and dense mitochondria rich in cristae. Note the smooth endoplasmic reticulum (SER). × 30,000.

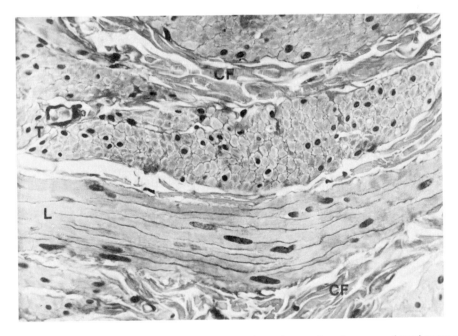

Figure 11 –17. Photomicrograph of a section of urinary bladder. Smooth muscle cells are sectioned transversely (T) and longitudinally (L). Note the collagen fibers (CF). H&E stain, × 400.

pear as straight lines or may exhibit a steplike morphology. Two regions can be distinguished in the
steplike junctions—a **transverse portion,** which
runs across the fibers at right angles, and a **lateral
portion** running parallel to the myofilaments. There
are 3 main junctional specializations within the
disk. **Fascia adherens,** the most prominent membrane specialization in transverse portions of the
disk, serves as anchoring sites for actin filaments of
the terminal sarcomeres. Essentially they represent **hemi (half) Z bands. Maculae adherentes**
(desmosomes) bind the cardiac cells together to
prevent their pulling apart under constant contractile activity. On the lateral portions of the disk, **gap
junctions** provide ionic continuity between adjacent cells. The significance of ionic coupling is that
chains of individual cells behave as a syncytium in
that the signal to contract passes in a wave from cell
to cell.

The structure and function of the contractile
proteins in cardiac cells is virtually the same as in
skeletal muscle (Fig 11–16). The T tubule system
and sarcoplasmic reticulum, however, are not as
regularly arranged in the cardiac myocytes. The T
tubules are more numerous and larger in ventricular muscle than in skeletal muscle. Cardiac T
tubules are found at the level of the Z band rather
than at the A-I junction, as in skeletal muscle. The
sarcoplasmic reticulum is not as well developed and
wanders irregularly through the myofilaments. As a
consequence, the actin and myosin are not carved
up into discrete myofibrillar bundles.

Triads are not common in cardiac cells, since
the T tubules are generally associated with only one
lateral expansion of sarcoplasmic reticulum cisternae. Thus, heart muscle characteristically possesses
diads composed of one T tubule and one sarcoplasmic reticulum cisterna.

In addition to large glycogen deposits and the
presence of lipofuscin (residual body) granules, the
cardiac sarcoplasm contains an abundance of
mitochondria clustered around each pole of the nucleus as well as in long chains intercalated among
the myofilaments (Figs 11–14, 11–15, and 11–16).

The rich nerve supply to the heart and the
rhythmic impulse-generating and conducting structures are dealt with in Chapter 12.

SMOOTH MUSCLE

Smooth muscle is composed of long (30–200
μm) spindlelike cells which in cross section appear
as narrow (5–10 μm) circular profiles (Figs 11–17
and 11–18). Each cell possesses a characteristic centrally located elongated nucleus. In contracted
cells, the nuclei are frequently folded or pleated. At
the poles of the nucleus lie numerous mitochondria,
a well-developed rough endoplasmic reticulum,

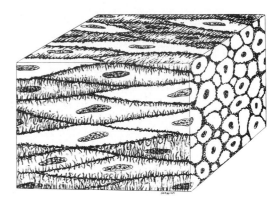

Figure 11–18. Diagram of a segment of smooth muscle. All
cells are surrounded by a net of reticular fibers. In cross
section, the cell exhibits variable diameters.

and a large Golgi body. Although most of the cytoplasm appears to be unstructured, at the electron
microscopic level it can be seen to consist of arrays
of myofilaments.

In bundles of smooth muscle, the fusiform cells
overlap one another along their length (Fig 11–18).
The bundles are normally organized into layers,
with cells in adjacent layers usually lying at right
angles to each other. Within the bundles, the cells
are enmeshed by a dense endomysial matrix consisting of a collagenous external lamina. Fascicles of
cells are delineated by perimysial connective tissue, while a thick epimysium separates the larger
bundles of muscle.

Smooth muscle cells can be dispersed in the
connective tissue of certain organs (eg, prostate,
seminal vesicles). They may group to form small
muscle bundles (eg, the arrector pili muscles in the
skin) or may be the predominant tissue of an organ
such as in the uterus. Unlike striated muscle, contraction of smooth muscle is relatively slow and the
cells may remain contracted for long periods without fatigue. In addition, individual smooth muscle
cells may undergo partial or "wavelike" contractions.

The characteristic contractile activity of
smooth muscle is related to the structure and organization of its actin and myosin filaments, which
do not exhibit the same paracrystalline organization
present in striated muscle. In smooth muscle cells,
bundles of myofilaments crisscross obliquely
through the cell, forming a latticelike network.
These bundles appeared to consist only of 5–7 nm
actin filaments until x-ray crystallography studies
on living smooth muscle cells revealed that thick ($\sim$
16 nm) myosin filaments were present in the
myofilament lattice. With improved fixation procedures, labile myosin filaments are now preserved
and visualized in smooth muscle cells. Unlike the
myosin filaments in skeletal muscle, which have a
bare central region with barbs (myosin heads) on
each end, smooth muscle myosin has barbs all along

its length with bare regions at the ends of the filaments. This morphology reflects polarity differences in the organization of the polymerized myosin molecules. Much greater actin "overlap" and a concomitantly greater degree of contraction are possible in smooth muscle as a result of the molecular organization of the myosin filaments. Both structural and biochemical studies reveal that actin and myosin contract by a sliding filament mechanism similar to that which occurs in striated muscle. During contraction, the entire myofilament lattice may contract all at once, or a "wave" of contraction may spread along the length of the cell.

Smooth muscle cells also exhibit an elaborate filamentous infrastructure. Networks of **10-nm intermediate filaments** crisscross through the cell, weaving a mesh matrix. **Dense bodies** are present where these filaments bind to the cell membrane and where they cross over one another. Presumably, the dense bodies represent sites of adhesion of intermediate filaments. Formerly, **dense bodies** were thought to represent actin binding sites analogous to Z disks present in striated muscle.

Owing to their narrow diameter and slow mode of contraction, smooth muscle cells do not need or have a T tubule system. Although present, the calcium-regulating sarcoplasmic reticulum is greatly reduced when compared to that in striated muscle. The numerous surface-associated pinocytotic vesicles (Fig 11–19) also play a role in the uptake and release of calcium ions.

The degree of innervation in a particular bundle of smooth muscle is dependent upon both the function and size of that muscle. Smooth muscle is innervated by both sympathetic and parasympathetic nerves of the autonomic system. Elaborate neuromuscular junctions similar to those in skeletal muscle are not present in smooth muscle. Frequently, autonomic nerve axons terminate in a series of dilatations in the endomysial connective tissue. Within these dilatations are vesicles containing either acetylcholine (cholinergic nerves) or norepinephrine (noradrenergic nerves). The dilatations may be as close as 10–20 nm to the surface of the muscle, or they may lie at greater distances (100 nm or more). In the latter case, excitation of the muscle depends upon long-range diffusion of the neurotransmitters through the intervening connective tissue.

In general, smooth muscle occurs in large

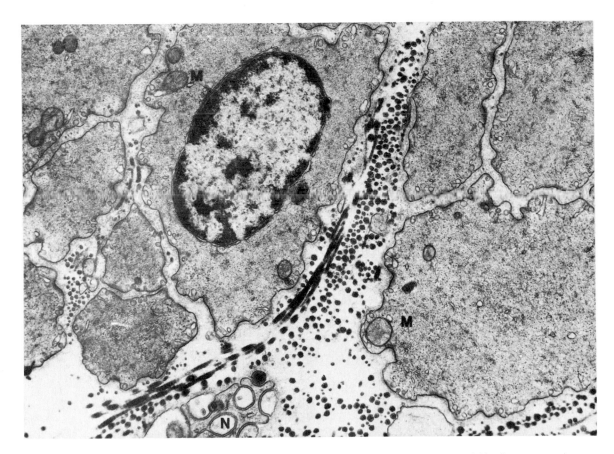

Figure 11 –19. Electron micrograph of a transverse section of smooth muscle. The cells have variable diameters and many pinocytotic vesicles on their surface. There are few mitochondria (M). Between the cells are collagen fibers and a small unmyelinated nerve (N). Reduced from × 7500.

sheets such as in the walls of hollow viscera, as in the intestines, uterus, and ureters. Their cells present abundant gap junctions and a relatively poor nerve supply. These muscles function in syncytial fashion and are called **visceral** or **unitary smooth muscles.** In contrast, the **multiunit smooth muscles** present a rich innervation and can produce very precise and graded contractions as occur in the iris of the eye.

Smooth muscle usually has spontaneous activity in the absence of nervous stimuli. Its nerve supply therefore has the function of modifying activity and not initiating it, as in skeletal muscle. Smooth muscle receives both adrenergic and cholinergic nerve endings that act antagonistically, stimulating or depressing its activity. In some organs, the cholinergic endings activate and the adrenergic nerves depress, while in others the reverse occurs.

In addition to contractile activity, smooth muscle cells have also been shown to synthesize collagen, elastin, and proteoglycans, extracellular products normally associated with the function of fibroblasts (see Chapter 5). The elaborate rough endoplasmic reticulum and well-developed Golgi are organellar correlates reflecting this synthetic behavior.

REGENERATION OF MUSCLE TISSUE

The 3 types of adult muscle exhibit varying potentials for regeneration after a destructive injury.

Cardiac muscle has practically no regenerative capacity beyond early childhood. Defects or damage (eg, infarcts) in heart muscle are generally replaced by proliferation of connective tissue, forming myocardial scars.

In skeletal muscle, although the nuclei in the syncytium are incapable of undergoing mitosis, the tissue undergoes extensive regeneration. The source of regenerating cells is believed to be the **satellite cell.** Satellite cells are a sparse population of mononucleated spindle-shaped cells which lie within the basal laminal sheath that surrounds each mature myofiber and, because of their intimate apposition with the myofiber surface, can be identified only with the electron microscope. Following injury or certain other stimuli, the normally quiescent satellite cells become activated, proliferate, and fuse to form new skeletal muscle fibers. A similar activity of satellite cells has been implicated with muscle hypertrophy, where they fuse with their "parent fibers" to increase muscle mass following extensive exercise.

Smooth muscle is capable of exhibiting a regenerative response. Following injury, viable mononucleated smooth muscle cells undergo mitosis and provide for the replacement of the damaged tissue.

●　　●　　●

References

Ballard FB & others: Myocardial metabolism of fatty acids. J Clin Invest 39:717, 1960.

Bennett T, Cobb JL: Studies on the avian gizzard: Morphology and innervation of the smooth muscle. Z Zellforsch Mikrosk Anat 96:173, 1969.

Bourne GH (editor): *The Structure and Function of Muscle.* Academic Press, 1972.

Burnstock G: Structure of smooth muscle and its innervation. Page 1 in: *Smooth Muscle.* Bülbring E & others (editors). Williams & Wilkins, 1970.

Challice CE, Viragh S (editors): *Ultrastructure of the Mammalian Heart.* Academic Press, 1973.

Cohen C: The protein switch of muscle contraction. Sci Am 233:36, Nov 1975.

Constantin LL, Franzini-Armstrong C, Podolsky RJ: Localization of calcium accumulating structures in striated muscle. Science 147:158, 1965.

Devine CE, Somlyo AV, Somlyo AP: Sarcoplasmic reticulum and mitochondria as calcium accumulation sites in smooth muscle. Philos Trans R Soc Lond [Biol] 265:17, 1973.

Ebashi S: Regulatory mechanism of muscle contraction with special reference to the Ca-troponin-tropomyosin system. Essays Biochem 10:1, 1974.

Fawcett DW: The sarcoplasmic reticulum of skeletal and cardiac muscle. Circulation 24:336, 1961.

Forssmann WG, Girardier L: A study of the T system in rat heart. J Cell Biol 44:1, 1970.

Gabella G, Blundell D: Nexuses between smooth muscle cells of the guinea-pig ileum. J Cell Biol 82:239, 1979.

Garamvölgyi N, Vizi ES, Knoll J: The regular occurrence of thick filaments in stretched mammalian smooth muscle. J Ultrastruct Res 34:135, 1971.

Gauthier GF, Padykula HA: Cytological studies of fiber types in skeletal muscle: A comparative study of the mammalian diaphragm. J Cell Biol 28:333, 1966.

Hanson J, Lowy L: Molecular basis of contractility in muscle. Br Med Bull 21:264, 1965.

Huxley HE: The mechanism of muscular contraction. Science 164:1356, 1969.

Huxley HE, Haman T: Changes in the cross striations of muscle during contraction and stretch and their structural interpretation. Nature 173:973, 1954.

Johnson PC: *Peripheral Circulation.* Wiley, 1978.

Jones PA, Scott-Burden T, Gevers W: Glycoprotein, elastin and collagen secretion by rat smooth muscle cells. Proc Natl Acad Sci USA 76:353, 1979.

Lipton BH, Schultz E: Developmental fate of skeletal muscle satellite cells. Science 205:1292, 1979.

MacLennan DH, Campbell KP: Structure, function and biosynthesis of sarcoplasmic reticulum proteins. Trans Int Biol Soc 4:148, 1979.

Mannherz HG, Goody RS: Proteins of contractile systems. Annu Rev Biochem 45:427, 1976.

McNutt NS: Ultrastructure of intercellular junction in adult and developing cardiac muscle. Am J Cardiol 25:169, 1970.

Murray JM, Weber A: The cooperative action of muscle proteins. Sci Am 230:58, Feb 1974.

Page S: Structure of the sarcoplasmic reticulum in vertebrate muscle. Br Med Bull 24:170, 1968.

Rash JE, Hudson CS, Ellisman MH: Ultrastructure of acetylcholine receptors at the mammalian neuromuscular junction. In: *Cell Membrane Receptors for Drugs and Hormones: A Multidisciplinary Approach.* Straub RW, Bolis L (editors). Raven Press, 1978.

Shoenberg CF, Needham DM: A study of the mechanism of contraction in vertebrate smooth muscle. Biol Rev 51:53, 1976.

Small JV: Studies on isolated smooth muscle cells: The contractile apparatus. J Cell Sci 24:327, 1977.

Somlyo AP, Somlyo AV: Ultrastructure of smooth muscle. In: *Methods in Pharmacology.* Daniel EE, Paton DM (editors). Plenum Press, 1975.

Somlyo AV: Bridging structures spanning the junctional gap at the triad of skeletal muscle. J Cell Biol 80:743, 1979.

Sommer JR, Johnson EA: A comparative study of Purkinje fibers and ventricular fibers. J Cell Biol 36:497, 1968.

Sommer JR, Waugh RA: The ultrastructure of the mammalian cardiac muscle cell—with special emphasis on the tubular membrane systems. Am J Pathol 82:192, 1976.

Taylor EW: Mechanism of actomyosin ATPase and the problem of muscle contraction. Curr Top Bioenerget 5:20, 1973.

Thaemert JC: Ultrastructure of cardiac muscle and nerve contiguities. J Cell Biol 29:156, 1966.

12 | Circulatory System

The circulatory system consists of the blood and lymphatic vascular systems. The blood vascular system comprises the following structures: (1) the heart, whose function is to pump the blood; (2) a series of efferent vessels, the arteries, which become smaller as they branch and whose function it is to carry the blood and, with it, nutrients and oxygen to the tissues; (3) a diffuse network of thin tubules—the capillaries—which anastomose profusely and through whose walls the interchange between blood and tissues takes place; and (4) the veins, the afferent vessels of the heart, which represent the convergence of the capillaries into a system of larger channels that convey into the vascular system products of metabolism, CO_2, etc.

The lymphatic vascular system begins in dead-end tubules, the lymphatic capillaries, which gradually anastomose in vessels of steadily increasing size and terminate in the blood vascular system, emptying into the large veins near the heart. The function of the lymphatic system is to return to the blood the fluid of the tissue spaces, which, on penetrating the lymphatic capillaries, contributes to formation of the liquid part of the lymph and, by passing through the lymphoid organs, contributes to circulation of lymphocytes and other immunologic factors.

The entire circulatory system is internally lined by a simple squamous epithelium, the **endothelium**, discussed in Chapter 4. The composition of the circulatory system, beginning with the simplest structures and proceeding to the more complex ones, is discussed in the following pages.

Capillaries

The capillaries are composed of a single layer of endothelial cells of mesenchymal origin, rolled up in the form of a tube, bounding a cylindric space. The average diameter of the capillaries is small, varying from 7 to 9 μm. When transversely cut, their walls are observed to consist of portions of 2 or 3 cells (Fig 12–1). The external surfaces of these cells rest on a basal lamina, a product of epithelial origin. Their margins are held together by occluding junctions, discussed in Chapter 3. The capillaries can be grouped into 3 types according to the structure of the endothelial cell walls. The type

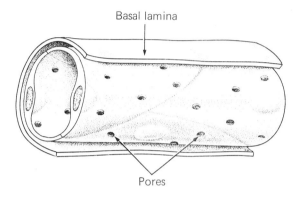

Figure 12–1. Diagram of the structure of a capillary with pores in its wall. The sectioned portion at left is composed of 2 endothelial cells. Not all capillaries have perforated walls. The basal lamina surrounds the capillary.

described above and illustrated in Fig 12–2 is a continuous capillary. A **fenestrated** or **perforated capillary** is characterized by the presence of pores **(fenestrae)** through the walls of the endothelial cells. These pores, closed by a diaphragm of complex structure and unknown chemical composition, are thinner than the cell membrane (Figs 12–1, 12–3, and 12–4). Perforated capillaries are usually encountered in tissues in which rapid interchange of substances occurs between the tissues and the blood, as is the case with the kidney, intestine, and endocrine glands. In some capillaries, the pores have a diaphragm with a sievelike structure, which suggests that they are the capillary pores described by physiologists. It has been shown that macromolecules injected into the bloodstream can and do cross the capillary wall through these orifices to enter the tissue spaces. This seems to be a more important means of transcapillary transport than that occurring as a result of pinocytosis as described in Chapter 4.

The third type of capillary, the **sinusoidal capillary** (Fig 15–19), has the following characteristics: (1) a tortuous path and a greatly enlarged diameter (30–40 μm), which slows the circulation of blood; (2) absence in the walls of a continuous lining of endothelial cells, leaving open spaces between cells

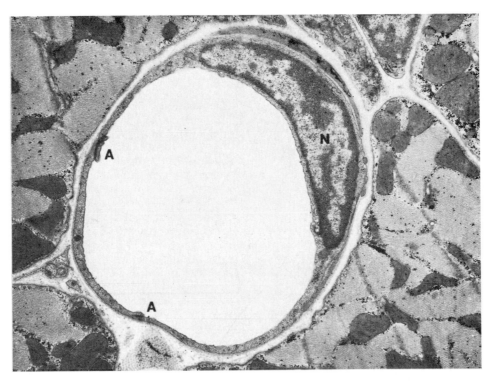

Figure 12 –2. Electron micrograph of a transverse section of a capillary from the myocardium. This is a continuous capillary. Note the nucleus (N) and the junction between neighboring cells (A). × 12,600. (Courtesy of J Rhodin.)

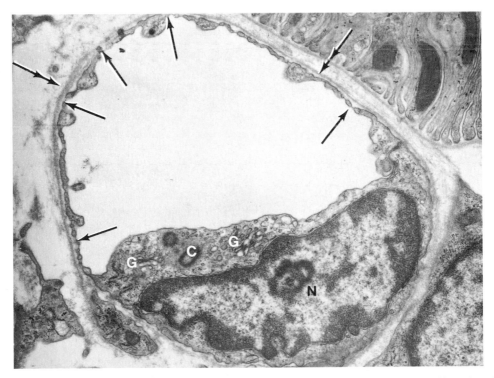

Figure 12 –3. A renal capillary with pores in its endothelial cell (arrows). In this cell the Golgi apparatus (G), nucleus (N), and 2 centrioles (C) can be seen. Note the continuous basal lamina on the outer surface of the endothelial cell (double arrows). × 20,000. (Courtesy of J Rhodin.)

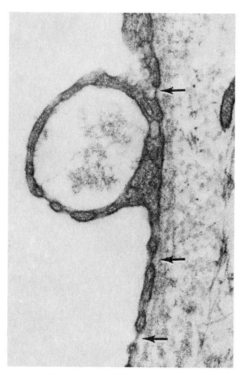

Figure 12–4. Electron micrograph of the endothelium of a fenestrated capillary. The arrows show the pores with their diaphragms. In the center is a large pinocytotic vesicle. Some blood vessels have many of these vesicles in different stages of evolution, causing a ruffled appearance of the endothelium (see also Fig 12–5).

through which the capillary communicates with the underlying tissue; (3) the presence in and around the wall—in addition to the usual endothelial cells—of cells with phagocytic activity; and (4) absence of a continuous basal lamina.

The sinusoidal capillaries are found mainly in the liver and in hematopoietic organs such as the bone marrow and spleen. These structural details suggest that in the sinusoidal capillaries the interchange between blood and tissues is greatly facilitated, so that blood fluids and macromolecules can easily pass back and forth between the 2 compartments.

In various locations along capillaries and small arteries, there are mesenchymal cells with long cytoplasmic processes that partially surround the endothelial cells. These adventitial cells or pericytes are enclosed in their own basal lamina. These perivascular cells have great potentiality for transformation into other cells. Whether they are contractile or not has been the subject of much controversy. Evidence from various sources strongly suggests that the endothelial cells can contract. The presence of abundant microfilaments in their cytoplasm is believed to be related to the proposed contractility of endothelial cells (Fig 12–5). Adjacent endothelial cells may possess gap junctions, which would provide for the exchange of information between cells. Junctions of the zonula occludens type are present between cells and are probably of physiologic importance, since such junctions may present a variable permeability to mac-

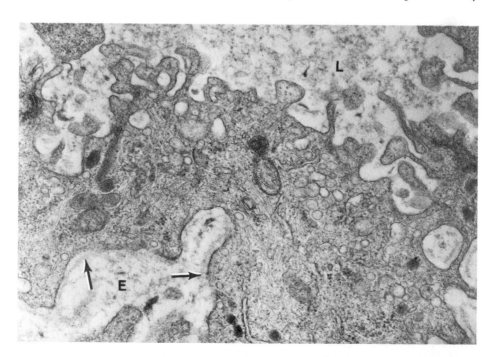

Figure 12–5. Electron micrograph of a section of a continuous capillary. Observe the ruffled appearance of its interior surface, the large and small pinocytotic vesicles, and numerous microfilaments in the cytoplasm. L, lumen of the capillary; E, its outer surface. The arrows show the basal lamina. Reduced slightly from × 30,000.

romolecules that play a significant role in normal physiologic or pathologic conditions.

As illustrated in Fig 12–6, the capillaries anastomose profusely, forming a rich network between the small arteries and veins. The arterioles branch into small vessels which present a discontinuous layer of smooth muscle, the **metarterioles.** These branch into capillaries that form an abundant network. The constriction of the metarterioles helps to regulate but does not completely stop the circulation in capillaries, and maintains pressure differences in the 2 systems. A simple ring of smooth muscle cells, the **sphincter,** exists at the point of origin of capillaries from the metarteriole. This precapillary sphincter can completely stop the blood flow within the capillary. The entire network does not always function simultaneously, and the number of functioning and open capillaries depends not only on the state of contraction of the metarterioles but also on arteriovenous anastomoses that enable the metarterioles to empty directly into small veins as illustrated in Fig 12–6. These interconnections are abundant in skeletal muscle and the skin of the hands and feet. When vessels of the

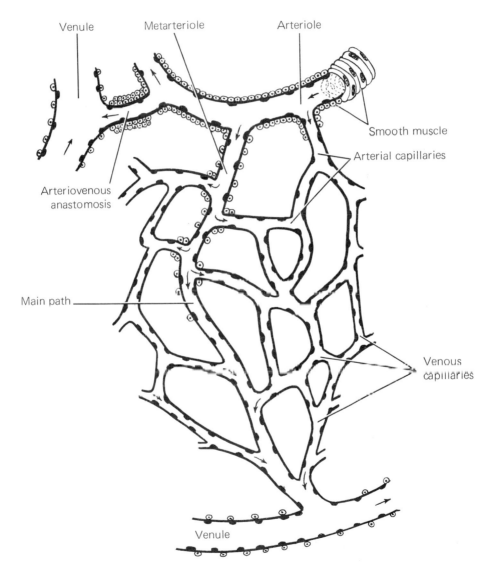

Figure 12–6. Branching of an arteriole to form a capillary network terminating in a venule. The continuous layer of smooth muscle from the arteriole becomes discontinuous in the metarterioles. In arteriovenous anastomosis, blood passes directly from the arterial to the venous system. When blood pressure is lowered—as a result of the opening of the arteriovenous anastomosis or of contraction of the metarterioles—blood flow may be restricted to the main paths as indicated by arrows in the drawing. It is thus possible to regulate the extension of the capillary network utilized in a given territory. (Reproduced, with permission, from Copenhaver WM, Bunge RP, Bunge MB: *Bailey's Textbook of Histology,* 16th ed. Williams & Wilkins, 1972.)

arteriovenous anastomosis contract, all the blood must pass through the capillary network. When it relaxes, some blood flows directly to a vein instead of circulating in the capillaries. Capillary circulation is controlled by neural and hormonal stimulation. The presence of locally liberated substances such as histamine can also play a conspicuous role during inflammatory processes. The position of the capillaries relative to the heart level also influences capillary circulation.

The wealth of the capillary network is a function of the metabolism of the tissues and represents a transition zone between the high-pressure system (arterial) and low-pressure system (venous). Tissues with high metabolic rates such as the kidney, liver, and cardiac and skeletal muscle have an abundant capillary network; the opposite is true of tissues with low metabolic rates such as smooth muscle and tendons.

An idea of the importance of the capillaries can be gained by noting that in the human body the surface area of the capillary network approaches 6000 m^2. Its total diameter is approximately 800 times larger than the aorta. A unit volume of fluid within a capillary is exposed to a larger surface area than the same volume in the other parts of the system. The flow of blood in the aorta averages 320 mm/s; in the capillaries, about 0.3 mm/s. The capillary system can thus be compared with a lake where a full-flowing river enters and leaves; because of their thin walls and slow blood flow, the capillaries are a favorable place for the interchange of water and solutes between blood and tissues.

Morphologic Basis of Capillary Permeability

The nature of the mechanism by which interchange of materials between blood and tissues occurs is highly controversial. Interpreting results of physiologic experiments, researchers have postulated the existence of 2 sizes of pores in the capillary walls. The smaller pores are thought to have a diameter of 9 nm and the larger pores a diameter of 40–70 nm. Three possible morphologic equivalents of these "physiologic pores" are (1) pores in the fenestrated capillaries (Figs 12–1, 12–3, and 12–4), (2) intercellular clefts where junctions occur between neighboring endothelial cells, and (3) large numbers of pinocytotic vesicles known to cross the endothelial cells of most capillaries. Currently available evidence indicates that substances can pass through the capillaries via these 3 structures. The relative importance of these 3 components under various physiologic and pathologic conditions is highly controversial.

The permeability of capillaries within various organs is significantly different. For example, in the kidney glomerulus, they are about 100 times more permeable than capillaries in muscle tissue. In abnormal states such as inflammation, injection of snake or bee venom, etc, capillary permeability is greatly increased. These conditions apparently alter the permeability of the junctions between endothelial cells. Under such circumstances, electron-dense colloidal substances can be observed to pass from capillary and small venule lumens into the surrounding tissues by traversing the endothelial cell junctions. Leukocytes may leave the bloodstream by passing between endothelial cells and entering the tissue spaces by a process called diapedesis. An increase in vascular permeability is considered to be mediated by the local liberation of such pharmacologically active substances as histamine and bradykinin.

The observation that some drugs given intravenously do not penetrate the brain whereas such penetration occurs in almost all other tissues of the body gave rise to the concept of the **blood-brain barrier.** This was initially studied by intravenous administration of dyes that readily escape from capillaries to surrounding tissues. Careful study of brain capillaries showed that not only do they lack pores and present few pinocytotic vesicles but that junctions between their endothelial cells do not permit the passage of macromolecules used as tracers. The behavior of the endothelial cells would appear to explain the barrier. Other blood-tissue barriers of physiologic importance are the blood-ocular barrier, blood-thymus barrier, blood-nerve barrier, and blood-testicular seminiferous tubule barrier.

GENERAL STRUCTURE OF THE BLOOD VESSELS

All blood vessels with lumens above a certain diameter present a number of structural features in common. To simplify a more detailed study of arteries and veins, a generalized description of the structural features found in both types of vessels is presented below. Depending on the organ studied, there are marked structural differences between the various types of blood vessels, although there exists a gradual transition from one structural type to another.

Blood vessels are usually composed of the following layers (Fig 12–7):

(1) **Tunica intima (internal tunic):** The **intima** consists of a layer of endothelial cells lining the vessel's interior surface. Beneath the endothelium is the **subendothelial layer,** consisting of delicate loose connective tissue that may contain an occasional smooth muscle cell. Owing to contraction of the vessel, this layer as seen in sections generally appears to have a scalloped morphology (Fig 12–8).

(2) **Tunica media (middle tunic):** The **media** consists chiefly of circumferentially arranged smooth muscle cells. Interposed among the smooth muscle cells are variable amounts of elastin, collagen, and proteoglycans. Smooth muscle cells, the

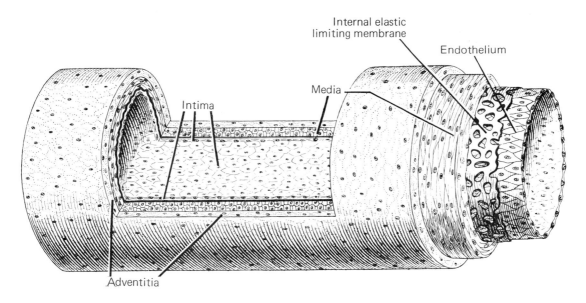

Figure 12 –7. Drawing of a medium-sized artery (muscular artery) showing its layers. In the usual histologic preparations, the layers appear thicker than shown here. Experimental work suggests, however, that the drawing is more closely similar to the in vivo architecture of the vessel. After death, the vessel contracts, the layers become thicker, and the lumen becomes smaller and corrugated.

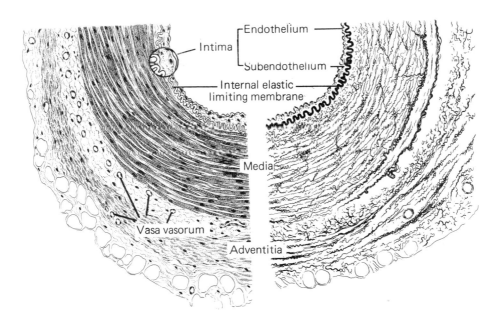

Figure 12 –8. Comparative diagrams of a medium-sized artery prepared by H&E staining *(left)* and by Weigert's staining method for elastic structures *(right).* The media is composed of a mixture of smooth muscle cells, collagen, and elastic membranes. The adventitia has small blood vessels (the vasa vasorum) and elastic and collagenous fibers.

chief sites of vascular metabolic activity, are the cellular source of this extracellular matrix. In arteries, the media is separated from the intima by an **internal elastic lamina.** This lamina, composed of elastin, is usually fenestrated, so that substances can diffuse through the holes in the lamina and nourish cells deep in the vessel wall. In larger vessels, a thinner **external elastic lamina** is often found separating the media from the outer **tunica adventitia.**

(3) **Tunica adventitia:** The **adventitia** consists principally of connective tissue with elastic fibers (Fig 12–9). Recent experimental observations reveal that collagen in the adventitia is only of type I, while the media collagen is of types I and III. This adventitia layer gradually fuses with the enveloping connective tissue of the organ through which the vessel is running. In larger vessels, **vasa vasorum** ("vessels of the vessel") branch profusely in the adventitia. The vasa vasorum provide metabolites to the adventitia and the media in larger vessels, since the layers are too thick to be nourished by diffusion from the bloodstream. In the arteries, these vessels are less frequent and reach only the adventitial layer, whereas in the veins they are more numerous, reaching the middle layer. The greater abundance of vessels in the veins can be attributed to lack of nutritional substances in venous blood. The nutrition of large arteries and of thicker medium-sized arteries comes from different sources. The adventitia receives metabolites from the vasa vasorum. Most of the middle tunic is supplied from arterioles that originate from the region where collateral branches emerge from the arteries. The intima and the most internal portion of media are avascular and receive metabolites by diffusion from the blood. In these avascular regions, changes in the organization and composition of the components (ground substance, fibers, and cells) may be of great importance in significantly affecting cellular nutrition.

Nonmyelinated vasomotor nerves form a network in the adventitial layer and end among the smooth muscle cells of the media. Myelinated fibers reach the intima, forming the sensory fibers of the veins.

Arteries

Arteries are classified according to their size into (1) arterioles; (2) arteries of medium size, or muscular arteries; and (3) large or elastic arteries, where elastic tissue predominates.

Arterioles are fine, generally less than 0.5 mm in diameter and have relatively narrow lumens. They exhibit a tunica intima with no subendothelial layer and generally lack an internal elastic limiting membrane. The media is muscular, generally composed of 1–5 circularly arranged layers of smooth muscle cells. The adventitia is narrow, poorly developed, and shows no external elastic limiting membrane (Fig 12–11).

Small and **medium-sized arteries** (muscular arteries) have the general structure of vessels illustrated in Figs 12–7 to 12–10. They are characterized by a thick muscular layer with as many as 40 layers of smooth muscle cells. These cells are intermixed with variable amounts of elastin, as well as collagen and proteoglycans, depending on the size of the vessel.

Large arteries (elastic arteries) include the aorta and its large branches. They have a yellowish color owing to the accumulation of elastin in the media. This type of artery presents the following characteristics: (1) The intima, thicker than the tunic of a muscular artery, is lined by endothelial cells. In the electron microscope, the endothelial cells show microvilli, pinocytotic vesicles, granular endoplasmic reticulum, microfilaments, intercellular junctions, and lysosomes. In large arteries,

Internal elastic limiting membrane

Media

Adventitia

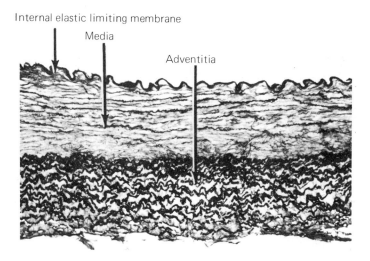

Figure 12 –9. Photomicrograph of a section of a medium-sized artery stained by Weigert's method for elastic structures. × 110.

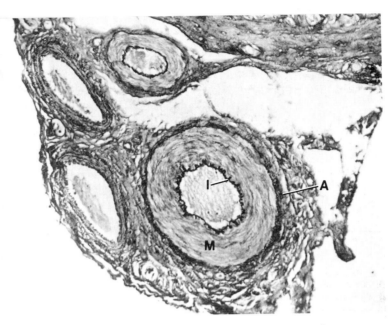

Figure 12 –10. Photomicrograph of 2 small arteries *(right)* and veins *(left).* The arteries have thicker walls than the veins. In the arteries, the elastin is present as an internal elastic lamina (I) and as dispersed elastic fibers in the adventitia (A). Between the elastin-containing structures is the thick muscular media (M), which is not evident in the veins. Weigert's stain, × 150.

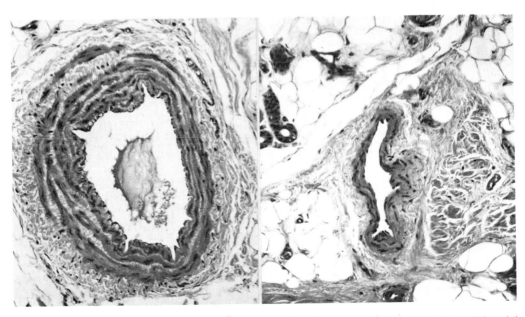

Figure 12 –11. Photomicrographs of sections of an arteriole *(left)* and a venule *(right).* Without special staining (eg, Weigert's), the elastin is not as apparent in the arteriole (Fig 12 –10). H&E stain, × 100.

a subendothelial basement membrane is sometimes not seen, but fibrillar connections between the basal plasma membrane and various components of the internal tunic are seen. Endothelial cells are in constant turnover and develop from preexisting ones by mitosis. In medium- and large-sized arteries, a folded endothelium whose cells bulge into the lumen of this vessel is often observed. This sometimes occurs as a result of postmortem contraction of the muscle of the arteries. The subendothelial layer is thick. The connective tissue fibers of the subendothelial layer display a longitudinal orientation and play an important role in the free play of the endothelial layer of cells during rhythmic contractions and dilatations of the vessel. An internal elastic limiting membrane is not always evident since it is confused with the membranes of the next layer. (2) The media consists of a series of concentrically arranged perforated elastic membranes whose number increases with age (40 in the newborn; 70 in the adult); elastic structures, once formed, usually become metabolically inert as shown by radioautographic studies, especially in older animals. The laminas exhibit a progressive increase in thickness by deposition of elastin composed of fibrils and amorphous material. Between these membranes are smooth muscle cells, thin collagen fibrils, and an amorphous substance consisting mainly of chondroitin sulfate, a structural compound similar to the extracellular matrix of loose connective tissue. (3) The adventitial tunic does not show an external limiting membrane, is relatively underdeveloped, and contains elastic and collagen fibers.

Histophysiology of the Arteries

The large arteries are also called **carriers** since their major function is transporting blood. The function of the medium-sized arteries, also known as **distributing arteries,** is to furnish blood to the various organs. The accumulation of elastic material is characteristic of the structure of the large arteries. This layer has an important function in regulating blood flow, for by dilating periodically it absorbs the intermittent impact of the cardiac pulse. During **diastole,** the large arteries return to normal size, impelling the blood forward. The consequence of this action is that arterial pressure and blood flow decrease and become less variable as the distance from the heart increases (Fig 12–12).

The muscular layer in the medium-sized or distributing arteries can, by contracting or not contracting, control the flow of blood to the various organs.

Blood vessels undergo progressive and gradual changes from birth to death, and it is difficult to say where the normal growth processes end and the processes of involution begin. Each artery exhibits its own aging pattern. The artery that changes most precociously, beginning at 20 years of age, is the coronary. Other arteries begin to be modified only after age 40. When the media of an artery is weakened by an embryologic defect or lesion, the wall of the artery gives way, dilating extensively. As this process progresses, it becomes an **aneurysm** and might result in rupture of the wall.

The alterations in arteriosclerosis generally begin in the subendothelial layer, passing to the media. The lesion of the intima and middle layer, with the destruction of the elastic tissue and the consequent loss of elasticity observed in arteriosclerosis, results in serious circulatory disturbances. Figure 12–12 illustrates the relationship between structure and biophysical characteristics of blood vessels.

Certain arteries irrigate only definite areas of specific organs, and obstruction results in necrosis (death of the tissues owing to lack of metabolites). These are **infarcts** that occur commonly in the heart, kidneys, cerebrum, and certain other organs. In other regions, such as the skin, arteries anastomose frequently, and the obstruction of one artery does not lead to tissue necrosis because blood flow is maintained.

The polypeptide angiotensin promotes hypertension by binding itself initially to vascular endothelial cells. It is believed that this initial endothelial stimulus is later transmitted to arterial smooth muscle cells, promoting their contraction and consequent increase in blood pressure. Support for this hypothesis comes from morphologic studies which reveal that endothelial cells exhibit processes that extend across the internal elastic limiting membrane and contact the smooth muscle cells.

Carotid & Aortic Bodies

Small structures encountered in the bifurcation of the common carotid artery and the aorta are believed to function as respiratory chemoreceptors. They are richly vascularized, exhibiting sinusoidal capillaries surrounded by clear cells, and have the function of detecting alterations in pH and CO_2 and oxygen tensions of the blood, transmitting this information to nearby nerve endings. They are specialized sense organs with the important homeostatic function of maintaining the partial pressures of CO_2 and oxygen in the blood at normal levels.

Arteriovenous Anastomosis

Direct communications between arterial and venous circulation are often observed. These arteriovenous anastomoses are distributed throughout the body and generally occur in small vessels. Lumens of these anastomoses vary depending on the physiologic condition of the organ, and changes in their diameter regulate the circulation in particular areas (Fig 12–6). Using the technic of injecting microspheres of a certain size that obliterate the capillaries, it is possible to calculate that about one-third of the blood flow in the ear of a rabbit can pass through arteriovenous anastomoses. Besides these

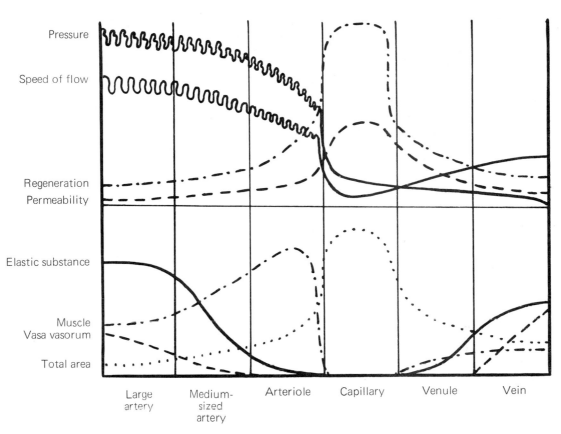

Figure 12–12. Relationship between the characteristics of blood circulation and the structure of the blood vessels. The arterial blood pressure and rapidity of flow decrease and become more constant as distance from the heart gradually increases. This coincides with a reduction in number of elastic fibers and an increase in the number of smooth muscle cells in the arteries. The graphs illustrate the gradual changes in vessel structure and their biophysical properties. Regenerative capacity and permeability are highly developed in the capillaries. (Reproduced, with permission, from Cowdry EV: *Textbook of Histology*. Lea & Febiger, 1944.)

direct communications, more complex structures, **glomera,** occur—mainly in fingerpads, fingernail beds, and ears. In these structures, the arterioles that establish continuity with venules lose their internal elastic membranes and acquire a thick layer of smooth muscle cells arranged longitudinally. This muscle layer forms a sheet that partially or completely surrounds the lumen of a vessel. Contraction of this layer can promote the complete or partial transitory closure of blood vessels. The systems have an important role in control of the circulation in various organs and participate in several physiologic phenomena such as menstruation, protection against low temperatures, and erection. The arteriovenous anastomoses are richly innervated by the sympathetic and parasympathetic nervous systems. Control of this activity appears to be mainly neural. Besides controlling the blood flow in the various organs, these anastomoses have a thermoregulatory function that is particularly evident in the skin of the extremities.

Veins

As with arteries, it is customary to arbitrarily classify the veins into venules and veins of small, medium, and large size.

Venules are small, with a diameter of 0.2–1 mm. They are characterized by an intima composed of endothelium; a thin media that may consist of from none to a few cell layers of smooth muscle; and an adventitial layer, which is the thickest layer and is composed of connective tissue rich in collagenous fibers. Venules have thin walls (Fig 12–11). Venules with luminal diameters up to 50 μm have the structure and other biologic features of capillaries and participate in inflammatory processes and interchange of metabolites between blood and tissues.

With the exception of the main trunks, most veins are **small** or **medium-sized veins** and have a diameter of 1–9 mm. The intima usually has a thin subendothelial layer, but this may at times be absent. The media consists of small bundles of smooth muscles intermixed with collagen fibers and a delicate network of elastic fibers. The collagenous adventitial layer is well developed (Fig 12–13).

Large veins have a well-developed tunica intima. The middle tunic is much smaller, with few smooth muscle cells and abundant connective tis-

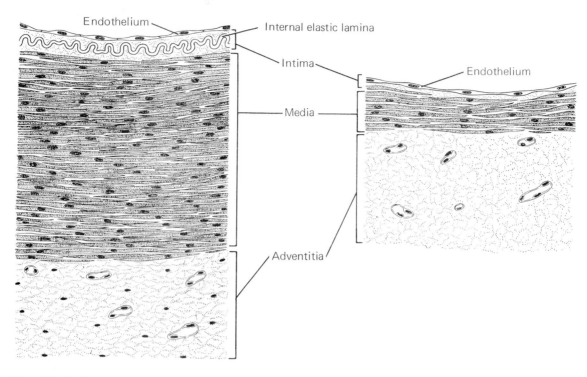

Figure 12 –13. Diagram comparing the structure of a medium-sized artery *(left)* and vein. Note that the tunica intima and tunica media are highly developed in the artery but not in the vein.

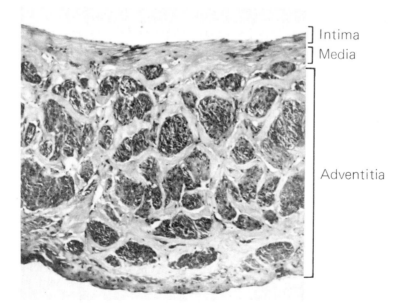

Figure 12 –14. Photomicrograph of a section of a large vein. Observe the well-developed adventitia with characteristic longitudinal smooth muscle bundles. H&E stain, × 100.

sue. The adventitia is the thickest layer and in the largest vessels may contain longitudinal bundles of smooth muscle (Fig 12–14). Besides these different layers, small or medium-sized veins exhibit valves in their interior. These structures consist of 2 semilunar folds of the internal layer of the vessel that project into the lumen. They are composed of elastic connective tissue and lined on both sides by endothelium.

The valves are especially numerous in the veins of the limbs (arms and legs). They propel the venous blood in the direction of the heart—thanks to contraction of skeletal muscles that surround these veins.

Heart

The heart is a muscular organ that contracts rhythmically, pumping the blood in the circulatory system. Its walls consist of 3 tunics: the internal, or **endocardium;** the middle, or **myocardium;** and the external, or **pericardium.** The heart has a fibrous central region, the **fibrous skeleton,** which serves as a support and site of origin and insertion of the cardiac myocytes. The heart contains cardiac valves and an impulse-generating and conducting system.

The **endocardium** is homologous with the intima of the veins. Lined with endothelium, it rests on a thin subendothelial layer of loose connective tissue. Uniting the myocardium with the subendothelial layer is a **subendocardial layer** of connective tissue containing veins, nerves, and branches of the impulse-conducting system.

Myocardium consists of cardiac muscle cells (see Chapter 11) arranged in layers that cover the heart chambers in a complex spiral manner. A large number of these layers insert themselves on the fibrous cardiac skeleton. The muscle cells of the heart are grouped into 2 populations: there are contractile cells and impulse-generating and conducting cells that generate and conduct the signal initiating the heartbeat. The arrangement of these muscle cells is extremely varied, so that in histologic preparations of a small area cells are seen oriented in many directions.

Epicardium is the serous membrane of the heart, forming the visceral lining of the pericardium. Externally, it is covered by simple squamous epithelium (mesothelium) supported by a thin layer of connective tissue. A subepicardial layer consisting of loose connective tissue contains veins, nerves, and nerve ganglia. The adipose tissue that generally surrounds the heart accumulates in this layer.

The **fibrous skeleton of the heart** is composed of dense connective tissue. Its principal components are the **septum membranaceum,** the **trigona fibrosa,** and the **annuli fibrosi.** These structures have the general appearance of an aponeurosis, with thick collagen fibers oriented in various directions. Certain regions contain nodules or areas of fibrous cartilage.

The **cardiac valves** consist of a central portion of dense fibrous aponeurosislike tissue lined on both sides by an endothelial layer.

Innervation of the Heart; Impulse-Generating & Conducting System of the Heart

The impulse-generating and conducting system of the heart consists of several structures that make it possible for the atria and ventricles to beat in succession and permit the heart to function as an efficient pump. The system is composed of 2 nodes: the **sinoatrial node** (of Keith and Flack) and the **atrioventricular node** (of Tawara) (Fig 12–15). There is also the atrioventricular bundle (or bundle of His), which originates in the atrioventricular node and is directed toward the ventricles, bifurcating and sending branches to both ventricles (Fig 12–15). The left branch divides into 2 main branches. The branches gradually divide in both ventricles into numerous anastomosing fine threads that end in the myocardium. The nodes consist of a mass of small spindle-shaped specialized muscle cells embedded in connective tissue. There is no visible connection between the 2 nodes in mammals.

The atrioventricular bundle originates in the node of the same name and at this site is composed of cells similar to those in the node. Distally, these cells enlarge and assume a characteristic shape; they are the **Purkinje fibers.** These have one or 2 central nuclei, as do cardiac muscle cells, but their cytoplasm is full of glycogen deposits interspersed with scarce myofibrils located mainly in the periphery of the cytoplasm (Fig 12–16). Gap junctions exist between these cells and provide a means of passing impulse signals from cell to cell. No nerve endings resembling motor end-plates exist in heart muscle cells.

Heart muscle has the capacity for autostimulation independent of nerve impulses. Tissue culture studies show that isolated cardiac cells beat with their own rhythm. In the cardiac muscle, however, these cells are closely united and exchange information owing to the presence of gap junctions at the intercalated disks (see Chapter 11). The cells that maintain a faster rhythm transmit their impulses to all the others and thus to the entire organ. In mammals, the sinoatrial node cells have a more rapid rhythm and the impulses generated in this region are rapidly transmitted to the rest of the heart. For this reason, the sinoatrial node is the **pacemaker** of the heart. If the conducting system fails, the heart may continue to function, although with a different rhythm.

Both the parasympathetic and the sympathetic divisions of the autonomic system contribute to innervation of the heart and form widespread plexuses at the base of the heart. In the regions close to the sinoatrial and atrioventricular nodes, ganglionic nerve cells and nerve fibers are present. It is known that these nerves do not affect generation of the

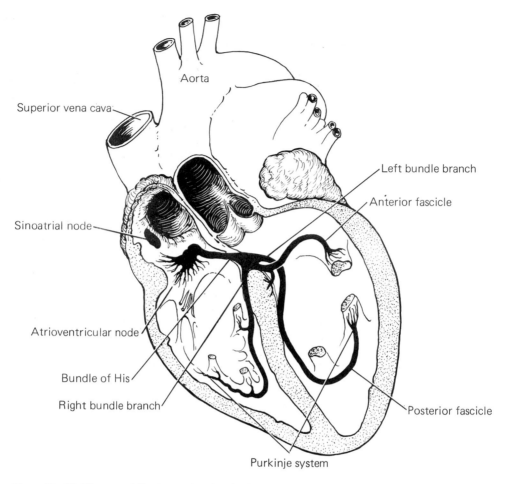

Figure 12 –15. Diagram of the heart showing the impulse-generating and impulse-conducting system.

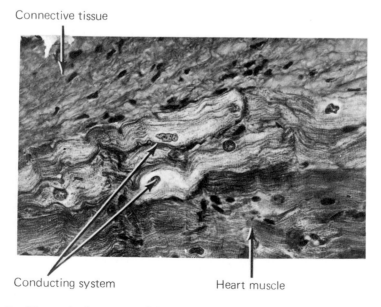

Figure 12 –16. The cells of the conducting system of the heart are characterized by a reduced number of myofibrils present mainly in the periphery of the muscle cell. The light area around the nuclei of the conducting cells is due to local accumulation of glycogen. H&E stain, × 400.

heartbeat, a process attributed to the sinoatrial (pacemaker) node. These nerves do affect heart rhythm, whereby stimulation of the parasympathetic division (vagus nerve) promotes a slowing of the heartbeat, whereas stimulation of the sympathetic nerve accelerates the rhythm of the pacemaker.

Lymphatic Vascular System

Besides blood vessels, the human body has a system of thin channels lined with endothelium that collects fluid from the tissue spaces and returns it to the blood. This fluid is called lymph; in contrast to the blood, it circulates in only one direction, ie, toward the heart.

The **lymphatic capillaries** originate in the various tissues as thin, blind-ended vessels. They consist of a single layer of endothelium. These thin vessels converge and end up as 2 large trunks, the **thoracic duct** and the **right lymphatic duct,** which empty into the junction of the internal jugular vein with the left subclavian vein and into the confluence of the subclavian vein and the right internal jugular vein. Interposed in the path of the lymphatic vessels are lymph nodes, whose morphology and functions are discussed in Chapter 15. With rare excep-

tions such as the nervous system and the bone marrow, a lymphatic system is found in almost all organs.

The **lymphatic vessels** have a structure similar to that of veins except they have thinner walls and lack a clear-cut separation between the 3 layers (intima, media, and adventitia). Like veins, they have numerous internal valves. These valves are, however, more numerous in lymphatic vessels. Between the valves the lymphatic vessels are dilated and assume a nodular appearance.

As in veins, lymphatic circulation is aided by the action of external forces (eg, contraction of surrounding muscle) on their walls. These forces act discontinuously, and lymph flow occurs mainly as a result of the presence of many valves in these vessels and the rhythmic contraction of the smooth muscle present in their walls.

The **lymphatic ducts** of large size have a structure similar to that of a vein with a reinforcement of smooth muscle in the middle layer. In this layer the muscle bundles are longitudinally and circularly arranged, with longitudinal fibers predominating. The adventitia is relatively underdeveloped. As with arteries and veins, large lymphatic ducts contain vasa vasorum and a rich neural network.

●   ●   ●

References

Abramson DL (editor): *Blood Vessels and Lymphatics.* Academic Press, 1962.

Becker RP, DeBruyn PP: The transmural passage of blood cells into myeloid sinusoids and the entry of platelets into the sinusoidal circulation: A scanning electron microscope investigation. Am J Anat 145:183, 1976.

Bennett HS, Luft JH, Hampton JC: Morphological classification of vertebrate blood capillaries. Am J Physiol 196:381, 1959.

Clementi F, Palade GE: Intestinal capillaries. 1. Permeability to peroxidase and ferritin. J Cell Biol 41:33, 1969.

Cliff WJ: The aortic tunica media in growing rats studied with the electron microscope. Lab Invest 17:599, 1967.

Edanaga M: Scanning electron microscope study on the endothelium of the vessels. Arch Histol Jpn 37:1, 1974.

Fernando NVP, Movat HZ: The smallest arterial vessels: Terminal arterioles and metarterioles. Exp Mol Pathol 3:1, 1964.

Fritz KE, Jarmolych J, Daoud AS: Association of DNA synthesis and apparent dedifferentiation of aortic smooth muscle cells in vitro. Exp Mol Pathol 12:354, 1970.

Fryer DG, Birnbaum G, Luttrell CN: Human endothelium in cell culture. J Atherosclerosis Res 6:151, 1966.

Giacomelli F, Wiener J, Spiro D: Cross-striated arrays of filaments in endothelium. J Cell Biol 45:188, 1970.

Hayes JR: Histological changes in constricted arteries and arterioles. J Anat 101:343, 1967.

Hinek A, Thyberg J: Electron microscopic observations on the formation of elastic fibers in primary cultures of aortic smooth muscle cells. J Ultrastruct Res 60:12, 1977.

Hofmann BF: Physiology of atrio-ventricular transmission. Circulation 24:506, 1961.

Hüttner I, Boutet M, More RH: Gap junctions in arterial endothelium. J Cell Biol 57:247, 1973.

Johnson PC: *Peripheral Circulation.* Wiley, 1978.

Karnovsky MJ: The ultrastructural basis of capillary permeability studied with peroxidase as a tracer. J Cell Biol 35:213, 1967.

Karnovsky MJ: The ultrastructural basis of transcapillary exchanges. J Gen Physiol 52:643, 1968.

Lauweryns JM, Boussauw L: The ultrastructure of lymphatic valves in the adult rabbit lung. Z Zellforsch 143:149, 1973.

Leak LV: Normal anatomy of the lymphatic vascular system. In: *Handbuch der Allgemeine Pathologie.* Meessen H (editor). Springer-Verlag, 1972.

Maul GG: Structure and formation of pores in fenestrated capillaries. J Ultrastruct Res 36:768, 1971.

Papp M & others: An electron microscopic study of the central lacteal in the intestinal villus of the cat. Z Zellforsch Mikrosk Anat 57:475, 1962.

Reynolds SRM, Zweifach BW: *The Microcirculation: A Symposium on Factors Influencing Exchange of Substances Across the Capillary Wall.* Univ of Illinois Press, 1959.

Rhodin JAG: Ultrastructure of mammalian venous capillaries, venules and small collecting veins. J Ultrastruct Res 25:452, 1968.

Rhodin JAG, Del Missier P, Reid LC: The structure of the specialized impulse-conducting system of the steer. Circulation 24:349, 1961.

Richardson JB, Beaulines A: The cellular site of action of angiotensin. J Cell Biol 51:419, 1971.

Scott MN, Fawcett DW: Myocardial ultrastructure. In: *The Mammalian Myocardium.* Langer GA, Brady TW (editors). Wiley, 1974.

Simionescu M & others: Morphometric data on the endothelium of blood capillaries. J Cell Biol 60:128, 1974.

Thaemert JC: Fine structure of the atrioventricular node as viewed in serial sections. Am J Anat 136:43, 1973.

Todd TW: The specialized systems of the heart. In: *Special Cytology.* Vol 2. Cowdry EV (editor). Hoeber, 1932.

Walford RL, Carter PK, Schneider RB: Stability of labeled aortic elastic tissue with age and pregnancy in the rat. Arch Pathol 78:43, 1964.

Willms-Kretschner K, Magno G: Ischemia of skin: Electron microscopic study of vascular injury. Am J Pathol 54:327, 1969.

Wissler RW: The arterial medial cell, smooth muscle or multifunctional mesenchyme? J Atherosclerosis Res 8:201, 1968.

Blood consists of the cells and fluid contained in the closed circulatory system that flow in a regular unidirectional movement, propelled mainly by the rhythmic contractions of the heart. Blood is made up of 2 parts: **formed elements,** or blood cells, and **plasma,** the liquid phase in which the former are suspended. The formed elements are **erythrocytes,** or red blood cells; **platelets;** and **leukocytes,** or white blood cells. Blood is a specialized connective tissue consisting of cells and an abundant extracellular interstitium.

If blood is removed from the circulatory system, it will clot. This clot contains formed elements and a clear yellow liquid called **serum,** which separates from the coagulum during the phenomenon of coagulation. Blood serum is equivalent in composition to plasma except that it lacks **fibrinogen** and some other protein factors necessary for clot formation and contains **serotonin** in increased amounts.

Blood collected and kept from coagulating by the addition of anticoagulants (heparin, citrate, etc) separates, when centrifuged, into layers that reflect its heterogeneity (Fig 13–1). The result obtained by this sedimentation, carried out in glass tubes of standard size, is the **hematocrit.**

The hematocrit permits estimation of the volume of packed erythrocytes per unit volume of blood. The normal value is 40–50% in the adult male, 35–45% in the adult female, approximately 35% in a child up to age 10 years, and 45–60% in the newborn. In pregnancy, this value is diminished by physiologic hemodilution. The hematocrit is normally higher in venous blood than in arterial blood because of the hydration of red cells and their increase in size. This value may vary in regard to the different compartments of the blood vascular system from which the samples are taken.

The translucent, yellowish, and somewhat viscous supernatant obtained when the hematocrit is measured is the plasma of the blood. The formed elements of the blood separate into 2 easily distinguishable layers. The lower layer represents 42–47% of the entire volume of blood present in the hematocrit tube. It is red and is made up of erythrocytes. The layer immediately above (1% of the blood volume), which is white or grayish in color, is called the **buffy coat** and consists of leukocytes. This

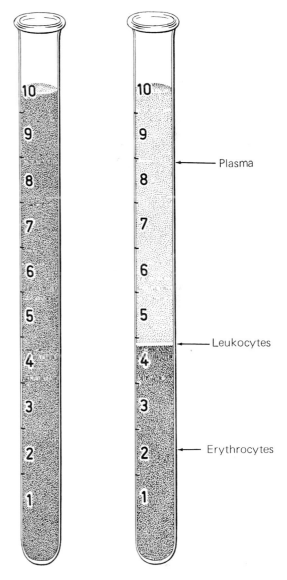

Figure 13–1. Hematocrit tubes with blood. **Left:** Before centrifugation. **Right:** After centrifugation. In the centrifuged tube, the red blood cells represent 43% of the blood volume. Between the sedimented red blood cells and the supernatant light-colored plasma is a thin layer of leukocytes called the buffy coat.

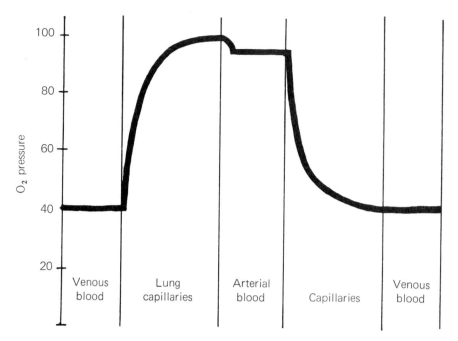

Figure 13 –2. Blood oxygen content in each type of blood vessel. The amount of oxygen (O_2 pressure) is highest in lung capillaries and in arteries and decreases in tissue capillaries, where exchange takes place between blood and tissues.

separation occurs because the leukocytes are less dense than the erythrocytes. Covering the leukocytes is a fine layer of platelets not distinguishable by the naked eye.

Leukocytes, some of which are phagocytic, constitute one of the chief defenses against infection and circulate through the body via the blood vascular system. By crossing the capillary wall, these cells become concentrated rapidly in the tissues and participate in inflammation. The blood vascular system is also the vehicle of transport of oxygen (O_2) (Fig 13–2) and carbon dioxide (CO_2); the former is mainly bound to the hemoglobin of the erythrocytes, whereas the latter, in addition to being bound to the proteins of the erythrocytes (mainly hemoglobin), is also carried in solution in the plasma as CO_2 or in the form of HCO_3^-.

The plasma transports metabolites from their site of absorption or synthesis, distributing them to different areas of the organism. It also transports the residues of metabolism, which are removed from the blood by the excretory organs. Blood, being the distributing vehicle for the hormones, permits the exchange of chemical messages between distant organs for normal cellular function. It further participates in the regulation of heat distribution and in acid-base and osmotic balance.

Composition of Plasma

Plasma is an aqueous solution containing substances of small or large molecular weight comprising 10% of its volume. The plasma proteins account for 7% and the inorganic salts for 0.9%; the remainder of the 10% consists of several organic compounds of different origin—amino acids, vitamins, hormones, lipids, etc.

Through the capillary walls, the plasma is in equilibrium with the interstitial fluid of the tissues. The composition of plasma is usually an indicator of the mean composition of the extracellular fluids in general.

Plasma proteins can be separated in the ultracentrifuge or by electrophoresis into **albumin; alpha, beta,** and **gamma globulins;** and **fibrinogen.** Albumin is the main component and has a fundamental role in maintaining the osmotic pressure of the blood. The gamma globulins are antibodies and are called **immunoglobulins.** Fibrinogen is necessary for the formation of fibrin in the final step of coagulation.

Several substances insoluble or only slightly soluble in water can be transported by the plasma because they combine with albumin or with the alpha and beta globulins. For example, lipids are insoluble in the plasma but combine with the hydrophobic portions of protein molecules. Since these molecules also have hydrophilic parts, the lipid-protein complex is soluble in water.

Staining of Blood Cells

Blood cells are generally studied in smears or films prepared by spreading a drop of blood thinly over a microscope slide (Fig 13–3). The blood should be evenly distributed over the slide and allowed to dry rapidly in air. In such films the cells are clearly visible and distinct from one another.

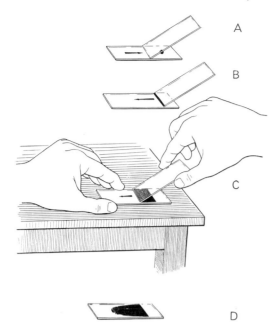

affinity for a complex dye present in the mixture—incorrectly thought to be neutral—is known as **neutrophilia** (salmon-pink to lilac).

FORMED ELEMENTS OF BLOOD

Erythrocytes

Mammalian erythrocytes have no nuclei, and in humans they are biconcave disks 7.2 μm in diameter (Fig 13–4). The biconcave shape provides the erythrocytes with a large surface, thus facilitating gas exchange.

Erythrocytes with diameters greater than 9 μm are called **macrocytes,** and those with diameters less than 6 μm are called **microcytes.** The presence of a high percentage of erythrocytes of abnormal variation in size is called **anisocytosis.**

The erythrocyte is quite flexible, and this property permits it to adapt to the irregular shape and small diameter of the capillaries. Observations in vivo show that when traversing the angles of capillary bifurcations the erythrocyte readily deforms and frequently assumes a cuplike shape.

The normal concentration of erythrocytes in blood is approximately 4.5–5 million/μL in women and 5 million/μL in men.

Figure 13 –3. Preparation of a blood smear. *A:* A drop of blood is placed on a microscope slide. A second slide is moved over the first at an angle of 45 degrees. *B:* When the slide edge touches the blood drop, the blood spreads along the edge. *C:* With a uniform movement of the oblique slide, a thin film of blood is spread on the horizontal fixed slide. *D:* After air drying, slides are stained and covered with coverslips.

Their cytoplasm is spread out, thus facilitating observation of their nuclei and cytoplasmic organization.

Blood smears are routinely stained with special dye mixtures first discovered by Dimitri Romanovsky and modified by other investigators. In 1891, Romanovsky observed that a mixture of solutions of methylene blue and eosin in certain proportions stained purple the nuclei of leukocytes and malaria parasites. This staining is due to the oxidation of the methylene blue and the formation in the mixture of new compounds called **azures.**

Stains currently used to study blood cells differ slightly in the proportion of their components and in the way methylene blue is oxidized. They are named for the investigator who first introduced the modification. Leishman's, Wright's, and Giemsa's stains are examples of modified stains collectively known as Romanovsky-type mixtures.

After application of a Romanovsky-type mixture, differentiation of the blood cells can be made based on 4 staining characteristics representing the affinity of cellular structures for the respective dyes of the mixture: (1) affinity for methylene blue (a basic dye) is known as **basophilia** (blue); (2) affinity for the azures is known as **azurophilia** (purple); (3) affinity for the eosin (an acid stain) is known as **acidophilia** or **eosinophilia** (yellowish-pink); and (4)

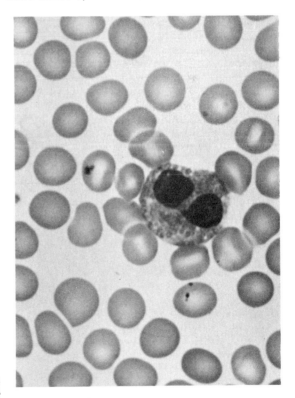

Figure 13 –4. Photomicrograph of a Leishman-stained human blood smear. There are numerous erythrocytes and one granulocyte (eosinophil).

Because of their richness in hemoglobin, a basic protein, erythrocytes are acidophilic. Besides hemoglobin, the erythrocytes contain a lipoprotein stroma. If placed in a hypotonic solution, they undergo tumefaction, become spherical, and lose hemoglobin to the surrounding liquid. This phenomenon is called **hemolysis.** The plasmalemma or empty shell that remains after this treatment is called the **ghost** and corresponds to the stroma. It is 50–60% protein and 35–40% lipid by weight. Since the ghost can reassume the biconcave disk shape, it is deduced that the stroma is responsible for the shape of the erythrocyte; this phenomenon requires the extrusion of Na^+ and water. The shape of the erythrocyte is maintained at the expense of energy; this process requires ATP, which is generated through glycolysis.

The red cell membrane, composed of proteins, carbohydrates, and lipids, gives to the cell its discoid appearance, and its structural flexibility allows great changes in the shape of the cell when it passes through capillaries. The cell membrane also acts as a semipermeable barrier, maintaining differences in the concentrations of sodium and potassium between the plasma and the interior of the cell and maintaining active transport systems for cation transfers against concentration gradients. Because red cells are not rigid particles, the viscosity of the blood remains low.

Erythrocytes recently released by the bone marrow into the bloodstream contain ribosomal RNA (rRNA), which, in the presence of supravital dyes (eg, brilliant cresyl blue), can be precipitated and stained. Under these conditions, the young erythrocytes, which are called **reticulocytes,** exhibit from a few granules up to a netlike structure (Fig 14–3). The reticulocytes normally constitute about 1% of the total number of circulating red blood cells since that is the rate at which erythrocytes are replaced daily by the bone marrow. The process by which the reticulocytes are released from the bone marrow into the circulation is not completely understood.

Sometimes—mainly in disease states—nuclear fragments (containing DNA) remain in the erythrocyte after extrusion of its nucleus, which occurs late in its development. These nuclear remnants are Feulgen-positive and stain with basic dyes. Often they take the form of one or 2 small granules (1 μm in size) and are called **Howell-Jolly bodies.** When they appear as circular filaments, they are called **Cabot rings.**

The hemoglobin molecule (a conjugated protein) consists of 4 subunits, each containing a heme group linked to a polypeptide. The heme group is a porphyrin derivative containing iron (Fe^{2+}).

Owing to variations in each polypeptide chain attached to the heme, various types of hemoglobin can be distinguished, several of which are considered normal: hemoglobins A_1 (HbA$_1$), A_2 (HbA$_2$), and F (HbF) are found normally in postnatal life.

HbA$_1$ represents 97% of the normal hemoglobin in adults; HbA$_2$ represents 2%. The third type (1%), fetal hemoglobin (HbF), represents the predominant hemoglobin of the fetus—around 80% of the hemoglobin in newborns—and decreases progressively to lower levels until the eighth postnatal month, when it represents a small percentage similar to that found in adults.

Combined with oxygen or CO_2, the hemoglobin forms **oxyhemoglobin** or **carbaminohemoglobin,** respectively. These combinations are unstable; however, the combination of hemoglobin with carbon monoxide, forming **carboxyhemoglobin,** is stable.

The erythrocytes of humans survive in the circulation for about 120 days. This is measured by labeling young erythrocytes with ^{14}C-glycine or ^{15}N-glycine and determining their survival. Worn-out erythrocytes are removed from the circulation by cells of the spleen and bone marrow.

Erythrocytes lose their mitochondria and ribosomes during maturation from reticulocytes to adult cells, a process which takes 24–48 hours. They depend continually on the system of anaerobic glycolysis and the pentose phosphate pathway for energy. They do not synthesize hemoglobin because they have no nucleus or other organelles necessary for protein synthesis.

Leukocytes

On the basis of specific granules in their cytoplasm as viewed in the light microscope, the white blood cells were classified into 2 groups: **granulocytes** and **agranulocytes.** Leukocytes can also be separated into **polymorphonuclear** and **mononuclear** cells in regard to nuclear morphology. In addition, they can be classified as myeloid or lymphoid cells depending their origin.

The granulocytes have irregularly shaped nuclei and, in their cytoplasm, the so-called **specific granules—neutrophils, eosinophils,** and **basophils.** These cytoplasmic granules have affinities for the specific stains characterizing the 3 types. Specificity of the granule is related to its own characteristics (dimensions, form, staining affinity, and ultrastructure), and a granule is considered specific when it is consistently present in a certain type of leukocyte and in most of its precursors.

Agranulocytes have nuclei with a regular shape; the cytoplasm does not possess specific granules but can have nonspecific granules characterized as azurophilic that are also present in the other leukocytes. Depending upon the appearance of their nuclei and the cytoplasmic staining characteristics, the agranulocytes can be classified as **lymphocytes** or **monocytes.**

The leukocytes are involved in the cellular and humoral defense of the organism against foreign material. They are spherical cells when in suspension in the circulating blood but are capable of becoming amebiform on encountering a solid sub-

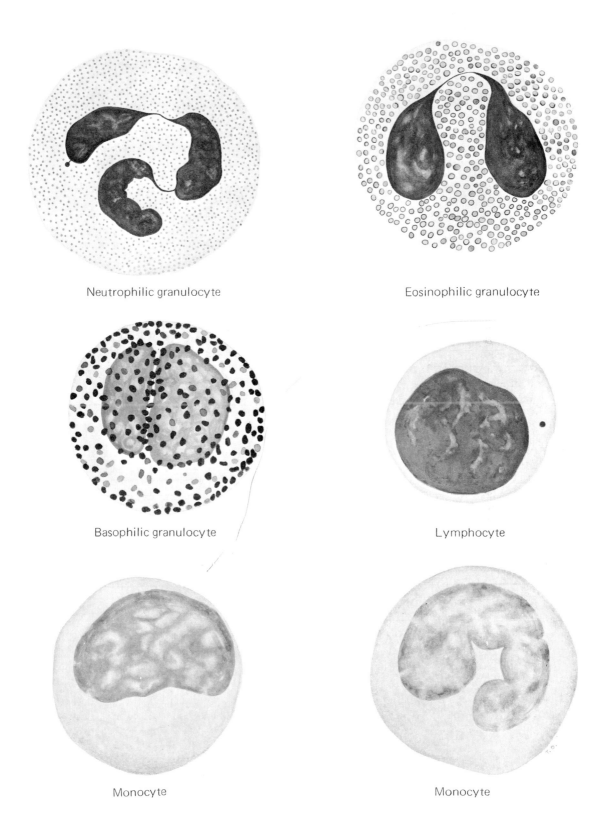

Neutrophilic granulocyte

Eosinophilic granulocyte

Basophilic granulocyte

Lymphocyte

Monocyte

Monocyte

Figure 13 –5. The 5 types of human leukocytes. The drawings were made from blood smears stained by the Romanovsky technic. (This illustration is reproduced in color on p xii.)

strate. Through the process of **diapedesis,** leukocytes may leave the capillaries by passing between
the endothelial cells and penetrating into the connective tissue. The population of leukocytes in connective tissue is so great that they are considered
normal cellular components of that tissue.

The number of leukocytes per microliter (μL)
of blood in the normal adult is 4–11 thousand; at
birth, it varies between 15 and 25 thousand, and by
the fourth day it falls to 12 thousand. At 4 years, the
average is around 8 thousand with a maximum normal limit of 12 thousand. The white count reaches
normal adult values at about 12 years of age. There
is a qualitative variation within the white cell population depending on age; thus, at birth there is a
preponderance of neutrophils, but by the second
week the lymphocytes constitute around 60% of the
leukocytes and predominate during infancy until
age 4, when the granulocytes and lymphocytes are
equal in number. There follows a progressive increase in the percentage of granulocytes, and at age
14–15 years the percentages typical of the adult
(50–70%) are reached. Not only the percentage but
also the absolute number of each cell type per unit
of blood volume must be taken into consideration
when studying physiologic and pathologic variations in the number of blood cells.

Neutrophils

These cells, which constitute 60–70% of circulating leukocytes, develop in the bone marrow
and are released into the circulation. They are about
12 μm in diameter, with a nucleus consisting of 2–5
sausage-shaped lobes (usually 3 lobes) linked to
each other by fine threads of chromatin (Fig 13–5).
The immature neutrophil has a nonsegmented nucleus in the shape of a horseshoe.

The nuclei of all granulocytes follow a similar
chromatin pattern in which dense masses of
heterochromatin are distributed at the periphery of

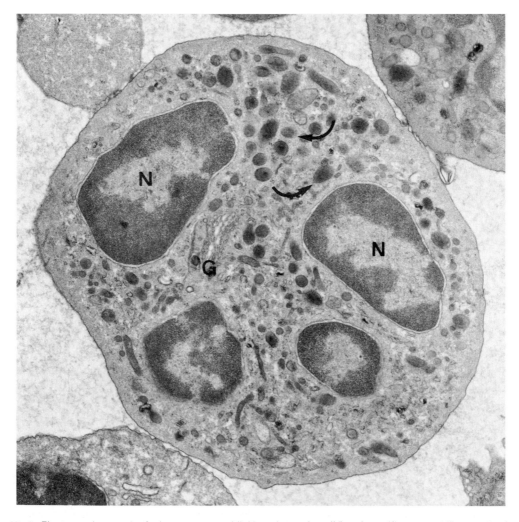

Figure 13 –6. Electron micrograph of a human neutrophil. Note the nucleus (N) and specific neutrophilic granules (arrows). The chromatin bridges that link the nuclear lobes do not appear in this section. G, Golgi apparatus. × 15,000.

the nuclear membrane (Fig 13–6). Zones of loosely arranged chromatin are located mainly in the center of the nucleus.

Neutrophils with more than 5 lobes are called **hypersegmented** and represent old cells. Although under normal conditions the maturation of the neutrophil parallels the increase in the number of nuclear lobes, this relationship is not absolute. In some pathologic conditions, young cells appear with 5 or more lobes.

In the living neutrophil, the shape of the nucleus is variable. The chromatin bridges that unite the nuclear lobes frequently change position and vary in number. Therefore, for the same cell, the number of lobes is variable from time to time depending on the moment when it is observed.

The abundant cytoplasm of the neutrophil is filled with specific granules whose dimensions (0.3–0.8 μm) lie close to the limit of resolution of the optical microscope. These granules are stained a salmon-pink color by Romanovsky-type mixtures (Fig 13–5). There are great differences in size and staining properties of the neutrophilic granules among mammals. For this reason, these granulocytes are also called heterophils. In the rabbit and guinea pig, heterophils have large acidophilic granules. Experimental results obtained with heterophils from other mammals cannot be assumed to be entirely valid for humans.

The granules present in the neutrophils (50–200 in each cell) are surrounded by a membrane and can be separated into 2 types: azurophilic and specific (Fig 13–6). In addition to their staining characteristics, the granules also differ in regard to the chronologic appearance of each type of granule during the development of the granulocytes in the bone marrow; the histologic appearance of the 2 types of granules in the electron microscope; and the enzymic content of each type, which accounts for the differences in their function. The azurophilic granules appear first in the promyelocyte stage of maturation and decrease in number with each successive division of the cell; they are present in mature cells, but most lose their staining characteristics; they are large and appear electron-dense under the electron microscope. They contain lysosomal enzymes and peroxidase.

Specific granules appear at the myelocyte stage; they are smaller and contain alkaline phosphatase and bactericidal substances (cationic proteins) called **phagocytins.** With Romanovsky-type stains, the azurophilic granules are stained reddish-purple, whereas the specific granules are salmon-pink. Both types of granules are formed in the Golgi apparatus but at different sites. Granules undergo Brownian movement or a rapid movement involving one or more granules showing small or great displacement.

After segmentation of its nucleus, the neutrophil is in the final stage of differentiation, possessing a limited capacity for protein synthesis. The mature neutrophil contains scarce profiles of the granular endoplasmic reticulum, a sparse population of free ribosomes, few mitochondria, a rudimentary Golgi apparatus, and a few granules of glycogen. It is a terminal cell for once it has performed its phagocytic function, it is unable to replace the used proteins and eventually dies.

Neutrophils constitute the first line of cellular defense against the invasion of microorganisms. They are active phagocytes of small particles, and this might be due to the specialization of their membrane for this process. These cells are inactive and spherical while circulating but change shape upon adhering to a solid substrate, over which they migrate via pseudopodia. The cells move at a speed of 19–36 μm/min. Following adhesion to a supporting surface, these granulocytes undergo a process

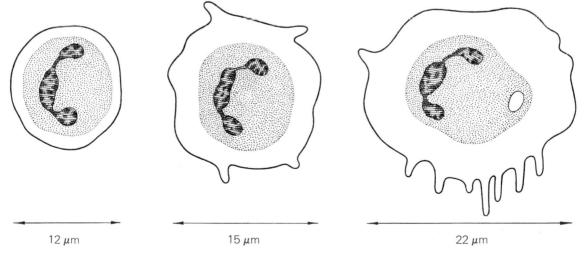

| 12 μm | 15 μm | 22 μm |

Figure 13 –7. Neutrophils undergo a process called "expansion" when in contact with a solid surface. Filopodial processes. spread out from the hyaloplasm; at the same time, the cell increases its diameter with no increase in volume as a result of flattening on the substrate.

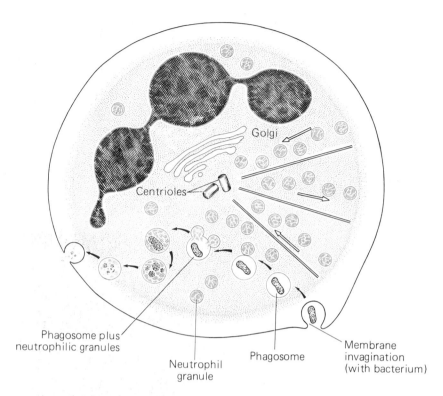

Figure 13–8. Some details of the neutrophil ultrastructure. Neutrophilic granules move constantly; microtubules radiate from the centrioles. The direction of this movement is indicated by white arrows. The lower part of the figure shows the process of intracellular digestion of a phagocytosed bacterium (black arrows). Neutrophilic granules fuse together with phagosomes. The bacterium may be digested in the secondary lysosomes thus formed. Later, the digestion products usually are expelled from the neutrophil.

called "expansion" or spreading, characterized by the emission of cytoplasmic processes in various directions that are transformed into fringes of hyaloplasm (cytoplasm without granules), attaining a diameter of 20 μm. It is interesting to note that the granules keep a distance of 3–5 μm from the cell boundary where ruffling of the membrane is occurring (Fig 13–7). In this process, the base of the cell does not adhere to the substrate but maintains itself above the surface and touches the substrate only with filamentous projections of the hyaloplasm.

The particle to be phagocytosed by the neutrophil is surrounded by pseudopodia that fuse around it (Fig 13–8); thus, the particle eventually occupies a vacuole (phagosome) delimited by a membrane derived from the cell surface and containing extracellular fluid within its contents. Immediately afterward, azurophilic and specific granules fuse their membrane to that of the phagosome and empty their contents into its interior, thus protecting the cytoplasm from exposure to enzymes present in the granules. In this process there is an expenditure of granules and consequent decrease in their number. The presence in the azurophilic granules of D-amino acid oxidase is important in the digestion of bacterial cell walls containing D-amino acids.

Lysozyme present in these granules is also important for the destruction of bacterial cell walls.

A third enzyme is also instrumental in the bactericidal effect of polymorphonuclear neutrophils. During the process of phagocytosis, peroxide is formed. Myeloperoxidase, which is present in the neutrophils, combines with the peroxide and halide to act on the tyrosine molecule of the bacterial cell wall and destroy it.

Under the action of certain toxic substances such as streptolysin (*Streptococcus* toxin), the neutrophils undergo rupture of the membranes of the granules, resulting in a tumefaction process followed by agglutination of the organelles and destruction of the neutrophils themselves.

Neutrophils are quite metabolically active and capable of both aerobic and anaerobic glycolysis. They depend mainly on the latter process for their energy supply. The Krebs cycle is less important, as might be expected in view of the paucity of mitochondria in these cells. The ability of neutrophils to survive in an anaerobic environment is highly advantageous, since they can kill bacteria and help clean up debris in necrotic tissue. Phagocytosis by the neutrophil stimulates hexose monophosphate shunt activity, increasing glycogenolysis.

Eosinophils

Eosinophils are much less numerous than neutrophils, constituting only 1–4% of leukocytes in normal blood. The eosinophil has a diameter of about 9 μm (slightly smaller than the neutrophil). Its nucleus is usually bilobate. The endoplasmic reticulum, mitochondria, and Golgi apparatus are poorly developed. The main identifying characteristic of the eosinophil is the presence of ovoid granulations that are stained by eosin (acidophilic granules). These granules are larger than those of the neutrophils, measuring 0.5–1.5 μm along their main axis (Fig 13–9). The granules are lysosomes containing acid phosphatase, cathepsin, and ribonuclease but not lysozyme.

Eosinophilic granules are surrounded by unit membrane. Parallel to the granule's longer axis, an electron-dense, elongated crystalloid or **internum** is found that is relatively resistant to mechanical trauma and osmotic lysis (Fig 13–9). The internum consists of phospholipids and unsaturated fatty acids. In humans, granules with more than one internum are rare, although this is a common characteristic in other species. The less dense layer surrounding the internum is called the **externum** or **matrix** and is rich in acid phosphatase. An increase in the absolute number of eosinophils in the blood (**eosinophilia**) is associated with allergic reactions in the organism.

The eosinophils have ameboid movement and are capable of phagocytosing, though they phagocytose in a slower but more selective way than the neutrophils. It was experimentally observed that the eosinophil does not phagocytose isolated bovine serum albumin (antigen) or its antibody (specific gamma globulin). However, the eosinophil phagocytoses the complex of this antigen with its antibody (see Chapter 5). It is a function of the

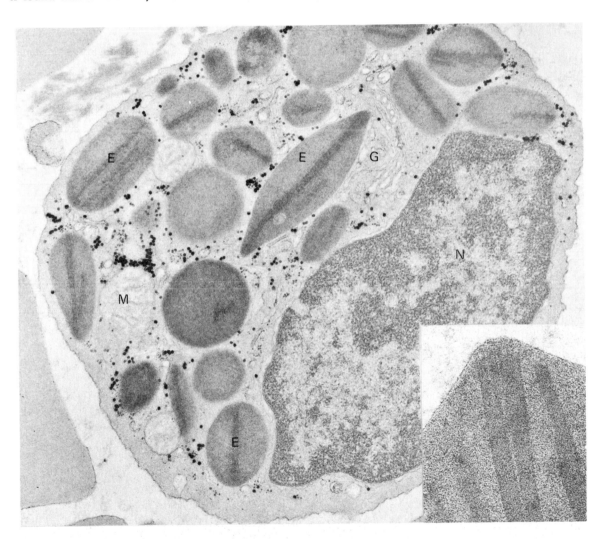

Figure 13–9. Electron micrographs of rabbit eosinophil. Observe a nuclear lobe (N), the Golgi complex (G), a mitochondrion (M), and the eosinophilic granules (E). × 21,500. The inset shows a higher magnification of an eosinophilic granule revealing its crystalloid organization. × 132,000. (Courtesy of DF Bainton and MG Farquhar.)

eosinophil to perform selective phagocytosis of antigen-antibody complexes.

In the same way as the neutrophil, the eosinophil exhibits the phenomenon of granule coalescence with the phagosomes, at which time the respective membranes fuse. In the eosinophil after fusion, it can be observed that only the network or **externum** of the granule appears to fulfill the function of destroying the engulfed material since the internum remains intact within the vacuole for a long time. Consequently, hydrolytic enzymes are localized in the externum of the granule.

Eosinophils contain profibrinolysin, which suggests that they play a role in keeping the blood from clotting, especially when its fluidity is altered by pathologic processes.

Corticosteroids (hormones from the adrenal cortex) produce a rapid fall in the number of blood eosinophils; however, these hormones have no effect on bone marrow eosinophils. Corticosteroids probably interfere with the release of granulocytes from the bone marrow to the bloodstream.

Basophils

Basophils number only 0–1% of blood leuko-

cytes. They measure about 12 μm in diameter and have a large nucleus with an irregular twisted shape, generally in the form of an S (Fig 13–5). The cytoplasm of the basophil is filled with granules larger than those seen in other granulocytes. Often the granules obscure the nucleus. These granules are irregular in size and shape and stain metachromatically. In smears stained by Romanovsky-type mixtures, they appear violet (Fig 13–5).

The granules of basophils are delimited by unit membrane and contain inclusions of uniform size in each granule (Fig 13–10). The size of these particles varies from one granule to another. It is suggested that variation in size may reflect different phases of a secretory cycle. Basophil secretions—histamine and heparin—are localized in the granules. There is some similarity between granules of basophils and those of mast cells (see Chapter 5). Both are metachromatic and contain heparin and histamine. In response to the action of certain antigens, the basophils can liberate their granules, as happens with the mast cell. Despite the similarities they present, mast cells and basophils are not the same, for in the same species they have different ultrastructural appearances. Under certain conditions,

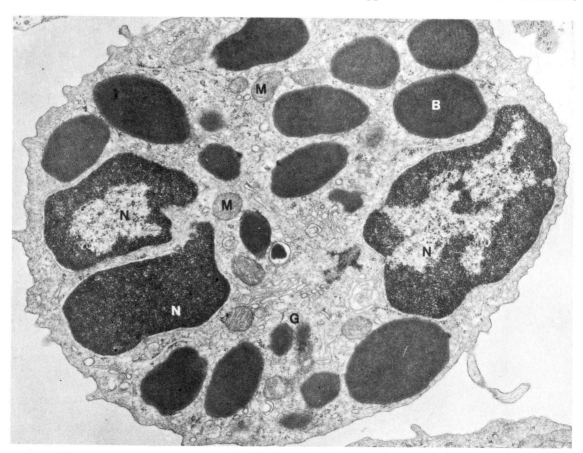

Figure 13–10. Electron micrograph of a rabbit basophil. The lobulated nucleus (N) appears as 3 separated portions. Note the basophilic granules (B), the mitochondria (M), and the Golgi apparatus (G). (Reproduced, with permission, from Terry RW, Bainton DF, Farquhar MG: Lab Invest 21:65, 1969.)

basophils constitute the major cell type in an inflammatory site. This condition has been called **cutaneous basophil hypersensitivity.** Like the other granulocytes, the basophils are capable of ameboid movement and phagocytosis, although they are not very active in this respect.

Lymphocytes

These are spherical cells with diameters of 6–8 μm. Lymphocytes with these dimensions are known as **small lymphocytes** (Fig 13–5). In the circulating blood there occurs a small percentage of **medium-sized lymphocytes** and **large lymphocytes.** This distinction is a holdover from the long period during which the role of the lymphocytes was poorly understood.

The small lymphocyte, predominant in the blood, has a spherical nucleus, sometimes with an indentation. Its chromatin is condensed and appears as coarse clumps, so that the nucleus is intensely stained in the usual preparations, a characteristic that facilitates the identification of the lymphocyte (Figs 13–5 and 13–11). In these preparations, the nucleolus of the lymphocyte is not visible, but it can be demonstrated by special staining technics and with the electron microscope.

The cytoplasm of the small lymphocyte is scanty, and in blood smears it appears as a thin corona around the nucleus. It is slightly basophilic, taking a light blue color in stained smears (Fig 13–5). Sometimes the cytoplasm is not visible. It may contain azurophilic granules that stain purple by Romanovsky-type mixtures. The granules are not exclusive to lymphocytes; they also appear in monocytes and in immature and mature granulocytes. The cytoplasm of the lymphocyte appears poor in organelles but contains many free ribosomes and polyribosomes (Fig 13–12).

The criteria that serve to distinguish large and small lymphocytes are that large ones have (1) an abundance of cytoplasm and greater numbers of polyribosomes; (2) fewer coarse heterochromatin clumps in their nuclei; (3) visible nucleoli within more euchromatic nuclei; and (4) more mitochondria and larger Golgi bodies. Both large and small lymphocytes show mobility both in vitro and in vivo.

Although morphologically similar, lymphocytes of blood constitute a heterogeneous cell population. They vary in size and in density. Experimental evidence, based on studies of electrophoretic mobility, surface topography, histologic localization, buoyant density, and responsiveness to mitogens, suggests the existence of at least 4 subgroups of lymphocytes with different and characteristic immunologic functions. They vary in life span, for some lymphocytes live only a few days while others survive in the circulating blood for many years.

A further classification of lymphocytes can be made by recognition of special molecular markers on the surface membrane of these cells. Some carry specific antigen-binding immunoglobulinlike receptors on their membranes that are absent from others, and they also show differences in the position and class of immunoglobulins they contain.

The simple appearance of the small lymphocytes gives little indication of the capacity of this cell to differentiate into other types of cells. This developmental modulation can be induced by many substances to which lymphocytes might be exposed in vitro. These nonspecific agents create molecular complexes that stimulate specific receptors on the membrane of the cell. In this latter case, only a part of the lymphocyte population responds to the agent. The specific or nonspecific agents probably activate different metabolic pathways or points on the pathways. The activated cells divide mitotically and give rise to large or small cells, as observed by following labeled blast cells and identifying the radioactivity in developing small cells. Small lymphocytes very seldom divide, although proliferation is common in large lymphocytes or blast forms.

There is a separation of functions among lymphocytes. Precursor cells originate in the bone marrow in late fetal and postnatal life and are capable of differentiating and becoming immunocompetent cells in sites outside the bone marrow. In birds, this differentiation occurs in 2 distinct areas: the **bursa of Fabricius** and the **thymus.** In the bursa of Fabricius, which is a mass of lymphoid tissue in the cloaca

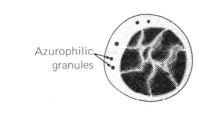

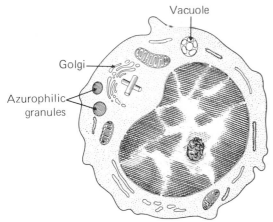

Figure 13–11. A medium lymphocyte as seen with the light microscope *(above)* and the electron microscope *(below).* Cytoplasmic organelles are scanty. Small lymphocytes exhibit even less cytoplasm.

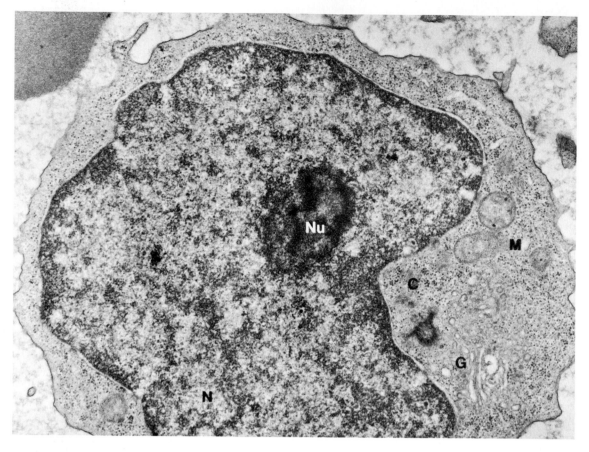

Figure 13–12. Electron micrograph of a human blood lymphocyte. This cell is poor in endoplasmic reticulum, containing a moderate quantity of free ribosomes. Observe the nucleus (N), the nucleolus (Nu), the centriole (C), the mitochondria (M), and the Golgi complex (G). Reduced from × 22,000. (Courtesy of DF Bainton and MG Farquhar.)

of birds, the undifferentiated cells of bone marrow origin are induced to become progenitor cells of lymphocytes that ultimately differentiate into plasma cells, which produce antibodies—**immunoglobulins**—to specific antigens. They are involved in the humoral immunity of the body. These lymphocytes are called **B (bursa-dependent) lymphocytes** (Fig 15–11).

In the thymus, undifferentiated lymphocytes of bone marrow origin are induced to become progenitor cells that function in the cellular immunity of the organism. These lymphocytes are called **T (thymus-dependent) lymphocytes** (Fig 15–11).

In mammals, the bursa of Fabricius does not exist, but the progenitor marrow cells differentiate into B cells in the bursa-equivalent, an area as yet unidentified that may be associated with the gastrointestinal tract or with the bone marrow itself. The thymus and the bursa-equivalent in mammals are called central lymphoid organs, and lymphocytes differentiated in these organs colonize other areas of the body where lymphoid tissue is found in encapsulated, diffuse, or organ form.

Under appropriate conditions, if a B lym-

phocyte recognizes an antigen, it can become activated and ultimately differentiate into plasma cells that synthesize antigen-specific antibodies secreted into the blood, intercellular fluid, and lymph.

In the blood, most lymphocytes are T cells and are responsible for the cell-mediated immune reactions not dependent on free circulating antibodies. Graft rejection is an example of a cell-mediated immune reaction. In this type of immune response, T lymphocytes directly bind to the foreign cells and produce factors that act on the grafted cells located around them. For this reason, cell-mediated reactions take place only when the T lymphocyte itself is present to elaborate these factors in the environment. T lymphocytes play a vital role in determining the type and amount of antibodies produced by some B lymphocytes.

B lymphocytes give rise to **memory cells.** These are lymphocytes that have been previously exposed to an antigen but have not differentiated into plasma cells. When they later come into contact with the same antigen again, these **activated** cells rapidly divide several times by mitosis and give rise to plasma cells which synthesize antibody against the antigen. Memory cells explain why the second injection of an antigen is followed by a higher and faster production of antibody than the first injection. There are also memory cells derived from T lymphocytes, which also react to and proliferate following contact with an antigen to which they have previously been exposed. In summary, both T and B lymphocytes contribute to **immunologic memory.**

Monocytes

These bone marrow-derived agranulocytes have diameters varying from 9–12 μm (Fig 13–5). The nucleus is oval, horseshoe-shaped, or kidney-shaped and is generally eccentrically placed. The chromatin is less condensed and exhibits a more fibrillar arrangement than in the lymphocytes, this being the most constant characteristic of the monocyte (Fig 13–13). Owing to the delicate distribution

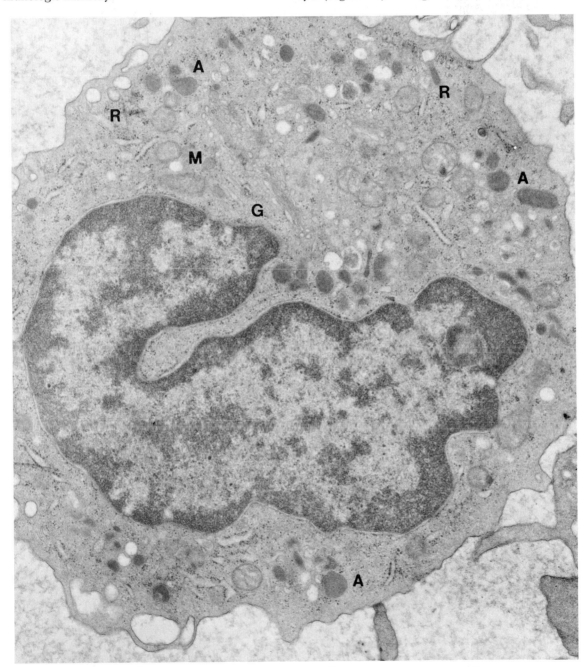

Figure 13–13. Electron micrograph of a human monocyte. Note the Golgi complex (G), the mitochondria (M), and the azurophilic granules (A). Endoplasmic reticulum is poorly developed. There are some free ribosomes (R). × 22,000. (Courtesy of DF Bainton and MG Farquhar.)

of their chromatin, the nuclei of monocytes are more lightly stained than those of large lymphocytes, which are the blood cells with which they may most easily be confused, although the monocytes are generally larger (Fig 13–5). The nucleus of the monocyte usually contains 2 or 3 nucleoli that can be seen in blood smears stained by Romanovsky-type mixtures.

The cytoplasm of the monocyte is basophilic and frequently contains very fine azurophilic granules, some of which are at the limits of optical microscopic resolution. These granules may be distributed throughout the cytoplasm, giving it a bluish-gray color in stained smears. The azurophilic granules of the monocytes are lysosomes. In the electron microscope, one or 2 nucleoli are seen in the nucleus and a small quantity of granular endoplasmic reticulum, ribosomes, polyribosomes, and many small elongated mitochondria are observed (Fig 13–13). A well-developed Golgi apparatus involved in the synthesis of the lysosomelike granules is present in the cytoplasm. Microfilaments and microtubules are usually observed in areas near the identation of the nucleus. Many microvilli and pinocytotic vesicles are found on the cell surface.

Monocytes are found in the blood, connective tissue, and body cavities. They belong to the **mononuclear phagocytic system (reticuloendothelial system)** and have receptor sites on their surface membrane for immunoglobulins and complement.

Monocytes circulate through the bloodstream and are capable of crossing the capillary wall, penetrating the connective tissues, and differentiating into phagocytic cells of the macrophage system. The half-life of the monocyte in the blood is a few days, and there is no strong evidence of recirculation after they enter the tissues. In the tissues they interact with lymphocytes and play an essential role in the recognition and interaction of the immunocompetent cells with antigen.

PLATELETS

Blood **platelets (thrombocytes)** are enucleated, disklike cell fragments 2–5 μm in diameter. Platelets originate from the budding of giant multinucleated **megakaryocytes** residing in the bone

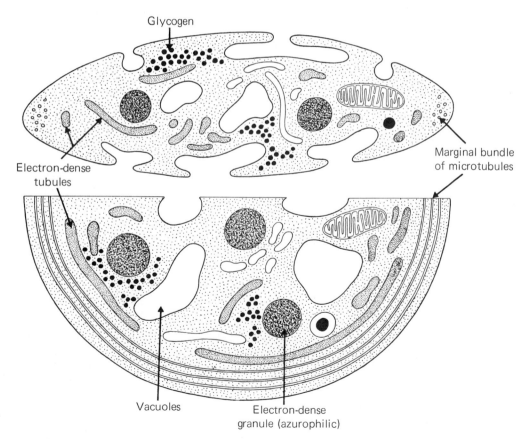

Figure 13–14. Ultrastructure of platelets in cross section *(above)* and in longitudinal section *(below)*. Infoldings of the plasma membrane give rise to numerous vacuoles. The large electron-dense granules are the azurophilic granules of light microscopy. Near the edge of the platelet, there is a marginal bundle of microtubules. Glycogen granules, mitochondria, and electron-dense tubules are present in the hyalomere.

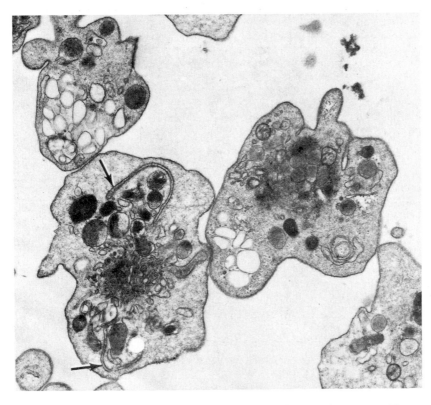

Figure 13–15. Electron micrograph of human platelets. Arrows indicate electron-dense tubules. The system of vacuoles and the electron-dense (azurophilic) granules are also seen. × 17,000.

marrow. Because of their tendency to agglutinate in clumps, platelet counts are difficult to derive; consequently, their reported normal concentration in human blood varies between wide extremes. Normal counts range from 150 to 300 thousand/μL of blood. Upon entering the bloodstream, platelets have a life span of about 8 days.

In stained blood smears, platelets often appear in clumps. Each platelet has a peripheral light blue-stained transparent zone, the **hyalomere,** and a central dense zone containing purple granules called the **granulomere.** Filopodialike processes extending from the hyalomere cause an irregular conformation of the platelet surface.

Platelet ultrastructure is diagrammatically illustrated in Fig 13–14. These cytoplasmic fragments exhibit a system of tubules and vesicles derived from invaginations of the platelet membrane (Fig 13–15). Consequently, the interior of the fragments communicates freely with the platelet surface. In the hyalomere zone, around the periphery of the platelet, lies a **marginal bundle** of microtubules that helps to maintain the platelet's ovoid shape. Actinlike microfilaments in the hyalomere function in the elaboration of filopodia and surface projections during platelet movement and aggregation. A cell coat rich in glycosaminogly-

cans and glycoproteins, 15–20 nm in diameter, lies outside the plasmalemma and is associated with platelet adhesion.

The dense granulomere possesses a variety of membrane-bound granules and a sparse population of mitochondria and glycogen particles (Fig 13–15). Some of the granules, which range in diameter from 0.5 to 1.5 nm, contain serotonin (5-hydroxytryptamine) and ADP, whereas others are lysosomes. The mitochondria, which function in calcium deposition, show structural changes during platelet aggregation.

Following rupture of a blood vessel, platelets in the area of the injury release their serotonin-containing granules. Serotonin, a vasoconstrictor, leads to contraction of vascular smooth muscle, slowing or stopping blood flow in the injured area. The platelets adhere readily to collagen exposed at the injured site and, along with damaged endothelial cells, release **thromboplastin.** In a chain reaction, thromboplastin enzymatically converts the plasma prothrombin into thrombin, which in turn converts fibrinogen into fibrin. Both prothrombin and fibrinogen are synthesized by the liver and released into the blood. Following its formation, fibrin polymerizes into a fibrillar matrix that entraps other platelets and blood cells and gives rise to the

hemostatic plug, the basis of the **blood clot (thrombus).**

Platelets also release **thrombosthenin,** a contractile protein that becomes incorporated into the clot and causes it to retract. Platelet lysosomes may subsequently play a role in lysis of the clot after healing.

• • •

References

Archer GT, Hirsch JG: Isolation of granules from eosinophil leukocytes and study of their enzyme content. J Exp Med 118:227, 1963.

Baggiolini M, Hirsch JG, de Duve C: Resolution of granules from rabbit heterophil leukocytes into distinct populations by zonal sedimentation. J Cell Biol 40:529, 1969.

Bainton DF: Sequential degranulation of the 2 types of polymorphonuclear leukocyte granules during phagocytosis of microorganisms. J Cell Biol 58:249, 1973.

Bainton DF, Farquhar MG: Origin of granules in polymorphonuclear leukocytes: Two types derived from opposite faces of the Golgi complex in developing granulocytes. J Cell Biol 28:277, 1966.

Bainton DF, Farquhar MG: Segregation and packaging of granule enzymes in eosinophilic leukocytes. J Cell Biol 45:54, 1970.

Barr RD, Whang-Peng J, Perry S: Hemopoietic stem cells in human peripheral blood. Science 190:284, 1975.

Becker RP, De Bruyn PP: The transmural passage of blood cells into myeloid sinusoids and the entry of platelets into the sinusoid circulation: A scanning electron microscope investigation. Am J Anat 145:183, 1976.

Behnke O: Electron microscopic observations on the membrane systems of the rat blood platelet. Anat Rec 158:121, 1967.

Bentfield ME, Nichols BA, Bainton DF: Ultrastructural localization of peroxidasis in leukocytes of rat bone marrow and blood. Anat Rec 187:219, 1977.

Bessis M: *Living Blood Cells and Their Ultrastructure.* Springer, 1973.

Campbell FR: Nuclear elimination from the normoblast of fetal guinea pig liver as studied with electron microscopy and serial sectioning techniques. Anat Rec 160:539, 1968.

Campbell FR: Ultrastructural studies of transmural migration of blood cells in the bone marrow of rats, mice and guinea pigs. Am J Anat 135:521, 1972.

Edelman GM: Antibody structure and cellular specificity in the immune response. Harvey Lect 68:149, 1974.

Gowans JL: Differentiation of the cells which synthesize the immunoglobulins. Ann Immunol (Paris) 125:201, 1974.

Gowans JL, Knight EJ: The route of recirculation of lymphocytes in the rat. Proc R Soc Lond [Biol] 159:745, 1965.

Hanifin JM, Cline MJ: Human monocytes and macrophages: Interaction with antigen and lymphocytes. J Cell Biol 46:97, 1970.

Marchalonis JJ: Lymphocyte surface immunoglobulins. Science 190:20, 1975.

McFarland W, Schecter GP: The lymphocyte in immunological reactions in vitro: Ultrastructural studies. Blood 35:683, 1970.

Miller F, de Harven E, Palade GE: The structure of eosinophil leukocyte granules in rodents and in man. J Cell Biol 31:349, 1966.

Nichols BA, Bainton DF: Differentiation of human monocytes in bone marrow and blood: Sequential formation of 2 granule populations. Lab Invest 29:27, 1973.

Nossal GJV: Genetic control of lymphopoiesis, plasma cell formation and antibody production. Int Rev Exp Pathol 1:1, 1962.

Polliack A & others: Identification of human B and T lymphocytes by scanning electron microscopy. J Exp Med 138:607, 1973.

Polliack A & others: Scanning electron microscopy of human lymphocyte–sheep erythrocyte rosettes. J Exp Med 140:146, 1974.

Roelants GE & others: Active synthesis of immunoglobulin receptors for antigen by T lymphocytes. Nature 247:106, 1974.

Simpson CF, Kling JM: The mechanism of denucleation in circulating erythroblasts. J Cell Biol 35:237, 1967.

Tanaka Y, Goodman JR: *Electron Microscopy of Human Blood Cells.* Harper & Row, 1972.

Ullyot JL, Bainton DF, Farquhar MG: Cytochemical studies of human neutrophilic leukocyte granules. J Histochem Cytochem 18:681, 1970.

Watanabe L, Donahue S, Hoggott N: Method for electron microscopic studies of circulating human leukocytes: An observation of their fine structure. J Ultrastruct Res 20:366, 1967.

Wintrobe M & others: *Clinical Hematology,* 7th ed. Lea & Febiger, 1974.

The Life Cycle of Blood Cells | 14

Mature blood cells exhibit a relatively short life span, and consequently the population must be continuously replaced by the progeny of stem cells produced in the **hematopoietic** organs. In the earliest stages of embryogenesis, erythrocytes arise from the yolk sac endoderm. However, with subsequent development, both erythrocytes and granular leukocytes are derived from stem cells localized in the bone marrow (myeloid tissue), and these cells comprise the **myeloid elements** of the blood. Although their stem cells initially arise from the marrow, circulating lymphocytes are mainly derived from the mitotic activity of stem cells that end up residing in the lymphatic organs. Lymphocytes therefore constitute the **lymphoid elements** of the blood.

Before attaining complete maturity and being released into the circulation, the blood cells go through specific stages of differentiation and maturation. Because these processes are continuous, cells with characteristics that are intermediate between 2 typical stages are frequently encountered in smears of blood or bone marrow.

It is probable that all of the formed elements of the blood originate from a single type of precursor cell (**unitarian** or **monophyletic theory**). In the past, some investigators favored the concept of more than one type of precursor cell (**polyphyletic theory**). The simplest polyphyletic theory assumes the existence of 2 stem cells, one for the cells that derive from myeloid tissue and the other for cells that derive from lymphatic tissue. The other extreme is the complete polyphyletic theory, which maintains that there is a primitive stem cell for each type of blood cell.

These theories represent an effort to resolve the difficulties of following the various stages of cell differentiation in bone marrow and lymphatic tissue. When cells at different stages of differentiation are arranged in a definite sequence—eg, in the stratified squamous epithelium (skin, esophagus) or in the seminiferous tubules (testis)—it is easy to follow each cell through its various stages of differentiation. In the hematopoietic organs, cells develop in clusters (groups of cells of the same origin). Because cells within the clusters do not exhibit any regular organization, cells in specific stages of differentiation can be recognized only by morphologic characterization. Since the immature cells of each blood cell type have more similarities among themselves than do the progeny that have reached a more highly differentiated stage, difficulties and controversies arise in relation to identifying these less mature cells.

According to the unitarian theory, all of the blood cells derive from the **hemocytoblast** or **stem cell**, a free cell which arises directly from the embryonic mesenchymal cell and has a strictly hematopoietic potential. The mitotic multiplication of the cells that derive from the stem cell, which are at the observed intermediate stages of differentiation, is almost sufficient to maintain the number of peripheral blood cells at a constant level. For this reason, the number of stem cells encountered in the hematopoietic organs is small and mitosis of these cells is very rare.

BONE MARROW

Bone marrow is found in the medullary canals of long bones and in the cavities of spongy bones. Two types have been described according to their appearance on gross examination: **red, hematogenous,** or **active bone marrow,** whose color is due to the presence of numerous erythrocytes and their precursors in several phases of maturation; and **yellow bone marrow,** rich in adipose cells, which does not produce blood cells except upon conversion or transformation into red bone marrow induced by severe bleeding or hypoxia. In newborns, all of the bone marrow is red and is therefore active in the production of blood cells. As the child grows, most of the bone marrow changes into the yellow variety; in adults, red bone marrow is primarily found only in the flat bones (sternum, vertebrae, ribs, clavicles, bones of the pelvis, and diploë of the skull bones); in young adults, red marrow is found also in the proximal epiphyses of the femur and humerus.

Active (Red) Bone Marrow
Like hematopoietic tissue in general, red bone marrow consists of reticular cells associated with

reticular fibers and cells of the erythroid series in different stages of maturation. These elements (cells and fibers) form a sponge traversed by numerous sinusoid capillaries whose lining contains endothelial cells. Among the above-mentioned cells there are macrophages and a variable number of adipose cells; in many cases, the boundary between red and yellow marrow is not clear.

The reticular cells, macrophages, and adipose cells are usually attached to the supporting stromal connective tissue. In the meshes of the myeloid tissue, there is a profusion of free cells consisting of blood elements (erythrocytes, granulocytes, monocytes, and platelets) and their precursors. The bone marrow may present still other cells—especially plasma cells—in different phases of maturation.

When they reach maturation, the blood cells enter the circulation by passing through the sinusoids of the marrow cavity. The sinusoids consist of an endothelial lining, a basement membrane, and adventitial cells that cover up to 60% of the outer surface of the sinusoid. Forming blood cells penetrate the sinusoids by passing between the adventitial cells, through the basement membrane, and through pores they create in the thin endothelial cells.

The adventitial cells extend from the periphery of the sinusoids and participate in the elaboration of a reticular matrix composed of cell processes and extracellular reticular fibers. This matrix serves as a support for the developing hematopoietic stem cells and their progeny.

The free cells of the myeloid tissue have a tendency to remain in groups. In each group, one type of cell predominates in different phases of its maturation.

The blood that comes from the arterioles penetrates into the sinusoids and is there enriched by the elements formed in the meshes of the myeloid tissue. From the sinusoids, the blood passes to veins that leave the bone marrow.

The main functions of the red bone marrow are in production of blood cells, destruction of erythrocytes and subsequent storage of iron, and production of undifferentiated B and T lymphocytes, which are carried by the blood to the central lymphatic organs.

By inoculating different bone marrow cells into animals whose lymphatic organs have been destroyed by irradiation, it is possible to show that lymphocyte precursors come from bone marrow. In general, only bone marrow cells are able to repopulate the destroyed central lymphatic organs. An exception to this rule would be the fact that cells taken from lymphatic tissues can temporarily repopulate these areas. All others—even cells from peripheral lymphatic tissue—lack the capacity to promote this regeneration except for a limited period of time.

Iron is stored in bone marrow as **ferritin** and **hemosiderin** in the cytoplasm of reticular cells and other macrophagic cells. However, large amounts of ferritin and hemosiderin are also stored outside the bone marrow in hepatocytes, skeletal muscle fibers, and spleen macrophages.

Ferritin contains iron and a protein with a molecular weight of 480,000 called **apoferritin.** This protein makes an envelope around a central core of colloid iron. The whole particle has a diameter of 12 nm, and the iron core has a diameter of 5.5 nm. Under the electron microscope, each ferritin particle shows 4–6 electron-dense subunits, which permits its identification in electron micrographs.

Hemosiderin is a heterogeneous complex containing apoferritin, other proteins, carbohydrates, lipids, and other molecules. The iron content is higher in hemosiderin than in ferritin. Hemosiderin exists in storage cells as granules 1–2 μm in diameter demonstrable by cytochemical reactions for iron.

Yellow Bone Marrow

In the yellow bone marrow there is a great predominance of adipose cells with an admixture of macrophages, undifferentiated mesenchymal cells, and reticular cells. Under stimulation, the undifferentiated cells may proliferate, giving rise to myeloid cells and transforming the yellow marrow into red marrow again.

The yellow bone marrow has 2 main functions: it is a storage organ, by virtue of its richness in fat; and it represents a reserve of hematopoietic tissue, becoming the site of production of cells in pathologic situations marked by frequent hemorrhages or excessive destruction of erythrocytes.

MATURATION OF ERYTHROCYTES

Stages in the differentiation and maturation of erythrocytic cells are the formation of **proerythroblasts, basophilic erythroblasts, polychromatophilic erythroblasts, normoblasts** (orthochromatic erythroblasts), **reticulocytes,** and finally **erythrocytes. A mature** cell is one that has differentiated to the state where it has acquired the capability to carry out all of its specific functions. The basic process in maturation is the synthesis of hemoglobin and the formation of a small corpuscle, the erythrocyte (red cell), which has the greatest possible area for the diffusion of oxygen (Fig 14–1).

During maturation of the cells of the erythrocytic series, the following major morphologic and histologic changes occur, corresponding to biochemical events of the developing erythroid cell: (1) cell volume decreases; (2) nucleoli diminish in size until they become invisible under the light microscope; (3) nuclear chromatin becomes increasingly more dense until the nucleus presents a pyknotic appearance and is finally extruded from the

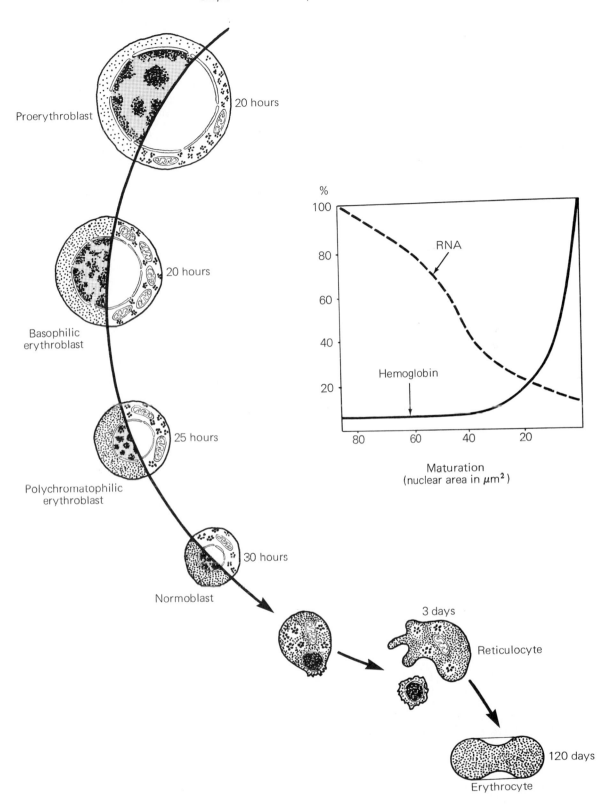

Figure 14–1. Summary of erythrocyte maturation. The stippled part of the cytoplasm shows that hemoglobin concentration increases continuously from the proerythroblast to the erythrocyte stage. There is also a decrease in nuclear volume and an increase in chromatin condensation, followed by extrusion of a pyknotic nucleus. In the graph, the higher concentrations of hemoglobin and RNA were considered to be 100%. The notations of times are average life spans.

cell; (4) there is a decrease in the number of polyribosomes (basophilia) and an increase in the amount of hemoglobin (acidophilia) within the cytoplasm; and (5) the quantity of mitochondria diminishes (Fig 14–1).

Proerythroblast (Pronormoblast)

The proerythroblast is a large cell (14–17 μm in diameter) that contains all of the elements characteristic of a cell undergoing intense protein synthesis. The nucleus is spherical and centrally located, occupying 80% of the cell, with a delicately structured chromatin and 1 or 2 large nucleoli. The cytoplasm is characteristically intensely basophilic, with a pale region around the nucleus. Electron microscopic examination demonstrates that this pale perinuclear halo contains mitochondria, the Golgi apparatus, and a pair of centrioles. The remaining cytoplasm contains numerous polyribosomes, but the endoplasmic reticulum is not well developed.

A main function of the proteins synthesized by the proerythroblast is to accommodate the increase in the cell's mass of protoplasm, since this cell divides rapidly. Hemoglobin synthesis also begins, since this protein can be detected by microspectrophotometry. Pinocytotic vesicles and ferritin can be seen in the cytoplasm. At this stage, the amount of hemoglobin is too small to be detected by the usual staining technics.

Basophilic Erythroblast (Basophilic Normoblast)

The basophilic erythroblast is slightly smaller (13–16 μm in diameter) than the proerythroblast and has a nucleus of the same shape as the proerythroblast that occupies three-fourths of the cell. The chromatin is more condensed, and the pattern of heterochromatin and euchromatin gives a clockface appearance. There are no visible nucleoli (Figs 14–2, 14–3, and 14–4) and little, if any, rough endoplasmic reticulum. Polyribosomes are present in the cytoplasm, and their large number accounts for the characteristic basophilia of this cell. The Golgi apparatus is well developed, and the cell exhibits an abundance of mitochondria. Mi-

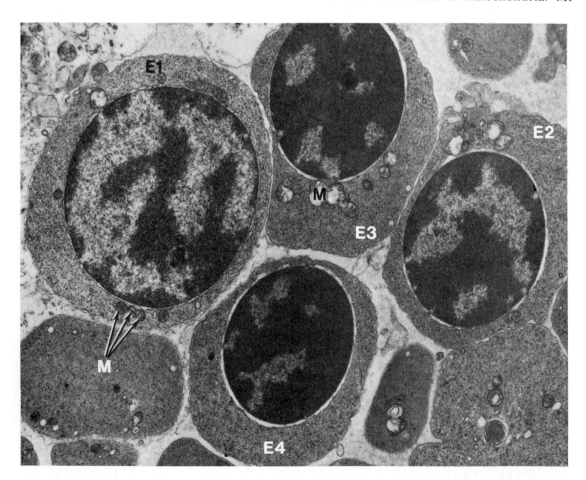

Figure 14–2. Electron micrograph of the bone marrow of a rat. Four erythroblasts in successive stages of maturation are seen (E1, E2, E3, and E4). As the cell matures, its chromatin becomes condensed and the accumulation of hemoglobin increases the electron density of the cytoplasm. Note the mitochondria (M). × 11,000.

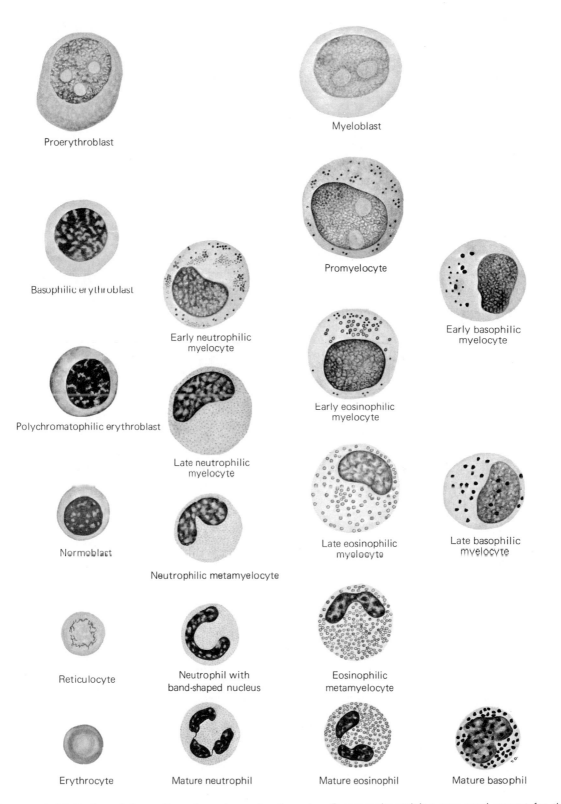

Figure 14 –3. Maturation of the erythrocytic and granulocytic series. Romanovsky staining was used except for the reticulocyte, which was treated additionally by cresyl blue in order to precipitate and stain the RNA found in this cell. (This illustration is reproduced in color on p xiii.)

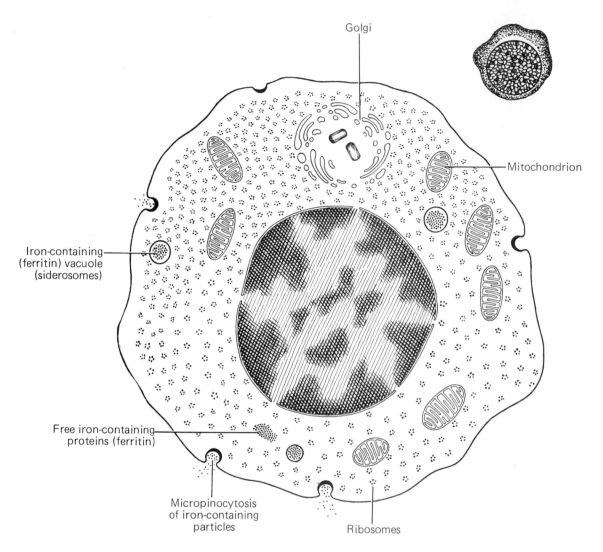

Figure 14–4. Ultrastructure of a basophilic erythroblast. Its cytoplasm contains many polyribosomes for the synthesis of hemoglobin. The upper right drawing shows the structure of the same cell as seen in bone marrow smears. The light area near the nucleus contains the Golgi complex and the centrioles.

crotubules and microfilaments are also present in the cytoplasm. The basophilic erythroblast undergoes one mitotic division. Hemoglobin continues to be formed.

Polychromatophilic Erythroblast
(Polychromatophilic Normoblast)

The polychromatophilic erythroblast is even smaller (12–15 μm in diameter) than the basophilic erythroblast, with a nucleus that occupies half of the cell or less and contains even more condensed chromatin in a checkerboard pattern. This polychromatophilic erythroblast contains hemoglobin in sufficient quantity to cause a cytoplasmic acidophilia (pink), which, added to the basophilia, gives a characteristic grayish-pink color to the cytoplasm (Figs 14–2 and 14–3). The

rest of the organelles decrease in size, but pinocytosis along the plasma membrane is still present. While in this stage, the cell undergoes a number of mitotic divisions each of which is followed by an increase in the degree of erythrocyte differentiation.

Normoblast (Orthochromatic Erythroblast)

The normoblast has a diameter of 8–10 μm. The nucleus shows condensed heterochromatin, has become smaller so that it occupies less than one-fourth of the cell area, and is disposed eccentrically. The cytoplasm of this cell is usually acidophilic because of the abundance of hemoglobin, but traces of basophilia (Fig 14–3) representing polysomes are still seen. Mitochondria and the Golgi apparatus become smaller and begin to degenerate. After 3 mitotic divisions, the pyknotic nucleus becomes incapable of further replication and is then extruded.

Reticulocytes

Microcinematography has demonstrated that at any given moment the normoblast puts forth a series of cytoplasmic protrusions. During this activity, the nucleus is expelled encased in a thin layer of cytoplasm containing hemoglobin. The extruded nuclei, separated from the normoblasts, are engulfed by bone marrow macrophages. Expulsion of nuclei may occur at an earlier maturation stage than the normoblast, in which case the erythrocyte will be larger than normal and is called a **macrocyte.** Following loss of its nucleus, the remaining part of the cell is called a **reticulocyte.** Under the electron microscope, it still presents 2 centrioles, some mitochondria, remnants of the Golgi apparatus, and polyribosomes. These last organelles synthesize the small quantity of hemoglobin (almost 20%) necessary to complete the total hemoglobin content of the mature erythrocyte. Polyribosomes cannot be renewed because of the absence of a nucleus, so protein synthesis ceases within a short time.

The reticulocyte is capable of contracting itself, forming folds at certain points and projections at others. The reticulocyte enters the circulation by sending forth a pseudopodium that penetrates the wall of the sinusoidal capillary and ultimately passes through into the lumen. The maturation period of the reticulocytes in the circulation is 24–28 hours, with a total life span of approximately 72 hours. During this period, autophagia and ejection of different organelles occur.

The reticulocyte differs from the erythrocyte in that it retains some RNA, thus showing a slight diffuse basophilia superimposed on the intense acidophilia of the hemoglobin. The reticulocytes are polychromatophilic red cells. In blood smears stained by the usual methods, the reticulocyte appears larger than the erythrocyte, measuring approximately 9 μm in diameter.

When treated with supravital dyes such as cresyl blue, the ribonucleoprotein of the reticulocytes precipitates, forming a reticulum of variable appearance and size that stains dark blue (Fig 14–3). During this period of maturation, all of the polyribosomes disperse into free single ribosomes.

The reticulocyte represents a young erythrocyte. An increase in the number of reticulocytes in the blood indicates increased production of erythrocytes as long as the number of reticulocytes in the bone marrow does not decrease. A high reticulocyte count in the blood accompanied by a decrease of their number in the bone marrow indicates more rapid liberation of these cells into the circulation without a corresponding increase in reticulocyte formation in the bone marrow.

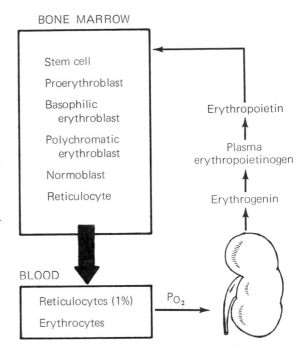

Figure 14–5. The erythron is composed of both the medullary and circulating blood compartments. Reticulocytes pass from the bone marrow to the blood, where they complete maturation into erythrocytes. A fall in blood oxygen tension (P_{O_2}) stimulates the kidney to produce erythrogenin, a renal factor interacting with a plasma globulin erythropoietinogen to produce an active hormone, erythropoietin, which accelerates the mitotic rate and the maturation of red cells in the medullary compartment. Thus, the number of liberated reticulocytes and erythrocytes in the blood increases.

Erythron (Fig 14–5)

The erythron is the total cell population of erythrocytes and their precursor cells and is a widely dispersed but functionally single organ. Its principal function is to supply the organism with the oxygen necessary for tissue metabolism. Moreover, it carries CO_2, a gas which is also transported dissolved in the plasma for elimination from the lungs.

The erythron can be divided into 2 functional compartments: (1) the **circulating** or **blood compartment,** represented by the erythrocytes in the blood; and (2) the **medullary compartment,** or **erythropoietic pool,** the bone marrow sites where formation of new elements takes place.

As ongoing synthesis and accumulation of hemoglobin-carrying cells occurs, continuous renewal of the cells released into the circulation is required since the mature erythrocyte in humans has a half-life of approximately 120 days.* Cell renewal depends upon the existence of another

*In other animals the red cell has a longer or shorter life span, but the measurement is always in days.

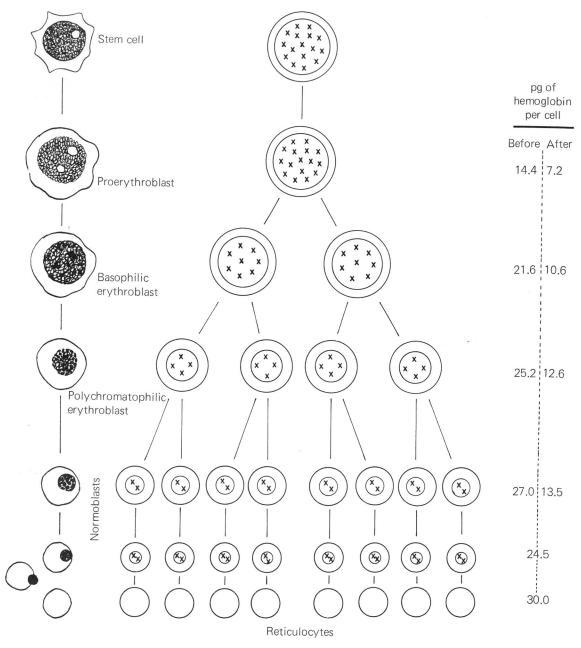

Figure 14 –6. Radioautographic data on the rate of erythrocyte maturation obtained after a single labeling injection of ³H-thymidine. Silver granules in the radioautographs are represented by crosses. In each mitotic division, the number of silver granules per nucleus is reduced by half. In adult bone marrow, stem cells (hemocytoblasts) are few in number, and they rarely divide. The erythrocytes are normally produced by multiplication of proerythroblasts, basophilic erythroblasts, and polychromatophilic erythroblasts.

cellular compartment which, via homeostatic mechanisms, makes immature forms of cells available for maturation (Fig 14–6). This can be easily shown by injecting ⁵⁹Fe and observing its incorporation into the hemoglobin molecule of maturing cells. Such experiments have demonstrated that the pool of proerythroblasts is increased by mitosis of existing proerythroblasts and by the emergence of

unlabeled erythroblasts from an early compartment. This precursor compartment is the committed stem cell compartment and depends on a multipotential cell compartment for maintaining its numbers of cells. The committed stem cell, according to some workers, is sensitive to erythropoietin, a hormone controlling the erythropoiesis. The same hormone also influences the differentiated compartment. A feedback mechanism exists between the multipotential and the committed cell compartments. These **stem cells** (formerly **hemocytoblasts**) appear to be small mononuclear cells similar to mature lymphocytes. The proponents of the **unitarian theory**—Maximow and, more recently, Yoffey—hold that these cells, which are similar to lymphocytes, act as precursors of proerythroblasts. Erythropoietin is essential for the maintenance of the precursor cells by enabling them to continue to proliferate into hemoglobin-synthesizing elements. It has been shown that erythropoietin might alter the hematopoietic internal microenvironment in order to provide optimal conditions for erythropoiesis. The cell cycle of these stem cells, or erythropoietin-responsive or sensitive cells, has a variable resting G_1 phase with an S phase of 6–12 hours and an M (mitotic) phase of 30–45 minutes. Erythropoietin acts on cells at the G_1 level and differentiates them into proerythroblasts. Experimentally, antibodies to erythropoietin can almost completely terminate erythrocyte production. It appears that, in humans, after an erythropoietic stimulus (eg, hemorrhage, high altitude), new reticulocytes enter the circulation within 5 days, which suggests that the time required for maturation in each stage is approximately 1 day. The erythropoietic pool accounts for approximately one-thirtieth of the circulating red cell volume.

The blood compartment consists of erythrocytes and a small percentage of reticulocytes. The medullary compartment contains principally nucleated elements (proerythroblasts, normoblasts) and a relatively small number of erythrocytes and reticulocytes (Fig 14–5). The latter remain in the bone marrow for 36–44 hours before entering the circulation.

Since the erythron has no large reserve compartment of mature forms, the concentration of erythrocytes in the blood reflects the rate of medullary production. An increase in the production of erythrocytes with no increase in their destruction results in a greater concentration of these cells in the blood.

Under conditions of hypoxia (deficient supply of oxygen to the tissues), the production of erythrocytes increases. This occurs, for example, in people who live at high altitudes where the atmospheric oxygen concentration is low. The same occurs after hemorrhage and in persons with chronic pulmonary dysfunction. Thus, hypoxia is a fundamental physiologic stimulus for erythropoiesis since oxygen supply and demand regulate the red cell production.

Erythropoietin is a glycoprotein hormone with a molecular weight of 45,800 when obtained from anemic sheep plasma. It contains 30% carbohydrate with a large component, 10.5%, being sialic acid. It is found in the plasma and urines of anemic and hypoxic experimental animals and humans and has a half-life of approximately 1–2 days in humans and a few hours in laboratory animals. Other organs must also produce erythropoietin, for this substance still appears in the blood of animals that have undergone bilateral nephrectomy. Thus, the feedback mechanism of production and release of erythropoietin is related to the need for oxygen in the tissues and the number of circulating erythrocytes carrying oxygen.

Numerous substances are essential for the proper functioning of the erythron and for the production of erythrocytes. Among these are iron, vitamin B_{12}, and folic acid.

Several hormones (eg, thyroxine, testosterone, cortisol) stimulate erythropoiesis, but the mechanisms of action are unknown and probably indirect. Injection of estrogens lowers the red cell count, and growth hormone acts directly upon the erythron; this has been demonstrated by perfusion of the femur of the dog, which is followed by an increase in the number of erythrocytes in the blood and in the percentage of erythroblasts in the bone marrow.

MATURATION OF GRANULOCYTES

The myeloblast is the most immature recognizable cell in this series and gives rise to the 3 types of granulocytes. The presence of azurophilic granules in the cytoplasm identifies a cell as a promyelocyte. When the various specific cytoplasmic granules are fully developed, the cell is called a **neutrophilic, eosinophilic, or basophilic myelocyte** according to the staining characteristics of the granules. The subsequent stages of maturation are from the **myelocyte** to the **metamyelocyte**, then to the **granulocyte with a band-shaped nucleus,** and finally to the mature granulocyte (neutrophilic, eosinophilic, or basophilic). Only the last 2 forms are normally seen in the circulation.

Myeloblast

The myeloblast is 10–15 μm in diameter, with a large spherical nucleus that has a delicate chromatin network and 1–3 nucleoli. Its cytoplasm is scanty and more basophilic than that of the stem cell (hemocytoblast) from which it is derived (Fig 14–3). Examination with the electron microscope shows many mitochondria, ribosomes, and dispersed granular endoplasmic reticulum.

Promyelocyte

The promyelocyte is the same size as or larger than the myeloblast (up to 20 μm or more). The nucleus is generally kidney-shaped; its chromatin is coarser than in the myeloblast; and nucleoli are prominent (Fig 14–3).

The cytoplasm of the promyelocyte is more basophilic than that of the myeloblast and contains

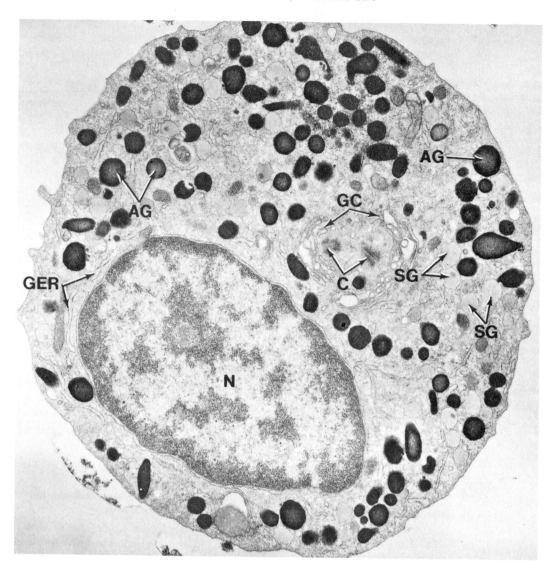

Figure 14–7. Neutrophilic myelocyte from normal human bone marrow treated with peroxidase. At this stage, the cell is smaller than the promyelocyte and the cytoplasm contains 2 different types of granules: (1) large, peroxidase-positive azurophilic granules (AG); and (2) the generally smaller specific granules (SG), which do not stain for peroxidase. Note that the peroxidase reaction product is present only in azurophilic granules and is not seen in the granular endoplasmic reticulum (GER) or Golgi cisternae (GC), which are located around the centriole (C). N, nucleus. × 15,000. (Courtesy of DF Bainton.)

azurophilic granules. These granules are different from the specific granules that appear in myelocytes, which develop in the next stage of maturation. They are derived from the fusion of dense-cored vesicles emerging from the **mature (concave) face** of the Golgi cisternae (Fig 14–8). They show a homogeneous density, are surrounded by a membrane, and contain lysosomal enzymes. Granular endoplasmic reticulum and Golgi complex are well developed.

Myelocyte

The myelocyte is 16–24 μm in diameter. The nucleus is ovoid and usually eccentric, with coarse chromatin. Different stages in the development of the myelocyte can be identified depending on the number of the specific granules, the appearance of the nucleus (from spherical to ovoid to kidney-shaped), and the relative size of its cytoplasm. A slight cytoplasmic basophilia and azurophilic granules are still encountered (Figs 14–3, 14–7, and 14–8). The origin of specific granules differs from that of azurophilic granules in that the former arise from the **immature (convex) face** of the Golgi body (Fig 14–8). During further differentiation of the granulocyte series, the percentage of azurophilic granules is constantly reduced since they are synthesized only in the promyelocyte stage.

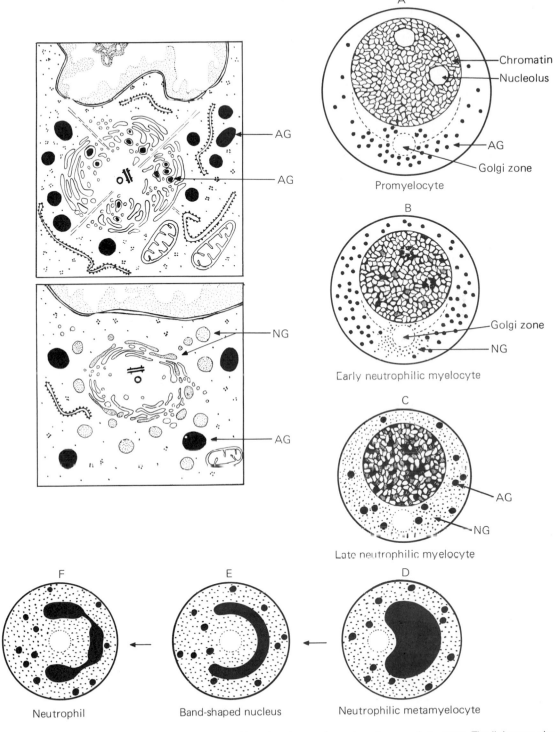

Figure 14–8. Several stages of neutrophil maturation. Note the changes in nuclear shape and structure. The light area close to the nucleus contains the Golgi complex and the 2 centrioles. This is the region where the neutrophilic granules (NG) and the azurophilic granules (AG) first appear. At upper left is shown the ultrastructure of the light juxtanuclear area. Both neutrophilic and azurophilic granules are formed in the cisternae of the Golgi complex. Observe that azurophilic granules are formed deep in the Golgi complex, close to the centrioles, whereas the neutrophilic granules are formed later in the maturation process in the outer cisternae of the Golgi complex. Note that during maturation the specific granules increase while the azurophilic granule population remains the same or is reduced.

What characterizes an immature cell of the granulocytic series as a myelocyte is the beginning of the appearance of the specific granules: **neutrophilic, eosinophilic,** and **basophilic.** The 3 different lines of granulocytes in the peripheral blood can be traced from this stage. The process of further maturation in each cell is characterized principally by changes in the size, shape, and appearance of the nucleus and by relative increases in the amount of cytoplasm. The granules appear first in the perinuclear region and later fill the cytoplasm. They are usually smaller than the azurophilic granules. Depending on the number of granules, the cytoplasm is bluish-pink in neutrophils to orange-salmon in eosinophils to dark purple and spotted in basophils. The cell still divides throughout the myelocyte stage.

Metamyelocyte

The metamyelocyte is characterized by a nucleus with a deep indentation, indicating the beginning of lobe formation. The cytoplasm is a deeper pink color. The nuclear pattern becomes denser, and azurophilic granules are still seen in the cytoplasm. During this stage of development, nuclear activity diminishes as the chromatin condenses into heterochromatin. Concomitantly, protein synthesis and related organelles (Golgi ribosomes and rough endoplasmic reticulum) are reduced. Glycogen accumulations are evident in the cytoplasm. The modifications that characterize the metamyelocytes are not easily identifiable in the basophilic cells, so that the basophilic metamyelocyte is not easily distinguished from mature basophils (Fig 14–3). The metamyelocyte does not divide.

Granulocyte With a Band-Shaped Nucleus

Before assuming the lobate form typical of a mature cell, the granulocyte goes through an intermediate stage in which the nucleus appears as a curved rod (Fig 14–3). This cell is found in the peripheral blood, and stimulation of granulocytopoiesis is associated with the appearance of larger than normal numbers of these cells in the peripheral blood. The normal percentage in blood is 3–5%. The appearance of large numbers of immature cells in the blood is called a "shift to the left" and is of clinical significance.

KINETICS OF THE NEUTROPHILS

The kinetics of the neutrophils are better understood than is the case with other granulocytes because these cells are more numerous in the blood and thus easier to study.

As shown in Fig 14–9, the neutrophils and their precursor cells occupy 4 different functional compartments: (1) the medullary formation com-

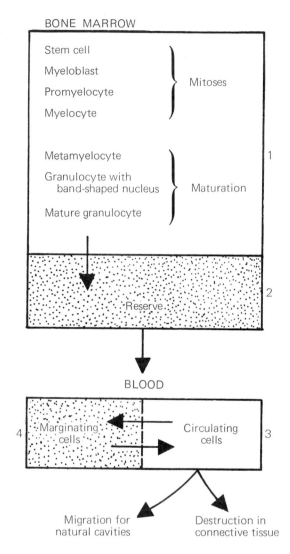

Figure 14–9. Functional compartments of neutrophils. *1:* Medullary formation compartment. *2:* Medullary reserve compartment. *3:* Circulating compartment. *4:* Marginating compartment. The size of each compartment is roughly proportionate to the number of cells.

partment, where new neutrophils are formed; (2) the medullary reserve compartment, in which mature neutrophils remain for a variable period before entering the blood; (3) the circulating compartment, consisting of neutrophils suspended in the plasma and circulating in the blood vessels; and (4) the marginating compartment, in which neutrophils are present but do not circulate. These latter neutrophils are in the capillaries, temporarily excluded from the circulation by vasoconstriction, or—especially in the lungs—at the periphery of the vessels, adhering to the endothelium, and not in the main bloodstream.

Neutrophils originate in the medullary formation compartment and enter first the medullary reserve compartment and then the circulating compartment. There is a constant interchange of cells between the circulating and marginating compartments. The marginating compartment and the circulating compartment thus contain equal numbers of neutrophils, and the medullary compartment contains more neutrophils than are present in the circulating blood. Thus **neutrophilia**, an increase in the number of neutrophils in the circulation, does not necessarily imply an increase in neutrophil production. Intense muscular activity or administration of epinephrine causes neutrophils in the marginating compartment to move into the circulating compartment, with an apparent neutrophilia even though neutrophil production has not increased.

Neutrophilia may also result from liberation of greater numbers of neutrophils of the medullary reserve compartment. This type of neutrophilia is transitory and is followed by a "recovery" period during which no neutrophils are liberated.

Increased production of neutrophils without neutrophilia occurs if there is an increase in the number of cells in the marginating compartment. An increase in the functional marginating compartment absorbs the excess production of cells by the bone marrow and maintains a normal level of circulating neutrophils.

The neutrophilia that occurs during the course of bacterial infections is due to an increase in neutrophil production and a shorter stay of these cells in the medullary reserve compartment. In such cases, immature forms such as neutrophils with band shaped nuclei, neutrophilic metamyelocytes, and even myelocytes may appear in the bloodstream. The neutrophilia that occurs during infection is of longer duration than that which occurs as a result of intense muscular activity.

Control of Neutrophilogenesis

There seems to be a mechanism which stimulates the production of neutrophils by the bone marrow that is set in motion by a decrease in the number of these cells. This conclusion arises from the observation that destruction of neutrophils (eg, by the injection of an antineutrophil antibody) immediately stimulates the production of these cells. Leukapheresis, which consists of withdrawing blood and reinfusing it after removal of most of the leukocytes, also causes neutrophilia, which rules out the possibility that a substance liberated by dead neutrophils (present in experiments with antineutrophil antibody) stimulates the production of these cells by the bone marrow. The production of neutrophils is controlled by a humoral mechanism not yet identified.

Destruction of Granulocytes

By various technics, including radioautography following the injection of labeled thymidine, it has been shown that the bone marrow of a man weighing 70 kg generates 150×10^9 granulocytes per day.

Because the number of these cells in the blood remains constant, an equivalent destruction of granulocytes must occur in the same period of time. The process by which this destruction is effected is not completely clear, though some of the means by which granulocytes are destroyed are known.

The granulocytes pass through the blood capillary wall and appear in the connective tissues. This phenomenon is widespread throughout the body. The granulocytes leave the vessels at random, regardless of their age, and after entering the connective tissue, they rarely return to the blood. There occurs, therefore, a constant and unidirectional flow of granulocytes into the connective tissues of all organs, where many of these cells die.

Destruction of granulocytes occurs also in the alimentary tract and lungs. These cells pass through the mucosa, principally where the epithelium is simple (stomach, intestines), to the lumen of the alimentary tract, where they die. Some authors contest this scheme but recognize that passage of lymphocytes occurs. Granulocytes also die in the lung alveoli after passing through the simple squamous epithelium. The half-life of circulating neutrophils is 6–7 hours.

MATURATION OF LYMPHOCYTES & MONOCYTES

Study of the precursor cells of lymphocytes and monocytes is difficult because these cells do not contain specific cytoplasmic granules or the nuclear lobulation that is present in the granulocytes, both of which facilitate the distinction between young and mature forms. Lymphocytes and monocytes are distinguished mainly on the basis of size, chromatin structure, and the presence of nucleoli in smear preparations. As lymphocytic cells mature, their chromatin becomes more compact, the nucleoli become less visible, and the cells decrease in size.

The circulating lymphocytes originate mainly in the lymphatic tissue of the central and peripheral lymphatic organs and, to a lesser extent, in the bone marrow. The precursor cell is the **lymphoblast**, which forms the mature **lymphocytes.** Many lymphocytes of the blood and lymph have a capacity for differentiation. It is not possible to distinguish the lymphocytes with this capacity by light microscopy, but electron and scanning microscopy have revealed differences between mature lymphocytes that appeared identical under the light microscope. It must be concluded that there is a circulating cell which is morphologically indistinguishable from a mature lymphocyte that is a stem cell of the lymphocytic series and in this way functionally similar to the lymphoblast. Many researchers maintain that this cell is comparable to the stem cell and can, after proper stimulation, give rise to any type of blood cell.

Lymphoblast

The lymphoblast is the largest cell of the lymphocytic series. It is spherical, with a basophilic cytoplasm and no azurophilic granules. The chromatin is relatively condensed and in blocks, foreshadowing the chromatin of a mature lymphocyte. The lymphoblast has 2 or 3 nucleoli.

Prolymphocyte

The prolymphocyte is smaller than the lymphoblast, has a basophilic cytoplasm, and may contain azurophilic granules. The chromatin of the prolymphocyte is condensed but to a lesser degree than that of the medium-sized and small lymphocytes. The nucleoli are not easily visible because of the condensed chromatin.

The prolymphocyte gives rise directly to the circulating lymphocyte.

Monocyte

As opposed to granulocytes, which are fully differentiated cells, monocytes are in an intermediate stage and ultimately differentiate into macrophages. The monocytic series starts in bone marrow; progeny enter the circulatory system as large monocytes and terminate in the connective tissues as macrophages. In some types of chronic inflammation, macrophages form epithelioid cells or multinucleated giant cells that represent their terminal differentiative stage.

Monocyte precursors cannot be identified accurately. It is possible to recognize the **promonocyte,** which is found in small numbers in normal bone marrow. The existence of a less differentiated cell called a **monoblast** is an open question. The fact that such cells are found in the circulation of patients with monocytic leukemia suggests that they may exist in normal bone marrow, although in very small numbers.

The promonocyte is 10–20 μm in diameter and is larger than the monocyte. It has a pale-staining nucleus, basophilic cytoplasm, abundant polyribosomes, and scanty rough endoplasmic reticulum. There are numerous fine azurophilic granules identified as lysosomes by their enzyme contents. Promonocytes divide frequently, and in 6 hours a promonocyte may differentiate into a monocyte, which can pass into the blood where it lasts from 8 to 12 hours.

Monocytes leave the blood through endothelial cell junctions in the walls of venules and capillaries, where the blood flow is slow. Immediately after penetrating the tissues, they increase their rate of protein synthesis, the size of their Golgi apparatus, and the number of microtubules and microfilaments, transforming themselves into typical macrophages.

Epithelioid inflammatory cells are a cystlike organization of macrophages organized into an epitheliumlike arrangement. In some cases, the macrophages fuse together, giving rise to a large syncytium known as a multinucleated giant cell. Fusion of macrophages is followed by a decrease in the synthesis of lysosomal enzymes and consequently a diminution in the number of lysosomes.

ORIGIN OF PLATELETS

In adults, the platelets originate in the red bone marrow by fragmentation of the cytoplasm of the mature **granular megakaryocytes.** These in turn arise by differentiation of the **megakaryoblasts.**

Megakaryoblast

The megakaryoblast is 15–50 μm in diameter and has a large ovoid or kidney-shaped nucleus with numerous nucleoli. The cytoplasm of this cell is homogeneous and intensely basophilic (rich in free ribosomes) (Fig 14–10).

Megakaryocyte

This is a giant cell (35–150 μm in diameter) with an irregularly lobulated nucleus, coarse chromatin, and no visible nucleoli. It has abundant and slightly basophilic cytoplasm. The megakaryocyte contains numerous azurophilic granules that at times occupy most of the cytoplasm. These granules will form the chromomeres of the platelets (Fig 14–10).

The cytoplasm of the megakaryoblast is rich in free ribosomes and contains little smooth and granular endoplasmic reticulum. Membrane-surrounded granules corresponding to the azurophilic granules seen under the light microscope appear during the process of maturation of the granular megakaryocyte. These granules are formed in the Golgi apparatus and later distributed throughout the cytoplasm. With maturation of the megakaryocyte there is an increase in the quantity of smooth membranes that will form **demarcation channels.** The membranes finally fuse and give rise to the membrane of the platelets.

In smear preparations of bone marrow, it is possible to observe platelets still bound to the cytoplasm of the megakaryocyte and in the various phases of separation. Furthermore, in cultures of megakaryocytes, the liberation of platelets can be observed under the microscope, which substantiates their megakaryocytic origin. In certain forms of **thrombocytopenic purpura,** a disease in which the number of blood platelets is reduced, platelets appear bound to the cytoplasm of the megakaryocytes, indicating a defect in the liberation mechanism of these corpuscles.

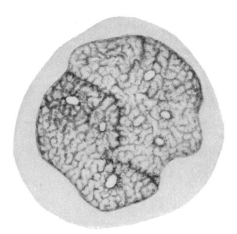

Megakaryoblast

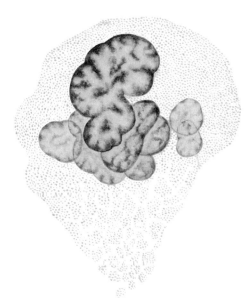

Megakaryocyte

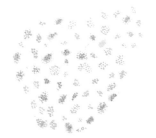

Platelets

Figure 14 –10. Cells of the megakaryocytic series. They are shown in bone marrow smear with Romanovsky staining.

In observations carried out using platelets marked in vitro with radioactive isotopes (^{32}P-labeled diisopropylfluorophosphate, ^{32}P, ^{35}S) and afterwards reinjected, the life span of these corpuscles was found to be approximately 10 days.

INTRAUTERINE HEMATOPOIESIS

There are 3 ill-defined stages of intrauterine hematopoiesis: a **primordial** or **prehepatic phase,** a **hepatosplenothymic phase,** and a **medullolymphatic** or **definitive phase.**

When one of these stages is initiated, the predominant processes of the previous phase persist for some time, though gradually decreasing in importance (Fig 14–11).

All formed elements of the blood are of mesenchymal origin. In organs of double embryonic origin such as the liver and thymus (endoderm and mesoderm), the cells originating in the mesoderm are responsible for hematopoiesis.

Primordial or Prehepatic Phase

In humans, the first blood cells appear in the mesoderm of the yolk sac during the third week of intrauterine life. The **blood islands** consist of elongated clusters of mesenchymal cells. The endothelium of the first vessels originates in the most superficial cells of these islands; the innermost cells become spherical and differentiate into blood stem cells.

By the association of the endothelial cells of contiguous islands, the first blood vessels are formed. These vessels soon establish communication with those in the body of the embryo. This permits cells formed in the yolk sac to penetrate and circulate in the body of the embryo.

The blood stem cells (hemocytoblasts) of the yolk sac divide within the vessels to form the **primitive erythroblasts,** which are larger than the **definitive erythroblasts.** Cells that arise by primitive red cell erythropoiesis are larger than those that develop as a result of definitive erythropoiesis, and this process is known as megaloblastic erythropoiesis. The majority of the erythroblasts formed in the yolk sac do not lose their nuclei, so that at this stage the red cells are predominantly nucleated. Only at the end of the primordial phase do enucleated erythrocytes appear as a result of extrusion of the erythroblast nucleus.

During the primordial phase, the blood contains only the above-mentioned red cell series. No leukocytes or platelets are present.

Hepatosplenothymic Phase

This period begins in the second month, with hematopoiesis taking place in the liver and spleen. Subsequently, the thymus starts producing **blood**

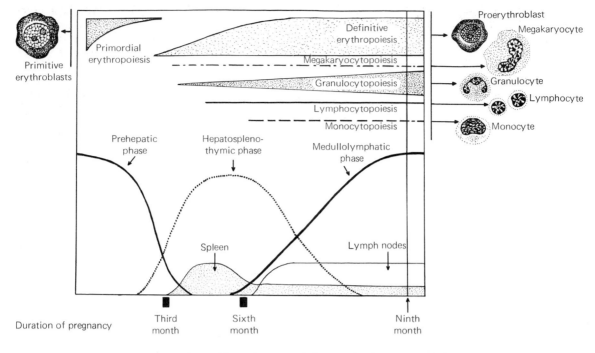

Figure 14–11. The main events in intrauterine hemocytopoiesis.

cells, almost exclusively lymphocytes. In the mesenchyme that invades the endodermal primordium of the liver appear precursor cells of the granulocytes, megakaryocytes, and definitive erythroblasts. Of the latter, a large number reach the blood without losing their nuclei. Although hepatic hematopoiesis begins to decline in the fifth month, it persists until some weeks after birth. In the adult, the liver is not a hematopoietic organ.

The spleen produces mainly cells of the red cell series and, in smaller quantity, granulocytes and platelets. Production of lymphocytes in the spleen becomes important as birth becomes imminent.

The thymus begins to form lymphocytes in the second month of intrauterine life and produces almost no other type of blood cell. The number of erythroblasts and granulocytes produced in the thymus is insignificant.

Medullolymphatic Phase

The clavicle is the first bone to show hematopoietic activity. Its bone marrow begins to function between the second and third month of intrauterine life. The marrow of other bones soon begins to function, and in the fourth month bone marrow hematopoiesis is significant.

The bone marrow shows great erythrocytic, granulocytic, and megakaryocytic activity. Lymphocytes and monocytes are also produced.

During this period—and close to birth—the lymph nodes (which since the beginning of their existence have been lymphocyte-producing organs) become very active. Before birth, the lymph nodes

may show discrete erythropoietic activity.

It is during this medullolymphatic period that a more functional separation is established between myeloid tissue (forming erythrocytes, platelets, and granulocytes) and lymphatic tissue (forming the lymphocytes).

MONONUCLEAR PHAGOCYTE SYSTEM (Reticuloendothelial System, RES)

Aschoff in 1924 introduced the concept of the existence of a group of mesynchymal cells distributed throughout the body with different morphologic characteristics and different names but sharing the important properties of phagocytosis and storage of vital dyes. In this so-called **reticuloendothelial system (RES)** were incorporated all of the macrophages described by Metchnikoff in 1893 and the phagocytic endothelia of sinusoids seen in the liver, adrenal, spleen, pituitary, and bone marrow. Many of these cells were associated with reticular fibers.

Recently, this concept has been modified by following the further development and movement within the body of radioactively labeled cells. It was found that the so-called phagocytic cells of the sinusoids are not more phagocytic than endothelia of other capillaries and that what was observed as phagocytosis in the light microscope was actually a function of the perivascular macrophages of

Table 14–1. The mononuclear phagocyte system.*

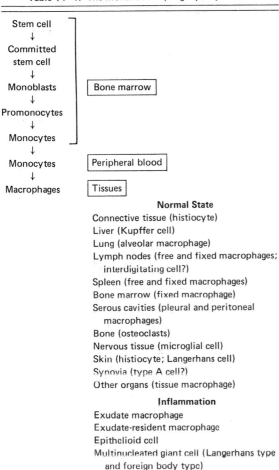

Stem cell
↓
Committed
stem cell
↓
Monoblasts   Bone marrow
↓
Promonocytes
↓
Monocytes
↓
Monocytes   Peripheral blood
↓
Macrophages   Tissues

Normal State

Connective tissue (histiocyte)
Liver (Kupffer cell)
Lung (alveolar macrophage)
Lymph nodes (free and fixed macrophages;
   interdigitating cell?)
Spleen (free and fixed macrophages)
Bone marrow (fixed macrophage)
Serous cavities (pleural and peritoneal
   macrophages)
Bone (osteoclasts)
Nervous tissue (microglial cell)
Skin (histiocyte; Langerhans cell)
Synovia (type A cell?)
Other organs (tissue macrophage)

Inflammation

Exudate macrophage
Exudate-resident macrophage
Epithelioid cell
Multinucleated giant cell (Langerhans type
   and foreign body type)

*Reproduced, with permission, from Van Furth R: In, *Mononuclear Phagocytes: Functional Aspects.* Martinus Nijhoff Publishers, 1980.

sinusoids. Since it has been shown that the Kupffer cells of the liver arise from the monocytes of blood or their precursors, which can also be transformed into macrophages, the concept of a reticuloendothelial system was abandoned in favor of a **mononuclear phagocyte system** originating in the monocyte and its precursors and including all of its derivatives in the tissues—fixed or free macrophages in connective tissue and lymphatic tissue, Kupffer cells, alveolar macrophages, macrophages of peritoneal and pleural cavities, and perivascular macrophages of sinusoids (Table 14–1). The cells of the mononuclear phagocyte system, which have receptor sites for immunoglobulins on their plasma membranes, originate in the bone marrow in the form of promonocytes and monocytes. Whether microglia cells of nerve tissue should be included as part of the mononuclear phagocytic system is still uncertain. Round phagocytic cells found in inflamed nerve tissue are believed to derive from microglia cells, but this view is not universally accepted. Most evidence shows that these phagocytic cells are macrophages derived from blood monocytes that migrate through the walls of blood vessels.

•   •   •

References

Bainton DF, Farquhar MG: Segregation and packaging of granule enzymes in eosinophilic leukocytes. J Cell Biol 45:54, 1970.

Bainton DF, Ullyot JL, Farquhar MG: The development of neutrophilic polymorphonuclear leukocytes in human bone marrow. J Exp Med 139:907, 1971.

Barr RD, Whang-Peng J, Perry S: Hemopoietic stem cells in human peripheral blood. Science 190:284, 1975.

Becker RP, DeBruyn PP: The transmural passage of blood cells into myeloid sinusoids and the entry of platelets into the sinusoidal circulation. Am J Anat 145:183, 1976.

Behnke O: An electron microscope study of the rat megacaryocyte. 2. Some aspects of platelet release and microtubules. J Ultrastruct Res 26:111, 1969.

Berman I: The ultrastructure of erythroblastic islands and reticular cells in mouse bone marrow. J Ultrastruct Res 17:291, 1967.

Bessis MC, Breton-Gorius J: Iron metabolism in the bone marrow as seen by electron microscopy: A critical review. Blood 19:635, 1962.

Bierman HR (editor): Leukopoiesis in health and disease. Ann NY Acad Sci 113:511, 1964.

Boyum A & others: Kinetics of cell proliferation of murine bone marrow cells cultured in diffusion chambers: Effect of hypoxia, bleeding, erythropoietin injections, polycythemia, and irradiations of the host. Blood 40:174, 1972.

Caffrey RW, Everett NB, Rieke WO: Radioautographic studies of reticular and blast cells in the hematopoietic tissues of the rat. Anat Rec 155:41, 1966.

Fedorko ME: Formation of cytoplasmic granules in human eosinophilic myelocytes: An electron microscope autoradiographic study. Blood 31:188, 1968.

Fedorko ME, Hirsch JG: Cytoplasmic granule formation in myelocytes: An electron microscope radioautographic study on the mechanism of formation of cytoplasmic granules in rabbit heterophilic myelocytes. J Cell Biol 29:307, 1966.

Glass J, Lavider LM, Robinson SH: Studies of murine erythroid cell development. J Cell Biol 65:298, 1975.

Gowans JL: Life-span, recirculation and transformation of lymphocytes. Int Rev Exp Pathol 5:1, 1966.

Leblond CP, Sainte-Marie G: Models for lymphocyte and plasmocyte formation. In: *Haemopoiesis: Cell Production and Its Regulation.* Wolstenholme GE, O'Connor M (editors). Little, Brown, 1960.

Marchesi VT, Florey HW: Electron microscopy on the emigration of leukocytes. Q J Exp Physiol 45:343, 1960.

Micklem HS, Anderson M, Ross E: Limited potential of circulating hemopoietic stem cells. Nature 256:41, 1975.

Moore MAS, Metcalf D: Ontogeny of the haemopoietic system: Yolk sac origin of in vivo and in vitro colony-forming cells in the developing mouse embryo. Br J Haematol 18:279, 1970.

Spinak JL, Marmor J, Dickerman HW: Studies on splenic erythropoiesis in the mouse. 1. Ribosomal ribonucleic acid metabolism. J Lab Clin Med 79:526, 1972.

Spitznagel JK, Dalldorf FG, Leffell MS: Characterization of azurophil and specific granules purified from human polymorphonuclear leukocytes. Lab Invest 30:774, 1974.

Thomas DB, Yoffey JM: Human fetal haemopoiesis. 1. The cellular composition of fetal blood. Br J Haematol 8:280, 1962.

Vietta ES, Uhr JW: Immunoglobulin-receptors revisited: A model for the differentiation of bone marrow–derived lymphocytes. Science 189:964, 1975.

Weiss L: *The Cells and Tissues of the Immune System.* Prentice-Hall, 1972.

Weiss L: The hematopoietic microenvironment of the bone marrow: An ultrastructural study of the stroma in rats. Anat Rec 186:161, 1976.

Weiss L, Chen L-T: The organization of hematopoietic cords and vascular sinuses in bone marrow. Blood Cells 1:617, 1975.

Yoffey JM, Courtice FC: *Lymphatics, Lymph and Lymphoid Tissue.* Harvard Univ Press, 1960.

The lymphoid system consists of cells and organs designed to protect the internal environment from invasion and damage by foreign substances. The cells of this system are therefore known as **immunocompetent cells** in that they have the capacity to distinguish self from nonself (foreign substances) and to provide for the inactivation or destruction of foreign material. This system consists chiefly of motile and fixed cells. Lymphocytes and macrophages constitute the principal motile cells, while reticuloendothelial and plasma cells are the primary constituents of the fixed cell population. Lymphatic organs generally consist of connective tissue–encapsulated networks of reticular cells and fibers within which lie lymphocytes, plasma cells, macrophages, and, to a lesser degree, other immunocompetent cells.

There are 3 types of lymphoid tissue: **loose lymphoid tissue,** in which the meshwork of fixed cells predominates; **dense lymphoid tissue,** where free cells (mainly lymphocytes) predominate; and **nodular lymphoid tissue,** which also contains a predominance of free cells but appears as typical spherical structures called **lymphatic nodules.** These immunologically active nodules are found in all of the lymphoid organs except the thymus.

The immune system consists of the lymphatic organs (thymus, spleen, tonsils, lymph nodes), lymphocytes of the blood and lymph, and collections of lymphocytes and plasma cells dispersed throughout the connective tissue but most prominent in the lining of the digestive and respiratory tracts. This system protects the body against foreign (nonself) materials that penetrate other defense barriers (eg, integument) and enter as either free molecules or as part of an invasive microorganism. It also recognizes as nonself aberrant structures that originate within the body, such as malignant cells. In response to an unfamiliar (nonself) macromolecule, this system initiates an **immune reaction.** An **antigen** is a molecule having the structural configuration to elicit an immune reaction. The part of the antigen molecule responsible for this property is called the **antigenic determinant.** Antigenic determinants are recognized by specific receptors found at the surface of lymphocytes to which they attach. This recognition triggers either a **cellular** or **humoral** immune response. A cellular response occurs when the recognition is made by a T lymphocyte and the subsequent destruction of the antigen-containing cell is initiated by cytotoxic substances produced by the activated T lymphocyte. In the cellular immune reaction the T lymphocytes act locally and directly with the antigen. A humoral immune response takes place when the antigenic determinant is recognized by B lymphocytes that, following activation, give rise to **plasma cells.** These cells have the capacity to synthesize and secrete antibodies (immunoglobulins) that are specific for and complex with the antigenic determinant.

In both cellular and humoral responses, the recognition of antigen by receptors present on the lymphocyte surface promotes changes in the morphology of the lymphocyte. Following activation, the cells enlarge and exhibit an abundant basophilic cytoplasm and large euchromatic nucleus. In this way, the lymphocyte is transformed into a less differentiated cell, called an **immunoblast** (or **pyroninophil cell** or **lymphoblast**). This cell divides several times, thereby increasing the number of cells with the capacity to react to the antigen determinant that first initiated the reaction (clonal expansion). This theory postulates that there are lymphocytes for all potential antigens. It is known that lymphocyte produces antibodies that recognize only one antigenic determinant. In normal conditions, when not stimulated by antigens, B lymphocytes produce very small amounts of antibodies, some of which remain attached to their surfaces. Antigens do not promote in the lymphocyte the ability to make the specific antibodies; they only stimulate the multiplication and synthetic activity of lymphocytes already capable of producing the antibody.

In humans there are 5 main types of antibodies or immunoglobulins, designated by the letters G, A, M, D, and E, and usually known as IgG, IgA, IgM, IgD, and IgE.

IgG is the most abundant and constitutes 75% of the serum immunoglobulins. Its molecular weight is 160,000. IgG is the only immunoglobulin that crosses the placental barrier and is incorporated into the circulatory system of the fetus, thus protecting the newborn against infection.

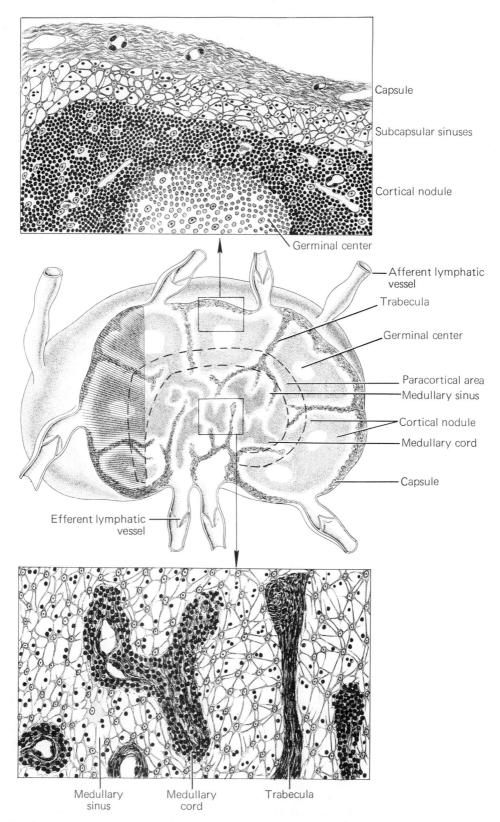

Capsule

Subcapsular sinuses

Cortical nodule

Germinal center

Afferent lymphatic
vessel

Trabecula

Germinal center

Paracortical area
Medullary sinus

Cortical nodule

Medullary cord

Capsule

Efferent lymphatic
vessel

Medullary
sinus

Medullary
cord

Trabecula

Figure 15–1. Histologic structure of a lymph node. The rectangular areas in the center drawing are magnified in the upper and lower drawings. The cortical layer is composed mainly of lymphatic nodules, whose germinal centers (lightly stained core of each nodule) are clearly seen in the center drawing.

IgA, with a molecular weight of 160,000 (monomere form), is found in small amounts in serum. It is the main immunoglobulin found in tears, colostrum, and saliva, in nasal, bronchial, intestinal, and prostatic secretions, and in the vaginal fluid. This secretory IgA (SIgA) is made of 2 molecules of monomeric IgA united by a polypeptide chain named **protein J** and combined to another protein known as the **secretory** or **transport component.** SIgA has a molecular weight of 400,000 and, being resistant to several enzymes, is suitable to provide protection against proliferation of microorganisms in body secretions and to aid in defense against penetration of foreign molecules into the body. IgA monomers and protein J are secreted by plasma cells of the mucous membranes lining the digestive, respiratory, and urinary passages, while the secretory component is synthesized by the mucosal epithelial cells.

IgM constitutes 10% of the serum immunoglobulins and usually exists as a pentamere with a molecular weight of 900,000. It is effective in activating the **complement system,** a group of plasma enzymes that has the capacity to lyse cells (including bacteria) and that participates in other aspects of the immune response. IgM is also found in small amounts in secretion, protected by a secretory component, as described for IgA.

IgE has a great affinity for receptors located in the surface membrane of mast cells and basophils. Immediately after its secretion by plasma cells, IgE attaches to those cells and practically disappears from the blood plasma. The complexing of antigens with the IgE bound to mast cells and basophils triggers the production and liberation of several biologically active substances, such as histamine, heparin, SRS-A (slow reacting substance of anaphylaxis) and ECF-A (eosinophil chemotactic factor of anaphylaxis). An **allergic reaction** is mediated by the activity of IgE and the antigens (**allergens**) that stimulate its production.

The properties and activities of IgD are not completely understood yet. It has a molecular weight of 160,000 and its concentration in blood plasma constitutes only 0.2% of the total of immunoglobulins.

LYMPHOID TISSUE

Lymphatic nodules—also called lymphatic follicles—can be found isolated in the loose connective tissue of several organs, mainly in the lamina propria of the digestive tract, the upper respiratory tract, and the urinary passages. Nodules do not have a connective tissue capsule and may occur in groups forming accumulations such as **Peyer's patches** in the ileum. Nodules are temporary structures and may disappear and reappear in the same place.

Each lymphatic nodule is a round structure that may attain a diameter of 0.2–1 mm (Figs 15–1 and 15–2). In histologic sections, nodules are strongly stained by hematoxylin as a consequence of the presence of a dense population of lymphocytes, which possess a basophilic nucleus with condensed chromatin and a narrow corona of basophilic cytoplasm. The interior of the nodule often shows a less densely stained region called the **germinal center** (Fig 15–1). This difference in staining of the central region of many nodules is due to the presence of activated lymphocytes (immunoblasts) that exhibit a large, pale-staining cytoplasm and large, active, euchromatic nucleus; for this reason, it contrasts with smaller lymphocytes, which have darker nuclei and predominate in the periphery of the nodule, which is not well defined. At times, many cells in the germinal center may exhibit mitotic figures. The presence of a germinal center may appear and disappear in a nodule according to its functional state.

In nodules in different phases of maturation, there is a predominance of free cells, principally **lymphoblasts;** small, medium, and large **lymphocytes; immunoblasts;** and **plasma cells.**

The activity of lymphatic nodules depends upon several factors including the effects of the bacterial flora. In animals kept in sterile conditions, nodules with germinal centers are rare. The opposite situation occurs in some infections, where the production of lymphocytes increases and germinal centers become frequent.

In newborns as well as in animals grown in aseptic environments, lymphatic nodules are very rare, which indicates that their formation depends on antigenic stimuli. In localized inflammations, there is an increase in the number of lymphatic nodules close to the inflamed site, and most nodules have a germinal center.

LYMPH NODES

The lymph nodes are encapsulated round or kidney-shaped organs composed of lymphoid tissue. They are distributed throughout the body, always along the course of the lymphatic vessels, which carry lymph into the thoracic and the right lymphatic ducts. They are found in the axillas and in the groin, along the great vessels of the neck, and in large numbers in the thorax, the abdomen, and especially in the mesentery. The lymph nodes constitute a series of in-line filters, whereby all tissue fluid–derived lymph is filtered by at least one node, prior to its return to the circulatory system. Kidney-shaped lymph nodes present a convex side and a depression, the hilum, through which the arteries and nerves penetrate and the veins leave the organ. The shape and internal structure of

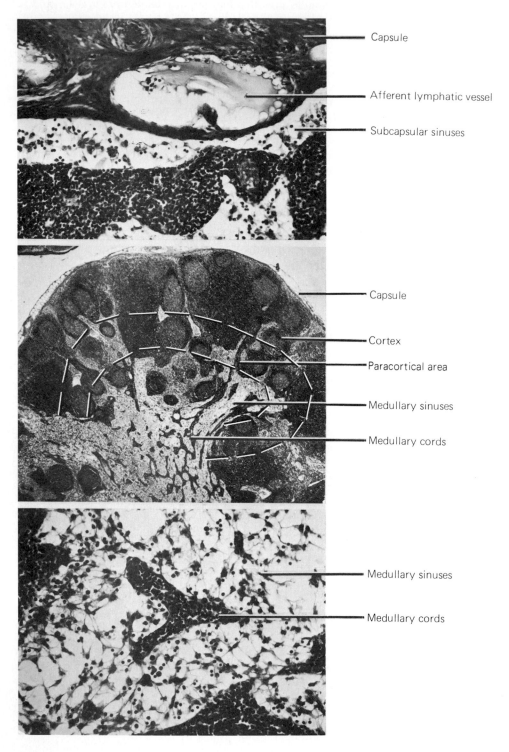

Figure 15 –2. Photomicrographs of lymph nodes, reduced from × 30 *(center)* and × 200 *(lower* and *upper)* magnification. H&E stain.

lymph nodes vary greatly, but all have the basic pattern of organization described below and illustrated in Figs 15–1 and 15–2.

The lymph penetrates the lymph node through the **afferent lymphatic vessels,** which enter on the convex surface of the organ, and it exits through the **efferent lymphatic vessels** of the hilum (Fig 15–1).

The capsule of dense connective tissue that covers the lymph nodes sends trabeculae to their interior, dividing the parenchyma into incomplete compartments. A reticular system, consisting of a network of reticular fibers ensheathed by the stellate reticular cells, unites with the connective tissue trabeculae and extends throughout the node, thus providing a network in which the cells are freely suspended.

Each lymph node has a **cortical region,** situated below the capsule (except at the hilum), and a **medullary region** that occupies the center of the organ and its hilum. The cortex of the lymph node contains dense aggregations of lymphocytes and reticular cells, known as lymphatic nodules (Figs 15–1 and 15–2).

Besides the cortical and medullary regions, which are the 2 regions classically described, there is the **paracortical zone,** poorly defined morphologically but functionally distinct. Basically, the paracortical zone consists of dense lymphoid tissue that lies in the **juxtamedullary region** (ie, in the cortex bordering the medulla). The lymphocytes of the paracortical zone—the **T lymphocytes**—have special properties that make them different from the other lymphocytes of the lymph node, the **B lymphocytes.**

The cortical region is composed of the **subcapsular** and **peritrabecular sinuses** and of lymphatic nodules (Figs 15–1 and 15–2) that may present germinal centers. The lymphatic sinuses are spaces incompletely lined by reticuloendothelial cells, with some reticular cells and fibers, forming part of the loose wall and containing, in the lumen, many lymphocytes and free macrophages. The sinuses receive the lymph brought by afferent vessels and carry it toward the medullary region. Within the cortex, the lymphatic nodules consist of dense aggregations of lymphocytes including a lesser population of macrophages and reticular cells that are enclosed by an incomplete lining of reticuloendothelial cells.

The medullary region consists of reticuloendothelium-lined **medullary cords** composed of dense lymphoid tissue, exhibiting many plasma cells, and the **medullary sinuses** (loose lymphoid tissue), which receive and circulate the lymph from the cortical sinuses (Fig 15–1). Medullary sinuses communicate with the efferent lymphatic vessels through which the lymph leaves the lymph node.

Lymphocytes found in the paracortical region disappear when an animal has its thymus removed, especially if this is done at birth. This shows that they are **thymus-dependent,** belonging to the population of **T lymphocytes.** They derive from precursor cells that migrate from the bone marrow to the thymus, where they divide by mitosis. T lymphocytes are most numerous in blood and lymph and are found also in the periarterial sheaths of the spleen and other lymphoid organs. They are responsible for cell-mediated immune responses such as delayed immune reactions and graft rejections. As explained in Chapter 13, these cells colonize the thymus-dependent zones in the peripheral lymphoid organs with long-lived lymphocytes that recirculate and are capable of further replication under proper stimulation. The remaining lymphocytes, which constitute the greater mass of cells in the cortex, are the B cells, responsible for the synthesis and secretion of immunoglobulins (antibodies).

Histophysiology

The lymph nodes are compared to filters through which the lymph flows and is cleared of foreign particles before its return to the circulating system. Because the lymph nodes are spread throughout the body, the lymph formed in the tissues must cross at least one lymph node before entering the bloodstream. Each node receives lymph from a limited region of the body of which it is said to be a **satellite node.** Malignant tumors often metastasize via satellite nodes.

The afferent lymph enters through the convex side of the nodes and percolates through the subcapsular sinuses, passes to the peritrabecular and medullary sinuses, and leaves the lymph nodes by the efferent lymphatic vessels. The lymph crosses the nodes through passageways created by the loose lymphoid tissue that constitutes the sinuses, which are much more permeable to lymph than is the dense lymphoid tissue of the nodules. As the lymph flows through the sinuses, 99% or more of the antigens and other debris are removed by the phagocytic activity of both macrophages and reticular cells that span the sinuses between the connective tissue capsule and trabeculae and the adjacent nodules and medullary cords.

As stated above, almost all of the lymph traverses the nodule by flowing through the sinuses. However, a small amount, less than 1% of the volume, will penetrate the nodules. As the lymph filters through the nodules, the bulk of the antigen is processed by macrophages. Some antigen, however, is trapped on the surface of specialized reticular cells known as **dendritic cells.** This bound antigen is not phagocytosed but is exposed on the dendritic cell surface where it may be recognized and acted upon by immunologically competent lymphocytes. If a B cell recognizes the antigen, under appropriate conditions (which may necessitate the involvement of T cells), the B lymphocyte may be **activated.** Activated B lymphocytes migrate to the germinal center and undergo a series of transitions and cell divisions that lead to the production of immature **immunoblasts.** These in turn divide and give rise to **plasma cells** and **activated B lymphocytes.** The plasma cells leave the germinal center and migrate into the medullary cords. Here, the cells actively synthesize specific antibodies and release them into the lymph flowing through the medullary sinuses. Activated B cells, which can secrete some antibody and also bind some to their surface, leave the nodule and flow with the lymph to reenter the circulatory system. If in its travels the B cell encounters more of the stimulating antigen, it may leave the blood, enter the connective tissue, and differentiate into an immotile, secretory plasma cell.

As a consequence of infection and antigenic stimulation, affected lymph nodes exhibit swelling, reflecting the formation of multiple germinal centers and active cell proliferation. In resting nodes, plasma cells constitute 1–3% of the cell population; however, their numbers are greatly increased and they partially account for the enlargement of stimulated lymph nodes.

Cells in the lymph are returned to the bloodstream via the thoracic duct. Blood-borne lymphocytes can repopulate the lymph nodes by leaving through specific venules in the paracortical zone of the lymph node. These vessels, **postcapillary venules,** exhibit an unusual endothelial lining consisting of tall cuboidal cells. Lymphocytes are capable of traveling between the endothelial cells of this vessel. It has been suggested that this migrating ability is related to a specific interaction of receptors (possibly polysaccharides) on the surfaces of both the lymphocytes and postcapillary venule endothelial cells. Lymphocytes which cross between the endothelial cells of the venules penetrate the paracortical zone and medullary sinuses and leave the node via efferent lymphatics together with newly formed lymphocytes. In this way, most T lymphocytes recirculate many times.

Recirculation of lymphocytes also occurs through venules found in the spleen and in Peyer's patches of the ileum. However, the participation of other lymphoid organs in lymphocyte recirculation is negligible.

TONSILS

Tonsils are organs composed of agglomerations of incompletely encapsulated lymphoid tissue that lie beneath but in contact with the epithelium of the gut. According to their location, tonsils in the mouth and pharynx are called the **palatine tonsils,** the **pharyngeal tonsil,** and the **lingual tonsils.** In the gut, lymph nodules beneath the intestinal epithelium, constituting a form of "intestinal ton-

Epithelium with   Heavily infiltrated
some infiltration   epithelium

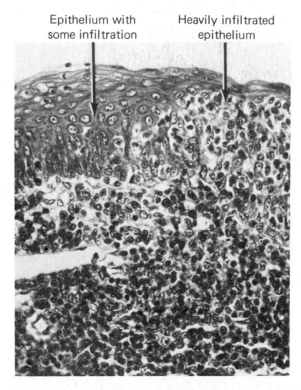

Figure 15–3. Photomicrograph of a palatine tonsil. The stratified squamous epithelium is infiltrated by lymphocytes. H&E stain, × 400.

sils," are known as **Peyer's patches.** The vermiform appendix, also consisting of epithelium-associated lymph nodules, represents another form of intestinal tonsils. In contrast to lymph nodes, the tonsils are not situated along the course of lymphatic vessels. Tonsils produce lymphocytes, many of which cross the epithelium and are deposited in the mouth, pharynx, and gut.

Palatine Tonsils

The 2 palatine tonsils are located in the oral part of the pharynx. The dense lymphoid tissue present in these tonsils forms, under the squamous stratified epithelium, a band that contains lymphatic nodules, generally with germinal centers. Each tonsil has 10–20 epithelial invaginations that penetrate deeply into the parenchyma, forming the **crypts,** which contain in their lumens desquamated epithelial cells, live and dead lymphocytes, and bacteria. They may appear like purulent spots in tonsillitis (Figs 15–3 and 15–4).

Separating the lymphoid tissue from subjacent organs is a band of dense connective tissue called the **capsule** of the tonsil. This capsule acts usually as a barrier against spreading tonsillar infections.

Pharyngeal Tonsil

This is a single tonsil situated in the superoposterior portion of the pharynx. It is covered by ciliated, cylindric, pseudostratified epithelium typical of the respiratory tract. Areas of stratified epithelium may also be observed.

The pharyngeal tonsil is composed of pleats of mucosa and shows diffuse lymphoid tissue and lymphatic nodules. It has no crypts.

The capsule of the pharyngeal tonsil is thinner than the capsules of the palatine tonsils.

Lingual Tonsils

The lingual tonsils are smaller and more numerous than the others. They are situated at the base of the tongue and are lined by squamous stratified epithelium. Each has a single crypt (Fig 16–1).

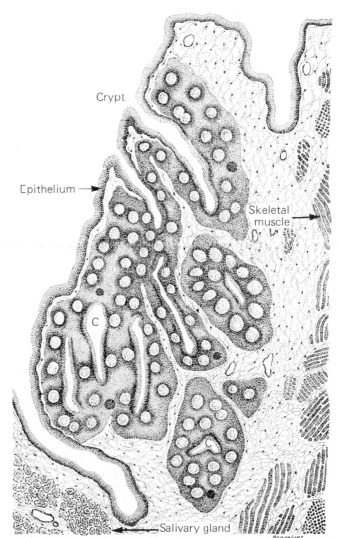

Figure 15–4 (at right). Palatine tonsil. There are numerous lymphatic nodules near the stratified squamous epithelium of the oropharynx. The light areas in the lymphoid tissue are germinal centers. Note the sections through the epithelial crypts (C).

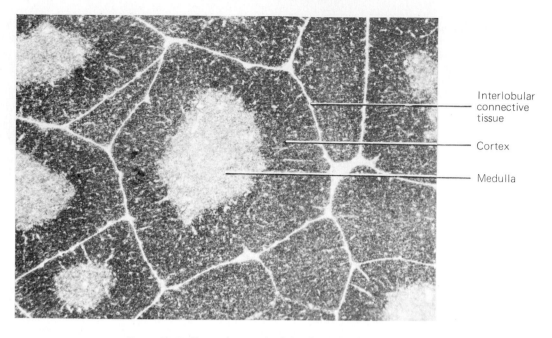

Figure 15 –5. Photomicrograph of the thymus. H&E stain, × 32.

Interlobular connective tissue

Cortex

Medulla

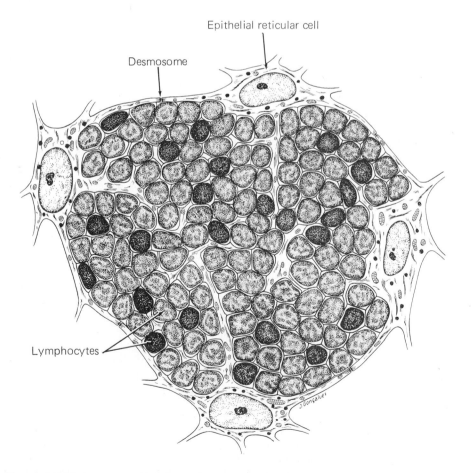

Epithelial reticular cell

Desmosome

Lymphocytes

Figure 15 –6. The relationship between epithelial reticular cells and thymus lymphocytes. Observe the long processes of epithelial reticular cells extending among the lymphocytes.

THYMUS

The thymus is a primary or central lymphoid organ situated in the mediastinum at about the level of the great vessels of the heart. It consists of incomplete lobules measuring about 0.5–2 mm in diameter and partially separated by septa of connective tissue of mesenchymal origin that envelops the organ (Fig 15–5).

In contrast to lymph nodes, the thymus has no afferent lymphatics or lymphatic nodules. Each lobule has a peripheral zone of dense **cortical** lymphoid tissue—consisting of a dense population of thymocytes or T lymphocytes—that surrounds a lightly staining central zone of loose lymphoid tissue, the **medullary zone** (Fig 15–5). Serial sections show that the cortical and medullary zones of a lobule are continuous with those of adjacent lobules. In the medulla are found **Hassall's corpuscles,** each consisting of 2 or more flattened, concentrically arranged epithelial cells. These apparently degenerative bodies are characteristic of the thymus (Fig 15–8).

Other lymphoid organs originate exclusively from mesenchyme, whereas the thymus has a double embryologic origin. Its lymphocytes arise from mesenchymal cells which invade an epithelial primordium that has its origin in the third and sometimes also the fourth pharyngeal pouch.

During intrauterine life, the thymus is colonized by lymphocyte-forming cells that come from the blood islands of the yolk sac and probably also from the hematopoietic tissue of the liver. After birth, it is believed that subsequent colonizing cells originate only in the bone marrow.

The intense lymphocytic proliferation that takes place during embryogenic through prepubertal development pushes apart the epithelial cells. Since these cells are bound with desmosomes, they remain attached to each other at the ends of their processes, creating an extensive network of stellate epithelial cells.

Thymus Cells

Both the cortical and the medullary zones have the same cellular types, although in different proportions. The most abundant are T lymphocytes and their precursor cells in various stages of differentiation and maturation and the **epithelial reticular cells** (Fig 15–6). Besides these cells, the thymus has a few mesenchymal reticular cells and many macrophages.

The **epithelial reticular cells** are morphologically very similar to the reticular cells of mesenchymal origin that occur in other lymphoid organs and also, though in smaller numbers, in the thymus. Unlike the mesenchymal cells, epithelial reticular cells have no reticular fibers, so that the reticulum existing in the thymus and in whose meshes the lymphocytes proliferate is composed almost exclusively of cell processes.

The epithelial reticular cells have large nuclei with fine chromatin and cytoplasm and numerous processes that are linked by desmosomes to the desmosomes of adjacent cells of the same type (Fig 15–6). Besides the desmosomes, these cells have tonofibrils that are also reminiscent of their epithelial origin (Fig 15–7). The electron microscope shows that in their cytoplasm are dense granules which may represent a secretion product.

In the cortical zone the epithelial reticular cells envelop groups of lymphocytes multiplying in isolation from circulating antigens. Furthermore, they seem to form a complete network in the periphery of the lobules and around the blood and lymphatic vessels. This network of epithelial cells joined by desmosomes forms a continuous layer that separates the thymic cortical parenchyma from the other histologic components of the organ, especially the vessels. Thus, between the epithelial cells and the capillaries, a space is encountered in which a basement membrane is seen and which also has macrophages. As a consequence of ensheathment of blood vessels by the epithelial reticular cells, antigenic material has difficulty in passing through this blood-thymus barrier and in coming into contact with the developing and programmed T lymphocytes, although some antigens eventually do pass through. It has also been suggested that the dynamics of flow in this space direct these antigens toward the medulla of the organ and away from the cortex.

The blood-thymus barrier is present only in the cortical zone. In the medullary zone the epithelial reticular lining of vessels is incomplete, and there is no special barrier to the passage of molecules from the blood to the thymic parenchyma.

Cortical Zone

In the cortical zone, mainly small lymphocytes predominate. These cells do not form nodules, as in other lymphoid organs, but are disposed in a continuous layer constituting a zone that passes from one lobule to the other. This area is a very active site of lymphocyte production. Many of the cells die in this area and are phagocytosed by cortical macrophages before their release. Plasma cells are not usually seen in the thymus. Epithelial reticular cells are less numerous at the cortical layer, and here their processes are generally very thin and long because of the distention that results from the intercalation of lymphocytes.

Medullary Zone

Lymphoblasts, young lymphocytes, and epithelial reticular cells predominate in the medulla. Normally, small lymphocytes are rare. The medulla also contains the Hassall corpuscles, which are a characteristic feature of the thymus (Fig 15–8).

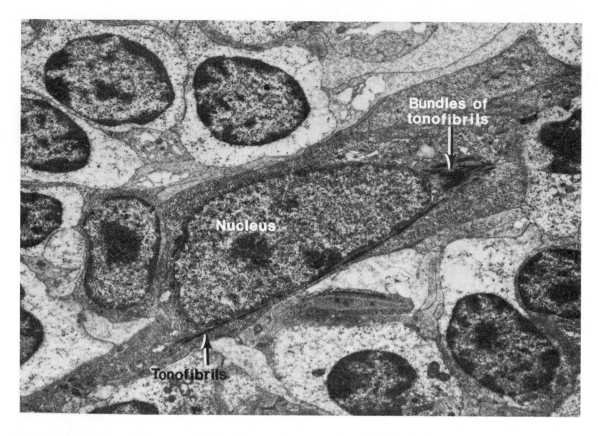

Figure 15 –7. Thymic medulla seen under the electron microscope. An epithelial reticular cell runs diagonally across the figure. It has fine chromatin and exhibits tonofibrils in the cytoplasm. × 7100.

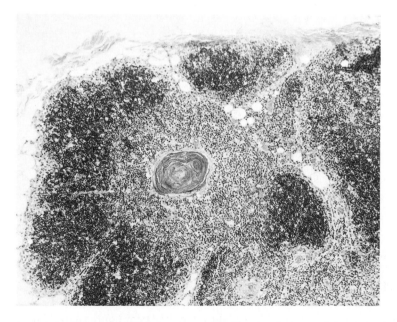

Figure 15 –8. Photomicrograph of a human thymus, showing the dense cortical and lighter medullary zones. Near the center, one Hassall corpuscle appears in the medulla. Connective tissue septa form incomplete lobules. H&E stain, × 118.

Hassall's bodies are 30–150 μm in diameter and consist of concentric layers of epithelial reticular cells. Some of these cells, mainly the innermost ones, degenerate and die. It is not rare to find Hassall's bodies with cores that consist only of cell remnants, sometimes calcified.

Development & Involution of the Thymus

In relation to body weight, the thymus shows its maximum development immediately after birth and undergoes accelerated involution after puberty. In the newborn, it weighs 12–15 g; at puberty, 30–40 g; and in old age, 10–15 g.

The thymus is very sensitive to radiation, infection, and disease. Thymuses observed at autopsies of children and adults who die after protracted illnesses are much smaller than normal.

Despite the processes of involution that accompany the passage of the years, the thymus remains capable of producing great numbers of lymphocytes when stimulated. The involuntary process of aging begins in the cortical zone, which gradually becomes thinner. The medulla begins its process of involution at puberty. Reticular cells of epithelial

origin and Hassall's corpuscles are more resistant to involution than lymphocytes. The thymus never disappears completely; it is still present even in very old people, represented by reticular cells, Hassall's corpuscles, some lymphocytes, and a great amount of connective tissue.

Vascularization

Arteries that penetrate the thymus through the capsule distribute blood first to the cortical area; the smaller branches then reach the medulla.

Thymic capillaries have an endothelium without pores and a very thick basement membrane (Fig 15–9). The endothelial cells have thin processes that perforate the basement membrane and may come in contact with epithelial reticular cells.

As mentioned earlier, cortical epithelial reticular cells surround all vessels of the thymus and constitute a layer that, although incomplete, separates the blood from the lymphocytes.

The medullary and cortical veins penetrate into the connective tissue septa and leave the thymus through its capsule.

The thymus does not have afferent lymphatic

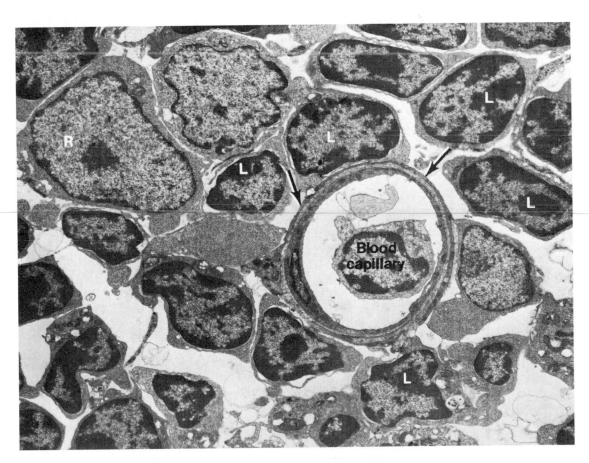

Figure 15–9. Electron micrograph of a thymic cortical layer. There is a blood capillary showing a thick basal lamina. Arrows point to epithelial reticular cells forming incomplete lining of blood vessel. Note the lymphocytes (L) annd the reticular cell (R). × 28,500.

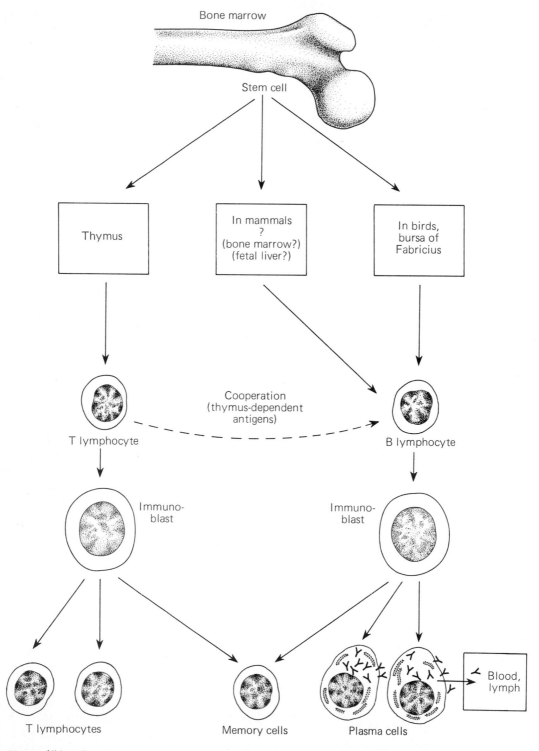

Figure 15–10. All lymphocytes originate from a stem cell, whose morphology is not clear. This cell migrates through the blood and invades the thymus, dividing many times to form T lymphocytes. (In birds, the stem cells are "conditioned" to become B lymphocytes in the bursa of Fabricius, a lymphatic organ located in the cloaca. The mammalian equivalent of the bursa of Fabricius is unknown. It may be the bone marrow itself, the fetal liver, or lymphoid areas of the digestive tract.) After encountering an antigen, the lymphocyte modulates into a larger cell—the immunoblast—which then proliferates and produces more T lymphocytes or plasma cells as the case may be. The so-called thymus-dependent antigens promote the transformation of B lymphocytes into plasma cells only when T lymphocytes are also present. This phenomenon is called cooperation between T cells and B cells in antibody production.

vessels and does not constitute a filter for the lymph as do lymph nodes. The few lymphatic vessels encountered in the thymus are all efferent and localized in the walls of blood vessels and in the connective tissue of the septa and the capsule.

Histophysiology

It was observed as long ago as 1961 that thymectomy in newborn rats caused atrophy of other lymphoid organs and a decrease in the number of circulating lymphocytes. We now know that undifferentiated cells whose morphology is little understood migrate through the blood from the bone marrow to the **thymus**, where they proliferate, giving rise to **T lymphocytes**. As explained in Chapter 13, these lymphocytes are responsible for cell-mediated immune reactions such as delayed hypersensitivity and graft rejection, whereas the **B lymphocytes** differentiate in plasma cells, which produce the humoral antibodies (Fig 15–10).

Leaving the thymus through the blood vessels in the medulla, T lymphocytes penetrate certain areas of other lymphoid organs called secondary or peripheral lymphoid organs. Those areas are called **thymus-dependent.** In mammals, thymus-dependent zones are the paracortical zone of lymph nodes, the periarterial sheaths in the white pulp of the spleen, and the loose lymphoid tissue found in Peyer's patches in the small intestine. The remaining lymphoid tissue of the body contains B lymphocytes.

Both in the light microscope and in the electron microscope, B and T lymphocytes are morphologically similar. For each type of lymphocyte (B or T), there is a difference in the type of marker present on the surface membrane. These differences in markers are used to identify the 2 types of lymphocytes. They are shown in Table 15–1.

T lymphocytes are long-lived cells and constitute a population of cells comprising a portion of the lymphocytes of the thymus, most lymph and blood lymphocytes, and the lymphocytes found in all thymus-dependent zones.

Mitotic proliferation of lymphocytes is much

Table 15–1. Surface markers of human T and B cells.

Marker	Method
T cells	
E rosettes	Binding of sheep red blood cells
Anti–T cell antibody	Direct or indirect immunofluorescence or cytotoxicity study
B cells	
Surface immunoglobulin	Direct immunofluorescence
EAC rosettes (complement receptor)	Binding of complement and IgM-coated sheep or ox red blood cells
Aggregated immunoglobulin	Direct or indirect immunofluorescence
Anti–B cell antibody	Direct or indirect immunofluorescence or cytotoxicity study

higher in the cortical than in the medullary zone, being 5–10 times higher than in other lymphoid organs. One milligram of mouse thymus produces 1 million lymphocytes per day. The thymic mitotic rate is at its maximum at birth and decreases with age. However, only a small number of the lymphocytes produced daily in the thymus leave this organ. Most are destroyed and phagocytosed within the thymus, a process whose significance is not yet fully understood.

Thymectomy at Birth

When newborn animals are thymectomized—or in cases where the thymus does not develop during embryonic life—the following effects are observed: (1) There is no formation of T lymphocytes, with a consequent decrease in the number of lymphocytes in blood and lymph as well as a depletion of all thymus-dependent zones of the lymphoid tissue. (2) There is no delayed hypersensitivity reaction, and graft rejection does not occur. (3) There is atrophy of all lymphoid organs. (4) Finally, after 3–4 months of age, the thymectomized animal becomes weak, loses weight, and dies. In humans, many diseases with symptoms that are related to these events have been described, and in such cases death usually occurs shortly after birth.

The pool of T lymphocytes does not exist in thymectomized animals. Consequently, they do not show cell-mediated immune responses since T lymphocytes probably synthesize specific factors and keep them attached to their membranes.

On the other hand, the pool of B lymphocytes in thymectomized animals is nearly normal. They react to most antigens, producing plasma cells which synthesize antibodies. However, there are some antigens which require both T and B lymphocytes for antibody formation. For these antigens, T lymphocytes are important for the differentiation of B lymphocytes into plasma cells. When injected into animals thymectomized immediately after birth, these antigens do not elicit the formation of antibodies and are thus called **thymus-dependent antigens** (Fig 15–10).

The generalized atrophy of lymphoid organs observed in animals thymectomized immediately after birth is believed to be due to lack of a humoral factor produced by the thymus, which stimulates the development of lymphoid tissue in general. This hypothesis is based on strong experimental evidence. For example, implantation of thymus fragments in a small box whose walls are permeable to fluids and small molecules but not to cells prevents the lymphoid atrophy of thymectomized newborn animals. It has been observed also that implantation of fragments of thymus whose lymphocytes have been destroyed by irradiation has the same protective effect. Epithelial reticular cells secrete a hormone, **thymopoietin**, which has a trophic action on the lymphoid system and appears to pro-

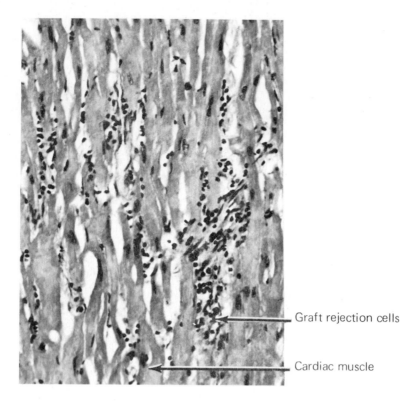

Figure 15–11. Photomicrograph of human myocardium from a transplanted heart. Among the cardiac muscle fibers that show degenerative changes there are many graft-rejecting cells. H&E stain, × 250.

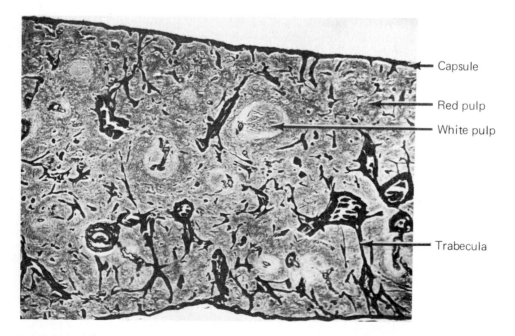

Figure 15–12. Photomicrograph of a silver-stained spleen section to show the general architecture of the organ. × 30.

mote the differentiation of T cells. The electron microscope shows, in the cytoplasm of these cells, small granules that are very similar to secretory granules of some endocrine glands. However, the thymus hormone has not yet been clearly identified.

Animals thymectomized just after birth develop in a few weeks a progressive, fatal wasting disease characterized by weakness, weight loss, lethargy, and diarrhea. Since it is believed that this disease is due to widespread infections which may take place simultaneously in several organs, this outcome can be prevented by continuous injection of antibiotics or by keeping the thymectomized animals in a sterile environment.

Thymectomy in Adults

In adult animals, the effects of thymectomy are not as pronounced as in younger animals. There is usually a slight decrease in the number of blood lymphocytes as well as in the weight of the lymphoid organs. Since they are long-lived, the T lymphocytes that exist at the time of thymectomy maintain the pool of these circulating cells at a nearly normal level. On the other hand, since the trophic activity of the thymus is important only for the development of the lymphoid system, the lymphoid organs, once formed, are able to maintain themselves.

Thymus Grafting

In animals of any age, thymus grafting avoids the adverse effects of thymectomy. Studies of graft recipients whose cells have been labeled by chromosome markers show that there is an initial proliferation of lymphocytes from the graft. However, after the third week, lymphocytes divide for a few days but soon disappear entirely. The donor thymus then would be populated with host stem cells.

Hormones Which Act on the Thymus

The thymus is subject to the effects of several hormones. Injections of some adrenocorticosteroids cause a reduction in lymphocyte number and mitotic rate. There is atrophy of the cortical layer of the thymus. Adrenocorticotropic hormone (ACTH) produced by the anterior pituitary achieves the same effect by stimulating the activity of the adrenal cortex.

Male and female sex hormones also accelerate thymic involution; castration has the reverse effect.

Pituitary growth hormone (somatotropin, STH) stimulates thymic development in a nonspecific way, having a general effect on body growth.

ORGAN TRANSPLANTATION

Transplants are classified as **autografts** when the transplanted tissue or organ is taken from a different site on the same individual; **isografts** when the tissue or organ is taken from an identical twin; **homografts** or **allografts** when it is taken from an unrelated individual of the same species; and **heterografts** or **xenografts** when it is taken from an animal of a different species.

Autologous and isologous transplants take easily as long as an efficient blood supply is established. In such cases, there is no rejection because the transplanted cells are genetically similar to those of the host and are composed of molecules that the organism recognizes as its own. For this reason, no antibodies are produced.

Homologous and heterologous transplants, on the other hand, contain cells whose membranes contain constituents that are foreign to the host and are therefore recognized and treated as such. Transplant rejection is due mainly to the activity of **graft rejection cells** (Fig 15–11). These cells are T lymphocytes that penetrate the transplant and act locally, destroying the transplanted cells.

Homologous transplants are normally rejected. However, when this type of transplant is carried out between fraternal twins who shared the same placenta, the graft is not rejected. This was verified after observing that fraternal twin calves that had shared a single placenta, although having different blood groups, had erythrocytes from each other and did not develop an immunologic reaction. What occurs in these cases is that during embryonic life there is an exchange of blood between the animals. It is now known that an organism will never form antibodies against an antigen that was present in it before its immune system started functioning. Only the molecules that enter the body after the organism has become **immunocompetent** and has begun to synthesize antibodies are recognized as foreign and treated as antigens. In humans, the synthesis of antibodies begins a few days after birth. The infant is protected during the first few days of life mainly by antibodies received from the mother through the placenta. This is, therefore, a passive immunity that protects against infection until the child's own cells begin to produce antibodies.

THE SPLEEN

The spleen is the largest accumulation of lymphatic tissue in the organism, and in humans it is the largest lymphatic organ in the circulatory system. Owing to its abundance of phagocytic cells and the close contact between the circulating blood and these cells, the spleen represents an important de-

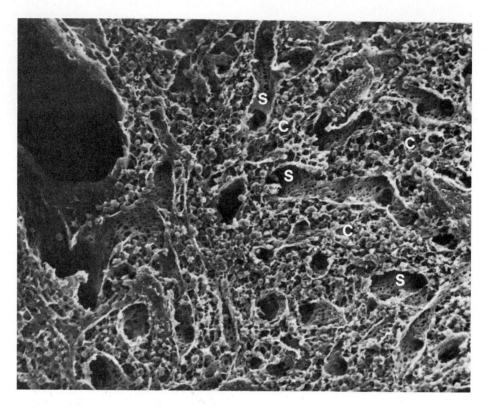

Figure 15–13. General view of splenic red pulp with a scanning electron microscope. Note the sinusoids (S) and the red pulp cords (C). × 360. (Reproduced, with permission, from Miyoshi M, Fujita T: Arch Histol Jpn 33:225, 1971.)

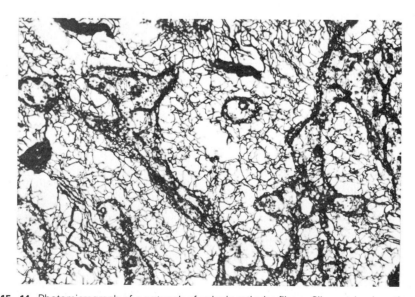

Figure 15–14. Photomicrograph of a network of splenic reticular fibers. Silver-stained section, × 200.

fense against microorganisms that penetrate the circulation and is also the site of destruction of many red cells. As is true of all other lymphatic organs, the spleen is a site of formation of activated lymphocytes, which pass into the blood. The spleen reacts promptly to antigens carried in the blood and is an important antibody-forming organ. While lymph nodes serve as immunologic filters of the lymph, the spleen is the immunologic filter of the circulatory system.

General Structure

The spleen is surrounded by a capsule of dense connective tissue which sends out trabeculae that divide the parenchyma or **splenic pulp** into incomplete compartments (Fig 15–12). The medial surface of the spleen presents a hilum at the level of which the capsule gives rise to a number of trabeculae through which the nerves and arteries penetrate. The veins derived from the parenchyma and the lymphatic vessels that originate in the trabeculae leave through the hilum. The splenic pulp has no lymphatic vessels.

The connective tissue of the capsule and of the trabeculae contains some smooth muscle cells. In humans, these cells are not numerous. In certain other mammals (cat, dog, horse) they are quite abundant, and their contraction causes the expulsion of accumulated blood from the spleen, which has a spongy structure and serves to store blood cells.

Splenic Pulp

On the surface of a fresh or fixed slice cut through the spleen, one can observe white spots in the parenchyma with the naked eye. These are lymphatic nodules and are part of the so-called **white pulp.** These nodules appear within the dark red tissue, rich in blood, called the **red pulp** (Figs 15–12, 15–13, 15–15, and 15–10).

Examination under a low-power microscope reveals that the red pulp is composed of elongated structures, the **splenic cords,** which lie between the sinusoids (Fig 15–13).

All of the splenic pulp consists of connective tissue containing reticular fibers. Fixed cellular elements of this tissue are the reticular cells and macrophages, and the function of the reticular fibers is that of support (Fig 15–14).

The relationship between the reticular cells and the reticular fibers has not been fully explained. Electron microscopy has demonstrated that the reticular fibers may be encased in extensions of reticular cells. These reticular fibers are composed of a collagen fibril associated with an amorphous PAS-positive polysaccharide material.

Blood Circulation

The splenic artery divides as it penetrates the hilum, branching out into vessels of various sizes that follow the course of the connective tissue trabeculae and are called **trabecular arteries.** When they leave the trabeculae to enter the parenchyma, the arteries are immediately enveloped in a sheath of lymphocytes. These vessels are known as the **central arteries** or **white pulp arteries.** Along its variable course, the lymphocytic sheath (white pulp) may thicken to form a number of lymphatic nodules in which the vessel, now an arteriole, occupies an eccentric position, although it is still called the central artery. During its course through the white pulp, the arteriole divides into numerous intercommunicating branches that will supply the lymphatic tissue surrounding it.

Before leaving the lymphatic tissue, the arteriole forms several more branches that reach into the red pulp and subdivide to form **penicilli,** arterioles with a diameter of approximately 25 μm. These penicilli, which possess smooth muscle in the first portion of these straight vessels, are called **pulp arteries.** They are composed of an endothelium supported by a thick basal lamina. Near their terminations, some of these branches present a typical thickening. These vessels are called the **sheathed arteries.** This sheath—cylindric, elliptic, or spherical in shape—consists of phagocytic cells that surround the endothelium. Although the endothelial layer in the area of the sheath may be continuous, its basement membrane is not and in some specimens is nonexistent.

Beyond the sheath, the vessels continue as simple arterial capillaries that transport blood to the **sinusoids** (red pulp sinuses). These sinusoids occupy the area between the red pulp cords (Fig 15–13). From the sinusoids, the blood proceeds to the red pulp veins that join together and enter the trabeculae, forming the **trabecular veins.** From these latter vessels originates the splenic vein, which emerges from the hilum of the spleen. The trabecular veins do not have individual muscle walls, ie, their walls are composed of trabecular tissue. They can be regarded as channels hollowed out in the connective trabecular tissue and lined by endothelium.

The manner in which blood flows from the arterial capillaries of the red pulp to the interior of the sinusoids has not yet been completely explained. Some investigators consider that the capillaries open directly into the sinusoids; others maintain that the blood passes through the spaces between the red pulp cord cells and then moves on to be collected by the sinusoids (Figs 15–15 and 15–18). In the first instance, this would mean a **closed** circulation, as proposed by the supporters of the "closed theory," who maintain that the blood always remains inside the vessels. In the second case, the circulation would **open** ("open theory") into the parenchyma of the organ between its cells and the blood would pass through the area between the cells in order to reach the sinusoids. Others maintain that in a distended spleen, full of blood, the circulation would be open, whereas in a spleen with

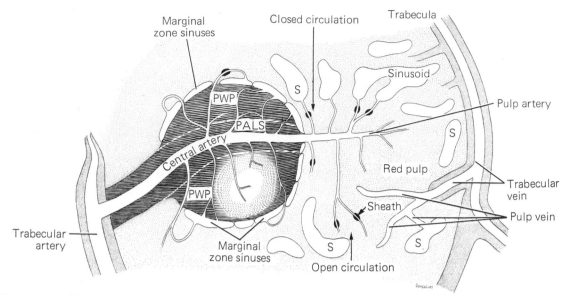

Figure 15–15. Schematic view of the blood circulation of the spleen. Theories of open and closed circulation are represented in this drawing. Splenic sinuses (S) are indicated. PALS, periarterial lymphatic sheath; PWP, peripheral white pulp. (Redrawn and reproduced, with permission, from Greep RO, Weiss L: *Histology,* 3rd ed. McGraw-Hill, 1973.)

little blood the arterial capillaries would connect directly with the sinusoids, establishing a closed circulation.

White Pulp

The white pulp consists of the lymphatic tissue arranged in sheaths around and sequential nodules along the arteries (Figs 15–15 and 15–16). As is the case with lymphatic tissue in general, reticular cells and reticular fibers are both encountered and form a 3-dimensional mesh. The spaces in this mesh are occupied mainly by lymphocytes and macrophages. The white pulp forms a sheath around the vessels and contains lymphatic nodules (Figs 15–15 and 15–16). These nodules are easily distinguished from other nodules encountered in the various lymphatic organs because of the presence of the central artery (Figs 15–15 and 15–17).

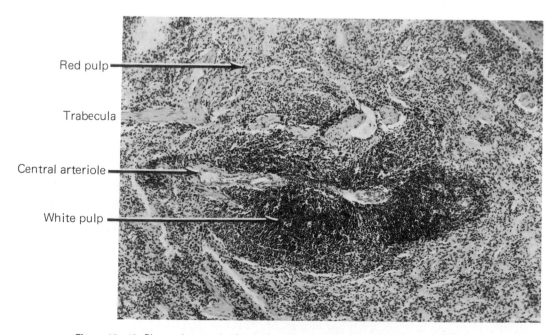

Figure 15–16. Photomicrograph of splenic white and red pulp. H&E stain, × 100.

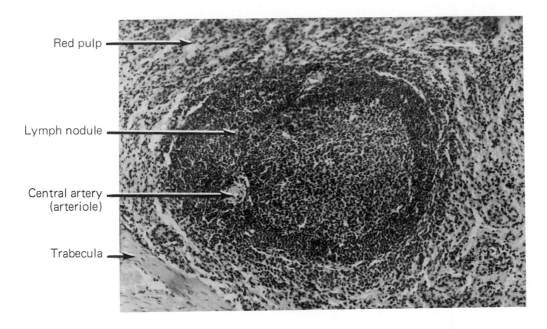

Red pulp

Lymph nodule

Central artery
(arteriole)

Trabecula

Figure 15–17. Photomicrograph of the spleen, showing a lymphatic nodule (white pulp) surrounded by red pulp.

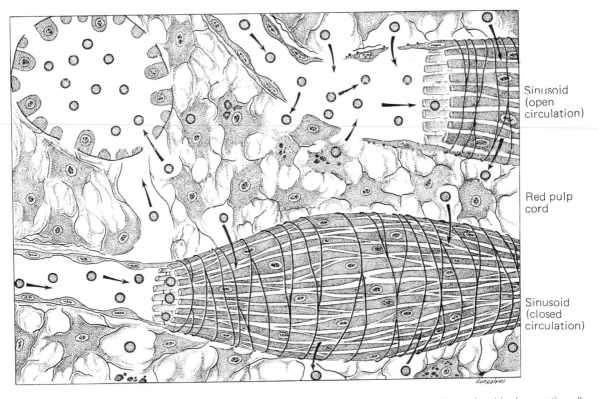

Sinusoid
(open
circulation)

Red pulp
cord

Sinusoid
(closed
circulation)

Figure 15–18. Structure of the red pulp of the spleen, showing splenic sinusoids and red pulp cords with phagocytic cells (some with phagocytosed material). The relationship between reticular fibers and sinusoid lining cells is also shown. A sinusoid in cross section is shown at upper left. Both the open and closed theories of spleen blood circulation are illustrated.

Between the lymphatic nodules and the red pulp lies a **marginal zone** consisting of many sinuses and of loose lymphoid tissue with few lymphocytes but with many macrophages having branching processes and showing active phagocytosis. The marginal zone retains great amounts of blood antigens and thus plays a major role in the immunologic activity of the spleen. Many of the pulp arterioles, derived from the central vein, extend out and away from the white pulp but then turn back and empty into the moatlike sinuses of the marginal zone that encircles the nodules. As a consequence of this drainage, which includes the added blood flow from vessels within the white pulp that also terminate in the marginal zone, this area plays a significant role in filtering the blood and launching an immune response. A large number of macrophages and reticuloendothelial cells serve to phagocytose and remove antigenic debris. Dendritic cells in the marginal zone trap and present antigens to immunologically competent cells. The marginal zone is an ideal site for this activity since not only the antigens are removed from the blood here but also the T and B lymphocytes. As these lymphocytes leave the systemic circulation to penetrate the white pulp, they pass by the dendritic cells, presenting exposed antigen. If the appropriate B cells, T cells, and antigen are present, an immune response will be initiated. Activated B cells migrate to the center of the white pulp nodule, the germinal center, and give rise to immunoblasts, plasma cells, and activated B cells. The latter 2 cells enter the red pulp, where the plasma cells remain in the cords and release antibody into the blood of the sinuses. The activated B cells leave the red pulp and return to the general circulation.

The lymphocytes of the **periarterial lymphatic sheath (PALS)** are **thymus-dependent,** whereas the marginal zones and periphery of the nodules—the **peripheral white pulp (PWP)**—are populated by B lymphocytes. Thus, the splenic white pulp has B and T lymphocytes segregated in 2 different sites.

Red Pulp

The red pulp is a reticular tissue with a special characteristic, ie, the presence of **splenic cords.** The cords appear only in histologic preparations since the red pulp actually is a sponge, the cavities of which are the sinusoids.

The cords are continuous and of varying thickness according to the local distention of the sinusoids. Besides the reticular cells, the splenic cords contain fixed and wandering macrophages, monocytes, lymphocytes, plasma cells, and many blood elements (erythrocytes, platelets, and granulocytes).

The **sinusoids** of the spleen differ from the common capillaries in 3 ways: (1) they have a dilated, large, irregular lumen; (2) between their lining endothelial cells are spaces that facilitate exchange between the sinusoids and adjacent tissues;

and (3) the basement membrane–like material is not continuous but forms barrel hooplike rings around the endothelial walls.

The endothelial cells that line the splenic sinusoids are elongated, with their long axis parallel to the sinusoids. These cells are enveloped in reticular fibers set mainly in a transverse direction, similar to the hoops of a barrel. The transverse fibers and those oriented in various directions join to form a network enveloping the sinusoid cells (Fig 15–18). It was formerly thought that the endothelial cells of sinuses were phagocytic; however, it appears that the observed phagocytosis was due to processes of macrophages that had penetrated into the spaces between adjacent endothelial cells.

The spaces between the cells of the splenic sinusoids can be 2–3 μm in diameter or even larger, so that the erythrocytes are able to pass easily from the lumen of the sinusoids to the red pulp cords (Fig 15–19).

Histophysiology

The spleen is a lymphatic organ with special characteristics. Its best-known functions are (1) formation of lymphocytes, (2) destruction of erythrocytes, (3) defense of the organism against foreign particles that enter the bloodstream, and (4) storage of blood.

A. Production of Blood Cells: The white pulp of the spleen produces lymphocytes that migrate to the red pulp and reach the lumens of the sinusoids, where they are incorporated into the blood that is present there. A constant flow of lymphocytes is observed from the splenic parenchyma to the bloodstream as well as in the opposite direction. Radioautography after intravenous injection of radioactive lymphocytes has demonstrated that many of these labeled lymphocytes appear in the white pulp of the spleen.

In the fetus, the spleen also produces granulocytes (neutrophils, basophils, and eosinophils) and erythrocytes, but this activity ceases at the end of the fetal phase. In certain pathologic conditions (eg, leukemia), the spleen may recommence the production of granulocytes and erythrocytes, thus undergoing a process known as **myeloid metaplasia** (pathologic transformation of one kind of cell into another).

B. Destruction of Erythrocytes: The red blood cells have an average life span of 120 days, after which time they are destroyed, mainly in the spleen. This phenomenon of the removal of degenerating erythrocytes (hemocatheresis) also occurs in the bone marrow.

The macrophages of the red pulp—in the red pulp cords—engulf entire pieces of the erythrocytes that frequently fragment themselves in the extracellular spaces.

The engulfed erythrocytes are altered and digested by the lysosomes of the phagocytes. The hemoglobin they contain is broken down, forming a

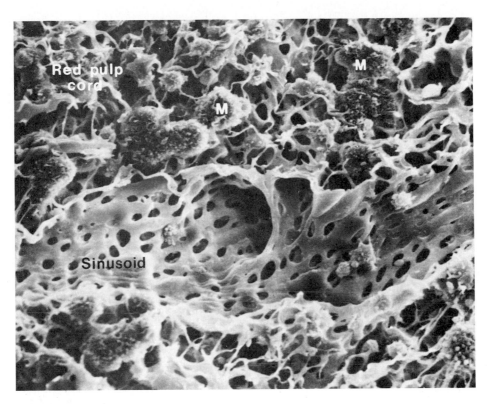

Figure 15 –19. Scanning electron micrograph of the red pulp of the spleen, showing sinusoids, red pulp cords, and macrophages (M). × 1600. (Reproduced, with permission, from Miyoshi M, Fujita T: Arch Histol Jpn 33:225, 1971.)

pigment, **bilirubin,** which contains no iron, and a protein, **ferritin,** which does contain iron. These compounds are then returned to the blood.

Bilirubin is excreted by the hepatic cells together with the bile. Ferritin, which represents a form of mobile iron, is used by the erythrocytes of the bone marrow, which draw iron from it for the synthesis of new hemoglobin.

C. Defense: Since it contains both B and T lymphocytes and macrophages, the spleen is important in body defense. In the same way that lymph nodes "filter" the lymph, the spleen is considered as a "filter" for the blood.

The T lymphocytes found in the periarterial sheaths of the white pulp proliferate and enter the bloodstream. They participate in cell-mediated immune mechanisms.

Radioautographic studies with labeled antigens injected into the blood show that the antigens are preferentially retained by the surface of cells found in the nodules and in the marginal zone. These cells have many long processes that branch profusely, thus increasing the cell surface. Because of their shape they are called **dendritic cells.**

Under the stimulus of antigens, splenic B lymphocytes proliferate and give rise to antibody-producing plasma cells.

Of all the macrophagic cells of the organism, those of the spleen are most active in the

phagocytosis of living particles (bacteria and viruses) and inert particles that find their way into the bloodstream. After the injection of trypan blue, the macrophages of the spleen are among the first to accumulate this dye.

When there is an excess of lipids in the blood plasma (hyperlipidemia), the macrophages of the spleen accumulate considerable quantities of these substances. In diabetes, hyperlipidemia is frequent, and for this reason large macrophages, their cytoplasm containing numerous lipid droplets, are common in the spleens of diabetics.

D. Blood Storage: Owing to the spongy structure of the red pulp, the spleen stores blood, which can be returned to the circulation to increase the volume of circulating blood. In animals with spleens composed of a capsule and trabeculae rich in smooth muscle, the organ is emptied by muscular contraction. Because the human spleen is poor in smooth muscle fibers, the storage and expulsion of blood depends on changes in the diameter of the blood vessels. It has been demonstrated that in humans the blood storage capacity of the spleen is very small.

Splenectomy

Although it has important functions, the spleen can be removed without serious damage to the individual. Other organs with cells similar to those found in the spleen will compensate for its loss.

After splenectomy, a temporary increase in the number of lymphocytes is observed in the blood. This is due to excessive compensatory lymphocyte production by other lymphatic organs (lymph nodes, isolated nodules, etc). The number of platelets also increases.

Splenectomy is beneficial in diseases where there is a deficiency in bone marrow function. In these cases, splenectomy is followed by bone marrow activation. This permits the conclusion that the spleen inhibits bone marrow function in such cases. This inhibiting effect has not been proved under normal conditions, but many investigators argue that the spleen has a regulating effect on bone marrow. This effect would be more pronounced in certain pathologic states.

●　　●　　●

References

Anderson AO, Anderson NJ: Studies on the structure and permeability of the microvasculature in normal rat lymph nodes. Am J Pathol 80:387, 1975.

Avrameas S, Leduc EH: Detection of simultaneous antibody synthesis in plasma cells and specialized lymphocytes in rabbit lymph nodes. J Exp Med 131:1137, 1970.

Binet JL, Mathe G: Optical and electron microscope studies of "immunologically competent cells" in graft reactions. Nature 193:992, 1962.

Bradfield JW, Born GV: The migration of rat thoracic duct lymphocytes through spleen. Br J Exp Pathol 54:509, 1973.

Chen LT, Weiss L: Electron microscope study of the red pulp of human spleen. Am J Anat 134:425, 1972.

Everett NB, Caffrey RW: Lymphopoiesis in the thymus and other tissues: Functional implications. Int Rev Cytol 22:205, 1967.

Fujita T: A scanning electron microscope study of the human spleen. Arch Histol Jpn 37:187, 1974.

Gowans JL, Knight EJ: The route of recirculation of lymphocytes in the rat. Proc R Soc Lond [Biol] 159:257, 1964.

Haar JL: Light and electron microscopy of the human fetal thymus. Anat Rec 179:463, 1974.

Hayes TG: The marginal zone and marginal sinus in the spleen of the gerbil: A light and electron microscope study. J Morphol 141:205, 1973.

Hirasawa Y, Tokuhiro H: Electron microscopic studies on the normal human spleen, especially on the red pulp and the reticuloendothelial cells. Blood 35:201, 1970.

Ito T, Hoshino T: Fine structure of the epithelial reticular cells of the medulla of the thymus in the golden hamster. Z Zellforsch Mikrosk Anat 69:311, 1966.

Joel DD, Hess MW, Cottier H: Thymic origin of lymphocytes in developing Peyer's patches of newborn mice. Nature 231:24, 1971.

Luk SC, Nopajaroonsri C, Simon GT: The architecture of the normal lymph node and hemolymph node: A scanning and transmission electron microscope study. Lab Invest 29:258, 1973.

Martin CR: T and B lymphocytes and immune responses. Nature 242:19, 1973.

Mellors RC, Korngold L: The cellular origin of human immunoglobulins. J Exp Med 118:387, 1963.

Metcalf D, Brumby M: The role of the thymus in the ontogeny of the immune system. J Cell Physiol 67 (Part 2):149, 1966.

Miller JFAP: Immunity and the thymus. Lancet 1:43, 1963.

Mishell RL, Dutton RW: Immunization of dissociated spleen cell cultures from normal mice. J Exp Med 126:423, 1967.

Osoba D, Miller JFAP: The lymphoid tissues and immune responses of neonatally thymectomized mice bearing thymus tissue in Millipore diffusion chambers. J Exp Med 119:177, 1964.

Raviola E, Karnovsky MJ: Evidence for a blood-thymus barrier using electron opaque tracers. J Exp Med 136:466, 1972.

Sainte-Marie G: Cytokinetics of antibody formation. J Cell Physiol 67 (Part 2):109, 1966.

Thomas CE: An electron and light microscope study of sinus structure in perfused rabbit and dog spleens. Am J Anat 120:527, 1967.

Trainen N, Smale M: Thymic humoral factors. Contemp Top Immunobiol 2:321, 1973.

Wagner H & others: Cell mediated immune response in vitro. J Exp Med 136:331, 1972.

Weiss L: *The Cells and Tissues of the Immune System*. Prentice-Hall, 1972.

Weiss L: A scanning electron microscopic study of the spleen. Blood 43:665, 1974.

Weissman IL: Development and distribution of immunoglobulin-bearing cells in mice. Trans Rev 24:159, 1975.

The digestive system consists of the digestive tract and its associated glands. Its function is to obtain from ingested food the metabolites necessary for the growth and energy needs of the body. Before stored or used as energy, food is digested and transformed into small molecules that can be easily absorbed through the lining of the digestive tract. However, a barrier between the environment and the internal milieu of the body must be maintained. The first step in the complex process known as digestion occurs in the mouth, where food is ground into smaller pieces by mastication and moistened by saliva, which also initiates the digestion of carbohydrates. Digestion continues in the stomach and small intestine. In the small intestine, the food—transformed into its basic components (amino acids, monosaccharides, glycerides, etc)—is absorbed. Water absorption occurs in the large intestine, and as a consequence the undigested contents become semisolid.

THE ORAL CAVITY

The oral cavity is lined with stratified nonkeratinized squamous (mucous) epithelium. Its superficial cells are nucleated and have scanty granules of keratin in their interior. In the lips, a transition from mucous to keratinized epithelium can be observed. The lamina propria presents papillae similar to those in the skin and is continuous with a submucosa containing diffuse small salivary glands.

The roof of the mouth is composed of the hard and soft palates, both covered with the same type of stratified squamous epithelium. In the hard palate, the mucous membrane rests on bony tissue. The soft palate has a center of striated skeletal muscle and numerous mucous glands in its submucosa.

The palatine **uvula** is a small conical process that extends downward from the center of the lower border of the soft palate. It has a core of muscle and areolar connective tissue covered by typical oral mucosa.

THE TONGUE

The tongue is a mass of striated muscle covered by a mucous membrane whose structure varies according to the region studied. The muscle fibers cross each other in 3 planes. They are grouped in bundles, usually separated by connective tissue. The mucous membrane is strongly adherent to the muscle because the connective tissue of the lamina propria penetrates into the spaces between the muscular bundles. On the lower surface of the tongue, the mucous membrane is smooth. The dorsal surface is irregular, covered anteriorly by a great number of small excrescences called **papillae.** The posterior region of the dorsal surface of the tongue is separated from the anterior portion by a V-shaped boundary. Behind this boundary, the surface of the tongue presents eminences composed mainly of small lymphatic aggregations of 2 types: (1) lymph follicles, which are small collections of lymph nodules; and (2) the lingual tonsils, where lymph nodules aggregate around invaginations of the mucous membrane (Fig 16–1).

The Papillae

The papillae are elevations or excrescences of the oral epithelium and lamina propria that assume different forms and functions. There are 4 types:

A. Filiform Papillae: These papillae have an elongated conical shape, are quite numerous, and are present over the entire surface of the tongue. Their epithelium, which does not contain taste buds, is frequently partially keratinized (Fig 16–1).

B. Fungiform Papillae: Fungiform resemble mushrooms in that they have a narrow stalk and smooth-surfaced, dilated upper part (Fig 16–1). These papillae, which contain scattered taste buds on their upper surfaces, are irregularly interspersed among the larger population of filiform papillae.

C. Foliate Papillae: Arranged as closely packed folds along the posterior lateral margins of the tongue, these papillae contain numerous taste buds. Ducts from serous glands drain through openings positioned around the bases of these papillae (Fig 10–3).

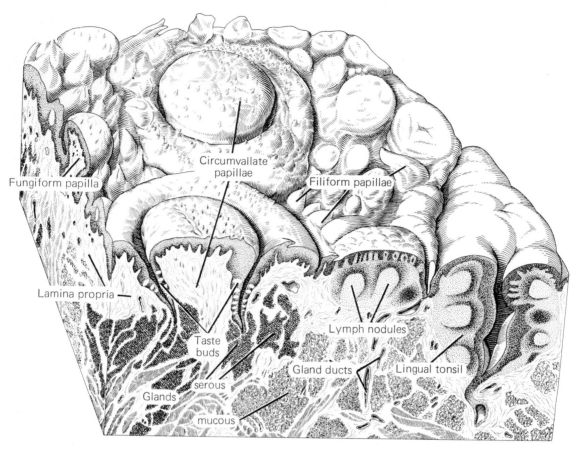

Figure 16–1. Surface of tongue on the region close to its V-shaped boundary between the anterior and posterior portions. Observe the lymph nodules, lingual tonsils, glands, and papillae. (After Braus.)

D. Circumvallate Papillae: These are extremely large circular papillae whose flattened surfaces extend above the other papillae (Fig 16–1). The 7–12 circumvallate papillae are distributed in the "V" region in the posterior portion of the tongue. Numerous mucous and serous (von Ebner) glands drain their contents into the deep groove that encircles the periphery of each papilla. This "moatlike" arrangement provides a continuous flow of fluid over the great number of taste buds present along the sides of this papilla. This flow of secretions is important in removing food particles from the vicinity of the taste buds so that they can receive and process new gustatory stimuli. In addition to the serous glands associated with this type of papilla, other small mucous and serous glands dispersed throughout the lining of the oral cavity act in the same way to prepare the taste buds in other parts of the oral cavity—epiglottis, pharynx, palate, etc—to respond to taste stimuli. The appearance and location of taste buds within the epithelium of the papillae are illustrated in Figs 10–3 and 10–4. The distribution of the various types of papillae on the surface of the tongue is illustrated in Fig 10–6.

THE PHARYNX

The pharynx represents a transition space between the oral cavity and the respiratory and digestive systems. It forms a communication between the nasal region and the larynx. The pharynx is lined by stratified squamous epithelium of the mucous type, except in those regions of the respiratory portions that are not subject to abrasion. In these latter areas, the epithelium is pseudostratified ciliated columnar with goblet cells.

The pharynx contains the tonsils (described in Chapter 15). The mucosa of the pharynx also has many small mucous glands in its dense connective tissue layer. Outside this layer are located the constrictor and longitudinal muscles of the pharynx.

THE TEETH & ASSOCIATED STRUCTURES

The teeth are disposed in 2 curved arches inserted in the maxillary and mandibular bones. Each

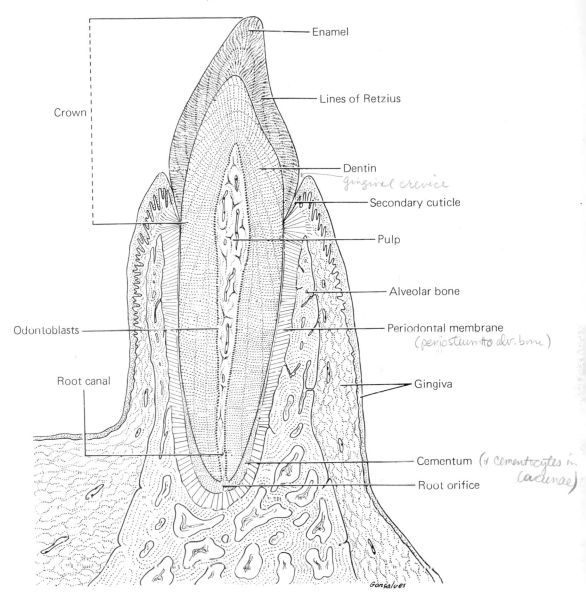

Figure 16–2. Diagram of a sagittal section from an incisor tooth in position in the mandibular bone. (Redrawn and reproduced, with permission, from Leeson TS, Leeson CR: *Histology,* 2nd ed. Saunders, 1970.)

tooth is composed of a portion that projects above the **gingiva** (or **gum**)—the **crown**—and a **root** below the gingiva which holds the tooth in a bony socket called the **alveolus,** one for the root of each tooth (Fig 16–2).

The point of transition from crown to root is the **neck.** The first **deciduous teeth** are gradually replaced by **permanent teeth.** Both are similar in structure and are composed of a nonmineralized portion—the **pulp**—and 3 mineralized portions—the **enamel, dentin,** and **cementum** (Fig 16–2).

Each tooth has a central cavity—the **pulp cavity**—which has roughly the same shape as the tooth. In the region of the roots, this cavity extends to the apex of the root and forms an orifice through which pass the blood vessels and nerves of the tooth. The **periodontal membrane** or **ligament** is a collagenous fibrous structure surrounding the cementum of the root, helping to fix the tooth firmly in its bony socket.

The dentin is covered by enamel in the crown of the tooth and by cementum in its roots (Fig 16–2).

Dentin

Dentin is a calcified tissue similar to bone but harder because of its higher content of calcium salts. It is composed mainly of collagen fibers, glycosaminoglycans, and calcium salts (80% of dry weight) in the form of crystals of hydroxyapatite. Its

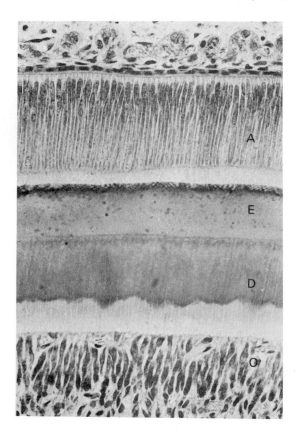

Figure 16–3 (at left). Photomicrograph of a section of an immature tooth, showing dentin (D) and enamel (E). The ameloblasts (A) and the odontoblasts (O) are both disposed as palisades. Masson's stain, × 350.

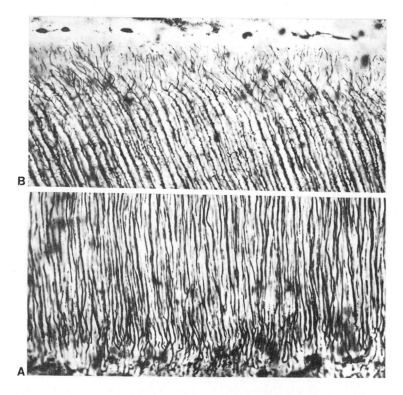

Figure 16 –4. Photomicrograph of a section of a tooth, showing the Tomes fibers of the dentin. *A:* Initial portion. *B:* Terminal portion. These fibers gradually get thinner and terminate by branching into delicate extensions. × 400.

organic matrix is synthesized by the **odontoblasts,** cells which line the internal surface of the tooth, separating it from the pulp cavity (Figs 16–3 and 16–5). Unlike the osteoblast, the odontoblast is a polarized, slender cell, producing organic matrix only at the dentinal surface. The cytoplasm of each of these cells contains a nucleus at its base, a large Golgi apparatus, and many ribosomes, both free and attached to granular endoplasmic reticulum, and has a slender extension that penetrates perpendicularly through the entire width of the dentin, forming the **Tomes fibers.** These fibers gradually become longer as the dentin becomes thicker, running in small canals called the **dentinal tubules.** The Tomes fibers initially have a diameter of 3–4 μm, gradually become thinner, and end by branching near the junction between the dentin and the enamel (Fig 16–4). The periodontoblastic space between the process of the cell and the tubule is full of tissue fluid.

The mineralization of the developing dentin begins by deposition of calcium salts in globules which gradually fuse together. This process is not complete, and noncalcified or partially calcified regions frequently remain between the globules as **interglobular spaces.** Dentin is sensitive to many stimuli such as heat, cold, acids, and trauma, and responds to all painful stimuli. Nerve fibers are very scarce in the dentin, and it may be that the Tomes fibers act as receptors and transmit the impulses to the pulp tissue, which is richly innervated. In contrast to bone, dentin persists as a mineral for a long time after destruction of the odontoblasts. It is thus possible to maintain teeth whose pulp and odontoblasts have been destroyed by infection. In adult teeth, destruction of the covering enamel due to erosion by wearing usually triggers a reaction in the dentin that causes it to resume the synthesis of its components. Thus, production of newly formed, usually irregular dentin can be observed on the wall of the pulp cavity.

Enamel

Enamel is the hardest structure of the body and the richest in calcium. It contains about 97% calcium salts and 3% organic material. It is of epithelial ectodermal origin, whereas the other structures of the teeth derive from mesoderm. The organic matrix is not composed of collagen fibers, and its main component is a protein in the cross β configuration, rich in proline. Mature enamel can only be studied in preparations obtained by grinding because the organic matrix collapses when decalcified and cannot be embedded and sectioned. However, it can be studied in growing teeth, where enamel is incompletely calcified.

Enamel matrix is secreted by cells called **ameloblasts.** The cells of the inner dental epithelium of the developing dental organ differentiate into ameloblasts (Fig 16–3), which have the organelles necessary for the secretion of the organic

matrix and which later become mineralized as in other hard tissues of the body. Dentin appears first between the ameloblasts and odontoblasts and extends down the dental papilla. This first soft fibrillar dentin is called **predentin.** A broad apical process of the cell (Tomes process) is embedded in the enamel matrix. When the enamel is fully calcified, the ameloblasts become small cuboidal cells and atrophy and disappear after forming the enamel cuticle that covers the external surface of the enamel.

Enamel is composed of elongated hexagonal rods or columns of structures in the shape of prisms—**enamel prisms**—bound together by an interprismatic substance. Each rod extends through the entire thickness of the enamel layer. Both enamel and cementing substance are heavily calcified. Starting from the dentin, they run perpendicular to the surface of the tooth. In the mid region, they are spiral and then become perpendicular again. In the lateral crown, prisms are disposed in horizontal planes.

Pulp

Tooth pulp consists of a loose type of connective tissue. Its main components are thin collagen fibers arranged asymmetrically plus a ground substance containing glycosaminoglycans. In young

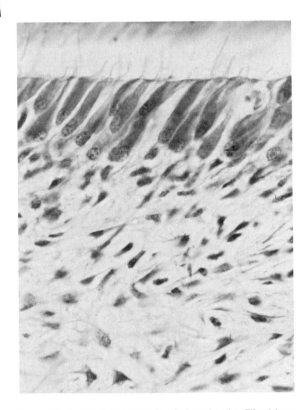

Figure 16–5. Photomicrograph of dental pulp. Fibroblasts are abundant. In the upper region are the odontoblasts, from which the Tomes fibers derive. H&E stain, × 400.

teeth, these fibers are nonexistent or scarce. Reticular fibers are present (Fig 16–5).

Pulp is a highly innervated and vascularized tissue. Numerous fibroblasts are present. Blood vessels and myelinated nerves extend through an orifice in the apex of the root and divide into numerous branches. Some nerve fibers lose their myelin sheath and extend for a short distance into the dentinal tubules. Surrounding the pulp and separating it from the dentin are the odontoblasts (Fig 16–5).

Associated Structures

The structures responsible for maintaining the teeth in the maxillary and mandibular bone consist of the **cementum, periodontal membrane, alveolar bone,** and **gingiva.**

A. Cementum: This tissue covers the dentin of the root and is similar in structure to bone, although Haversian systems and blood vessels are absent. It is thicker in the apical region of the roots, and in this area there are cells with the appearance of osteocytes, the **cementocytes.** Like osteocytes, they are encased in lacunas that communicate through canaliculi. Like bony tissue, cementum is labile and reacts by resorption or production of new tissue according to the stresses to which it is subjected. When periodontal membrane is destroyed, the cementum undergoes necrosis and may be resorbed. Continuous production of cementum compensates for the normal growth which teeth undergo. This process maintains a close contact between the roots of the teeth and their sockets.

B. Periodontal Membrane: Periodontal membrane is composed of a special type of dense connective tissue whose fibers penetrate the cementum of the tooth and bind it to the bony walls of its socket—permitting, however, limited movements of the tooth. It serves as periosteum to the alveolar bone. Its fibers are so organized that the pressures exerted during mastication are supported by them. This avoids transmission of pressure directly to the bone—a process that would cause localized resorption of this structure.

The collagen of the periodontal membrane has characteristics that resemble those of immature tissue. It has a high protein turnover rate (as demonstrated by radioautography) and a large content of soluble collagen. The space between its fibers is filled with glycosaminoglycans. This high rate of collagen renewal in the periodontal membrane allows processes affecting protein or collagen synthesis—eg, protein or vitamin C deficiency—to cause atrophy of this membrane. As a consequence, teeth become loose in their sockets and in extreme cases may fall out. This relative plasticity of the periodontal membrane is important because it allows orthodontic intervention, which can produce extensive changes in the disposition of teeth in the mouth.

C. Alveolar Bone: This portion of bone is in immediate contact with the periodontal membrane. It is an immature bone in which the collagen fibers are not arranged in the typical lamellar pattern present in adult bone. Many of the collagen fibers of the periodontal membrane are arranged in bundles that penetrate into this bone and the cementum, forming a connecting bridge between these structures. The bone closest to the roots of the teeth forms the socket. Vessels and nerves run through this alveolar bone and foramens of the root to enter the pulp.

D. Gingiva: The gingiva is mucous membrane firmly bound to the periosteum of the maxillary or mandibular bone. It is composed of stratified squamous epithelium and numerous connective tissue papillae. This epithelium binds itself to the tooth enamel by means of its basement membrane and forms the **epithelial attachment of Gottlieb.** Between the enamel and the epithelium is a small deepening surrounding the crown called the gingival crevice. These epithelial cells are fixed to the basement membrane by hemidesmosomes.

GENERAL STRUCTURE OF THE DIGESTIVE TRACT

The entire gastrointestinal canal presents certain common structural characteristics. The digestive tract is composed of 4 principal layers: the **mucous layer (mucosa),** the **submucosa,** the **muscle layer,** and the **serous layer.** The structure of these layers is summarized below and illustrated in Fig 16–6.

The **mucous layer** is composed of (1) an **epithelial lining;** (2) a **lamina propria** of loose connective tissue rich in blood and lymph vessels and smooth muscle cells, sometimes containing also glands and lymphoid tissue; and (3) **muscularis mucosae,** a continuous thin layer of smooth muscle separating the mucosa from the submucosa.

Submucosa is composed of loose connective tissue with many blood and lymph vessels and a **submucosal** (also called **Meissner's) nerve plexus.** It may also contain glands and lymphoid tissue.

The **muscle layer** contains the following elements: (1) Smooth muscle cells, spirally oriented, divided into 2 sublayers according to the main direction the muscle cells follow. In the internal sublayer (close to the lumen), the orientation is generally circular; in the external sublayer, mostly longitudinal. (2) The myenteric (or Auerbach's) nerve plexus, which lies between the 2 muscle sublayers. (3) Blood and lymph vessels in the connective tissue between the muscle sublayers.

The **serosa** is a thin layer composed of (1) loose connective tissue, rich in blood and lymph vessels

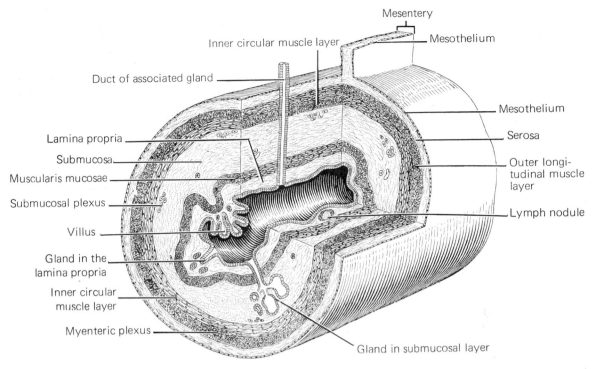

Figure 16–6. Schematic structure of a portion of the digestive tract with various possible components. (Redrawn and reproduced, with permission, from Bevelander G: *Outline of Histology,* 7th ed. Mosby, 1971.)

and adipose tissue; and (2) simple squamous covering epithelium (mesothelium).

The main functions of the mucosal epithelial lining of the digestive tract are (1) to provide a selectively permeable barrier between the contents of the tract and the tissues of the body; (2) to facilitate the transport and digestion of food; and (3) to promote the absorption of the products of this digestion. Cells in this layer either produce mucus or are involved in digestion or absorption of food.

The abundant lymphoid nodules present in the lamina propria and in the submucosal layer protect the organism (in association with the epithelium) from bacterial invasion. The necessity of this immunologic support is obvious if one considers that—with the exception of the oral cavity, esophagus, and anal canal—the entire digestive tract is lined by a simple thin and vulnerable epithelium. Careful study of the lamina propria has demonstrated that there is a a zone rich in macrophages and lymphoid cells just below the epithelium. Some of these lymphoid cells actively produce gamma globulins, ie, antibodies. These antibodies are mainly of immunoglobulin class A (IgA) and are bound to a secretory protein present in the epithelial cells of the intestinal lining and secreted into the intestinal lumen. This complex is thought to have a protective activity against viral and bacterial invasion. It is significant that the population of secretory, IgA-producing cells in this region is much higher (180,000/μL of lamina propria) than the population of IgG- and IgM-producing cells (18,000–30,000/μL).

The muscularis mucosae promotes the movement of the mucous layer independently of other movements of the digestive tract and, as a consequence, increases its contact with the food. The contractions of the muscle layer propel and mix the food in the digestive tract. Nerve plexuses coordinate this muscular contraction. They are composed mainly of nerve cell aggregates (multipolar visceral neurons) forming small parasympathetic ganglia. A rich network of pre- and postganglionic fibers of the autonomic nervous system and some visceral sensory fibers in these ganglia permit communication between them. The number of these ganglia along the digestive tract is variable. They are more numerous in regions where motility is greatest.

In certain diseases such as Hirschsprung's disease or *Trypanosoma cruzi* infection (Chagas' disease), the digestive tract plexuses are severely injured and most of their neurons are destroyed. This results in disturbances of digestive tract motility with frequent dilatations in some areas. The fact that the digestive tract receives abundant innervation from the autonomic nervous system provides an anatomic explanation of the widely observed action of emotional disturbances on the digestive tract—a phenomenon of importance in psychosomatic medicine.

ESOPHAGUS

This part of the gastrointestinal tract is a muscular tube whose function is to transport foodstuffs from the mouth to the stomach. It is covered by nonkeratinized stratified squamous epithelium (Fig 16–7). In general, it has the same layers as the rest of the digestive tract. In the submucosa are groups of small mucus-secreting glands, the **esophageal glands.** In the lamina propria of the region proximal to the stomach are groups of glands called **esophageal cardiac glands.** At the distal end of the esophagus the muscular layer consists of only smooth muscle cells; in the mid portion, a mixture of striated and smooth muscle cells; and at the proximal end, only striated muscle cells.

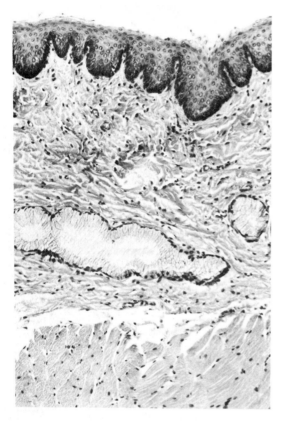

Figure 16–7. Photomicrograph of a section of the upper region of the esophagus. Mucous glands are in the submucosa; striated muscle in the muscle layer. H&E stain, × 20.

STOMACH

The stomach is a dilated segment of the digestive tract whose main function is to add fluid to the ingested food, transforming it into a viscous pulp and continuing the process of digestion. Three regions with different histologic structures can be observed in this organ: the **cardiac body** and **fundus** and the **pylorus** (Fig 16–8). The lining epithelium of all 3 regions consists of columnar mucus-secreting (PAS-positive) cells distinguished from goblet cells by their nuclei, which are not flattened at the base of the cells but are round and in the center. The surface of the stomach is characterized by the presence of ridges or folds called **rugae.** Within the folds, depressions or invaginations of its lining epithelium penetrate the lamina propria, forming microscopic furrows called **gastric pits** or **foveolae gastricae.** Throughout the entire mucosa, a number of small gastric glands, deeply situated in the lamina propria, open into the bottom of these pits. Each of the 3 regions of the stomach contains gastric glands of different structure, whereas the gastric pits have the same morphology in all parts of the stomach. The gastric glands lie in the lamina propria and never extend through the muscularis mucosae into the submucosa. The lamina propria of the stomach is composed of loose connective tissue interspersed with smooth muscle and lymphoid cells.

Various organizations of the mucosa lining the different parts of the stomach are discussed below.

Cardiac Region

The cardia is a narrow circular band at the transition between the esophagus and the stomach (Fig 16–8). Its lamina propria contains simple or branched tubular cardiac glands. The terminal portion of these glands is frequently coiled and often presents a large lumen. Their secretory cells produce mucus. These glands are similar in structure to the cardiac glands of the terminal portion of the esophagus and contain (and probably secrete) the enzyme lysozyme.

Body & Fundus

The lamina propria of these areas is filled with characteristic branched tubular **gastric glands** opening into the bottom of the gastric pits. Cellular population and organization within these glands are not uniform (Figs 16–8 and 16–9). It is customary to regard them as consisting of 3 regions from the end of the gastric pit to the base of the gland: the isthmus, the neck, and the base. Six different types of cells are present whose aspect, function, and location in the gland will be described: (1) isthmus mucous cells, (2) parietal (oxyntic) cells, (3) mucous neck cells, (4) chief (zymogenic) cells, (5) argentaffin cells, and (6) cells producing glucagonlike substance.

(1) **Isthmus mucous cells** (Figs 16–8 and 16–9) are present in the upper region of the gland in the transitional region between the neck and the gastric pits. These cells are continuous with and similar to the covering epithelium of the stomach, but they are lower and have fewer mucous granules in their cytoplasm. They secrete a neutral mucus that lines

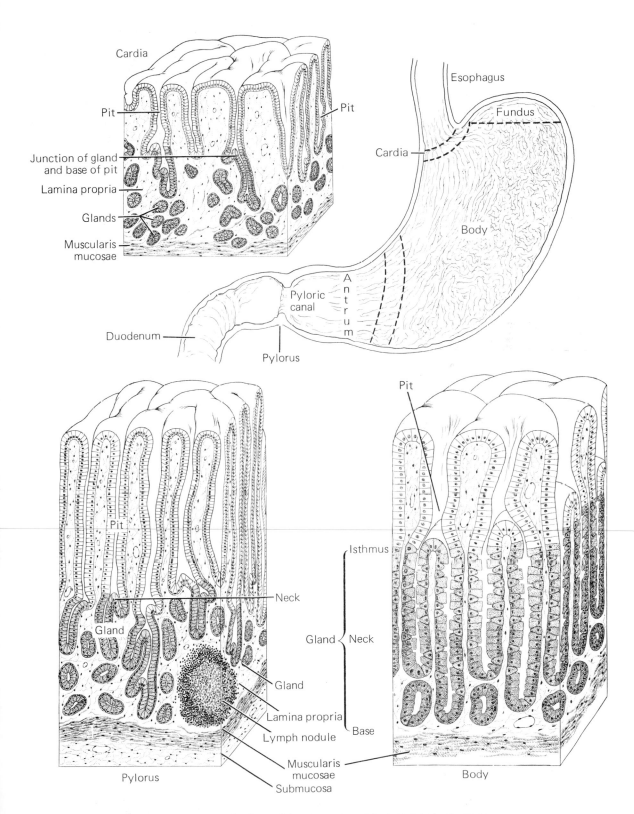

Figure 16–8. Regions of the stomach and their histologic structure.

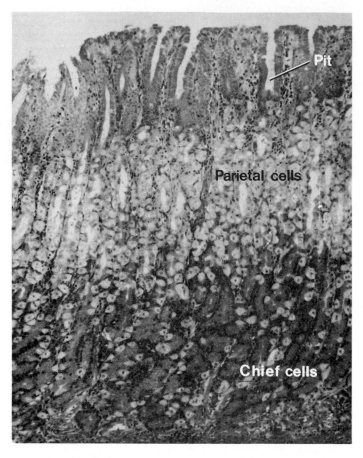

Figure 16 –9. Photomicrograph of a section of a gastric gland in the fundus of the stomach. Parietal (light) cells predominate in the upper region of the gland; chief (dark) cells (zymogenic cells) predominate in the lower region. H&E stain, × 100.

and protects the surface from secreted acid. They probably derive from mitotic activity of small undifferentiated cells in the neck region.

(2) The **parietal (oxyntic) cells** are present mainly in the upper half of the gland and are intercalated between mucous neck cells (Figs 16–8 and 16–9). They are scarcer in the gland's base. They are rounded or pyramidal cells with central spherical nuclei and intensely eosinophilic cytoplasm. When observed in the electron microscope, they present the following characteristics: (a) A deep circular invagination into the apical cytoplasm provides for the presence of **intracellular canaliculi.** (b) The eosinic cytoplasm possesses a great number of mitochondria with abundant cristae, a discrete Golgi apparatus near the cell base, and no secretory granules (Figs 16–10 and 16–11). (c) In the resting cell a number of tubulovesicular structures can be seen in the apical region of the cell just below its plasmalemma (Fig 16–10, left side). When stimulated to produce hydrochloric acid, these tubulovesicles fuse with the cell membrane and form microvilli that bulge into the cytoplasmic invagination (Fig 16–10, right side). Actin filaments, present between these tubulovesicles, probably

play a role in the extrusion of these structures.

Parietal cells produce the hydrochloric acid present in gastric juice. In human disease, the number of parietal cells is correlated with the acid-producing capacity of the stomach. In cases of atrophic gastritis, both parietal and chief cells are much less numerous, and the gastric juice has little or no acid or pepsin activity.

Parietal cells secrete 0.16 M hydrochloric acid, 0.07 M potassium chloride, traces of other electrolytes, and practically no organic matter. They deal mainly, therefore, with ions. There is evidence that the acid secreted originates from chlorides present in the blood plus a cation (H^+) resulting from the action of an enzyme—**carbonic anhydrase.** Carbonic anhydrase acts on CO_2 to produce carbonic acid, which dissociates into bicarbonate and one H^+. Both the cation and the chloride ion are actively transported across the cell membrane whereas water would diffuse passively along the osmotic gradient (Fig 16–13). The presence of abundant mitochondria in the parietal cells indicates that their metabolic processes are highly energy-consuming. As a matter of fact, this cell type presents histochemical pecularities that characterize it

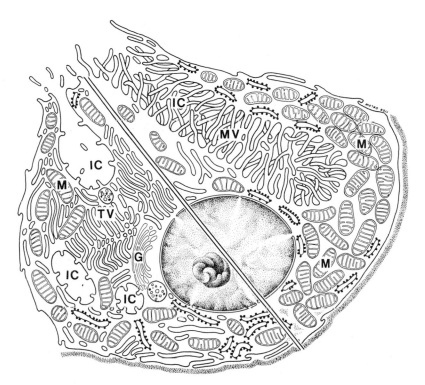

Figure 16–10. The parietal cell. Composite diagram showing the ultrastructural differences between a resting (left) and active (right) cell. Observe that the tubulovesicles (TV) present in the cytoplasm of the resting cell fuse with the plasmalemma to form the microvilli (MV) that extend into the intracellular canaliculi (IC). Golgi apparatus (G). Mitochondria (M). (Based on the work of Ito S, Schofield GC: J Cell Biol 63:346, 1974.)

as one of the cells with the highest observable energy metabolism.

Radioautographic studies performed with labeled vitamin B_{12} suggest that the parietal cells are, in humans, the site of production of **intrinsic factor**, a glycoprotein that binds avidly to vitamin B_{12}. In other species, however, this substance may be present in other cells.

The presence of intrinsic factor is normally required for vitamin B_{12} absorption, and this vitamin binds strongly in the lumen of the stomach with intrinsic factor. This complex is absorbed by the cells in the ileum. This explains why lack of intrinsic factor can lead to vitamin B_{12} deficiency—a disease that results in a disorder of the red blood cell-forming mechanism known as **pernicious anemia** and is usually caused by **atrophic gastritis.** In a high percentage of cases, pernicious anemia seems to be an autoimmune disease, since antibodies against parietal cell proteins are often detected in the blood of patients with the disease.

The secretion of parietal cells is activated by different mechanisms. One is through cholinergic nerve endings. Histamine and a polypeptide **gastrin,** both secreted in the gastric mucosa, act strongly to stimulate the production of hydrochloric acid.

(3) **Mucous neck cells** are present in clusters or as single cells between parietal cells in the necks of the gastric glands. Despite being mucous cells, they have morphologic and histochemical characteristics that make their mucous secretions quite different from that of the surface-lining epithelial mucous cells. They are irregular in shape, having their nuclei at the base of the cell. In the electron microscope, they show interdigitations of their lateral surfaces and desmosomes. Their ovoid or spherical granules are near the apical surface and are stained intensely with PAS or mucicarmine. Unlike the neutral mucous secretions of the surface cells, the mucous neck cells secrete an acid mucus rich in glycosaminoglycans.

(4) **Chief (zymogenic) cells** (Fig 16–12) predominate in the lower region of the tubular glands and have all the characteristics of a protein-synthesizing and exporting cell. The granules present in their cytoplasm contain the inactive enzyme pepsinogen. Their basophilia is due to the large number of ribosomes present in the cytoplasm and on the granular endoplasmic reticulum (see Chapter 4). In humans, these cells produce the enzymes pepsin and lipase. When the inactive pepsinogen granule is released into the acid environment of the stomach, the enzyme is converted into the highly active proteolytic enzyme pepsin. Their lipolytic activity, however, is weak and of doubtful physiologic importance.

(5) **Argentaffin cells** are also called **entero-chromaffin cells** because of their affinity for chromium as well as silver salts. These cells are less numerous and are located at the base of the gland interspersed between zymogenic cells (Fig 16–12). In electron micrographs, they are characterized by the presence of abundant dense secretory granules that have a loosely fitting membrane (Fig 16–14). These granules are basally located and consequently close to the basal lamina and blood vessels. From their location, it appears that these granules are released into the lamina propria and not the gastric lumen. Their secretory product contains, at least in some cases, **5-hydroxytryptamine.** Their exact function is a matter of speculation. Cer-

tain tumors called **carcinoids** that derive from these cells have a high content of 5-hydroxytryptamine and produce symptoms similar to those of overdosage with this compound. The argentaffin cells are spread throughout the digestive tract and are endocrine unicellular glands. One might consider them as a diffuse endocrine gland. Evidence has been presented to support the concept of the existence of different types of argentaffin cells with different functions.

(6) Other endocrine cells that can be classified as **APUD** (amine precursor uptake and decarboxylation) **cells** are discussed in Chapter 4. The nature of these cells in the gastrointestinal tract (based on our current understanding) is discussed later in this

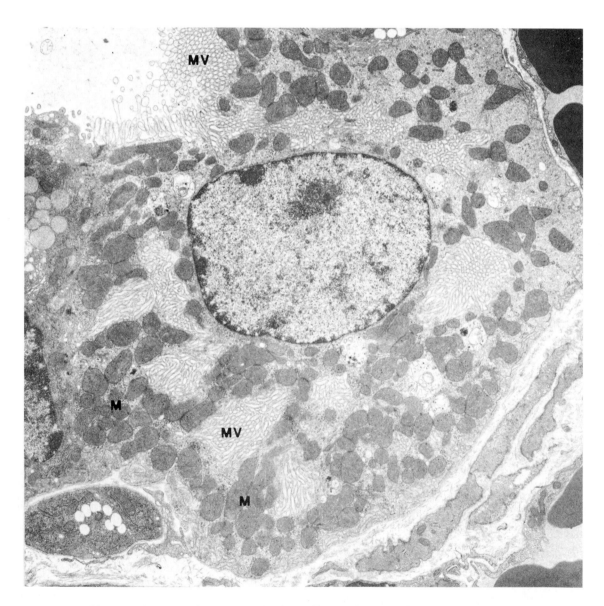

Figure 16–11. Electron micrograph of an active parietal cell. Observe the microvilli (MV) protruding into the intracellular canaliculi and abundant mitochondria (M). × 300. (Courtesy of S Ito.)

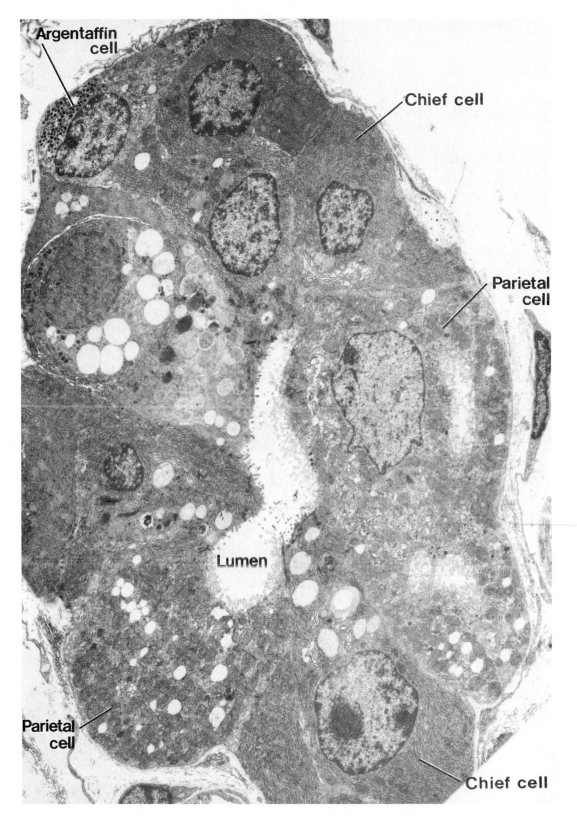

Figure 16–12. Electron micrograph of a section of gastric gland in the fundus of the stomach. Note the lumen and the parietal (containing abundant mitochondria), chief (extensive rough endoplasmic reticulum), and argentaffin (with secretory granules) cells. × 5300.

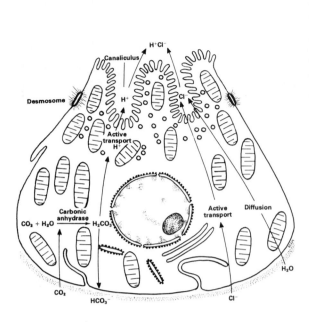

Figure 16–13. Diagram of a parietal cell, showing the main steps in the synthesis of hydrochloric acid. Blood CO_2 under the action of carbonic anhydrase produces carbonic acid, which dissociates into bicarbonate ion and a proton, H^+, which reacts with the chloride ion to produce hydrochloric acid. The tubulovesicles of the cell apex seem to be related to hydrochloric acid secretion since they decrease after parietal cell stimulation. The bicarbonate ion returns to the blood and is responsible for a measurable increase in blood pH during digestion.

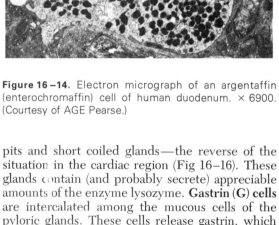

Figure 16–14. Electron micrograph of an argentaffin (enterochromaffin) cell of human duodenum. × 6900. (Courtesy of AGE Pearse.)

chapter (see Endocrine Cells of the Gastrointestinal Tract).

Pylorus

The pylorus presents deep gastric pits into which open tubular or ramified tubular glands, the **pyloric glands,** which are similar to the glands of the cardiac region. In the pyloric region are found long pits and short coiled glands—the reverse of the situation in the cardiac region (Fig 16–16). These glands contain (and probably secrete) appreciable amounts of the enzyme lysozyme. **Gastrin (G) cells** are intercalated among the mucous cells of the pyloric glands. These cells release gastrin, which leads to release of acid secretions in the stomach glands.

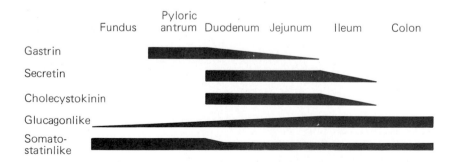

Figure 16–15. Distribution of gastrointestinal endocrine cells along the digestive tract. (Based on Grossman MI: Distribution of gastrointestinal APUD cells along the digestive tract. Proc Int Cong Endocrinol 2:1, 1976.)

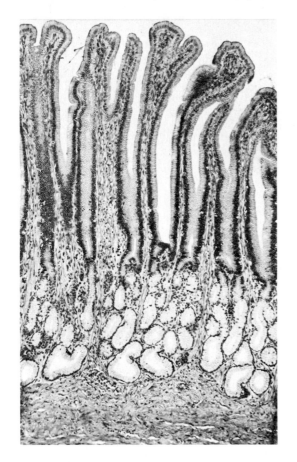

Figure 16–16. Photomicrograph of a section of the pyloric region of the stomach. Observe the deep gastric pits with short pyloric glands in the lamina propria. H&E stain. × 40.

Other Layers of the Stomach

The muscularis mucosae of the stomach is composed of 2 or 3 different layers. From this layer, perpendicular muscle fibers penetrate into the lamina propria; when they contract, folds are produced in the organ's internal surface. This contraction may also be important in compressing the glands of the stomach and eliminating their secretion.

The submucosa is composed of loose connective tissue and blood and lymph vessels and is infiltrated by lymphoid cells and mast cells. The muscularis externa is composed of spiral fibers oriented in 3 main directions: The external layer is longitudinal, the middle layer is circular, and the internal layer is oblique. The serous layer is thin and covered by mesothelium.

Turnover of Gastric Mucosa

In addition to replacing daily sloughed epithelial cells, the mucous membrane of the stomach can regenerate when injured. Mitotic activity is confined mainly to cells of the necks of the glands. From this region arise 2 lines of cells. One is directed toward the surface of the mucous membrane and becomes differentiated into the mucous epithelial lining. This process is constant and relatively rapid. The rate of renewal of these epithelial cells is about 5 days. The epithelial lining of the stomach is short-lived, and cells are constantly shed into the lumen.

The other line of cells derived from mitosis of neck cells flows in an opposite direction. These slowly differentiate into parietal and chief (zymogenic) cells. This is a slow process, and regeneration of the secretory portion of the gastric glands is correspondingly slow.

THE SMALL INTESTINE

In the small intestine, the processes of digestion are completed and the products of digestion are absorbed. The small intestine is relatively long—approximately 6 m—and this permits prolonged contact between food and digestive enzymes, as well as between the digested products and the absorptive cells of the epithelial lining. The small

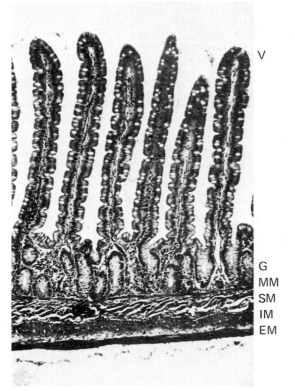

Figure 16–17. Photomicrograph of the small intestine. Observe the villi (V), the intestinal glands (G), muscularis mucosae (MM), submucosa (SM), and the external and internal muscle layers (EM and IM). H&E stain. × 40.

intestine consists of 3 segments: **duodenum,
jejunum,** and **ileum.** The 3 segments have many
characteristics in common and will be discussed
together.

Mucous Membrane of the Small Intestine

Grossly, the lining of the small intestine shows
a series of permanent folds, <u>plicae circulares</u> or
valves of Kerckring, consisting of mucosa and submucosa and having a semilunar, circular, or spiral
form. The plicae are most developed in, and consequently a characteristic of, the jejunum. Although frequently present, they do not constitute a
significant feature of the duodenum and ileum.
Under magnification, **intestinal villi** are seen.
These structures, 0.5–1.5 mm long, are outgrowths
of the mucosa (epithelium plus lamina propria) projecting into the lumen of the small intestine. In the
duodenum they are leaf-shaped, gradually assuming the form of a finger as the ileum is reached (Figs
16–17 and 16–20).

Between the areas where villi insert into the

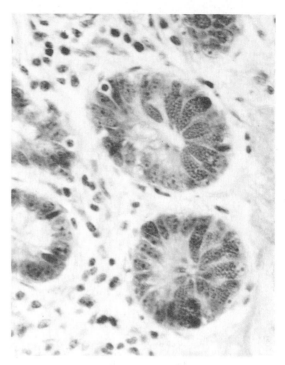

Figure 16–19. Section of the basal portion of the intestinal
glands showing the Paneth cells with their typical coarse
secretory granules.

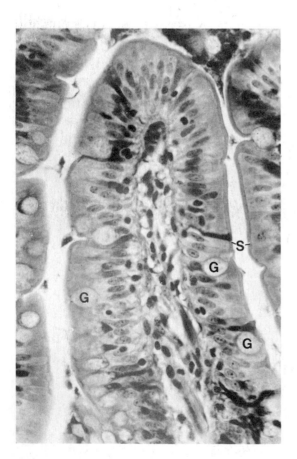

Figure 16–18. Photomicrograph of the tip of a villus of the
human ileum. Observe the connective tissue core with
blood and lymph vessels surrounded by the epithelial layer,
in which goblet cells (G) frequently occur. At right, the
striated border (S) formed by microvilli present on the surface of the cell is clearly visible. H&E stain, × 450.

mucous membrane are small openings of simple
tubular glands called **intestinal glands (crypts or
glands of Lieberkühn)** (Figs 16–17 and 16–20).
Analysis of transverse sections of the intestine
shows that there exists a continuity between the
epithelium of these glands and the epithelium that
covers the villi. The rate of renewal of the
epithelium of the villi is rapid, and the lining is
completely renewed every 2–4 days. The cells thus
formed gradually migrate upward in the direction of
the tips of the villi to be desquamated individually
(Fig 16–20). About 30 g of epithelium are shed
every day.

The epithelial cells of the entire gastrointestinal tract respond to certain stimuli (hormones, cholinergic neural activity) by production of new cells.
Cells of the basal layer of the esophageal
epithelium, of the isthmus between the gastric pits
and the glands, of the lower half of the Lieberkühn
glands, and of the lower third of the crypts of the
large intestine are easily labeled with tritiated
thymidine and consequently identified as proliferating cells. The villus increases or decreases in
size depending on the number of cells produced
and desquamated in the lumen (Fig 16–20A). From
this proliferative zone in each of the regions, the
cells move to the maturation area where they
undergo normal structural and enzymic maturation, providing the functional cell differentiation of
each region.

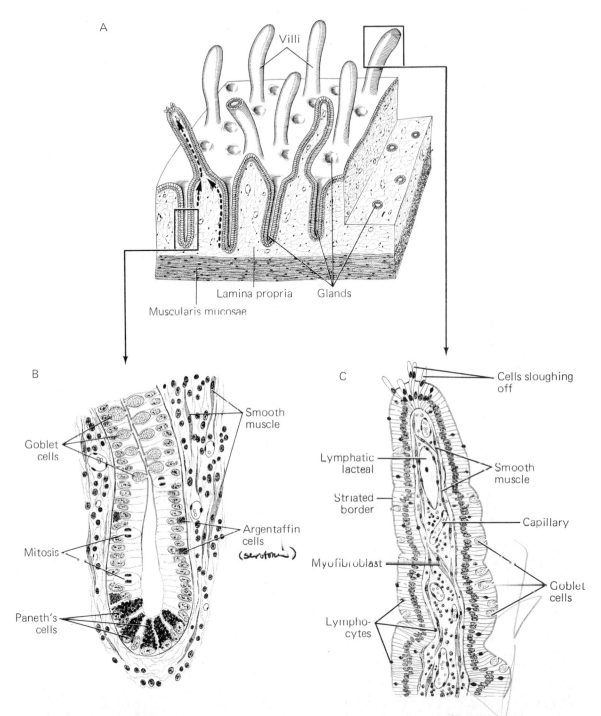

Figure 16–20. Schematic diagrams illustrating the structure of the small intestine. *A:* The small intestine under low magnification. In the villus to the left, observe the desquamation of epithelial cells. Because of constant mitotic activity of the cells from the blind end of the glands and the upward migration of these cells (dotted arrows), the intestinal epithelium is continuously renewed. Observe the glands of Lieberkühn. *B:* The intestinal glands present a lining of intestinal epithelium and goblet cells (upper portion). At a lower level, the immature epithelial cells are frequently seen in <u>mitosis</u>; note also the presence of Paneth and argentaffin cells. As the immature cells progress upward, they differentiate and develop microvilli seen as cuticle in the light microscope. Thus, in the blind end of these glands, cell proliferation and cell differentiation occur simultaneously. *C:* A villus tip seen with medium magnification, showing the columnar covering epithelium with its striated border and a moderate number of goblet cells. In the connective tissue core of the villus, capillaries, a lymphatic lacteal, smooth muscle cells, myofibroblasts, and leukocytes can be seen. Lymphocytes are in the epithelial layer in great numbers. (Redrawn and reproduced, with permission, from Ham AW: *Histology,* 6th ed. Lippincott, 1969.)

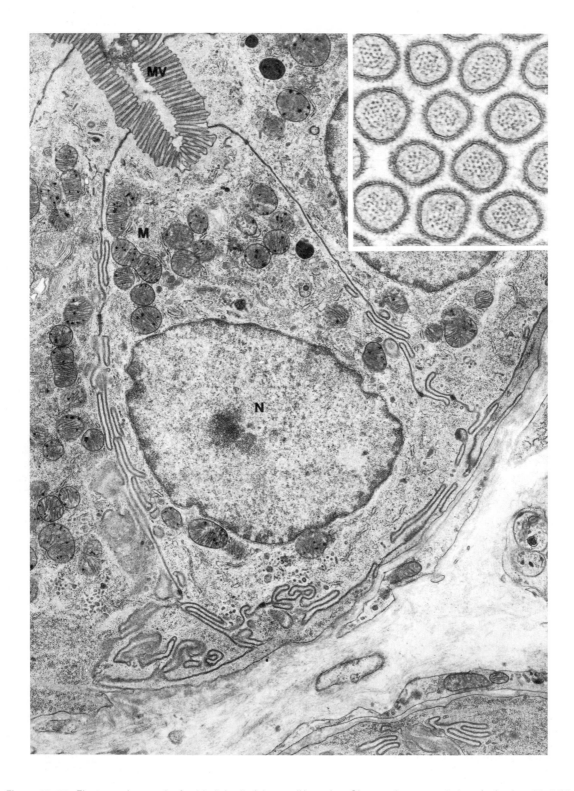

Figure 16–21. Electron micrograph of epithelial cell of the small intestine. Observe the accumulation of mitochondria (M) in their apexes. The luminal surface is covered with microvilli (MV) (shown in transverse section in the inset). Actin filaments, sectioned transversely, constitute the only structural feature in the core of the microvilli. N, nucleus. Reduced from × 8000. (Courtesy of KR Porter.)

In humans, the renewal rate of the epithelium in the esophagus is approximately 2–3 days; in the epithelial lining of the remainder of the intestinal tract, it is less than 5 days. This is probably one of the fastest rates of cell renewal in the body and explains why the intestine is promptly affected by the administration of antimitotic drugs, as in cancer chemotherapy. This replacement time contrasts with that of the parietal and chief cells of the stomach, which ranges from 1 year to many years.

The mucosa of the small intestine is lined with several types of cells. The most common are **columnar (absorptive) intestinal** epithelial cells, followed by **goblet cells, argentaffin cells, Paneth cells,** and **endocrine polypeptide-secreting cells.**

The **absorptive cells** are columnar cells characterized by the presence of a specialized apical surface called the **striated border** (Fig 16–18). With the aid of the electron microscope, the striated border can be seen to be a layer of densely grouped microvilli (Figs 16–21 and 16–22). It is estimated that each of these cells has an average of about 3000 microvilli and that 1 sq mm of mucosa contains about 200 million of these structures. Microvilli have the important physiologic function of considerably increasing the area of surface contact of the intestines with food. Studies performed by isolating the striated border of these cells by differential centrifugation and then applying immunofluorescence technics suggest that the striated border is the site of activity of the disaccharidases of the small intestine. These enzymes, bound to microvilli, hydrolyze the disaccharides into monosaccharides, which are easily absorbed. Deficiencies of these disaccharidases have been described in human diseases characterized by digestive disturbances. Some of these enzymatic deficiencies seem to be of genetic origin. An analogous localization has been postulated for dipeptidases that hydrolyze dipeptides into their component amino acids.

A more important function of the columnar intestinal cells is to absorb the metabolites that result from the digestive process. This is discussed further below.

Goblet cells are interspersed between the absorptive cells. They are less abundant in the duodenum and increase in number as the ileum is approached. They produce acid glycoproteins whose main function is to protect and lubricate the lining of the intestine.

Argentaffin cells (Fig 16–22) have already been described in the section on the stomach. More numerous in the basal portion of the intestinal glands, these cells may release 5-hydroxytryptamine, which stimulates the smooth muscle layer of the intestines and would greatly increase the motility of this organ.

Paneth cells in the basal portion of the intestinal glands are exocrine serous cells that synthesize a complex of protein and polysaccharide (described in Chapter 4). They have a well-developed granular

endoplasmic reticulum and Golgi apparatus. Researchers utilizing immunocytochemical methods have detected lysozyme—an enzyme that digests the cell wall of some bacteria—in the coarse secretory granules of these cells (Figs 16–19 and 16–20). It is postulated that lysozyme possesses antibacterial activity and may play a role in controlling the intestinal flora. Radioautographic studies have shown that the renewal rate of the Paneth cells is about 30 days—much slower than the rate of 5 days noted in the case of the mucous and absorptive cells of the intestinal lining.

Endocrine Cells of the Gastrointestinal Tract

In addition to the cells discussed above, the gastrointestinal tract contains a series of widely distributed **polypeptide-producing endocrine cells.** These have the characteristics of APUD cells (see Chapter 4) and are always located near the basal lamina of the gastrointestinal tract epithelium; their secretory granules are in the pole of the cell in contact with the basal lamina.

For the purpose of simplification, all of these cells will be considered at one time, without regard to location in the gastrointestinal tract. This subject is being actively studied at present. Better localization of several cell types will undoubtedly be achieved and new cell types discovered. The experimental results reported are summarized in Fig 16–15 and Table 16–1. It is apparent that cells having the characteristics of the APUD series and producing glucagon can be found throughout the mucosal lining of the stomach, whereas gastrin-producing cells are restricted to the pylorus. Cells with APUD characteristics but containing no identifiable peptide can be found in all parts of the stomach and intestines.

In the intestinal tract, cells have been identified that produce the following hormones: secretin (Fig 16–23), glucagon, somatostatin, and a gastric inhibitory peptide. Figure 16–23 illustrates a secretin-producing cell. The cells that produce **cholecystokinin**—a polypeptide known to be present in the intestine and of physiologic importance in stimulating contraction of the gallbladder and pancreatic secretion—have not been clearly identified. Although the picture of gastrointestinal endocrinology is still incomplete, it is clear that the activity of the digestive system is controlled by the nervous

Table 16—1. Polypeptide-secreting cells in the gastrointestinal tract.

Cell Type and Location	Hormone Produced
AL of the stomach	Glucagonlike substance
G of the stomach	Gastrin
S of the duodenum	Secretin
K of the duodenum	Gastric inhibitory polypeptide
EG of the intestine	Glucagonlike substance
D of the intestine	Somatostatin

Chapter 16. Digestive Tract

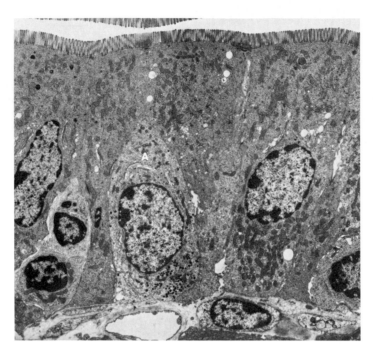

Figure 16 –22. Section of epithelium of small intestine. With the light microscope, abundant microvilli at the cell apex can be seen to form the striated border. At left are 2 lymphocytes migrating through the epithelium. In the center is shown an argentaffin absorptive cell (A) with its basal secretory granules. Reduced from × 3000.

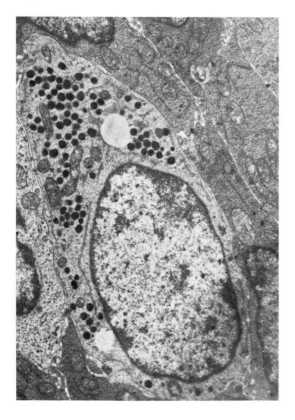

Figure 16 –23 (at left). A secretin-producing cell from dog duodenum. × 10,250. (Courtesy of AGE Pearse.)

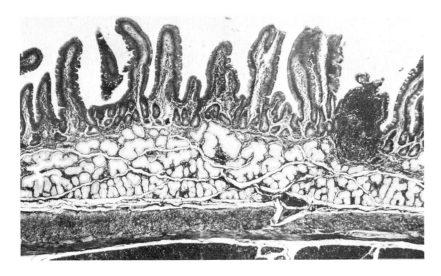

Figure 16–24. Photomicrograph of the duodenum, showing villi and duodenal glands in the submucosa. Dark structure at right is an intestinal tonsil; at the bottom are 2 smooth muscle layers of the muscularis. H&E stain, × 30.

system and modulated by a complex and efficient system of peptide hormones produced in cells derived embryologically from nerve tissue.

Lamina Propria Through Serosa

The lamina propria of the small intestine is composed of loose connective tissue and blood and lymph vessels, nerve fibers, and smooth muscle cells. Just below the basement membrane, a continuous layer of antibody-producing lymphoid cells and macrophages exists, forming an immunologic barrier at this region.

The lamina propria penetrates into the core of the intestinal villi, taking along blood and lymph vessels, nerves, connective tissue, myofibroblasts, and smooth muscle cells. The latter 2 cell types are responsible for the rhythmic movements of the villi, which are important for absorption.

The **muscularis mucosae** does not present any peculiarities in this organ. The **submucosa** contains, in the initial portion of the duodenum, clusters of ramified, coiled tubular glands that open into the intestinal glands. These are the **duodenal** (or **Brunner**) **glands** (Figs 16–24 and 16–25). Their cells are of the mucous type and produce in humans a neutral glycoprotein. The product of secretion of the glands is distinctly alkaline (pH 8.1–9.3), and it probably acts to protect the duodenal mucous membrane against the effects of the acid gastric juice and to bring the intestinal contents to the optimum pH for pancreatic enzyme action. By using immunofluorescence, it has been possible to show that Brunner gland cells contain **urogastrone,** a hormone that inhibits gastric hydrochloric acid secretion.

Besides the duodenal glands, the intestinal submucosa contains frequent isolated lymph nodules. Aggregations of these nodules form structures called **Peyer's patches**, intestinal tonsils wherein the nodules lie in direct contact with the intestinal epithelium. Peyer's patches are found in the ileum.

Vessels & Nerves of the Small Intestine
(Fig 16–26)

The blood vessels that nourish the intestine and serve to remove absorbed products of digestion penetrate the muscle layer and form a large plexus in the submucosa. From the submucosa, branches

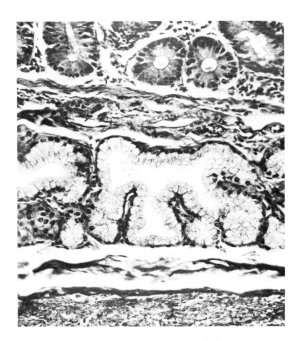

Figure 16–25. Details of the submucosal duodenal glands under higher manigification than that shown in Fig 16–24. H&E stain, reduced from × 200.

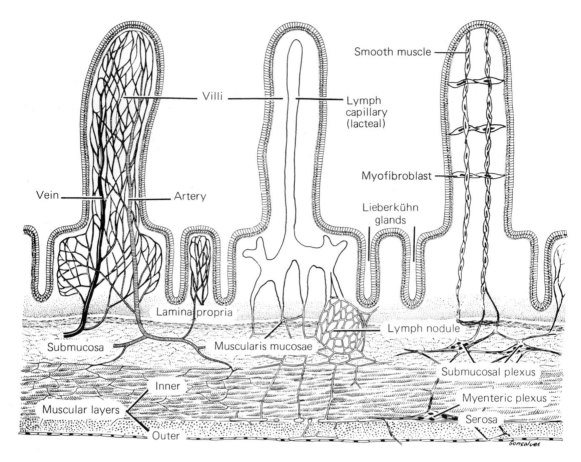

Figure 16–26. Diagram showing the blood circulation *(left)*, lymphatic circulation *(center)*, and innervation *(right)* of the small intestine. The smooth muscle–myofibroblast system for contracting and reextending the villi is illustrated in the villus on the right.

extend to the muscle layer, lamina propria, and villi. Each villus receives, according to its size, one or more branches that form a capillary network just below its epithelium. At the tips of the villi, one or more venules arise from these capillaries and run in the opposite direction, reaching the veins of the submucosal plexus. The lymph vessels of the intestine begin as blind tubes in the core of the villi. These structures, despite being larger than the blood capillaries, are difficult to observe because their walls are usually collapsed. These vessels run to the region of lamina propria above the muscularis mucosae, where they form a plexus. From there they are directed to the submucosa, where they surround lymph nodules. These vessels anastomose repeatedly and leave the intestine with the blood vessels.

The innervation of the intestines is formed mainly by an intrinsic and an extrinsic component. The intrinsic component is constituted by groups of neurons that form the **myenteric (Auerbach's) plexus,** present between the outer longitudinal and the inner circular muscle layers, and the **submucosal (Meissner's) plexus** in the submucosa. The

plexuses contain some sensory neurons that receive information from nerve endings near the epithelial layer and in the smooth muscle layer regarding the composition of the intestinal content (chemoreceptors) and the intestinal wall (mechanoreceptors). The other nerve cells are effectors and innervate the muscle layers and hormone-secreting cells. The intrinsic innervation formed by these plexuses is responsible for the intestinal contractions that occur in the total absence of the extrinsic innervation. The extrinsic innervation is formed by preganglionic parasympathetic cholinergic nerve fibers that stimulate the activity of the intestinal smooth muscle and by postganglionic sympathetic adrenergic nerve fibers that depress the intestinal smooth muscle activity.

HISTOPHYSIOLOGY

In the small intestine, the digestive process is completed and its products are absorbed. Lipid digestion occurs mainly as a result of the action of pancreatic lipase and bile. In humans, most of the lipid absorption occurs in the duodenum and upper jejunum. Figures 16–27 and 16–28 illustrate present concepts of this process of absorption.

The amino acids and monosaccharides derived from digestion of the proteins and carbohydrates are absorbed by the epithelial cells by active transport without visible morphologic correlates. In newborn animals, but apparently not in humans, transfer of undigested proteins from colostrum occurs as a result of pinocytotic processes in the cell apex. In this way, antibodies secreted into the colostrum can be transferred to the young animal—an important aspect of the immune defense mechanism. This capacity to transfer proteins is almost completely lost after a few days and is minimal in adults. In diseases marked by severe damage to epithelial cells, the transfer of undigested proteins to the blood increases considerably. The presence of folds, villi, and microvilli greatly increases the surface of the intestinal lining—an important characteristic in an organ where absorption occurs so intensely. It has been calculated that the presence of villi increases the intestinal surface 8-fold whereas the microvilli increase it 20-fold. Both of these processes are thus responsible for a 160-fold increase in the intestinal surface.

Another process that is probably of importance for intestinal function is the rhythmic movement of the villi. This is the result of the contraction of 2 separate cell systems. Smooth muscle cells running vertically between the muscularis mucosa and the tip of the villi can contract and shorten the villi (see villus at right in Fig 16–26). In order to extend the contracted villi, a network of contractile myofibroblasts span the villi from side to side (Fig 16–26). When these cells contract, the formerly contracted, squat villus extends to its original height. These asynchronous movements occur at the rate of several strokes per minute. During digestion, their rate increases; in fasting animals, the rate is much lower. These contractions also tend to empty the lymph vessels and propel the lymph and absorbed metabolites to the mesenteric lymphatics.

The filaments found in the microvilli (Figs 16–21 and 16–29) are composed of actin. Movement of the microvilli plays an important role in mixing the microenvironment—an important event in the process of metabolite absorption.

In disorders marked by atrophy of the intestinal mucosa due to infections or nutritional deficiencies, the absorption of metabolites is greatly hindered, producing the **malabsorption syndrome.**

Frequently, lymphocytes are seen between the intestinal epithelial cells. The widely held view that these cells migrate to the intestinal lumen where they are digested has been challenged, and some authors think that the lymphocytes in the intestinal epithelium migrate back to the lamina propria and from there return to the lymph vessels.

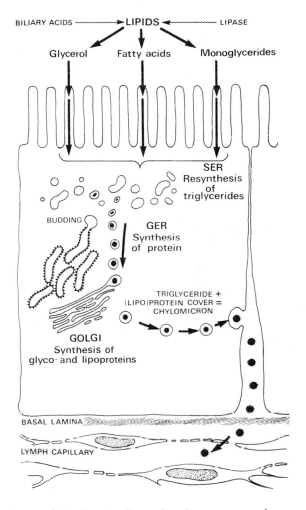

Figure 16–27. Drawing illustrating the sequence of processes that promote lipid absorption in the small intestine. Lipase promotes the hydrolysis of lipids to monoglycerides and fatty acids in the intestinal lumen. These compounds are stabilized in an emulsion by the action of biliary acids. The products of hydrolysis cross the microvilli membranes passively and are collected in the cisternae of the smooth endoplasmic reticulum, where they are synthesized back to triglycerides. These triglycerides are surrounded by a thin layer of proteins forming particles called chylomicrons (0.2–1 μm in diameter). These chylomicrons are transferred to the Golgi apparatus, and from there they migrate to the lateral membrane, cross it by a process of membrane fusion (reverse pinocytosis), and flow in the extracellular space in the direction of the blood and lymph vessels. Most chylomicrons go to the lymph and a few to the blood vessels. The long chain lipids (more than C_{12}) go mainly to the lymph vessels. Fatty acids of less than 10–12 carbon atoms are not reesterified to triglycerides but leave the cell directly and enter the blood vessels. GER, granular endoplasmic reticulum; SER, smooth endoplasmic reticulum. (Based on results published by Friedman HI, Cardell RR Jr in Anat Rec 188:77, 1977.)

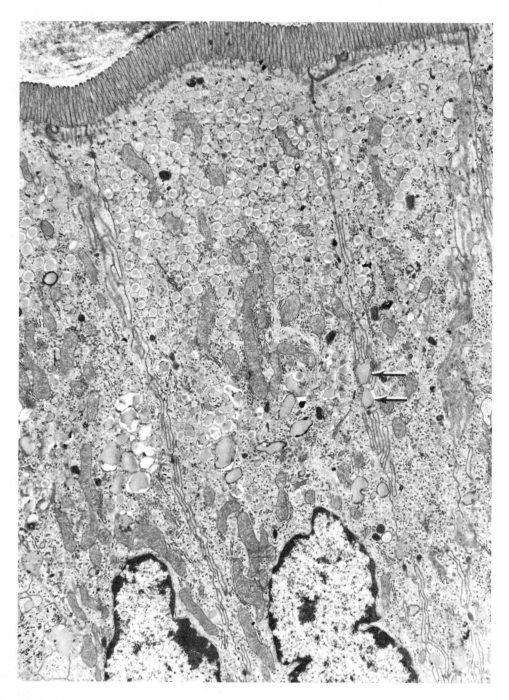

Figure 16–28. Electron micrograph of the intestinal epithelium in the lipid absorption phase. Observe the accumulation of lipid droplets in vesicles of the smooth endoplasmic reticulum. (Compare with Fig 16–21.) These vesicles fuse near the nucleus, forming larger lipid droplets that migrate laterally and cross the cell membranes to the extracellular space (arrows). × 5000. (Courtesy of HI Friedman.)

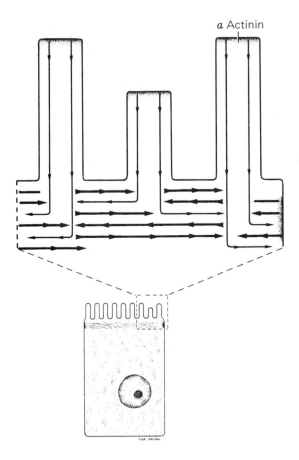

α Actinin

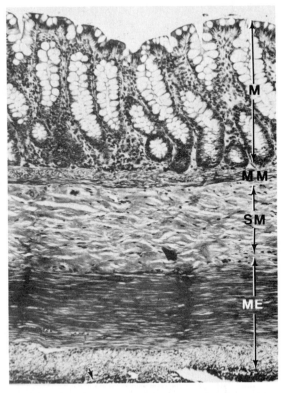

M

MM

SM

ME

Figure 16-30. Photomicrograph of a section of large intestine with its various layers. Observe the absence of villi. Mucosa (M), muscularis mucosa (MM), submucosa (SM), muscularis externa (ME), serosa (S). H&E stain, × 30.

Figure 16-29. Diagram illustrating the concept explaining the movements of microvilli. Upper drawing is an enlargement of part of the surface of an intestinal cell. The microvilli contain actin filaments (thin arrows) that interact with myosin filament (thick arrows) in the cell apex. The dense regions in the upper lateral wall contain α actin and are the probable site of insertion of the actin filaments. The localization of these 3 proteins was identified by using immunofluorescent cytochemistry. (Based on studies by Rodenwald R & others in J Cell Biol 70:541, 1976.)

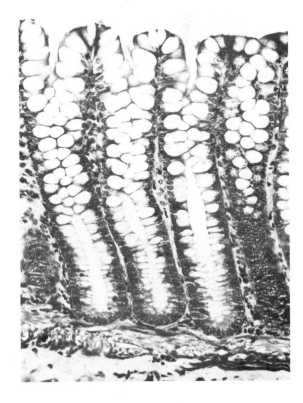

Figure 16-31 (at right). Photomicrograph of a section of large intestine. Observe the intestinal glands with abundant goblet cells. H&E stain, reduced from × 100.

THE LARGE INTESTINE

The large intestine consists of a smooth mucosal membrane with no folds except in its distal (rectal) portion. No villi are present in this portion of the intestine. The epithelial lining is columnar and has a thin cuticular region. The **intestinal glands of Lieberkühn** are long and characterized by a great abundance of goblet cells and a small number of argentaffin cells (Figs 16–30, 16–31, and 16–32). This organ is well suited to its main functions: water absorption and formation of the fecal mass plus production of mucus and lubrication of the mucosal surface.

The lamina propria is rich in lymphoid cells and nodules. The nodules frequently extend into and invade the submucosa. The muscle layer is composed of longitudinal and circular strands. This layer differs from the small intestine since fibers of the outer longitudinal layer congregate in 3 thick longitudinal bands called **teniae coli.** In the free portions of the colon, the serous layer is characterized by small pendulous protuberances composed of adipose tissue—the **appendices epiplociae** (Fig 16–33).

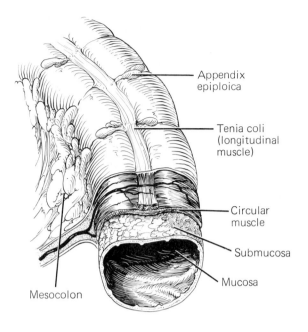

Figure 16 –33. Cross section of colon. (Reproduced, with permission, from Dunphy JE, Way LW [editors]: *Current Surgical Diagnosis & Treatment,* 4th ed. Lange, 1979.)

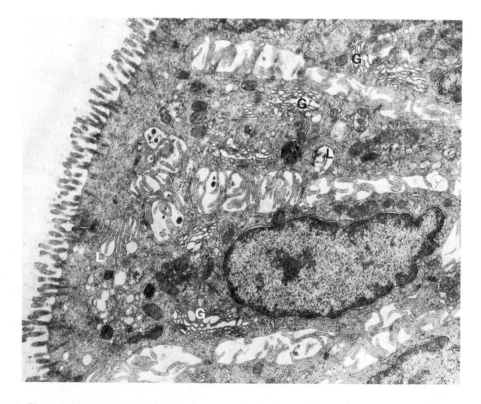

Figure 16 –32. Electron micrograph of epithelial cells of the large intestine. Observe the luminal surface of the microvilli, the well-developed Golgi apparatus (G), lysosomes (L), and dilated intercellular spaces filled by microvilli. Reduced from × 5000.

In the anal region, the mucous membrane presents a series of longitudinal folds, the **rectal columns of Morgagni.** About 2 cm above the anal opening, the intestinal mucosa is replaced by stratified squamous epithelium. In this region, the lamina propria contains a plexus of large veins that, when excessively dilated and varicose, produce hemorrhoids.

THE APPENDIX

The appendix is an evagination of the cecum characterized by a relatively small, narrow, and irregular lumen due to the presence of abundant lymphoid follicles in its wall. Its general structure is similar to that of the large intestine. However, it contains fewer and shorter intestinal glands and has no teniae coli (Fig 16–34).

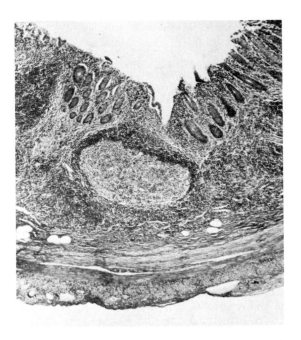

Figure 16 –34. Photomicrograph of a section of appendix. There are few glands and abundant lymphoid modules. H&E stain, × 20.

● ● ●

References

Anderson JH, Taylor AB: Scanning and transmission electron microscopic studies of jejunal microvilli of the rat, hamster, and dog. J Morphol 141:281, 1973.

Bortoff A: Myogenic control of intestinal motility. Physiol Rev 56:418, 1976.

Cardell RR Jr, Bandenhausen S, Porter KR: Intestinal triglyceride absorption in the rat. J Cell Biol 34:123, 1967.

Creamer B: Variations in small-intestinal villous shape and mucosal dynamics. Br Med J 2:1371, 1964.

Croft DN & others: DNA and cell loss from normal small-intestinal mucosa: A clinical method of assessing cell turnover. Lancet 2:70, 1968.

David H: The mechanism of desquamation of cells from the intestinal villi: An electron microscopic study. Virchows Arch [Pathol Anat] 342:19, 1967.

Deane HW: Some electron microscopic observations on the lamina propria of the gut, with comments on the close association of macrophages, plasma cells, and eosinophils. Anat Rec 149:453, 1964.

Doell RG, Rosen G, Kretchmer N: Immunochemical studies of intestinal disaccharidases during normal and precocious development. Proc Natl Acad Sci USA 54:1268, 1965.

Elder JB & others: Cellular localization of human urogastrone-epidermal growth factor. Nature 271:466, 1978.

Freeman JA: Goblet cell fine structure. Anat Rec 154:121, 1966.

Friedman HI, Cardell RR Jr: Alterations in the endoplasmic reticulum and Golgi complex of intestinal epithelial cells during fat absorption and after termination of this process. Anat Rec 188:77, 1977.

Fujita T, Kobayashi S: Structure and function of gut endocrine cells. Int Rev Cytol (Suppl):187, 1977.

Greco V & others: Histochemistry of the colonic epithelial mucins in normal subjects and in patients with ulcerative colitis. Gut 8:491, 1967.

Grossman MI: The gastrointestinal hormones: An overview. Proc Int Cong Endocrinol 2:18, 1976.

Hoedemseker PJ & others: Further investigations about the site of production of Castle's gastric intrinsic factor. Lab Invest 15:1163, 1966.

Hugon J, Borgers M: Fine structural localization of lysosomal enzymes in the absorbing cells of the duodenal mucosa of the mouse. J Cell Biol 33:212, 1967.

Ito S, Schofield GC: Studies on the depletion and accumulation of microvilli and changes in the tubulovesicular compartment of the mouse parietal cells in relation to gastric acid secretion. J Cell Biol 63:364, 1974.

Ito S, Winchester RJ: The fine structure of the gastric mucosa in the rat. J Cell Biol 16:541, 1963.

Klockars M, Reitamo S: Tissue distribution of lysozyme in man. J Histochem Cytochem 23:932, 1975.

Leaming DB, Cauna N: A qualitative and quantitative study of the myenteric plexus of the small intestine of the cat. J Anat 95:160, 1961.

Leblond CP, Messier B: Renewal of chief cells and goblet cells in the small intestine as shown by radioautography after injection of thymidine H[3] into mice. Anat Rec 132:247, 1958.

Leeson TS, Leeson CR: The fine structure of Brunner's glands in man. J Anat 103:263, 1968.

Lipkin M: Proliferation and differentiation of gastrointestinal cells. Physiol Rev 53:981, 1973.

Lorenzsonn V, Trier JS: The fine structure of human rectal mucosa: The epithelial lining of the base of the crypt. Gastroenterology 55:88, 1968.

MacDonald WC, Trier JS, Everett NB: Cell proliferation and migration in the stomach, duodenum, and rectum of man: A radioautographic study. Gastroenterology 46:405, 1964.

Marsh MN: Studies of intestinal lymphoid tissue. (2 parts.) Gut 16:665, 675, 1975.

Mattern CFT, Daniel WA, Henkin RI: The ultrastructure of the human circumvallate papilla. I. Cilia of the papillary crypt. Anat Rec 167:175, 1970.

McGuigan JE: Gastric mucosal intracellular localization of gastrin by immunofluorescence. Gastroenterology 55:315, 1968.

Mjör IA, Pindberg JJ: Histology of the Human Tooth. Munksgaard, 1973.

Mooseker MS, Tilney LG: Organization of an actin filament-membrane complex: Filament polarity and membrane attachment in the microvilli of intestinal epithelial cells. J Cell Biol 67:725, 1975.

Pearse AGE, Polak YM: Endocrine tumours of neural crest origin: Neurolophomas, apudomas and the APUD concept. Med Biol 52:3, 1974.

Pearse AGE, Riechen ED: Histology and cytochemistry of cells of small intestine. Br Med Bull 23:217, 1967.

Pfeiffer CJ, Rowden G, Weibel J: Gastrointestinal Ultrastructure. Academic Press, 1974.

Pick J, De Lemos C, Cianella A: Fine structure of nerve terminals in the human gut. Anat Rec 159:131, 1966.

Potten CS, Allen TD: Ultrastructure of cell loss in intestinal mucosa. J Ultrastruct Res 66:272, 1977.

Robertson RN: The separation of protons and electrons as a fundamental biological process. Endeavour 26:134, 1967.

Rodenwald R & others: Contraction of isolated brush borders from intestinal epithelium. J Cell Biol 70:541, 1976.

Rubin W & others: The normal human gastric epithelia: A fine structural study. Lab Invest 19:598, 1968.

Schade SG: Studies on antibody to intrinsic factor. J Clin Invest 46:615, 1967.

Solcia E & others: Endocrine cells of the gastric mucosa. Int Rev Cytol 42:223, 1975.

Tagaki T & others: Scanning electron microscopy on the human gastric mucosa; fetal, normal and various pathological conditions. Acta Pathol Jpn 24:233, 1974.

Troughton WD, Trier JS: Paneth cell and goblet cell renewal in mouse duodenal crypts. J Cell Biol 41:251, 1969.

Ugolev AM, Kooschuck KI: Hydrolysis of dipeptides in cells of the small intestine. Nature 212:859, 1966.

Glands Associated With the Digestive Tract | 17

The subjects of this chapter are the salivary glands, pancreas, liver, and gallbladder. The functions of the salivary glands are to wet and lubricate the oral cavity and its contents; to initiate the digestion of food; to promote the excretion of certain substances such as urea and thiocyanate; and to reabsorb sodium and excrete potassium.

The main functions of the pancreas are to produce digestive enzymes which act in the small intestine and to secrete the hormones insulin and glucagon into the bloodstream. The liver produces bile, an important fluid in the digestion of fats; plays a major role in lipid, carbohydrate, and protein metabolism; inactivates and metabolizes many toxic

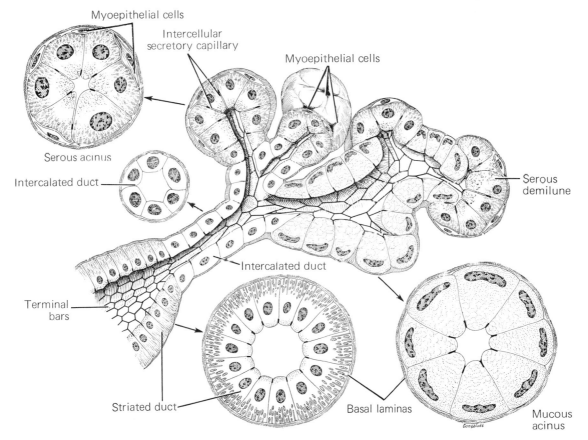

Figure 17–1. The structure of the submandibular (submaxillary) gland. In the secretory portion, acini are composed of pyramidal serous and mucous cells and tubules of mucous cells. In serous cells, the nuclei are euchromatic and rounded, and in the basal third of the cell an accumulation of granular endoplasmic reticulum (ergastoplasm) is evident. The cellular apex is filled with proteinaceous secretory granules. The nuclei of mucous cells are flattened with condensed chromatin and located near the bases of the cells; they have no ergastoplasm and present distinct secretory granules. The intercalated ducts are short and are lined by cuboidal epithelium. The striated ducts are composed of columnar cells with characteristics of ion-transporting cells (see Fig 17–6 and Chapter 4), such as basal membrane invaginations and mitochondrial accumulation. (After Braus.)

substances and drugs; and participates in iron metabolism and the synthesis of blood proteins and factors necessary for blood coagulation. The gallbladder reabsorbs water from the bile and stores the bile in a concentrated form.

THE SALIVARY GLANDS

Besides the small glands scattered throughout the oral cavity described in the previous chapter, 3 pairs of large salivary glands are present: the **parotid, submandibular (submaxillary)**, and **sublingual** glands.

They are composed of morphologic and functional units called **adenomeres.** An adenomere of the submandibular gland is illustrated in Fig 17–1. It has a secretory portion composed of glandular cells, conducting **intercalated** ducts, and **striated** ducts. Near the bases of the cells of the secretory portion and of the intercalated ducts, myoepithelial cells (described in Chapter 4) are present.

The large salivary glands are not mere collections of adenomeres but contain other components such as connective tissue, blood and lymph vessels, and nerves organized in a definite pattern.

These glands are surrounded by a capsule of connective tissue rich in collagen fibers. From this capsule, septa of connective tissue penetrate into the gland, dividing it into lobules. From these septa are derived fibers of connective tissue that individ-

ually involve the components of the adenomeres. Between these fibers and the cells, a distinct basal lamina can be observed under the electron microscope (Fig 17–1). The vessels and nerves enter the gland at the **hilum** and branch gradually to the lobules and adenomeres. A rich capillary network surrounds the components of the adenomeres. The striated ducts present in the lobules—also called **intralobular ducts**—converge and fuse into ducts in the septa separating the lobules, at which point they become **extralobular ducts.** These are characterized by an abundant sheath of connective tissue and a lining of stratified columnar epithelium that is gradually transformed into stratified squamous epithelium.

The specific characteristics of each of the major salivary glands will be considered individually.

Parotid Glands

The parotid gland is a branched acinous gland. Its secretory portion is composed almost exclusively of seromucous cells (Fig 17–2). These cells have a moderate amount of ribosomal RNA in their basal regions as compared to the pancreatic exocrine cell. In humans, in addition to having the characteristics of a serous cell, the secretory granules of these seromucous cells exhibit a positive periodic acid-Schiff (PAS) reaction indicating the presence of polysaccharides (sialomucin and sulfomucin) in these structures. The secretory granules (Fig 17–3) are rich in proteins and have a high amylase activity. The other components of this gland are similar to the general description just given. In humans, se-

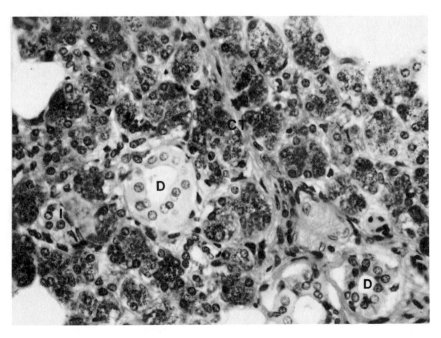

Figure 17–2. Photomicrograph of a human parotid section, showing acini and striated ducts (D). An intercalated duct (I) consisting of pale-staining cuboidal cells is present in the lower left of the section. A portion of the connective tissue septum (CT) separates the lobules. H&E stain, × 360.

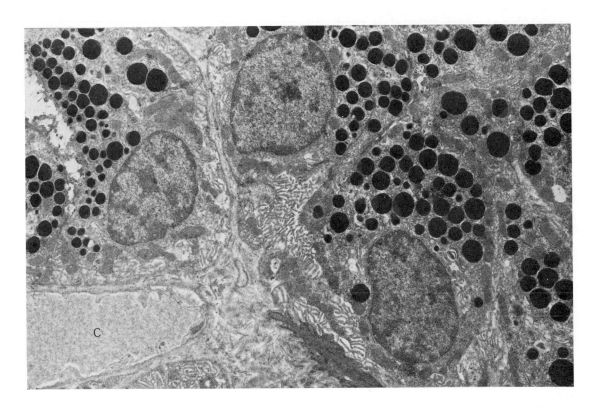

Figure 17 –3. Section of a parotid gland showing 3 nuclei of secretory cells and their characteristic secretory granules. At lower left is a fenestrated capillary (C). (Courtesy of LL George.)

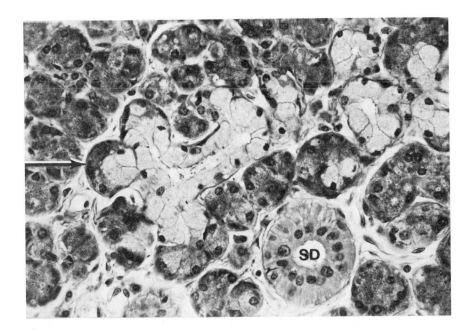

Figure 17 –4. Photomicrograph of a section of human submandibular gland. Observe the presence of dense serous and pale-staining mucous cells. In the lower right region is a striated duct (SD). The arrow shows a demilune where serous cells are eccentrically displaced, assuming the form of a crescent. H&E stain, × 360.

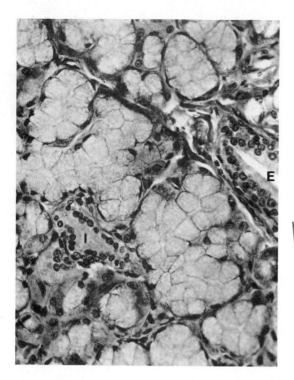

Figure 17–5. Photomicrograph of a human sublingual gland showing the predominance of mucous cells. Examples of an interlobular (I) and connective tissue–ensheathed extralobular (E) duct are also present. H&E stain, × 600.

cretory cells represent about 90% of the gland's cell volume; striated ducts account for about 5%; and the remainder consists of excretory ducts, connective tissue, vessels, nerves, etc. The encapsulating connective tissue is of the reticular type and contains many plasma cells and lymphocytes. The plasma cells secrete an immunoglobulin, IgA, which complexes with a proteinaceous **secretory piece,** probably synthesized by the seromucous acinar cells. The IgA-secretory piece complex released into the saliva is apparently resistant to enzymatic digestion and may constitute an immunologic defense mechanism against orally introduced pathogens. The bases of the cells of the striated ducts in salivary glands described in this chapter have the characteristics of ion-transporting cells (Figs 17–1 and 17–6).

Submandibular (Submaxillary) Glands

The submandibular gland is a branched tubuloacinar gland. Its secretory portion contains both pure mucous and seromucous cells. The seromucous cells contain protein secretory granules that are PAS positive due to the presence of carbohydrate moieties (sialomucin and sulfomucin). The seromucous cells are the main component and are easily distinguished from pure mucous cells by their rounded, euchromatic nuclei and basophilic, PAS-positive cytoplasm. The presence of extensive lateral and basal membrane infoldings toward the vas-

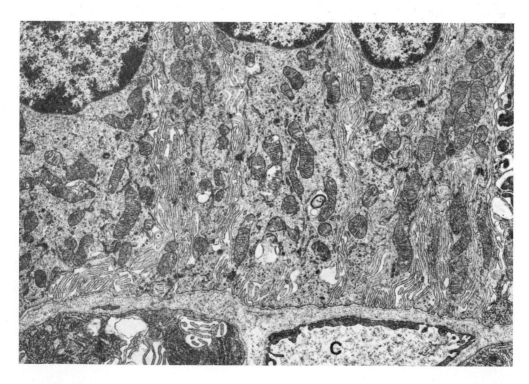

Figure 17–6. Electron micrograph of the basal portion of cells of a striated duct. Observe the membrane invaginations and mitochondria disposed in palisades, characteristics of ion-transporting cells. At the lower right is a fenestrated capillary (C). × 6000. (Courtesy of LL George.)

cular bed increase the ion-transporting surface area 60 times, thus facilitating electrolyte and water transport during primary secretion. As a consequence of these folds, the cell boundaries are indistinct. These cells are responsible for the weak amylolytic activity present in this gland and its saliva. The cells that form the demilunes in both the submandibular and sublingual glands contain and secrete the enzyme lysozyme, whose main activity is to hydrolyze the wall of bacteria. In humans, this gland consists of 80% serous cells, 5% mucous cells, and 5% striated ducts; the remainder consists of vessels, nerves, and other ducts.

Sublingual Gland

The sublingual gland is (like the submandibular gland) a branched tubulo-acinar gland. It presents, however, no acini formed exclusively by serous cells, and mucous cells predominate in the sublingual gland. Serous cells form demilunes on mucous acini. This gland consists of 60% mucous cells, 30% serous cells, and 3% striated ducts (Fig 17–5); the remainder consists of vessels, nerves, and other ducts.

Histophysiology of the Salivary Glands

Moistening and lubricating functions of the salivary glands are performed by the water and glycoproteins of saliva. The latter are synthesized mainly by the mucous cells and to a lesser degree by the serous cells of the glands. Human saliva consists of secretions from the parotid glands (25%), the submandibular glands (70%), and the sublingual gland (5%).

Another important function of these glands is the digestion of carbohydrates. The major part of the hydrolysis of ingested carbohydrates is due to salivary amylase activity. This digestion begins in the mouth but takes place also in the stomach before the gastric juice acidifies the food, thereby decreasing considerably amylase activity.

The function of the intercalated ducts, other than transport of saliva to larger ducts, is unknown, although in some species their cells contain secretory granules.

Studies performed by inserting micropipettes into the striated and excretory ducts strongly suggest that the saliva produced by the secretory cells—called **primary saliva**—has the same ionic

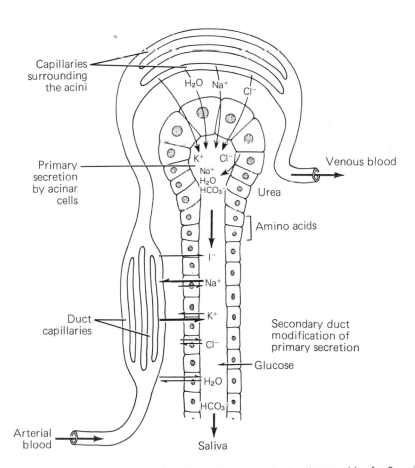

Figure 17–7. Schematic illustration of the characteristic blood vessel organization that provides for 2 capillary nets around the ducts and acini in the parotid. Primary saliva secretion occurs in the acini and subsequently becomes modified as it passes through the duct system. (From Davenport HW: *Physiology of the Digestive Tract*. Year Book, 1977.)

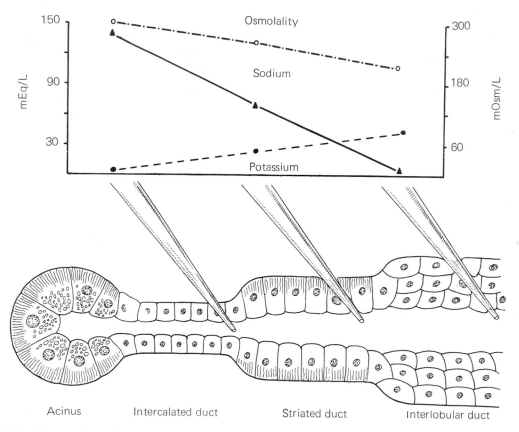

Figure 17 –8. Diagram illustrating the results obtained from micropuncture experiments in the salivary gland. When the puncture is close to the secretory portion in the intercalated duct, the sodium and potassium content and the osmolality of the saliva are equal to that observed in the blood. With gradual movement away from the intercalated ducts, the potassium content increases and sodium content and osmolality decrease. This strongly suggests that these changes are mediated by the epithelial lining of the ducts.

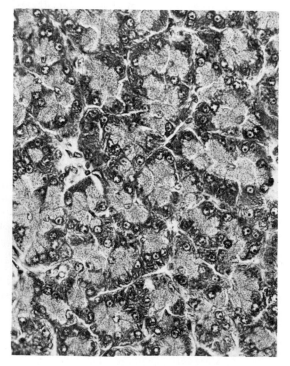

composition and is therefore isosmotic with blood. As it progresses through the striated and excretory ducts, the duct cells actively reabsorb sodium and excrete potassium (Fig 17–8). The ionic modification of saliva is facilitated by the double capillary network associated with the secretory and duct portions of the gland (Fig 17–7). This explains why saliva is hypotonic and has a higher concentration of potassium and a lower concentration of sodium than blood. The striated ducts bear morphologic and functional similarities to the renal tubules (Figs 17–6 and 20–9). Both have cells with characteristics of ion-transporting cells, and both are sensitive to aldosterone.

Human salivary glands, although sensitive to hormones, are controlled mainly by the sympathetic and parasympathetic nervous systems, both of which have nerve endings in these glands.

Figure 17 –9 (at left). Photomicrograph showing the appearance of the acinar portion of the pancreas with its secretory cells. H&E stain, × 400.

THE PANCREAS

The pancreas is a mixed exocrine and endocrine gland. The endocrine portion is composed of the **islets of Langerhans** (see Chapter 22). The exocrine portion is a compound acinar gland (Fig 17–9), similar in structure to the parotid. In histologic slides, a differential diagnosis can be made based on the absence of striated ducts and the presence of the islets of Langerhans in the pancreas. Another characteristic detail is that the initial portion of the intercalated ducts penetrate into the lumen of the acini. The central nuclei, diagnostic for the pancreatic acini, belong to the **centro-acinar cells** that constitute the intra-acinar portion of the intercalated duct (Fig 17–10). The intercalated ducts are tributary to larger interlobular ducts lined by columnar epithelium in which goblet cells can be observed.

The acinar cell in the human is a serous cell. It has all the characteristics of a protein-synthesizing cell as described in Chapter 4. In terms of RNA content, it is one of the richest cells of the body—a characteristic that coincides with its active protein-synthetic activity. Following their synthesis in the basal portion of the cell, the proenzymes leave the rough endoplasmic reticulum and enter the Golgi apparatus. The inactive enzymes are then concentrated in secretory vesicles known as **prozymogen granules.** Mature secretory granules, the **zymogen granules,** are membrane-bound and accumulate in the apical portion of the cell. In the rat, under conditions of maximal stimulation, the pancreas can produce up to 1.5% of its total proteins in 1 hour. The number of zymogen granules in its cells is variable and depends on the digestive phase, attaining its maximum in fasted animals.

The pancreas is covered by a thin capsule of connective tissue that sends septa into it, separating the pancreatic lobules. The acini are surrounded by a basal lamina supported by a delicate sheath of reticular fibers. It has a rich capillary network.

The human exocrine pancreas secretes, besides water and ions, the following enzymes and proenzymes: trypsinogen, chymotrypsinogen, carboxypeptidase, ribonuclease, deoxyribonuclease, lipase, and amylase.

The control of pancreatic secretion is performed mainly through 2 hormones—**secretin** and **cholecystokinin** (previously called pancreozymin)—produced by the duodenal mucosa. Stimulation of the vagus nerve will also produce pancreatic secretion.

Secretin promotes secretion of an abundant fluid, poor in protein and enzyme activity and rich in bicarbonate. Its function is mainly in promoting water and ion transport, which is probably derived from the duct cells and not the acinar cells. This secretion product serves to neutralize the acidic **chyme** (partially digested food) so that pancreatic enzymes can function at their optimal neutral pH range. Cholecystokinin promotes secretion of a less abundant but protein- and enzyme-rich fluid. This hormone acts mainly in the process of extrusion of the zymogen granules. The integrated action of both of these hormones provides for a heavy secretion of the enzyme-rich pancreatic juices. In conditions of extreme malnutrition such as kwashiorkor, the pancreatic cells undergo atrophy and lose much of their granular endoplasmic reticulum, and the production of digestive enzymes is hindered.

THE LIVER

With the exception of the skin, the liver is the largest organ of the body. It is situated in the abdominal cavity beneath the diaphragm. Most of its blood (about 70%) comes from the portal vein; the smaller percentage is supplied by the hepatic artery. Through the portal vein, all the material absorbed via the intestines reaches the liver except the lipids, which are transported mainly by the lymph vessels. The position of the liver is convenient for gathering, transforming, and accumulating metabolites and for neutralizing and eliminating toxic substances. This elimination occurs in the bile, an exocrine secretion of the liver of importance in lipid digestion.

In addition to these main functions, other important functions of the liver will be discussed later.

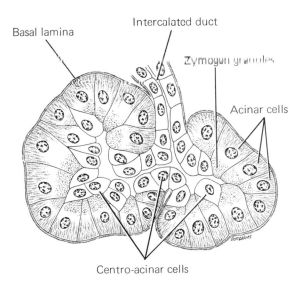

Figure 17–10. Schematic drawing of the structure of the pancreatic acini. Acinar cells are pyramidal, with granules at their apex and ergastoplasm at the cell base. The intercalated duct penetrates partially into the acini forming the centro-acinar cells.

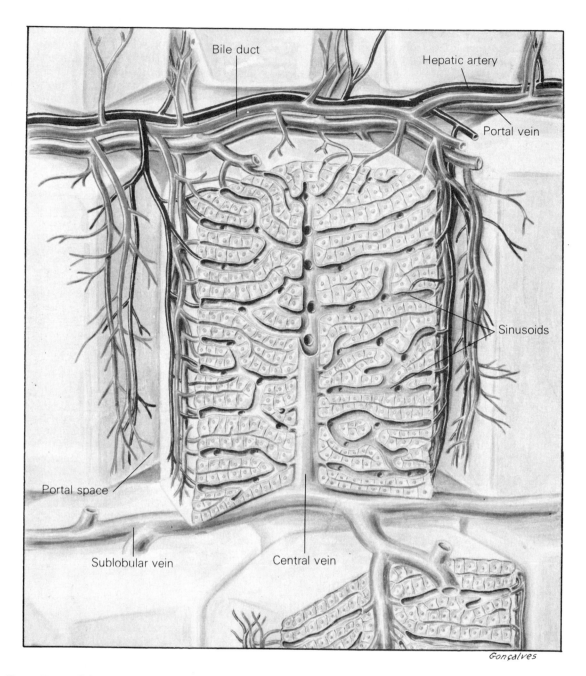

Figure 17 –11. Schematic drawing of the structure of the liver. In the center, the liver lobule is surrounded by the portal space. The portal spaces are shown dilated here for the sake of clarity; in the human liver, these spaces are much smaller and in some places nonexistent. Arteries, veins, and bile ducts occupy the portal spaces. Lymph vessels and connective tissue are also present but are not shown in this illustration. Observe in the lobule the radial disposition of the plates formed by liver cells. The sinusoid capillaries separate cords of liver cells. The bile canaliculi can be seen between the liver cells. The sublobular (intercalated) veins derive from the lobules. (Redrawn and reproduced, with permission, from Bourne G: *An Introduction to Functional Histology.* Churchill, 1953.)

The Liver Lobule

The main structural component of the liver is the liver cell or hepatocyte. These epithelial cells are grouped in plates that are interconnected in such a way as to show, in light microscope sections, structural units called by early investigators **liver lobules** (Fig 17–11). The liver lobule forms a prismatic polygonal mass of liver tissue about 0.7×2 mm in size (Figs 17–11 and 17–12). In certain animals (eg, the pig), these lobules are separated from each other and sharply delimited by a layer of connective tissue. This does not occur in humans, where the various lobules are in close contact along most of their extent, making it difficult to establish precisely the exact limits between different lobules. In some regions, however, the lobules are separated by connective tissue and blood vessels. These regions, the so-called **portal spaces,** are present at the corners of the polygons and are occupied by the **portal triads** (also called **portal canals** or **portal tracts**). The human liver contains 3–6 portal triads per lobule, each containing a venule (a branch of the portal vein); an arteriole (a branch of the hepatic artery); a duct (part of the bile duct system); and lymphatic vessels. The venule is usually the largest of these tubular structures, containing blood coming from the superior and inferior mesenteric and splenic veins. The arteriole contains blood from the celiac trunk of the abdominal aorta. The duct, lined by cuboidal epithelium, carries bile from the parenchymal cells and eventually empties into the hepatic duct. One or more lymphatics carry lymph

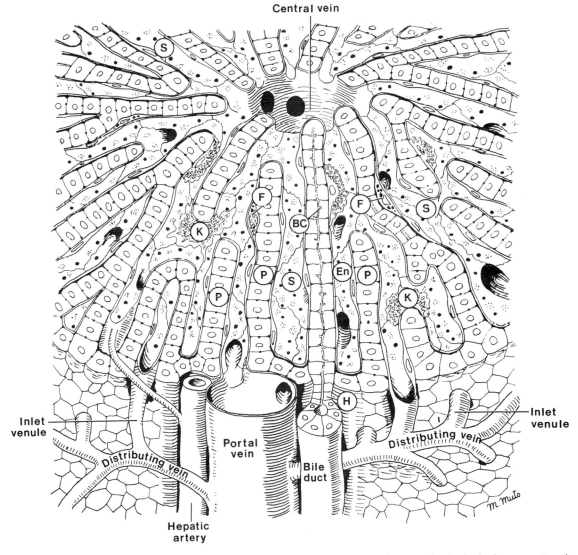

Figure 17 –12. Three-dimensional aspect of the normal liver. In the upper center, the central vein; in the lower center, the portal vein. BC, bile canaliculi; P, liver plates; H, Hering canal; K, Kupffer cells; S, sinusoid; F, fat-storing cell; En, sinusoid endothelial cell. (Courtesy of M Muto.)

that eventually enters the blood circulation. All of these structures are embedded in a sheath of connective tissue (Fig 17–13).

The hepatocytes are radially disposed in the liver lobule. They are piled up, forming a layer one cell thick in a fashion similar to the bricks of a wall. These plates are directed from the periphery of the lobule to its center and anastomose freely, forming a complex labyrinthine and spongelike structure (Fig 17–11). The space between these plates constitutes the sinusoid capillaries, the so-called liver sinusoids (Figs 17–11, 17–12, and 17–13). As seen in Chapter 12, sinusoids are irregularly dilated vessels composed of only one discontinuous layer of endothelial cells.

In addition to large fenestrations, gaps or discontinuities also exist between adjacent endothelial cells. The endothelial cells are separated from the underlying hepatocytes by a subendothelial space known as the space of Disse, which is virtually collagen and basal lamina–free (Figs 17–15 and 17–18). Consequently, blood fluids readily percolate through the endothelial wall and make intimate contact with the microvillar-lined hepatocyte surface (Fig 17–14A). In addition to the endothelial cells, the sinusoids also contain phagocytic cells of the reticuloendothelial series known as

Kupffer cells. These cells are found on the luminal surface of the endothelial cells, spanning the sinusoidal space and intercalated among other lining cells of the endothelial wall. Kupffer cells have definite cytologic characteristics such as clear vacuoles, lysosomes, and granular endoplasmic reticulum scattered throughout the cytoplasm that distinguish them from the endothelial cells. Evidence shows that these cells derive from bone marrow, as do other macrophages. The fat-storing cells (Fig 17–12) are star-shaped cells located in the perisinusoidal spaces (spaces of Disse; see below and Fig 17–12). They have the capacity to accumulate exogenously administered vitamin A in lipid droplets, but their physiologic function, if any, is obscure.

The liver sinusoid capillaries have an incomplete lining (Fig 17–15) and permit easy flow of macromolecules from the lumen to the liver cells and vice versa (Fig 17–14A). The sinusoid is surrounded and supported by a delicate sheath of reticular fibers important in maintaining its form. The sinusoids arise in the periphery of the lobule, fed by the inlet venules, terminal branches of the portal veins, and hepatic arterioles, and they run in the direction of its center, where they drain into the central vein (Figs 17–12 and 17–13).

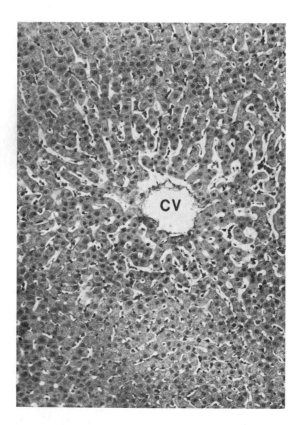

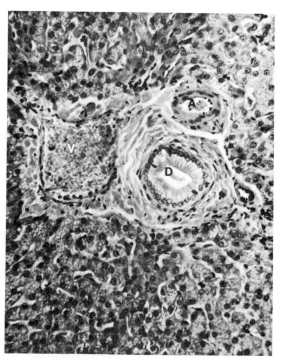

Figure 17–13. Photomicrograph of the liver. **Left:** A central vein (CV). Observe the liver plates that anastomose freely, limiting the space occupied by the sinusoids. H&E stain, × 200. **Right:** A portal space with its characteristic artery (A), vein (V), and bile duct (D) surrounded by connective tissue. Masson's stain, × 300.

Liver Blood Supply

Blood circulation through the liver occurs in the following ways (Figs 17–11 and 17–12):

A. Portal Vein System:

1. The portal vein branches repeatedly and sends small venules, the **portal venules,** to portal triads. These are sometimes called the **interlobular branches.**

2. The portal venules branch into **distributing veins** that run around the periphery of the lobule. From the distributing veins, small terminal **inlet venules** penetrate the hepatocyte wall and drain into the **sinusoids.**

3. These sinusoids run radially and converge in the center of the lobule to form the **central** or **centrolobular vein.** This vessel has thin walls consisting of only endothelial cells supported by a sparse population of collagen fibers. Numerous sinusoids in the wall of the central vein collect the blood from the surrounding sinusoids.

4. As the central vein progresses along the lobule, it receives more and more sinusoids and gradually increases in diameter. At its end, it leaves the lobule at its base by merging into the larger **sublobular vein.**

5. These **sublobular veins** gradually converge and fuse, forming the 2 or more large hepatic veins that end in the inferior vena cava.

B. Arterial System: The hepatic artery branches repeatedly and forms the **interlobular arteries;** some irrigate the structures of the portal canals and others end directly in the sinusoids at varying distances from the portal tracts, thus promoting a mixture of arterial and portal venous blood (Fig 17–12).

Blood therefore flows from the periphery to the center of the classic hepatic lobule. Consequently, the metabolites and all other toxic or nontoxic substances absorbed in the intestines reach first the peripheral cells and then the central cells of the lobule. This peculiarity partly explains why the cytologic and physiologic behavior of the perilobular cells is different from those of the centrolobular cells. This duality of behavior of the hepatocyte is particularly evident in pathologic specimens, where certain changes occur preferentially either in the central or in the peripheral cells of the lobule.

The description just given of the liver lobule with its blood supply corresponds to the classic concept of this subject in which the centrolobular veins constitute the axis of these structures. (See the hexagons limited by portal spaces [PS] with the central vein [CV] in the center in Fig 17–16.)

Other points of reference may be used in analyzing possible functional units of the liver's structure. Thus, another unit can be visualized, the **portal lobule,** which has at its center the portal triad and at its periphery the regions of adjoining hepatic lobules, all of which drain bile into the bile duct of the central portal triad. A portal lobule would be triangular, as opposed to the polygonal appearance of the classic liver lobule; it would have a central vein at the tip of each of its angles; and it would contain parts of 3 adjoining liver lobules. (See the dashed triangle in Fig 17–16 with the portal space [PS] at its center.)

Another way of subdividing the liver into functional lobules is to regard as a unit of liver parenchyma that region which is irrigated by a terminal branch of the distributing veins. This unit is called the **hepatic (Rappaport) acinus.** These appear diamond-shaped in section (see dotted area CV, PS, CV, PS in Fig 17–16). In addition to the terminal branches of the portal vein, an arterial branch and a bile ductule are in the center of this subdivision of hepatic parenchyma, which is situated in adjacent areas of 2 different classic hepatic lobules (Fig 17–16). This suggests that the liver is made up of diamond-shaped acini.

In relation to their proximity to the distributing veins, cells in the hepatic acinus can be subdivided into zones (Fig 17–16). Cells in zone I would be those closest to the vessel and consequently the first to be affected by or to alter the incoming blood. Cells in zone II would be second to respond to the blood, while those in zone III would see portal vein blood that had been previously altered by cells in both zones I and II. For example, after feeding, cells in zone I would be the first to receive incoming glucose and subsequently store it as glycogen. Any glucose passing the cells in zone I would likely be picked up by cells in zone II. In the event of fasting, cells in zone I would be the first to respond to glucose-poor blood by breaking down glycogen and releasing it as glucose. In this event, the cells in zones II and III would not respond to the fasting condition until glycogen was depleted from zone I cells. This zonal arrangement would account for some of the differences in the selective damage of hepatocytes by various noxious agents or in different disease conditions.

The Hepatocyte

Liver cells are polyhedral, with 6 or more surfaces, and have a diameter of approximately 20–30 μm. In sections stained with hematoxylin and eosin, the cytoplasm of the hepatocyte is eosinophilic mainly because of the presence of large numbers of mitochondria and to some extent smooth endoplasmic reticulum. The hepatocytes located at different distances from the portal triads show variations in structural, histochemical, and biochemical parameters. The surface of each liver cell is in contact with the wall of the sinusoids, through the space of Disse, and with the surfaces of other hepatocytes. Wherever 2 hepatocytes abut, they delimit a tubular space between them known as the **bile canaliculus** (Figs 17–14C, 17–15, 17–17, and 17–18).

These canaliculi are the first portions of the bile duct system. They are tubular spaces limited by

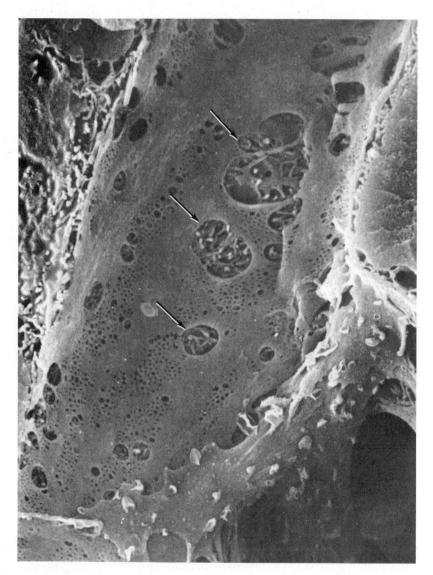

Figure 17 –14A. Portion of a liver lobule observed by scanning electron microscope. A sinusoid runs parallel to the picture. Observe the irregular fenestrations of the endothelial cell and, through the larger fenestrations, the hepatocyte microvilli that protrude in the space of Disse (arrows). (From Motta P, Andrews PM, Porter KR: *Microanatomy of Cell and Tissue Surfaces: An Atlas of Scanning Electron Microscopy.* Lea & Febiger, 1977.)

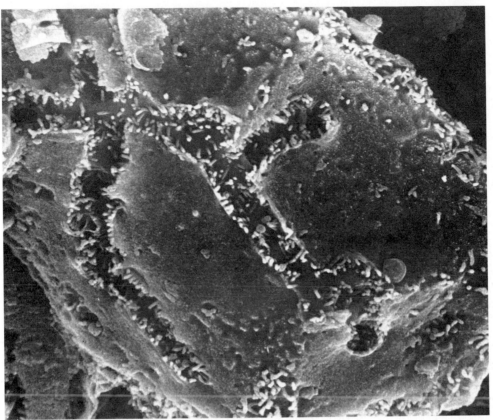

Figure 17 –14C. Branching bile canaliculi observed in liver by scanning electron microscope. Observe the microvilli lining its internal surface. (From Motta P, Andrews PM, Porter KR: *Microanatomy of Cell and Tissue Surfaces: An Atlas of Scanning Electron Microscopy.* Lea & Febiger, 1977.)

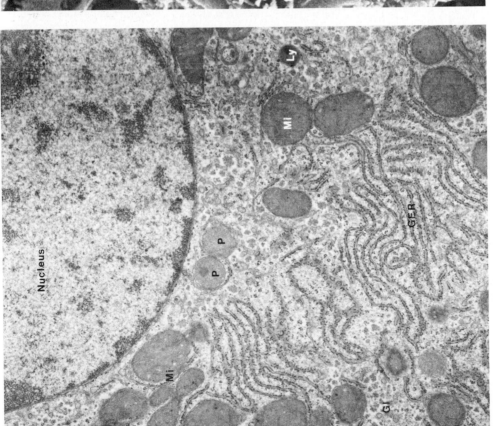

Figure 17 –14B. Electron micrograph of a hepatocyte. In the cytoplasm, below the nucleus, are mitochondria (Mi), granular endoplasmic reticulum (GER), glycogen (Gl), lysosomes (Ly), and peroxisomes (P). × 6600.

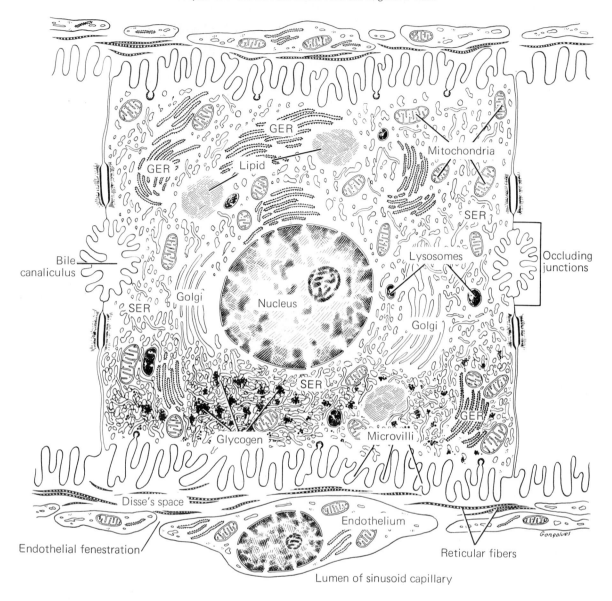

Figure 17–15. Diagram of the ultrastructure of a hepatocyte. GER, granular endoplasmic reticulum. SER, smooth endoplasmic reticulum. × 10,000.

only the plasma membranes of 2 hepatocytes and have a small number of microvilli in their interior (Figs 17–15, 17–17, and 17–18). The cell membranes near these canaliculi are firmly bound by occluding junctions as described in Chapter 4. Gap junctions are frequent in this region and are sites of intercellular communication, an important process for the coordination of the physiologic activities of these cells. The bile canaliculi form a complex anastomosing network progressing along the plates of the liver lobule and terminating in the region of the portal canals (Fig 17–12). The bile flow therefore progresses in a direction opposite to that of the blood, ie, from the center of the lobule to its periphery. At the periphery, the bile enters the **bile**

ductules or **Hering's canals** (Fig 17–19). These are composed of cuboidal cells with a clear cytoplasm and few organelles. After a short distance, these bile ductules cross the limiting hepatocytes of the portal lobule and end in the **bile ducts** in the portal triads (Figs 17–12 and 17–13). These ducts are lined by a cuboidal or columnar epithelium and have a distinct connective tissue sheath. They gradually enlarge and fuse, forming the right and left **hepatic ducts,** that subsequently leave the liver. The surface of the hepatocyte which faces the space of Disse presents many microvilli protruding in that space but always leaving a space between them and the cells of the sinusoidal wall (Figs 17–15 and 17–18). The liver cell presents one or 2 rounded nuclei with one or 2

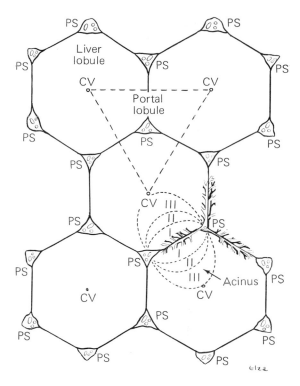

Figure 17 –16 (at right). Schematic drawing illustrating the territories of the classic liver lobules, hepatic acini, and portal lobules. The classic lobule has a central vein (CV) and is outlined by lines that connect the portal spaces (PS) (solid lines). The portal lobules have their center in the portal space and are outlined by lines that connect the central veins (upper triangle). They comprise the portion of the liver from which bile flows to a portal space. Finally, the hepatic acinus comprises the region irrigated by one distributing vein (lower triangles). Zonation of the hepatic acinus is indicated by Roman numerals I, II, and III. (Redrawn and reproduced, with permission, from Leeson TS, Leeson CR: *Histology,* 2nd ed. Saunders, 1970.)

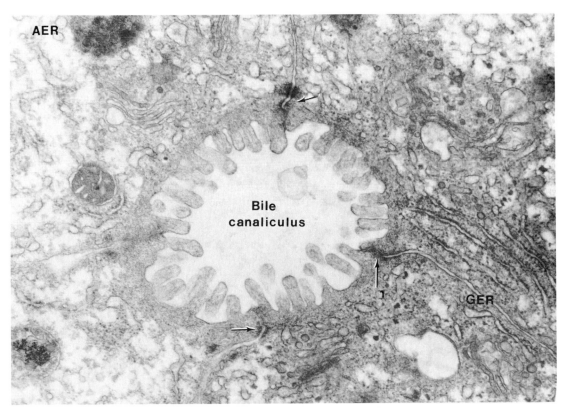

Figure 17 –17. Electron micrograph of frog liver bile canaliculus showing the microvilli in its lumen and the junctional structures (arrows). GER and AER are granular (rough) and agranular (smooth) endoplasmic reticulum of adjoining hepatocytes. × 35,000.

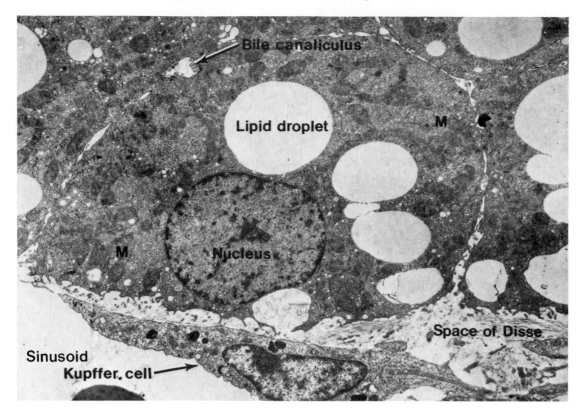

Figure 17 –18. Electron micrograph of the liver of a monkey. Note a hepatocyte containing lipid droplets and mitochondria (M). At upper left is a bile canaliculus with microvilli. Below are a Kupffer cell and Disse's space. × 6300.

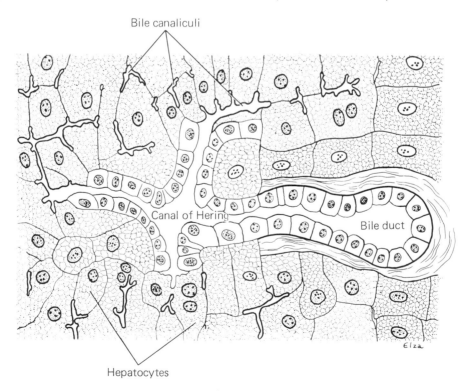

Figure 17 –19. The passage of bile canaliculi to the Hering canals lined by cuboidal epithelium. These structures merge with the bile ducts of the portal spaces.

typical nucleoli. It has an abundant endoplasmic reticulum both in its smooth and granular varieties (Figs 17–14B and 17–15). In this cell, the granular endoplasmic reticulum forms aggregates dispersed in the cytoplasm, called **basophilic bodies** by classic microscopists. Several proteins—eg, blood albumin and fibrinogen—are synthesized in these structures. Various important processes occur in the smooth endoplasmic reticulum that is distributed diffusely throughout the cytoplasm. This organelle seems to be responsible for the process of conjugation in which various substances are bound to sulfate or glucuronide during the process of inactivation or detoxification before excretion from the body. The smooth endoplasmic reticulum of the hepatocyte is a labile system that reacts promptly to changes in the environment. Administration of certain drugs, such as barbiturates, to laboratory animals promotes in a short time an in-

crease in the smooth endoplasmic reticulum of the liver cell, with a parallel increase in the activity of enzymes responsible for conjugation of these drugs. This reaction of the smooth endoplasmic reticulum has led to the use of barbiturates in the treatment of a disease caused by a deficiency of glucuronyl transferase, an enzyme normally present in the endoplasmic reticulum.

Another typical component of the liver cell is glycogen. This polysaccharide appears in the electron microscope as coarse, electron-dense granules that frequently collect near areas of smooth endoplasmic reticulum, assuming the form of berries (Figs 3–23, 17–15, and 17–20). The amount of glycogen present in the liver conforms to a diurnal rhythm and depends also upon the nutritional state of the animal. The liver glycogen pool is a depot of glucose and is mobilized if the blood glucose level falls below normal. In this way, hepatocytes main-

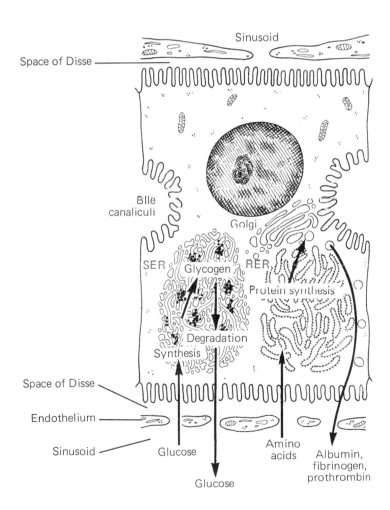

Figure 17 –20. Protein synthesis and carbohydrate storage in the liver. Protein synthesis occurs in the granular (rough) endoplasmic reticulum, which explains why liver cell lesions lead to a decrease in the amounts of albumin, fibrinogen, and prothrombin in a patient's blood. In several diseases, glycogen degradation is depressed with abnormal intracellular accumulation of this compound. SER, smooth endoplasmic reticulum; RER, rough endoplasmic reticulum.

tain a steady level of blood glucose, the main metabolite used by the body.

The liver cell has many mitochondria (approximately 2000) with a spherical or ovoid form. Their cristae are not so numerous or closely packed as mitochondria of the muscle cell, a characteristic consistent with the moderate oxygen consumption observed in this organ. Similar to what occurs in most cellular components, the proteins of the liver mitochondria are constantly being renewed. The average life span of the structural proteins of this organelle is calculated to be about 10 days. Other frequent cellular components are the lipid droplets, whose quantity varies greatly (Fig 17–18). Lysosomes and peroxisomes are abundant in the hepatocytes, although their exact function in this cell is still a subject of speculation. Administration of the pancreatic hormone glucagon promotes the appearance of many autophagosomes in the liver cell. They might be related to processes of turnover of the hepatocyte. The Golgi system consists of several aggregates, usually near the bile canaliculi. Its function in the hepatocyte is not clear, although it may participate in the formation of lysosomes and in the secretion of blood proteins. The presence of variable quantities of lipids, glycogen, and granular endoplasmic reticulum in the liver cell is due to the multiple potential functions of hepatocytes and is responsible for its great morphologic variability.

HISTOPHYSIOLOGY & LIVER FUNCTION

The liver cell undoubtedly is the most versatile cell in the body. It is at the same time a cell with endocrine and exocrine functions, and it synthesizes and accumulates certain substances, detoxifies others, and transports still others. We shall now examine the main activities of this cell.

Protein Synthesis

Besides synthesizing the proteins for its own maintenance, the liver cell produces various pro-

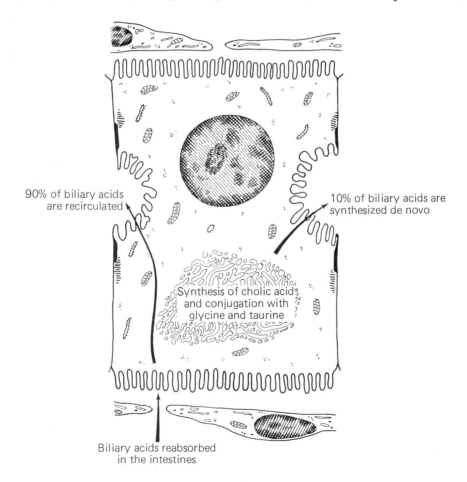

90% of biliary acids are recirculated

10% of biliary acids are synthesized de novo

Synthesis of cholic acid and conjugation with glycine and taurine

Biliary acids reabsorbed in the intestines

Figure 17–21. Mechanism of secretion of biliary acids. About 90% of these compounds derive from bile acids reabsorbed in the intestinal epithelium and recirculated to the liver. The remainder are synthesized in the liver by conjugating cholic acid with the amino acids glycine and taurine. This process occurs in the smooth endoplasmic reticulum.

teins for export—among them albumin, prothrombin, and fibrinogen of the blood plasma. These proteins are synthesized on the granular endoplasmic reticulum. Contrary to what is observed in other glandular cells, the hepatocyte does not store proteins in its cytoplasm as secretory granules but gradually releases the protein produced into the bloodstream. Thus it functions as an endocrine gland during this activity (Fig 17–20).

Radioautographic studies using the electron microscope show that protein is synthesized in the granular endoplasmic reticulum of the hepatocyte. The protein migrates to the Golgi region and is subsequently extruded into the blood. About 5% of the protein exported by the liver is produced by the cells of the macrophage system (Kupffer cells); the remainder is synthesized in the hepatocytes.

Bile Secretion

Bile production is an exocrine secretion in the sense that the hepatocytes transform and transport blood components into the bile canaliculi. Besides water, bile has 2 main components: bile acids and bilirubin. The secretion of bile acids is illustrated in Fig 17–21. About 90% of these substances are derived by absorption from the intestinal lumen through the intestinal epithelium, being transported as such by the hepatocyte from the blood to the bile canaliculi. About 10% of these compounds are synthesized in the smooth endoplasmic reticulum of the hepatocyte by conjugation of cholic acid with the amino acids glycine and taurine. Thus, glycocholic and taurocholic acids are produced. Cholic acid is also synthesized at this level from cholesterol. The bile acids have an important func-

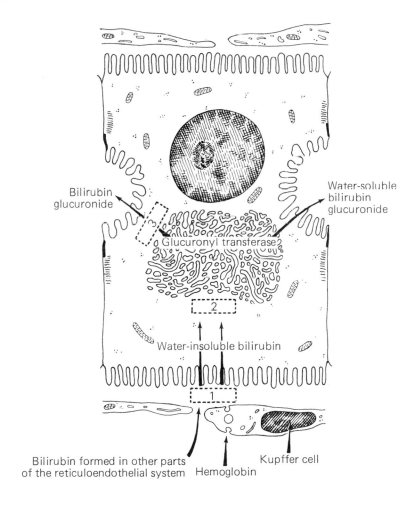

Figure 17–22. The secretion of bilirubin. This water-insoluble compound derives from the metabolism of hemoglobin in the macrophages of the macrophage system (or reticuloendothelial system), including the Kupffer cells of the liver sinusoids. In the hepatocytes, by means of glucuronyl transferase activity, bilirubin is conjugated in the smooth endoplasmic reticulum with glucuronide, forming a soluble compound. When bile secretion is blocked by one of several possible mechanisms, the yellow bilirubin glucuronide accumulates in the blood and jaundice appears. Several mechanisms can produce jaundice: (1) a defect in the capacity of the cell to trap and absorb bilirubin (rectangle 1); (2) inability of the cell to conjugate bilirubin because of deficiency in the enzyme glucuronyl transferase (rectangle 2); or (3) problems in the transfer and excretion of bilirubin into the biliary canaliculi (rectangle 3). One of the most frequent causes of jaundice, however, is obstruction of bile flow.

tion in emulsifying the lipids in the digestive tube and promoting easier digestion by lipase and subsequent absorption.

Bilirubin is formed in the macrophage system (this includes the Kupffer cells of the liver sinusoids) and is transported to the hepatocyte. In the smooth endoplasmic reticulum of the hepatocyte, hydrophobic (water-insoluble) bilirubin is conjugated to glucuronic acid, forming a water-soluble **bilirubin glucuronide** (Fig 17–22). In a further step, the bilirubin glucuronide is secreted into the bile canaliculi.

The hepatocyte also has the ability to actively transport several dyes. This ability to eliminate dyes is used as a test of liver function. One of the dyes classically used for this purpose is sulfobromophthalein (Bromsulphalein, BSP).

Storage of Metabolites

Lipids and carbohydrates are stored in the liver in the form of fat and glycogen (Figs 17–18 and 17–20). This capacity to store energetic metabolites is important because it supplies the body with energy between meals. Figure 17–20 shows how this is done for the carbohydrates. The liver also serves as the major storage compartment for vitamins.

Metabolic Function

The hepatocyte is also responsible for converting lipids and amino acids into glucose by means of a complex enzymatic process called **glyconeogenesis.** It is also the main site of amino acid deamination, resulting in the production of urea. This compound is transported by the blood to the kidney and excreted by that organ.

Detoxification & Inactivation

Various drugs and substances can be inactivated by oxidation, methylation, and conjugation. The enzymes participating in these processes are considered to be located mainly in the smooth endoplasmic reticulum. Glucuronyl transferase, an enzyme that conjugates glucuronic acid to bilirubin, causes conjugation of several other compounds such as steroids, barbiturates, antihistamines, and anticonvulsants. Conjugation is an important function of the smooth endoplasmic reticulum of the hepatocyte.

Liver Regeneration

Despite being an organ whose cells are renewed at a slow rate, the liver has an extraordinary capacity for regeneration. The loss of hepatic tissue due to the action of toxic substances or surgical removal triggers a mechanism by which liver cells begin to divide, and this continues until restoration of the original mass of tissue is achieved. In rats, the liver can regenerate a loss of 75% of its weight in 1 month. In humans, this capacity is said to be considerably restricted. The process of regeneration is probably controlled by circulating substances called **chalones,** which inhibit the mitotic division of a certain cell type. When a tissue is injured or partially removed, the amount of chalones it produces decreases; consequently, a burst of mitotic activity occurs in this tissue. As regeneration proceeds, the amount of chalones produced is increased and mitotic activity decreases. It is a self-regulating process. There is evidence that this mechanism is present in different tissues and is a generalized phenomenon.

The regenerated liver tissue is usually similar to the removed tissue. However, in the case of continuous or repeated damage to this organ, an abundant production of connective tissue occurs simultaneously with liver cell regeneration. This exaggerated connective tissue production can disorganize the regeneration and produce a condition called **cirrhosis.**

THE BILIARY TRACT

The bile produced by the liver cell flows through the **biliary canaliculi, bile ductules,** and **bile ducts.** These structures gradually fuse, forming a rich network that converges to form the **hepatic duct.** The hepatic duct, after receiving the **cystic duct** from the gallbladder, continues to the duodenum as the **common bile duct** (or **ductus choledochus**).

The hepatic, cystic, and common bile ducts are lined by a mucous membrane that presents a columnar epithelium composed of cells with abundant mitochondria. The lamina propria is thin and surrounded by an inconspicuous layer of smooth muscle. This muscle layer becomes thicker near the duodenum and finally forms, in the intramural portion, a sphincter that regulates bile flow.

THE GALLBLADDER

The gallbladder is a hollow, pear-shaped organ attached to the lower surface of the liver. It communicates with the common hepatic duct through the cystic duct. The wall of the gallbladder consists of the following layers (Fig 17–23): (1) a mucous layer composed of columnar epithelium and lamina propria, (2) a layer of smooth muscle, (3) a well-developed perimuscular connective tissue layer, and (4) a serous membrane.

The mucous layer presents folds that are particularly evident in the empty bladder. The epithelial cells are rich in mitochondria and have their nuclei in their basal third (Fig 17–24). Microvilli are frequent in the apical region. Near the cystic duct, the epithelium invaginates into the lamina propria,

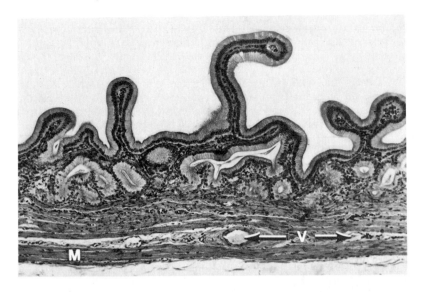

Figure 17 –23. Photomicrograph of a section of gallbladder. Observe the lining columnar epithelium, the smooth muscle layer (M), and the blood vessels (V). H&E stain, × 30.

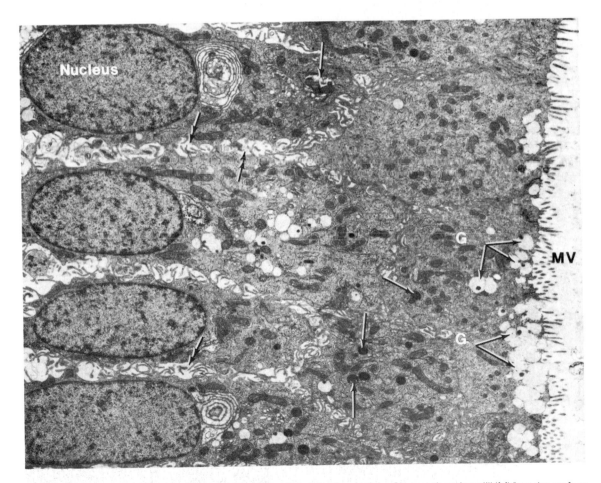

Figure 17 –24. Electron micrograph of a section from the gallbladder of a monkey. Observe the microvilli (MV) on the surface of the cell and secretory granules (G) containing glycoprotein complexes. The single arrows indicate the lysosomes; the double arrows show the ample intercellular spaces. These are cells that transport sodium chloride from the lumen to the blood vessels, secrete mucous substances, and digest particles reabsorbed from the bile. × 6500.

forming tubulo-acinar glands with a wide lumen. Cells of these glands have characteristics of mucus-secreting cells and are responsible for the production of the mucus present in bile.

The muscular layer is thin and irregular. A thick connective tissue layer binds the superior surface of the gallbladder to the liver. The opposite surface is covered by a typical serous layer, the peritoneum.

The main function of the gallbladder is to store bile and concentrate it by reabsorbing its water. This process depends upon an active sodium- and chloride-transporting mechanism in its epithelium.

The water reabsorption is considered to be an osmotic consequence of the sodium pump. Because sodium and chloride ions are transported in equal amounts, no potential difference is evident between the 2 surfaces of this organ. The sodium, chloride, and water cross the membrane of the cell apex and move laterally to the intercellular spaces and from there to the blood vessels of the lamina propria. Contraction of the smooth muscle of the gallbladder is induced by **cholecystokinin,** a hormone produced in the mucosa of the small intestine.

• • •

References

Pancreas & Salivary Glands

Amsterdam A & others: Concomitant synthesis of membrane protein and exportable protein of the secretory granule in rat parotid gland. J Cell Biol 40:187, 1971.

Castle JD, Jamieson JD, Palade GE: Radioautographic analysis of the secretory process in the parotid acinar cell of the rabbit. J Cell Biol 53:290, 1972.

Junqueira LCU: Control of cell secretion. In: *Secretory Mechanisms of Salivary Glands.* Schneyer LH, Schneyer CA (editors). Academic Press, 1967.

Junqueira LCU, de Moraes FF: Comparative aspects of the vertebrate major salivary glands' biology. In: *Functionelle und Morphologische Organization der Zelle: Sekretion und Exkretion.* Wohlfarth-Buttermann KE (editor). Springer, 1965.

Junqueira LCU, de Moraes FF, Toledo AMS: Action of vasopressin on salivary secretion. Acta Physiol Lat Am 17:36, 1967.

Leeson CR: Structure of salivary glands. In: *Handbook of Physiology.* Vol 2. Code CF, Heidel W (editors). American Physiological Society, 1967.

Munger BL: Histochemical studies on seromucous and mucous-secreting cells of human salivary glands. Am J Anat 115:411, 1964.

Opie EL: Cytology of the pancreas. In: *Special Cytology,* 2nd ed. Cowdry EV (editor). Hoeber, 1932.

Stormont DL: The salivary glands. In: *Special Cytology,* 2nd ed. Cowdry EV (editor). Hoeber, 1932.

Tandler B: Ultrastructure of the human submaxillary gland. 1. Architecture and histological relationship of the secretory cells. Am J Anat 111:287, 1962.

Tomasi TB, Bienenstock J: Secretory immunoglobins. Adv Immunol 9:11, 1968.

Young JA & others: A microperfusion investigation of sodium resorption and potassium secretion by the main excretory duct of the rat submaxillary gland. Pfluegers Arch 295:157, 1967.

Liver & Biliary Tract

Ashley CA, Peters T Jr: Electron microscopic radioautographic detection of sites of protein synthesis and migration in liver. J Cell Biol 43:237, 1969.

Babcock MB, Cardell RR Jr: Hepatic glycogen patterns in fasted and fed rats. Am J Anat 140:299, 1974.

Becker FF: The normal hepatocyte in division: Regeneration of the mammalian liver. In: *Progress in Liver Diseases.* Vol 3. Popper H, Schaffner F (editors). Grune & Stratton, 1970.

Bolender RP, Weibel ER: A morphometric study of the removal of phenobarbital-induced membranes from hepatocytes after cessation of treatment. J Cell Biol 56:746, 1973.

Braner RW: Liver circulation and function. Physiol Rev 43:115, 1963.

Bruni C, Porter KR: The fine structure of the parenchymal cell of the normal rat liver. 1. General considerations. Am J Pathol 46:691, 1965.

Diamond JM, Tormey JM: Studies on the structural basis of water transport across epithelial membranes. Fed Proc 25:1458, 1966.

Elias H, Sherrick JC: *Morphology of the Liver.* Academic Press, 1969.

Greenway CV, Stark RD: Hepatic vascular bed. Physiol Rev 51:23, 1971.

Howard JG: The origin and immunological significance of the Kupffer cells. In: *Mononuclear Phagocytes.* Van Furth R (editor). Blackwell, 1970.

Ito T, Shibasaki S: Electron microscopic study on the hepatic sinusoidal wall and the fat-storing cells in the human normal liver. Arch Histol Jpn 29:137, 1968.

Jones AL, Fawcett DW: Hypertrophy of the agranular endoplasmic reticulum in hamster liver induced by phenobarbital. J Histochem Cytochem 14:215, 1966.

Kaye GI & others: Fluid transport in the rabbit gallbladder: A combined physiological and electron microscopic study. J Cell Biol 30:237, 1966.

Lin C, Chang JP: Electron microscopy of albumin synthesis. Science 190:465, 1975.

McMinn RMH, Kugler JH: The glands of the bile and pancreatic ducts: Autoradiographic and histochemical studies. J Anat 95:1, 1961.

Motta P: A scanning electron microscopic study of the rat sinusoids. Cell Tiss Res 164:371, 1975.

Mueller JC, Jones AL, Long JA: Topographical and subcellular anatomy of the guinea pig gallbladder. Gastroenterology 63:856, 1972.

Onstad GR, Schoenfield LJ, Higgins JA: Fluid transfer in the everted human gallbladder. J Clin Invest 46:608, 1967.

Orrenius S, Ericsson JLE, Ernster L: Phenobarbital-induced synthesis of the microsomal drug-metabolizing enzyme system and its relationship to the proliferation of endoplasmic membranes: A morphological and biochemical study. J Cell Biol 25:627, 1965.

Peters T Jr: The biosynthesis of rat serum albumin. 2. Intracellular phenomena in the secretion of newly formed albumin. J Biol Chem 237:1186, 1962.

Rappaport AM: Acinar units and the pathophysiology of the liver. In: *The Liver: Morphology, Biochemistry, Physiology*. Vol 1. Rouiller C (editor). Academic Press, 1963.

Rouiller C (editor): *The Liver: Morphology, Biochemistry, Physiology*. 2 vols. Academic Press, 1963, 1964.

Sasse D, Schenk A: A 3-dimensional presentation of the functional liver unit. Acta Anatomica 93:78, 1975.

Simon FR, Arias IM: Alterations in liver plasma membranes and their possible role in cholestasis. Gastroenterology 62:341, 1972.

Wisse E, Knook DL (editors): *Kupffer Cells and Other Sinusoidal Cells*. Elsevier/North-Holland, 1977.

18 | Respiratory System

The function of the respiratory system is to provide oxygen to the blood and remove CO_2. The respiratory system includes the lungs and a system of tubes that link the pulmonary tissue with the external environment. It is customary to separate the respiratory system into 2 principal divisions (Fig 18–1): a **conducting portion**, consisting of the nasal cavity, nasopharynx, larynx, trachea, bronchi, and bronchioles; and a **respiratory portion**, which consists of the alveoli and their associated structures. The exchange of gases occurs between the air and the blood only within the alveoli, specialized saclike structures that make up the greater part of the lung.

The conducting portion serves 2 main functions: (1) to provide a conduit through which air can travel to and from the lungs, and (2) to condition the inspired air. To carry out these functions, each subdivision of the conducting portion exhibits several structural features in common with the others. In order to ensure an uninterrupted supply of air, a combination of cartilage, elastic fibers, and smooth muscle provide the conducting portion with a rigid structural support and a necessary flexibility and extensibility. The cartilages, primarily hyaline (with some elastic cartilage in the larynx), are found in the periphery of the lamina propria, and they exhibit various forms ranging from irregular plates to complete rings. The cartilages generally serve to support the walls of the conducting portion, preventing a collapse of the lumen and thereby ensuring continuous access of air to the lungs. Both the conducting and respiratory portions are richly endowed with elastic fibers that provide the structures with flexibility and allow them to "spring back" after distention. In the conducting portion, the elastic fibers are found in the lamina propria and are mainly longitudinally oriented. Elastic fiber concentration is inversely proportionate to the diameter of the conducting tubule (ie, the smallest bronchioles have the highest proportion of elastic fibers). Bundles of smooth muscle are found extending from the trachea to the alveolar ducts (a subdivision of the respiratory portion). Constriction of the smooth muscle serves to reduce the diameter of the conducting tubules and thereby regulates air flow during inspiration and expiration.

Conditioning of Air

A major function of the conducting portion is to "condition" the inspired air. Before it enters the lungs, inspired air is cleansed, moistened, and warmed. To carry out these functions, the mucosa of the conducting portions is lined by a specialized respiratory epithelium (described below), and there is a heavy investment of mucous and serous glands as well as a rich superficial vascular network in the lamina propria.

As the air enters the nose, large vibrissae serve to remove coarse particles of dust and other substances. Once the air reaches the nasal fossae, par-

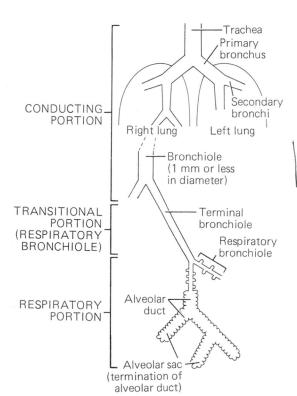

Figure 18–1. The main divisions of the respiratory tract. For instructional purposes, the natural proportions of these structures have been altered; thus, for example, the respiratory bronchiole is in reality a short transitional structure.

ticulate and gaseous impurities are trapped in a layer of mucus. This mucus, in conjunction with serous secretions, also serves to moisten the incoming air, which protects the delicate alveolar lining from desiccation. In addition, the incoming air is warmed by a rich superficial vascular network.

Respiratory Epithelium

Most of the conducting portion is lined by pseudostratified columnar ciliated epithelium containing a rich population of goblet cells. Deeper in the bronchial tree, this epithelial cell population is modified as the epithelium undergoes a transition into simple squamous epithelium. As the bronchi subdivide into the bronchioles, the pseudostratified organization gives way to a simple columnar epithelium, which is further reduced to a simple cuboidal layer in the smallest (terminal) bronchioles. The rich goblet cell population tapers off in the smaller bronchi and is totally absent from the epithelium in the terminal bronchioles. It is important to note that ciliated cells, which accompany the goblet cells, continue through the finer bronchioles in the absence of goblet cells. The continuation of the ciliated cells beyond the goblet cells serves to prevent mucus from accumulating in the respiratory portion of the system. The mucus, which entraps particulate matter and absorbs water-soluble gases (eg, SO_2 and ozone), is continually propelled by ciliary action toward the pharynx, where it is either swallowed or expectorated. The movement of the mucous layer is generated and directed by a subjacent stream of serous secretions in which the cilia beat. In addition to clearing pollutants, the mucous and serous layers also serve to moisten the inspired air.

Typical respiratory epithelium consists of 6 cell types as seen in the electron microscope. **Ciliated columnar cells** constitute the most abundant type.

Each cell possesses about 300 cilia on its apical surface (Figs 18–2, 18–3, and 18–4), while beneath the cilia, in addition to basal bodies, there are numerous small mitochondria. From experimental studies, it has been demonstrated that adenosine triphosphate (ATP) is required for ciliary beating, an observation that is consistent with the apical localization of mitochondria. Evidence has been presented that a disorder characterized by sterility and chronic respiratory tract infection—Kartagener's syndrome—is due to immobility of cilia and flagella induced by deficiency of a protein called **dynein,** normally present in the cilia. This protein is responsible for sliding of the microtubules, a process necessary for ciliary movement.

The next most abundant cells are the **mucous goblet cells** (Fig 18–4). The apical portion of these cells (described in Chapter 4) contains the polysaccharide-rich mucous droplets. The remaining columnar cells are known as "**brush cells**" owing to the numerous microvilli present on their apical surface. Two types of brush cells are present. One has the cytologic characteristics of an immature cell and most likely represents replacements for dead or dying ciliated or goblet cells. The other brush cells exhibit dendritic synapses on their basal surfaces and are considered to be sensory receptors. **Basal (short) cells** are small rounded cells that lie on the basal lamina but do not extend to the apical surface of the epithelium. These cells are believed to be the generative cells that undergo mitoses and subsequently differentiate into the other cell types. The remaining cell type is the **small granule cell,** which resembles a basal cell except that it possesses numerous granules 100–300 nm in diameter with dense cores. Histochemical studies reveal that these cells constitute a population of APUD cells (see Chapter 4). These endocrinelike granule cells may act as effectors in the integration of the mucous

Table 18–1. Structural changes in the conducting portions of the respiratory tract.

	Nasal Fossae	Naso-pharynx	Larynx	Trachea	Bronchi Large	Bronchi Small	Bronchioles Regular	Bronchioles Terminal	Bronchioles Respiratory
Epithelium	Pseudostratified columnar ciliated*†						Pseudo-stratified columnar ciliated →	Transition → Simple columnar ciliated →	Simple cuboidal ciliated
Goblet cells	Abundant				Present	Few	Scattered	None	
Glands	Abundant			Present		Few	None		
Cartilage			Complex (hyaline and elastic)	C rings	Complete rings	Plates and islands	None		
Smooth muscle	None			Spanning open ends of C rings	Crisscrossing spiral bundles				
Elastic	None		Present				Abundant		

*Stratified squamous in regions of direct air flow or abrasion.
†Vestibule of nose shows transition from keratinized stratified squamous to pseudostratified columnar ciliated epithelium.

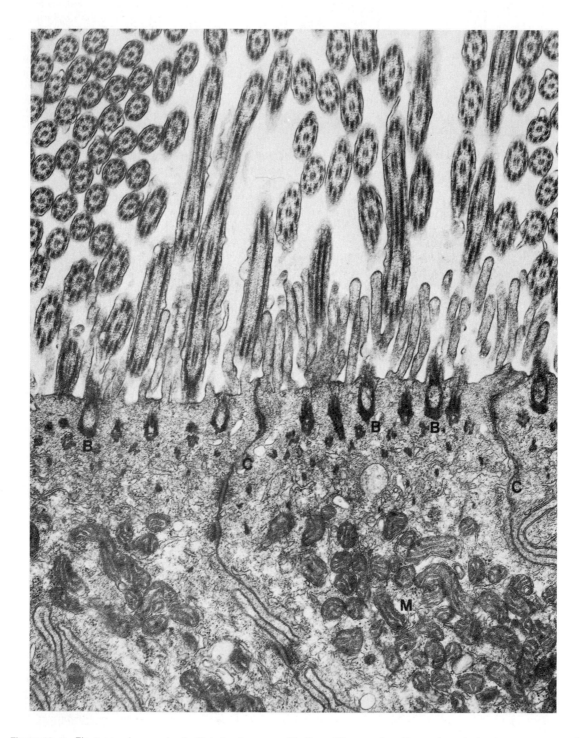

Figure 18–2. Electron micrograph of ciliated columnar epithelium. Observe the ciliary microtubules in transverse and oblique section. In the cell apex are the U-shaped basal bodies (B) where the cilia insert themselves. At (M), local accumulation of mitochondria is probably related to energy production for ciliary movement. At (C), observe junctional complexes. Note the emergence of microvilli between the ciliary roots. Reduced from × 10,000.

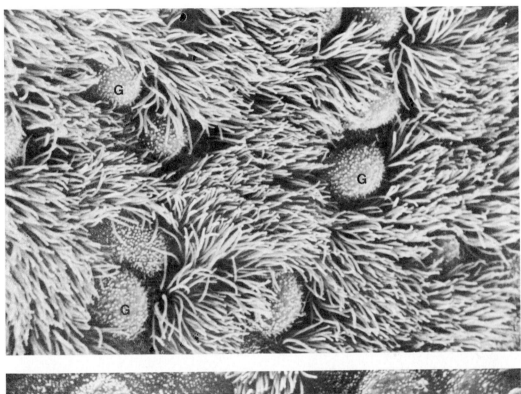

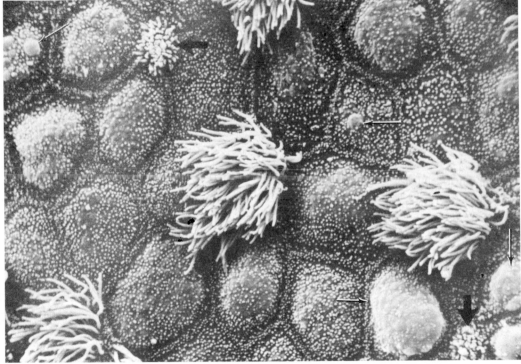

Figure 18 –3. Scanning electron micrograph of the surface of rat respiratory mucosa. G, goblet cells. Most of the surface is covered by the cilia. In the lower micrograph, subsurface accumulations of mucus are evident in the goblet cells (arrows). (Reproduced, with permission, from Andrews P: A scanning electron microscopic study of the extrapulmonary respiratory tract. Am J Anat 139:421, 1974.)

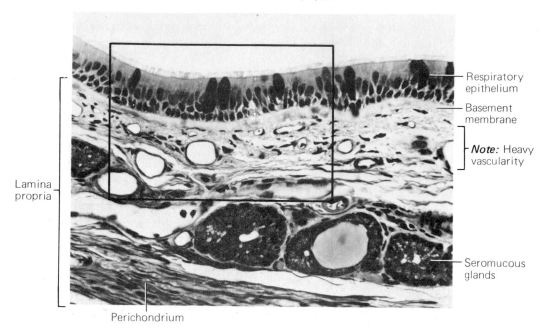

Respiratory
epithelium

Basement
membrane

Note: Heavy
vascularity

Lamina
propria

Seromucous
glands

Perichondrium

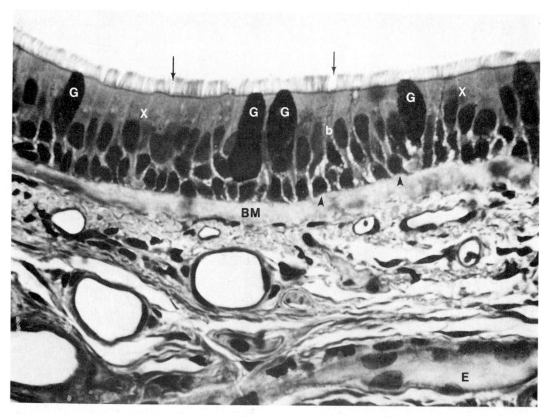

Figure 18 –4. *Top:* Section of monkey trachea revealing typical respiratory epithelium, thick basement membrane, heavily vascularized connective tissue of the lamina propria, and the presence of seromucous glands. Beneath the glands lies the dense connective tissue of the perichondrium, which surrounds the supporting hyaline cartilage (not visible). *Bottom:* Enlargement of the rectangular area shown above. The tracheal lumen is lined by typical pseudostratified columnar ciliated epithelium with goblet cells. This epithelium plays a significant role in conditioning the inspired air. Beneath the unusually thick basement membrane (BM) lies the lamina propria, whose rich vascularity aids in warming the incoming air. G, goblet cells containing mucous secretion; X, ciliated columnar cells; b, nonciliated brush cell; arrowheads, rounded basal cell; ↓, cilia; E, en face view of venule endothelial cells.

and serous secretory processes. All cells of the pseudostratified columnar ciliated epithelium touch the basal layer, and the epithelium is adherent to a prominent basement membrane (Fig 18–4, bottom).

From the nasal cavity through the larynx, portions of the epithelium are stratified squamous. This type of epithelium is evident in regions exposed to direct air flow or physical abrasion (eg, oropharynx, epiglottis, vocal folds) since it provides more protection from attrition than typical respiratory epithelium. If air flow currents are altered or new abrasive sites develop, the affected areas can convert from typical pseudostratified columnar ciliated epithelium to a stratified squamous epithelium. Similarly, in smokers, the proportion of ciliated cells to goblet cells is altered in order to aid in clearing the increased particulate and gaseous (eg, CO, SO_2) pollutants. Although the greater number of goblet cells in a smoker's epithelium provide for a more rapid clearance of pollutants, the reduction of ciliated cells due to excessive CO results in a decrease in the movement of the mucous layer and frequently leads to congestion of the smaller airways. These **reversible** changes in cellular organization are referred to as **metaplasia.**

NASAL CAVITY

The nasal cavity consists of 2 different structures: the external **vestibule** and the internal **nasal fossae.**

Vestibule

The vestibule is the most anterior and dilated portion of the nasal cavity. The outer integument of the nose enters the **nares** (nostrils) and continues part way up the vestibule. Around the inner surface of the nares are numerous sebaceous and sweat glands in addition to the thick short hairs or **vibrissae** that serve to filter out large particles from the inspired air. Within the vestibule, the epithelium loses its keratinized nature and then undergoes a transition into typical respiratory epithelium before entering the nasal fossae.

Nasal Fossae

Within the skull lie 2 cavernous chambers separated by the osseous **nasal septum.** Extending from each lateral wall are 3 bony shelflike projections known as **conchae.** Of the superior, middle, and inferior conchae, only the middle and inferior projections possess respiratory epithelium. The superior conchae are covered by a specialized olfactory epithelium. The structure and function of this olfactory region is discussed in Chapter 10. The narrow ribbonlike passages created by the conchae improve the conditioning of the inspired air (1) by increasing the surface area containing the respi-

ratory epithelium and (2) by creating turbulence in the air flow that results in increased contact between air streams and the mucous layer. Within the lamina propria of the conchae are large venous plexuses known as **swell bodies.** Every 20–30 minutes, the swell bodies on one side of the nasal fossae become engorged with blood, which results in distention of the conchal mucosa and a concomitant decrease in the flow of air. During this time, most of the air is directed through the other nasal fossa. These periodic intervals of occlusion reduce air flow, so that the respiratory epithelium can recover from desiccation. Allergic reactions can cause abnormal engorgement of swell bodies in both fossae and result in severely restricted air flow.

In addition to swell bodies, the nasal cavity has a rich and complexly organized vascular system. Large vessels form a close-meshed latticework next to the periosteum, from which arcading branches lead toward the surface. Smaller vessels branch from the arcading vessels and run perpendicular to the surface. These smaller vessels form a rich capillary bed beneath the epithelium. Blood flows forward from the rear to each fossa. In each arcading loop, the flow of blood counters the flow of inspired air. As a result, the incoming air is efficiently warmed by a countercurrent system.

PARANASAL SINUSES

The paranasal sinuses are cavities in the frontal, maxillary, ethmoid, and sphenoid bones that are lined with a lower respiratory epithelium containing few goblet cells. The lamina propria contains only a few small glands and is continuous with the underlying periosteum. The mucus produced in these cavities drains into the nasal passages as a result of the activity of its ciliated epithelial cells.

NASOPHARYNX

The nasopharynx is the first part of the pharynx, continuing caudally with the oral portion of this organ, the **oropharynx.** It is lined with respiratory-type epithelium in the portion that is in contact with the soft palate.

LARYNX

The larynx is an irregular tube that connects the pharynx to the trachea. Within the lamina propria lie a number of laryngeal cartilages, structurally the most complex in the respiratory tree. The larger cartilages (thyroid, cricoid, and most of the arytenoids) are hyaline cartilage, and some are subject to calcification in old people. The smaller cartilages (epiglottis, cuneiform, corniculate, and the tips of the arytenoids) are elastic cartilage. Ligaments bind the cartilages together, and most are articulated by the intrinsic muscles of the larynx, which in themselves are unusual in that they are striated skeletal muscle. In addition to their supporting role (maintenance of an open airway), these cartilages serve as a valve to prevent swallowed food or fluid from entering the trachea. They also serve as a means of producing tone for phonation.

The **epiglottis,** which projects from the rim of the larynx, extends into the pharynx and therefore has both a lingual and laryngeal surface. The entire lingual surface and the apical portion of the laryngeal side are covered by stratified squamous epithelium. Toward the base of the epiglottis on the laryngeal side, the epithelium undergoes a transition into pseudostratified columnar ciliated epithelium. Mixed mucous and serous glands, mainly found beneath the columnar epithelium, make deep excursions that create characteristic pockmarks in the underlying elastic cartilage.

Below the epiglottis, the mucosa forms 2 pairs of folds that extend into the lumen of the larynx. The upper pair constitute the **false vocal cords** (or vestibular folds), and they possess typical respiratory epithelium below which lie numerous seromucous glands within the lamina propria. The lower pair of folds constitute the **true vocal cords.** Within the vocal folds, which are covered by a stratified squamous epithelium, lie large bundles of parallel aligned elastic fibers that compose the **vocal ligament.** Parallel to the ligaments are bundles of skeletal muscle, the **vocalis muscles,** which regulate the tension of the fold and its ligaments and consequently, as air is forced between the folds, provide for production of sounds with different tones.

TRACHEA
(Fig 18–4)

The trachea is a thin-walled tube that extends from the base of the larynx (the cricoid cartilage) to the point at which it bifurcates into the 2 primary bronchi. The trachea is lined with a typical respiratory mucosa. Sixteen to 20 C-shaped rings of hyaline cartilage found in the lamina propria serve to keep the tracheal lumen patent. A fibroelastic ligament and bundle of smooth muscle (trachealis muscle) bind to the perichondrium and bridge the open ends of these C-shaped cartilages. The ligament prevents overdistention of the lumen, while the muscle allows the cartilage to close down. Contraction of the muscle and the concomitant narrow-

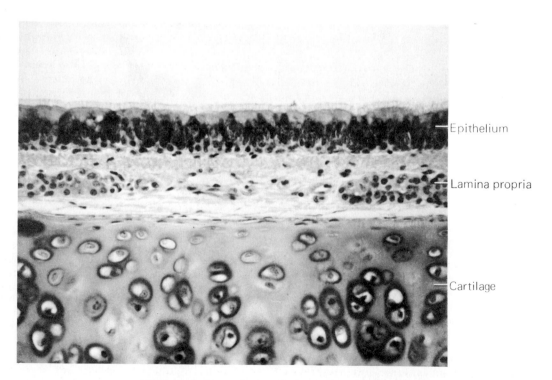

Epithelium

Lamina propria

Cartilage

Figure 18–5. Photomicrograph of a section of dog trachea.

ing of the tracheal lumen are used in a cough response. Following contraction, the resulting smaller bore of the trachea will provide for increased velocity of expired air, which aids in clearing the air passage.

BRONCHIAL TREE

The trachea divides into 2 **primary bronchi,** which enter the lungs at the hilum (Fig 18–7). In addition, at each hilum, the arteries enter and the veins and lymphatic vessels leave the lungs. These structures are surrounded by dense connective tissue and form a unit called the **pulmonary root.**

After entering the lungs, the primary bronchi course downward and outward, giving rise to 3 bronchi in the right lung and 2 in the left lung, each of which supplies a pulmonary lobe (Fig 18–1). These **lobar bronchi** divide repeatedly, giving rise to smaller bronchi the terminal branches of which are called **bronchioles.** Each bronchiole enters a pulmonary lobule, where it branches to form 5–7 **terminal bronchioles.**

The pulmonary lobules are pyramid-shaped, with the apex directed toward the pulmonary surface. Each lobule is delimited by a thin connective tissue septum, best seen in the fetus. In adults, these septa are frequently incomplete, resulting in a poor delineation of the lobules. In lobules nearest the **pleura** (the outer lining of the lungs), the lobules are frequently delineated as a result of the accumulation of carbon and dust particles deposited in the connective tissue of the interlobular septa.

The primary bronchi generally possess the same histologic picture as the trachea. As we proceed toward the respiratory portion, we can observe a simplification of the histologic organization of both the epithelium and underlying lamina propria. It must be stressed, however, that this simplification is slow and gradual, and no abrupt transition can be observed between the bronchi and bronchioles. For this reason, the division of the bronchial tree into bronchi, bronchioles, etc, is to some extent artificial despite the fact that it has teaching and practical value.

Bronchi (Figs 18–6 and 18–7)

With 2 exceptions, the mucosa of the bronchi is structurally similar to that in the trachea. Unlike those found in the trachea, the bronchial cartilages are more irregular in shape; in the larger portions of the bronchi, the cartilage rings completely encircle the lumen. As bronchial diameter decreases, the cartilage rings are replaced by isolated "plates" or "islands" of hyaline cartilage. Beneath the epithelium, in the bronchial lamina propria, one can observe the presence of a smooth muscle layer con-

sisting of crisscrossing bundles of **spirally arranged** smooth muscle (Fig 18–7). Bundles of smooth muscle become a more prominent feature in the walls of the conducting portion as one approaches the respiratory zone. In histologic sections, this muscular layer may appear to be discontinuous. The contraction of this muscle after death is responsible for the folded aspect of the bronchial mucosa observed in histologic section. The lamina propria is rich in elastic fibers and exhibits an abundance of mucous or seromucous glands whose ducts open into the bronchial lumen. Numerous free lymphocytes are found both within the lamina propria and among the epithelial cells. Lymphatic nodules are present and are particularly numerous at the branching points of the bronchial tree.

Bronchioles (Fig 18–7)

These are intralobular segments with diameters of 1 mm or less. Bronchioles have neither cartilage nor glands in their mucosa and show only scattered goblet cells within the epithelium of the initial segments. In the larger bronchioles, the epithelium is pseudostratified ciliated columnar, which decreases in height and complexity to become a simple ciliated cuboidal epithelium in the smaller **terminal bronchioles.** In addition to ciliated cells, terminal bronchioles also possess **Clara cells** with dome-shaped apical surfaces that project into the lumen. Studies on human Clara cells suggest that they are secretory cells; at present, however, their function is unknown.

A large part of the lamina propria is smooth muscle and elastic fibers. The musculature of both the bronchi and bronchioles is under the control of the vagus nerve and the sympathetic nervous system. Stimulation of the vagus nerve decreases the diameter of these structures, whereas sympathetic stimulation produces the opposite effect. This explains why epinephrine and other sympathomimetic drugs are frequently employed to relax smooth muscle during asthmatic attacks. When the thicknesses of the bronchial and bronchiolar walls are compared, it can be seen that the bronchiolar muscle layer is proportionally better developed than that of the bronchi. Increased airway resistance in asthma is believed to be due mainly to contraction of bronchiolar muscle.

Respiratory Bronchioles (Figs 18–9 and 18–10)

Each terminal bronchiole subdivides into 2 or more **respiratory bronchioles** that serve as regions of transition between the conducting and respiratory portions of the respiratory system. The respiratory bronchiolar mucosa is structurally identical to that of the terminal bronchioles except that their walls are interrupted by numerous saccular alveoli (Figs 18–1 and 18–9). Portions of the respiratory bronchioles may be lined with ciliated cuboidal epithelium, but at the rim of the alveolar openings the bronchiolar epithelium becomes continuous

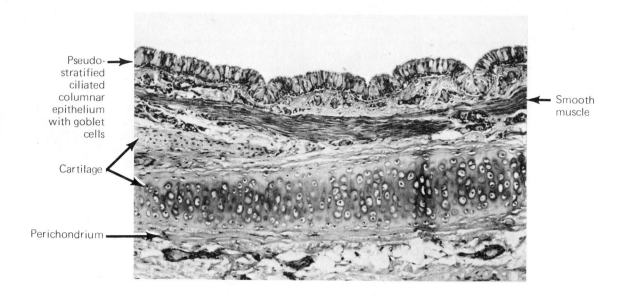

Pseudo-
stratified
ciliated
columnar
epithelium
with goblet
cells

Cartilage

Perichondrium

Smooth
muscle

Figure 18 –6. Photomicrograph of a large bronchus. Observe the ciliated pseudostratified epithelium with many goblet cells, 2 cartilaginous plates, and smooth muscle. H&E stain, reduced from × 200.

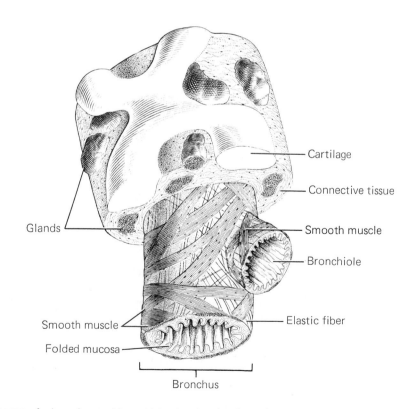

Cartilage

Connective tissue

Smooth muscle

Bronchiole

Glands

Smooth muscle

Folded mucosa

Elastic fiber

Bronchus

Figure 18 –7. Diagram of a bronchus and bronchiole showing the discontinuous smooth muscle layer. The contraction of this muscle induces folding of the mucosa. Smooth muscle is present in all of the bronchiolar tree, up through the respiratory bronchiole. The elastic fibers present in the bronchus continue into the bronchiole. An irregular cartilaginous plate sectioned in 2 regions is shown in white. The adventitia is not represented in this drawing.

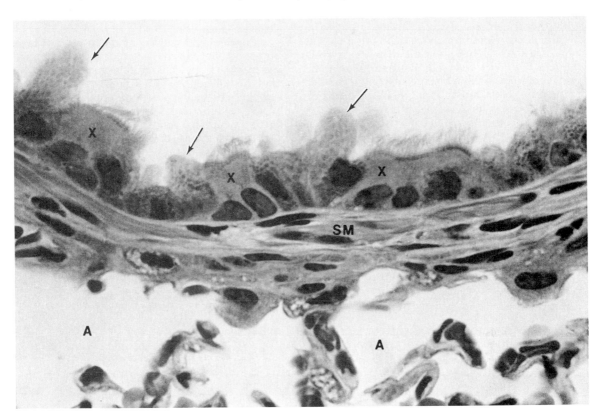

Figure 18–8. Portion of terminal bronchiole in mouse lung. In addition to the ciliated cuboidal cells (X) are the larger secretory Clara cells (arrows). Bundles of smooth muscle (SM) cells lie beneath the epithelium. Surrounding the terminal bronchiole are alveoli (A).

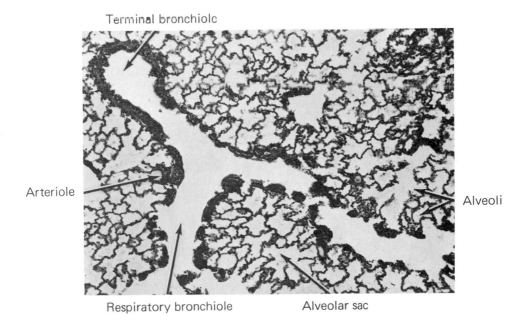

Terminal bronchiole

Arteriole

Alveoli

Respiratory bronchiole

Alveolar sac

Figure 18–9. Photomicrograph of a thick lung section showing a terminal bronchiole dividing into 2 respiratory bronchioles in which alveoli appear. The spongelike aspect of the lung is due to the abundance of alveoli and alveolar sacs. H&E stain, × 80.

with the squamous alveolar lining. Proceeding distally along these bronchioles, the number of alveoli increases greatly, and the distance between them is markedly reduced. Between alveoli, the bronchiolar epithelium consists of ciliated cuboidal epithelium; however, in more distal portions, the cilia may be absent. Along walls heavily populated with alveoli, bronchiolar characteristics are evident only between the alveoli and consist of small groups of cuboidal cells overlying bands of smooth muscle and elastic connective tissue. Since the alveoli are sites of gas exchange, the term "respiratory bronchiole" aptly describes the dual function of this segment of the respiratory tree.

Alveolar Ducts (Fig 18–10)

Proceeding distally along the respiratory bronchioles, it is noted that the number of alveolar openings into the bronchiolar wall becomes ever greater until the wall consists of nothing else. Although the branches still retain a conduit appearance, in histologic section the alveolar duct presents a very discontinuous wall. Both the alveolar ducts and alveoli are lined by extremely attenuated squamous epithelial cells. In the lamina propria surrounding the rim of the alveoli is an interwoven network of smooth muscle cells. These sphincterlike smooth bundles appear as knobs between adjacent alveoli. A rich matrix of elastic and collagen fibers provides

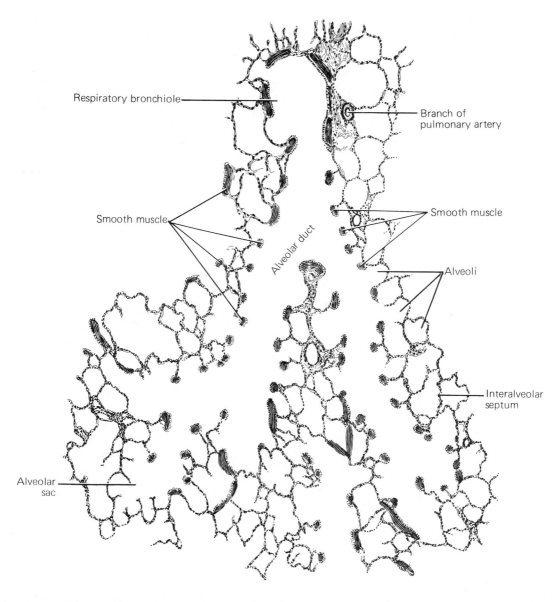

Figure 18–10. Diagram of a portion of the bronchial tree. Observe that smooth muscle present in the alveolar ducts disappears in the alveoli. (Redrawn from Baltisberger.)

the only support for the duct and its alveoli.

Alveolar ducts open into **atria,** vestibules that communicate with **multilocular alveolar sacs.** Two or more alveolar sacs arise from each atrium. A heavy investment of elastic fibers and collagen forms a complex network encircling the openings of atria, alveolar sacs, and alveoli. The elastic fibers enable the alveoli to expand upon inspiration and to passively contract during expiration. The collagen serves as a support that prevents overdistention and damage to the delicate capillaries and thin alveolar septa.

Alveoli

Alveoli are small saclike evaginations of the respiratory bronchioles, alveolar ducts, and alveolar sacs. Alveoli are the terminal portions of the bronchial tree and are responsible for the spongy structure of the lungs. Structurally, alveoli resemble small pockets open on one side, similar to the

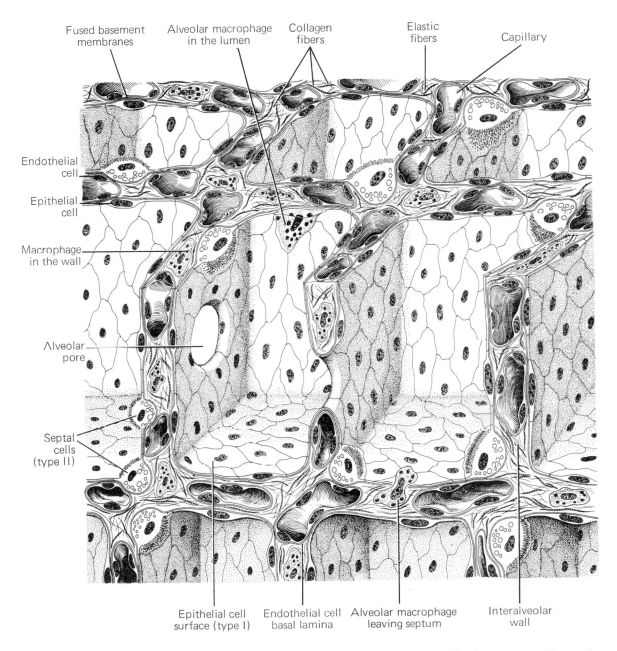

Figure 18–11. Three-dimensional diagram of pulmonary alveoli showing the interalveolar wall and its structure. Observe the capillaries, connective tissue, and macrophages. These cells can also be seen in the alveolar lumens or passing into them. Alveolar pores are numerous. The septal cells are identified by their abundant apical microvilli. The alveoli are lined by a continuous epithelial layer.

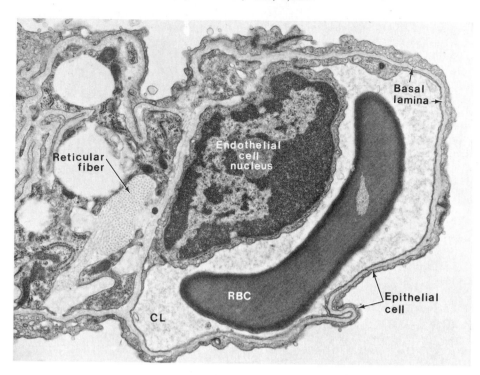

Figure 18–12. Electron micrograph of the alveolar wall. Observe a capillary containing a red blood cell (RBC), the capillary lumen (CL), basal lamina, and epithelial cell (type I cell) cytoplasm. × 17,000. (Reproduced, with permission, from Schneeberger EE: *Lung Liquids*. Ciba Foundation Symposium No. 38. Elsevier/North-Holland, 1976.)

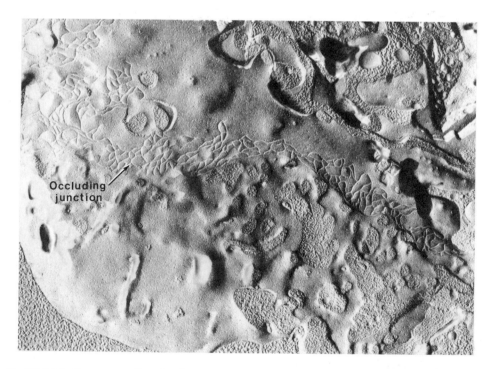

Figure 18–13. Freeze fracture preparation showing an occluding junction between 2 epithelial cells (type I) of the alveolar lining.× 25,000. (Reproduced, with permission, from Schneeberger EE: *Lung Liquids*. Ciba Foundation Symposium No. 38. Elsevier/North-Holland, 1976.)

honeycombs of a beehive. Within these cuplike structures, oxygen and CO_2 are exchanged between the air and the blood. The structure of the alveolar walls is specialized for promoting diffusion between the external and internal environments. Generally, each wall is common to 2 neighboring alveoli and is thus termed an **interalveolar septum** or **wall.** An alveolar septum consists of 2 thin squamous epithelial layers between which lie capillaries, elastic and collagen fibers, and fibroblasts. The capillaries and connective tissue matrix constitute the **interstitium.** Within the interstitium of the alveolar septa are the richest capillary networks in the body (Fig 18–11).

The air in the alveoli is separated from capillary blood by 4 layers of cells and membranes: the cytoplasm of the epithelial cells, the basal lamina of the epithelium, the basal lamina of the endothelial cells, and the cytoplasm of the endothelial cells (Figs 18–12 and 18–13). To reduce dimensions of the air-blood barrier, the 2 basal laminas are generally fused into one thin lamina. The total thickness of these 4 layers varies from 0.2 to 0.5 μm. Within the interalveolar septa, the anastomosing pulmonary capillaries are supported by a meshwork of collagen and elastic fibers. These fibers, which are arranged to permit expansion and contraction of alveolar walls, are the primary means of structural support of the alveoli. Within the interstitium of the septa, leukocytes, macrophages, and fibroblasts can also be found (Fig 18–11).

The oxygen of the alveolar air passes into the capillary blood through the above-mentioned membranes (Fig 18–14); CO_2 diffuses in the opposite direction. Liberation of CO_2 from H_2CO_3 is catalyzed by the enzyme carbonic anhydrase present in red blood cells. It is not surprising, therefore, that the erythrocyte contains more of this enzyme than any other cell in the body. The lungs contain approximately 300 million alveoli, thus increasing considerably their internal exchange surface, which has been calculated to be approximately 70–80 m².

The interalveolar wall is composed of 3 main cell types: capillary endothelial cells, squamous (type I) epithelial cells, and great alveolar (type II or septal) cells (Figs 18–12 and 18–15).

Endothelial cells of the capillaries are extremely thin and may have a smaller, more elongated-appearing nucleus than the epithelial lining cells with which they are frequently confused. The endothelial lining of the capillaries is continuous and not fenestrated (Fig 18–12). Cytologically, the nuclei and other organelles are clustered to allow the remaining areas of the cell to become extremely thin in order to increase the efficiency of gas exchange. The most prominent feature of the cytoplasm in the flattened portions of the cell are numerous pinocytotic vesicles.

Squamous alveolar cells, also called **type I cells,** are extremely attenuated cells that line the alveolar surfaces. These cells are so thin, sometimes

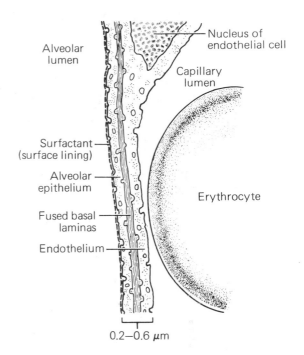

Figure 18–14. The alveolo-capillary membrane. To reach the red cell, O_2 traverses the surface lining, the alveolar epithelial cytoplasm, the basal lamina, the endothelial cell cytoplasm, and the plasma. In some locations, there is loose interstitial tissue between the epithelium and the endothelium. (Approximate magnification × 20,000.) (Modified and reproduced, with permission, from Ganong WF: *Review of Medical Physiology,* 8th ed. Lange, 1977.)

only 25 nm in diameter, that electron microscopic analysis was needed to prove that all capillaries were covered by an epithelial lining (Figs 18–9 and 18–12). To reduce the thickness of the air-blood barrier, the nuclei and organelles of the squamous cells are clustered, while around the nuclei the cytoplasm fans out, forming a thin lining layer. The cytoplasm in the thin portion consists mainly of pinocytotic vesicles, which play a significant role in the turnover of surfactant (described below) and the removal of small particulate contaminants from the outer surface. Cytologically, squamous epithelial and capillary endothelial cells are virtually mirror images of each other. In addition to desmosomes, which bind adjacent cells, all epithelial cells have occluding junctions that serve to prevent the leakage of tissue fluid into the alveolar air space (Fig 18–12). The main role of this cell is to provide a barrier of minimal thickness that is readily permeable to gases.

Great alveolar cells or **type II cells,** also called **septal cells,** are found interspersed among the squamous epithelial cells, with which they have occluding and desmosomal junctions (Figs 18–11 and 18–14). Great alveolar cells are roughly cuboidal cells that are usually found in groups of 2 or 3 along the alveolar surface at points where the alveo-

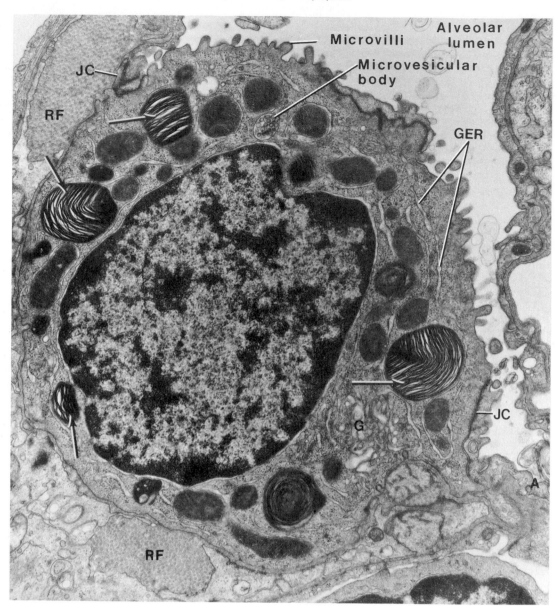

Figure 18–15. Septal cell from rat lung protruding into the alveolar lumen. Arrows point to lamellar bodies containing newly synthesized pulmonary surface-active material. GER, granular endoplasmic reticulum; G, Golgi body. At A, the cytoplasm of an epithelial lining cell. Note the microvilli of the septal cell and the junctional complexes (JC) with the epithelial lining cell. × 17,000. (Courtesy of M Williams.)

lar walls unite and form angles. These cells, which sit on the basal lamina, are part of the epithelium, for they have the same origin as the squamous epithelial cells that line the alveolar walls. Cytologically, these cells resemble typical secretory cells. They have mitochondria, granular endoplasmic reticulum, a well-developed Golgi apparatus, and microvilli on their free apical surface. In histologic sections, they exhibit a characteristic vesicular or foamy cytoplasm. The vacuoles are due to the presence of **multilamellar bodies** or **cytosomes** that are preserved and evident in tissue prepared for elec-

tron microscopy. The multilamellar bodies, which average about 0.2 μm in diameter, contain granules possessing concentric or parallel lamellas limited by a unit membrane. Histochemical studies reveal that these bodies, which contain phospholipids, mucopolysaccharides, and proteins, are continuously synthesized and released at the apical surface of the cell. The multilamellar bodies, which are extruded singly, give rise to a material that spreads over the alveolar surfaces, providing an extracellular coating, **surfactant,** that possesses an unusual surface activity. The secretory processes of the type II cell have been elucidated by the aid of electron microscopy and radioautography and are summarized in Fig 18–13.

The surfactant layer consists of an aqueous proteinaceous hypophase covered by a monomolecular phospholipid film, primarily composed of **dipalmitoyl lecithin.** Surfactant serves several major functions in the economy of the lung. Primarily, surfactant aids in reducing the surface tension of the squamous alveolar cells. Without surfactant, these extremely flattened cells would tend to round up, a general phenomenon exhibited by cells in response to the need to reduce the energy expenditures required to maintain the more extensive surface area present on flattened cells. Reduction of surface tension means that less inspiratory force is needed to inflate the alveoli, thus reducing the work of breathing. In fetal development, surfactant appears in the last weeks of gestation and coincides with the appearance of multilamellar bodies in the great alveolar cells. In cases of premature birth, infants frequently exhibit labored breathing that results in respiratory distress. **Hyaline membrane disease** in newborns has been shown to be the result of insufficient surfactant production, so that the infant has difficulty in expanding the alveoli. Fortunately, surfactant synthesis can be induced, so that the respiratory distress syndrome usually represents a short-term management problem. In addition to its surface-active properties, surfactant facilitates the transport of gases between the air and liquid phases. Recently, surfactant has also been demonstrated to have a bactericidal effect which aids in the removal of potentially dangerous bacteria that reach the alveoli.

The surfactant layer is not static but is constantly being turned over. The lipoproteins are gradually removed from the surface by the pinocytotic vesicles of the squamous epithelial cells. These vesicles transport the material through the cell and release it into the interstitium, where it is eventually removed by lymphatics. These substances therefore undergo a continuous cycle of secretion and reabsorption.

Alveolar lining fluids are also removed via the conducting passages as a result of ciliary activity. As the secretions pass up through the airways, they combine with bronchial mucus, forming a **broncho-alveolar fluid.** This fluid aids in the removal of particulate and noxious components from the inspired air. Within the fluids are several lytic enzymes (eg, lysozyme, collagenase, and β-glucuronidase) that are probably derived from the alveolar macrophages.

Alveolar Macrophages (Fig 18–11)

The thinnest barrier between blood plasma and inspired air is reduced to an alveolar epithelium, a fused basal lamina, and the capillary endothelium. Although seemingly susceptible to bacterial and viral infection, chronic inflammation does not exist, since a barrier to infection is provided by the **alveolar macrophage.** These macrophages, also called **dust cells,** are derived from monocytes that originate in bone marrow. They are found in the interior of the alveolar septum or are often seen protruding from the alveolar walls into the lumen. Although it is commonly considered that these macrophages can reenter the interstitium after being in the alveolar lumen, recent evidence suggests that macrophages do not recross the alveolar wall. Numerous carbon- and dust-laden macrophages in the connective tissue around major blood vessels or in the pleura probably represent cells that have never passed through the epithelial lining. The phagocytosed debris within these cells was probably passed from the alveolar lumen into the interstitium by the pinocytotic activity of the squamous epithelial cells. The alveolar macrophages that scavenge the outer surface of the epithelium, within the surfactant layer, are carried to the pharynx where they are swallowed.

In heart failure, the lungs become congested with blood and the red cells pass into the alveoli (diapedesis), where they are phagocytosed by the alveolar macrophages. In such cases, these macrophages are called **cardiac failure cells** and are identified by a positive histochemical reaction for iron pigment (hemosiderin).

In addition to the cells discussed above, the alveolar septum also contains fibroblasts, mast cells, and a recently identified contractile cell. Interstitial fibroblasts synthesize collagen, elastic fibers, and ground substance glycosaminoglycans. The collagen constitutes 15–20% of the parenchymal mass and consists primarily of types I and III collagen. Type III fibers probably correspond to the alveolar reticular fibers (Fig 18–12), whereas type I collagen is probably concentrated in the walls of the conducting passages and in the pleura. Lung collagen proliferation is common, and more than 100 disease entities are known to be associated with lung fibrosis.

Contractile cells in the septum are found bound to the basal surface of the alveolar epithelium and not to the endothelial cells. These cells, which react with antiactin and antimyosin, contract and reduce the volume of the alveolar lumen. In vitro, it has been demonstrated that lung parenchymal tissue will contract when exposed to pharmacologic agents such as epinephrine and histamine.

Alveolar Pores (Figs 18–11 and 18–17)

The interalveolar septum may contain one or more pores, 10–15 μm in diameter, connecting neighboring alveoli. They might equalize pressure in the alveoli or might make possible collateral circulation of air when a bronchiole is obstructed.

Alveolar Lining Regeneration

It has been observed that inhalation of NO_2 promotes destruction of most of the cells lining the

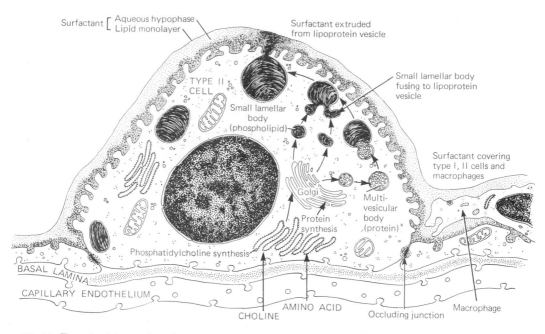

Figure 18–16. The physiology of surfactant secretion by the septal cell. The surfactant consists of an overlying monomolecular film of lipid and an underlying aqueous hypophase. When present in the alveolar lumen, macrophages lie outside of the epithelium but within the surfactant layer. Occluding junctions around the margins of the epithelial cells prevent leakage of tissue fluid into the alveolar lumen.

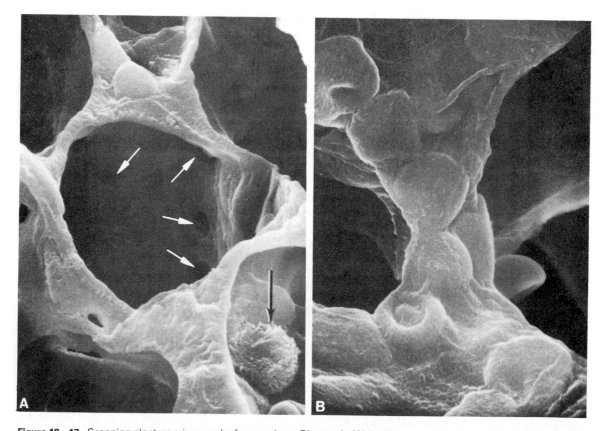

Figure 18–17. Scanning electron micrograph of mouse lung. Observe in *(A)* the thin septa and alveolar pores (white arrows). At the black arrow, a macrophage with its typical ruffled membrane. × 3200. In *(B)*, the alveolar wall is so thin that one can see the shape of the red blood cells in a capillary. × 6700. (Courtesy of Greenwood MF, Holland P: Lab Invest 27:296, 1972.)

alveoli (type I and type II cells). The action of this compound or other toxic substances with the same effect is followed by a drastic increase in the mitotic activity of the remaining cells, producing great numbers of type II cells. In the second step of alveolar lining regeneration, most of the type II cells are transformed into type I cells, and the alveolar lining regains its normal appearance. The normal turnover rate of type II cells is estimated to be 1% per day, maintaining a continuous renewal of its own type and also of type I cells.

PULMONARY BLOOD VESSELS

Circulation in the lungs includes nutrient and functional vessels.

The functional circulation is represented by pulmonary arteries and veins. The pulmonary artery is elastic in type and contains venous blood to be oxygenated in the pulmonary alveoli. Within the lung this artery branches, accompanying the bronchial tree (Fig 18–18). Its branches are surrounded by adventitia of the bronchi and bronchioles. At the level of the alveolar duct, the branches of this artery

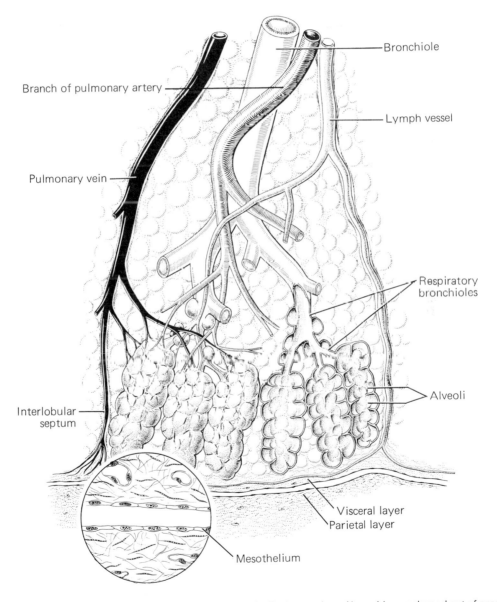

Figure 18–18. Blood and lymph circulation in a pulmonary lobule. Both vessels and bronchi are enlarged out of proportion in this drawing. In the interlobular septa, only the vein (left) or lymph vessel (right) has been represented, although both actually coexist in this region. At lower left, an enlargement of the pleura showing its mesothelial lining. (Based partially on Ham AW: *Histology,* 6th ed. Lippincott, 1969.)

form a capillary network in close contact with the alveolar epithelium. The lung has the best-developed extremely fine capillary network in the body. The capillaries occur in all alveoli, including those present in the respiratory bronchioles.

Venules that originate in the capillary network occur singly in the parenchyma; they are supported by a thin covering of connective tissue and enter the interlobular septa (Fig 18–18). After veins leave a lobule, they follow the bronchial tree toward the hilum; until then, they are found singly in the pulmonary parenchyma.

Nutrient vessels include bronchial arteries and veins, which are smaller than the pulmonary artery and veins. The branches of the bronchial arteries also accompany or follow the bronchial tree, but only to the respiratory bronchioles, at which point they anastomose with the pulmonary artery.

PULMONARY LYMPHATIC VESSELS

The lymphatic vessels (Fig 18–18) follow the bronchi and the pulmonary vessels; they also occur in the interlobular septa, and all drain into the lymph nodes in the region of the hilum. This lymphatic network is called the deep network to distinguish it from the superficial network, which includes lymphatic vessels present in the visceral pleura. The lymphatic vessels of this region drain toward the hilum. They either follow the entire length of the pleura or penetrate the lung tissue via the interlobular septa.

In the terminal portions of the bronchial tree and beyond the alveolar ducts, lymphatic vessels do not occur.

PLEURA

The pleura (Fig 18–18) is the serous membrane covering the lung. It consists of 2 layers, parietal

and visceral, which are continuous in the region of the hilum. Both membranes are covered by mesothelial cells that rest on a fine connective tissue layer containing collagen and elastic fibers. The elastic fibers of the visceral pleura are continuous with those of the pulmonary parenchyma.

These 2 layers, therefore, delimit a cavity entirely lined by mesothelial squamous cells. Under normal conditions, this pleural cavity contains only a film of liquid that acts as a lubricating agent, permitting the smooth sliding of one surface over the other during respiratory movements. In certain pathologic states, the pleural cavity can become a real cavity, containing liquid or air in its interior. The walls of the pleural cavity, like all serosal cavities (peritoneal and pericardial), are quite permeable to water and other substances—thus the high frequency of fluid accumulation in this cavity in pathologic conditions. This fluid is derived from the blood plasma by exudation. Conversely, under certain conditions, liquids or gases present in the pleural cavity can be rapidly reabsorbed.

RESPIRATORY MOVEMENTS

During inhalation, contraction of the intercostal muscles elevates the ribs and contraction of the diaphragm lowers the bottom of the thoracic cavity, increasing its diameter and resulting in pulmonary expansion. The bronchi and bronchioles increase in diameter and length during inhalation. The respiratory portion also enlarges, mainly as a result of expansion of the alveolar ducts; the alveoli enlarge only slightly. The elastic fibers of the pulmonary parenchyma are stretched by this expansion, so that during exhalation caused by muscle relaxation the retraction of the lungs is passive, mainly because of the elastic fibers, which were under tension.

• • •

References

Adamson IYR, Bowden DH: Adaptive responses of the pulmonary macrophagic system to carbon. 2. Morphologic studies. Lab Invest 38:430, 1978.

Ali MY: Histology of the human nasopharyngeal mucosa. J Anat 99:657, 1965.

Andrews PM: A scanning electron microscopic study of the extrapulmonary respiratory tract. Am J Anat 139:399, 1974.

Bertalanffy FD: Respiratory tissue: Structure, histophysiology, cytodynamics. 1. Review and basic cytomorphology. Int Rev Cytol 16:233, 1964.

Bouhuy SA: *Lung Cells in Disease*. Elsevier/North-Holland, 1976.

Camner P, Mossberg B, Afzelius BA: Evidence for congenital nonfunctional cilia in the tracheobronchial tract in two subjects. Am Rev Respir Dis 112:807, 1975.

Chevalier G, Collet AJ: In vivo incorporation of choline-^{3}H, leucine-^{3}H and galactose-^{3}H in alveolar type two pneumocytes in relation to surfactant synthesis: A quantitative radioautographic study in mice by electron microscopy. Anat Rec 174:289, 1972.

Cutz E & others: Ultrastructure and fluorescence histochemistry of endocrine (APUD-type) cells in tracheal mucosa of human and various animal species. Cell Tissue Res 158:425, 1975.

Dermer GB: The pulmonary surfactant content of the inclusion bodies found within type II alveolar cells. J Ultrastruct Res 33:306, 1970.

Etherton JE, Conning DM, Corrin B: Autoradiographic and morphological evidence for apocrine secretion of dipalmitoyl lecithin in the terminal bronchiole of mouse lung. Am J Anat 138:11, 1973.

Evans MJ: Transformation of type II cells to type I cells following exposure to NO_2. Exp Mol Pathol 22:142, 1975.

Goerke J: Lung surfactant. Biochim Biophys Acta 344:241, 1979.

Goldberg VE, Buckingham S, Sommers SC: Pilocarpine stimulation of granular pneumocyte secretion. Lab Invest 20:147, 1969.

Greenwood M, Holland P: The mammalian respiratory tract surface: A scanning electron microscope study. Lab Invest 27:296, 1972.

Hatasa K, Nakamura T: Electron microscopic observations of lung alveolar epithelial cells of normal young mice, with special reference to formation and secretion of osmiophilic lamellar bodies. Z Zellforsch Mikrosk Anat 68:266, 1965.

Heineman HO, Fishmann AP: Nonrespiratory functions of mammalian lungs. Physiol Rev 49:1, 1969.

Hung KS & others: Ultrastructure of nerves and associated cells in bronchial epithelium of the mouse lung. J Ultrastruct Res 43:426, 1973.

Juers JA: Enhancement of bactericidal capacity of alveolar marcophages by human alveolar living material. J Clin Invest 58:271, 1976.

Kapanci Y & others: Contractile interstitial cells in pulmonary alveolar septa: A possible regulator of ventilation/perfusion ratio. J Cell Biol 60:375, 1974.

Kikkawa Y & others: The type II epithelial cells of the lung. 2. Chemical composition and phospholipid synthesis. Lab Invest 32:295, 1975.

Kuhn C III: The cells of the lung and their organelles. In: *The Biochemical Basis of Pulmonary Function*. Crystal RG (editor). Marcel Dekker, 1976.

Kuhn C III, Finke EH: The topography of the pulmonary alveolus: Scanning electron microscopy using different fixations. J Ultrastruct Res 38:161, 1972.

Nagaishi C: *Functional Anatomy and Histology of the Lung*. University Park Press, 1972.

Ryan JW, Ryan US: Pulmonary endothelial cells. Fed Proc 36:2683, 1977.

Schneeberger EE: *Lung Liquids*. Ciba Foundation Symposium No. 38. Elsevier/North-Holland, 1976.

Sorokin SP: A morphologic and cytochemical study on the great alveolar cells. J Histochem Cytochem 14:884, 1966.

Sorokin SP, Brain JD: Pathways of clearance in mouse lungs exposed to iron oxide aerosols. Anat Rec 181:581, 1975.

Thomas ED & others: Direct evidence for a bone marrow origin of the alveolar macrophage in man. Science 192:1016, 1976.

Thurlbeck WM, Abell MR (editors): *The Lung: Structure, Function, and Disease*. Williams & Wilkins, 1978.

Tobin CE: Human pulmonic lymphatics. Anat Rec 127:611, 1957.

Weibel ER: Morphological basis of alveolar capillary gas exchange. Physiol Rev 53:419, 1973.

19 | Skin

Skin is the heaviest single organ of the body, accounting for about 16% of total body weight. It is composed of an epithelial layer of ectodermal origin, **epidermis,** and a layer of connective tissue of mesodermal origin, **dermis** or **corium.** The junction of dermis and epidermis is irregular, and projections of the dermis called **papillae** interdigitate with invaginations of the epidermis called **epidermal ridges** (Fig 19–1). Beneath the dermis lies the **hypodermis** or **subcutaneous tissue,** a loose connective tissue containing many adipose cells, the **panniculus adiposus.** The hypodermis, not considered part of the skin, binds skin loosely to the subjacent tissues. Epidermal appendages include hairs, nails, and sebaceous and sweat glands.

The external layer of the skin is relatively impermeable to water, which prevents extreme water loss by evaporation and allows for terrestrial life. The skin functions as a receptor organ in continuous communication with the environment (see Chapter 10) and protects the organism from impact and friction injuries. A pigment called **melanin,** produced and stored in the cells of the epidermis, provides further protective action against ultraviolet rays.

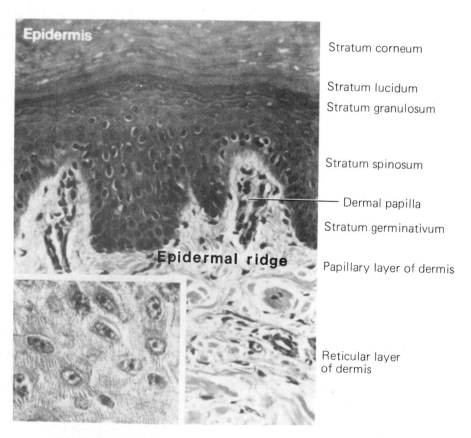

Stratum corneum

Stratum lucidum
Stratum granulosum

Stratum spinosum

Dermal papilla

Stratum germinativum

Papillary layer of dermis

Reticular layer of dermis

Figure 19–1. Photomicrographs of a section of human thick skin from the sole of the foot. Observe the papillae of the papillary layer and the thickness of the stratum corneum. The inset, at higher magnification, shows cells of the stratum spinosum with characteristic "spiny" intercellular bridges. H&E stain, × 100 and × 600.

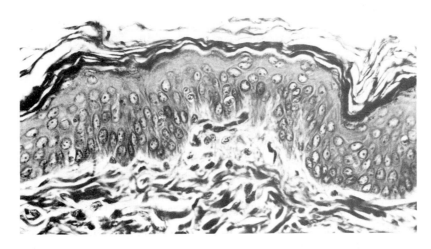

Figure 19 –2. Photomicrograph of a section of human abdominal (thin) skin. Compare with Fig 19–1 and note the thinness of the whole epidermis and, specifically, the stratum corneum. The strata are not as clearly seen as in Fig 19–1. H&E stain, × 310.

Glands of the skin, blood vessels, and adipose tissue participate in thermoregulation, body metabolism, and excretion of various substances. Because skin is endowed with elasticity, it can cover large areas in conditions associated with swelling.

Upon close observation, certain portions of human skin show lines arranged in definite patterns which are distinctive and never exactly alike in any 2 individuals. These ridges appear first during intrauterine life at 13 weeks in the tips of the digits (fingerprints) and later in the volar surfaces of the hands and feet. Ridges and sulci and their configuration are known as **dermatoglyphics**. They are unique for each individual and used for personal identification, appearing as loops, arches, whorls, or combinations of these forms. These configurations are probably determined by multiple genes, and dermatoglyphics (fingerprints) is a field that has recently come to be of considerable medical and anthropologic as well as legal interest.

EPIDERMIS

The epidermis consists essentially of stratified squamous keratinized epithelium, but it contains 3

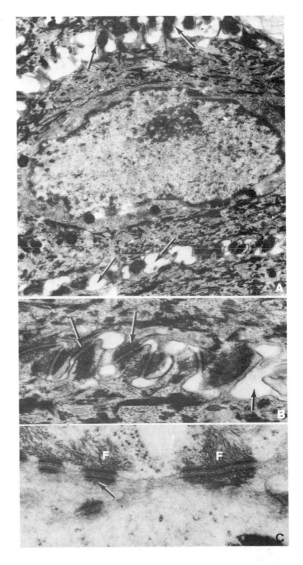

Figure 19 –3 (at right). Electron micrograph of the stratum spinosum of human skin. *A:* A cell of the stratum spinosum with its cytoplasm full of tonofibrils and with melanin granules. The arrows show the "intercellular bridges" with their desmosomes. Reduced from × 14,000. *B* and *C:* Desmosomes in greater detail. Observe that a dense substance appears between the cell membranes and that bundles of cytoplasmic filaments (F) (tonofibrils) insert themselves on the desmosomes. Reduced from × 60,000 and × 75,000. (Courtesy of C Barros.)

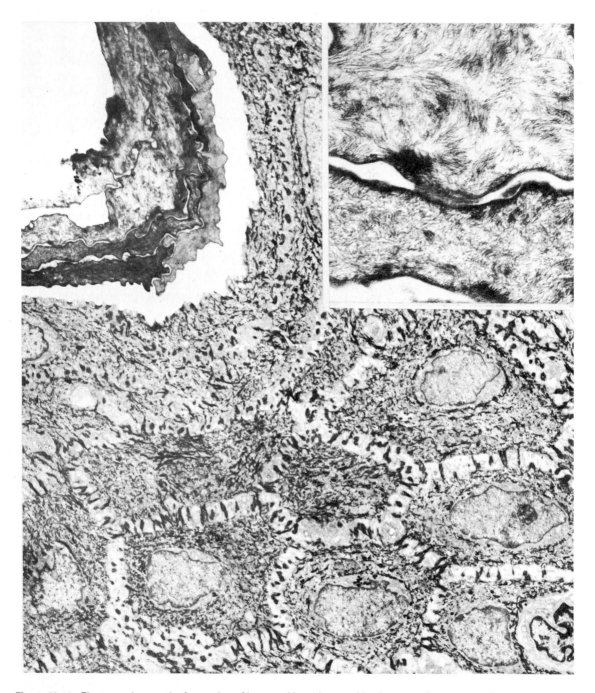

Figure 19–4. Electron micrograph of a section of human skin at the transition between the stratum spinosum and stratum corneum. Observe the cells with their typical cytoplasmic expansions, "intercellular bridges," and cytoplasmic tonofibrils. At upper left is the stratum corneum, seen in detail in the inset at upper right. Observe that these cells are packed with 10-nm intermediate filaments. × 5500 and × 36,000. (Courtesy of C Barros.)

less abundant cell types: **melanocytes, Langerhans cells,** and **Merkel cells.** The keratinizing epidermal cells are called **keratinocytes. Melanocytes** produce the pigment melanin and are derived from the embryonic neural crest and invade the epidermis during the 12th and 14th weeks of human pregnancy.

The thickness of the epidermis varies in different parts of the body. **Thick skin** on the palms of the hands and the soles of the feet may be as thick as 1.5 mm (Figs 4–2, 19–1, and 19–2).

From the dermis outward, the epidermis consists of 5 layers as follows:

(1) The **stratum basale (stratum germinativum)** consists of basophilic columnar or cuboidal cells which rest on the dermal-epidermal junction that separates the dermis from the epidermis. Their long axes are perpendicular to the skin surface. Desmosomes in great quantity bind the cells of this layer in their lateral and upper surfaces. Hemidesmosomes, found in the basal plasmalemma, help bind these cells to the basal lamina (or basement membrane). The stratum basale is characterized by intense mitotic activity and is responsible, in conjunction with the initial portion of the next layer, for constant renewal of epidermal cells. The human epidermis is renewed about every 15–30 days depending on the region of the body, age, and other factors. In vitro cultivation of living human epidermis, in contact with dermis which is killed by repeated freezing and thawing, demonstrates the emergence of a clear-cut basal lamina, indicating an epidermal origin for this extracellular structure. All cells in the stratum basale have filaments about 10 nm in diameter. As the cells progress upward, the number of filaments increases until they represent, in the stratum corneum, half of its total protein.

(2) The **stratum spinosum** consists of cuboidal, polygonal, or slightly flattened cells with a central nucleus and a cytoplasm with processes filled with bundles of filaments. These bundles converge into many small cellular extensions, terminating with desmosomes located at the end of these expansions (Figs 19–1 and 19–3). The cells of this layer are firmly bound together by this system of filament-filled cytoplasmic expansions and desmosomes that cover its whole surface, giving a prickle-studded appearance in the light microscope (Fig 19–4). Such bundles, visible under the light microscope, are called **tonofibrils.** At one time they were believed to cross the intercellular bridges that united cell to cell; however, they are now known to end and insert in the cytoplasmic densities of the desmosomes. It is believed that the filaments play an important role in maintaining cohesion among cells and in resisting the effects of abrasion, especially at the sites of the desmosomes. The epidermis of areas subject to continuous friction and pressure (such as the soles of the feet) has a thicker stratum spinosum with more abundant tonofibrils.

The term **malpighian layer** denotes the stratum basale and stratum spinosum considered together.

(3) The **stratum granulosum** is characterized by 3–5 layers of flattened polygonal cells containing centrally located nuclei and cytoplasm filled with coarse basophilic granules called **keratohyaline granules.** Biochemical studies show that keratohyaline granules contain a histidine-rich protein. These granules are not membrane-bound, and they become part of the interfilamentous matrix in the cells of the stratum corneum. PAS-positive nonglycogen substances are usually found in the intercellular spaces of this layer.

Another characteristic structure found with the electron microscope in the cells of the granular layer of epidermis is the **membrane-coating granule,** ovoid or rodlike in appearance. These granules, formed in association with the Golgi apparatus, move near the upper part of the cell near its plasma membrane. They fuse with the membrane and discharge their contents into the intercellular spaces of the granular layer. Under high magnification in the electron microscope, these granules show a lamellar arrangement. Histochemical reactions indicate that they contain acid mucopolysaccharides and phospholipids. The function of this extruded material is similar to that of an intercellular cement substance which acts as a barrier to the penetration of foreign materials and provides in the skin a very important sealing effect. Studies made in keratinized and nonkeratinized human oral epithelium show that penetration of peroxidase and lanthanum tracers does not occur in the regions where this material fills the extracellular space. Formation of this barrier, which appeared first in reptiles, was one of the important evolutionary events that permitted development of terrestrial life.

(4) The **stratum lucidum,** usually present in thick skin, is translucent and composed of a thin layer of extremely flattened eosinophilic cells (Fig 19–1). The organelles and nuclei are no longer evident, and the cytoplasm consists primarily of densely packed filaments embedded in an electron-dense matrix. Desmosomes are still evident between adjacent cells.

(5) The **stratum corneum** contains flattened nonnucleated keratinized cells whose cytoplasm is filled with a birefringent filamentous scleroprotein, **keratin** (Figs 19–1 and 19–4). This protein consists of elongated protein chains, rich in disulfide bonds, present as bundles of 7–8 nm packed filaments embedded in a dense amorphous matrix. In this stage, the cell membrane becomes 15 nm thick and a unit membrane structure cannot be seen.

After keratinization, the cells consist of only fibrillar and amorphous proteins and thickened plasma membranes and are called **horny cells.** Lysosomal hydrolytic enzymes play a role in the disappearance of the cytoplasmic organelles. At the surface of the stratum corneum, cells are continuously shed.

This description of the epidermis corresponds to its most complex structure in areas where it is very thick, as on the soles of the feet. In other areas the epidermis is much thinner; the stratum granulosum and stratum lucidum are often less well developed; and the stratum corneum may be quite delicate.

Renewal of the epidermis under normal conditions every 15–30 days is due to mitotic activity, observed mainly in the germinativum and spinosum layers. Mitosis is related to epinephrine, a potent mitotic inhibitor present in the bloodstream in greater amounts during periods of activity. During the process of keratinization, gradual cytoplasmic deposition of protein as filaments and an amorphous substance occurs in the cells as they migrate from the base to the surface of the epidermis. Keratinization consists of the synthesis and deposition of a specific fibrous scleroprotein, kera-

tin, that fills the cytoplasm of the cells of this layer. During this process, the structure of keratin is reinforced by formation of several disulfide bonds derived from preexistent sulfhydryl groups. Keratin, which shows great insolubility and resistance to enzymes, gives an α-diffraction pattern similar to that of myosin or fibrinogen. This α type of keratin is present in the epidermis of all vertebrates. Reptilian scales and bird feathers contain protein that gives a β-diffraction pattern. Lysosomes increase considerably in keratinization, during which time their enzymes act in the cytoplasm, digesting cellular organelles. This explains the loss of cell structure and the hyaline appearance of keratinized cells.

Melanocytes

The color of the skin results from several factors, but the most important are its content of melanin and carotene, the number of blood vessels, and the color of the blood flowing in them.

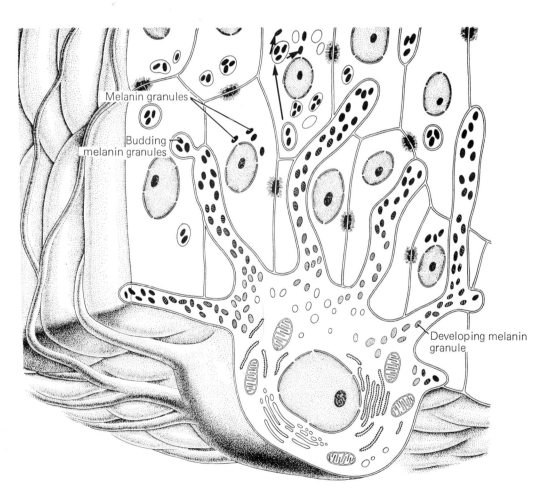

Melanin granules

Budding
melanin granules

Developing melanin
granule

Figure 19–5. Diagram of a melanocyte. Its arms extend upward into the interstices between the epithelial cells. The melanin granules are synthesized in these cells, migrate to its arms, and are transferred into the cytoplasm of epithelial cells. Ribosomes, Golgi apparatus, granular endoplasmic reticulum, and mitochondria are also present. (Based on the work of Fitzpatrick & Szabó, 1959.)

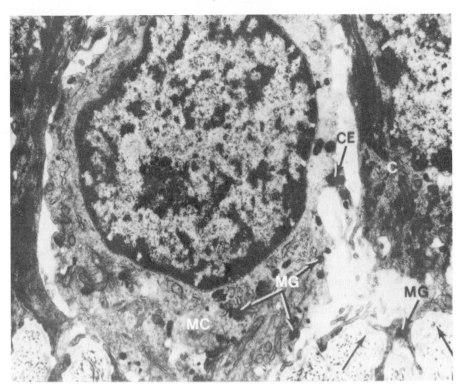

Figure 19 –6. Electron micrograph of a melanocyte (MC) between 2 epidermal epithelial cells. Observe the presence of melanin granules (MG) in its cytoplasmic extensions (CE) and in the neighboring epithelial cells (C). Desmosomes are not present between melanocytes and epithelial cells. The arrows are within the basement membrane. × 14,000. (Courtesy of C Barros.)

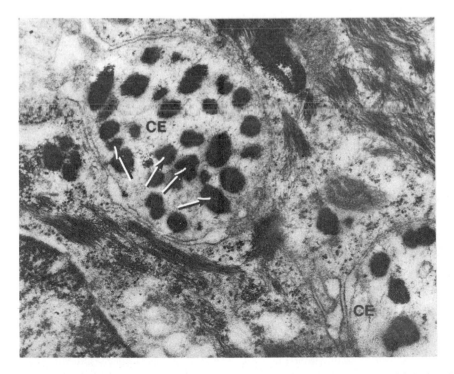

Figure 19 –7. Electron micrograph showing 2 melanocyte extensions sectioned transversely and full of melanin granules. The cytoplasm of the surrounding cells contains tonofibrils. × 40,000. CE, cytoplasmic extensions. (Courtesy of C Barros.)

Melanin is a dark brown pigment produced by a specialized cell of the epidermis, the **melanocyte,** usually found beneath or between the cells of the basal layer and the upper layers of the epidermis. Melanocytes can be found in the hair follicle. They have rounded cell bodies from which long irregular extensions branch into the epidermis, running between the cells of the germinativum and spinosum layers. Tips of these extensions terminate in invaginations of the cells present in the 2 layers. The electron microscope shows a lack of desmosomal attachments and a paucity of tonofibrils in these cells (Figs 19–5, 19–6, and 19–7). Synthesis of melanin occurs in the interior of the melanocyte, and tyrosinase plays an important role in this process. As a result of its activity, tyrosine is transformed first into 3,4-dihydroxyphenylalanine (dopa) and then into dopaquinone, which is converted, after a series of transformations, into melanin. Tyrosinase is synthesized on the ribosomes, transported in the lumen of the granular endoplasmic reticulum of melanocytes, and accumulated in vesicles formed at the Golgi zone (Fig 19–8). These tyrosinase-filled vesicles are **stage II melanosomes** (formerly **premelanosomes**) and are the sites where synthesis of melanin begins. Melanin gradually accumulates in these vesicles and forms **stage III melanosome,** where tyrosinase coexists with melanin (Fig 19–8). In the last stage (stage IV), the synthesis of melanin ceases, the vesicle is filled with melanin, and no tyrosinase activity can be detected in it. It is then a **melanin granule** (Figs 19–5 to 19–8). Thus, in the development of the mature melanin granule, there are 4 developmental stages:

Stage I: A vesicle surrounded by a membrane, showing beginning of tyrosinase activity and formation of fine granular material; at its periphery, electron-dense strands show an orderly arrangement of tyrosinase molecules on a protein matrix.

Stage II: The vesicle is ovoid now and shows, in its interior, parallel filaments with a definite periodicity of about 10 nm or cross-striations of about the same periodicity. Melanin is deposited on the protein matrix.

Stage III: As a result of increased melanin formation, the internal periodic fine structure is less visible.

Stage IV: The mature melanin granule is visible in the light microscope, and the melanin completely fills the vesicle. No ultrastructure is visible.

When no tyrosinase activity exists in the melanocyte or when this activity is defective, no pigment is produced, resulting in **albinism.**

Once formed, the melanin granules migrate within cytoplasmic extensions of the melanocyte and are transferred to cells of the germinativum and

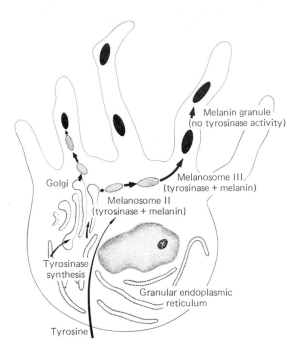

Figure 19–8. Diagram of a melanocyte, illustrating the principal process occurring during melaninogenesis. Tyrosinase is synthesized in the granular endoplasmic reticulum and is accumulated in vesicles of the Golgi apparatus. The free vesicles are now called melanosomes. Melanin synthesis begins in the stage II melanosomes, where this compound is accumulated and forms stage III melanosomes. Later, this structure loses its tyrosinase activity and becomes a melanin granule. Melanin granules migrate to arm tips and are then transferred to the epithelial cells of the malpighian layer.

spinosum layers of the epidermis. This transfer process has recently been shown, with the aid of cinematography in skin tissue culture. Melanin granules are essentially "injected" into other epithelial cells in a process called **cytocrine secretion.** Whereas melanocytes synthesize melanin, epithelial cells act as a depot for this pigment and contain more than melanocytes. Inside the keratinocytes, the melanin granules are linked with lysosomes and their enzymes. In this interaction between keratinocytes and melanocytes, which results in the pigmentation of the skin, the important factors are the rate of formation of melanin granules within the melanocyte, their transfer into the keratinocytes, and the ultimate disposition of the granules by the keratinocytes. A feedback mechanism may exist between melanocytes and keratinocytes.

Melanocytes can be easily visualized by incubating fragments of epidermis in dopa. This compound, under the action of tyrosinase, produces in the melanocyte an insoluble deposit of dark brown melanin. It is possible to count the number of melanocytes of the epidermis per unit area. Such studies show that these cells are not distributed at random among keratinocytes; rather, there is a definite pattern in their distribution called the epidermal-melanin unit. In humans, the ratio of dopa-positive melanocytes to keratinocytes in the stratum basale is constant for each specific area of the body but varies from one region to another. The number of melanocytes per unit area is not influenced by sex or race, and skin color differences are due mainly to differences in the number of melanin granules in the keratinocytes.

Darkening of the skin after exposure to ultraviolet light of the sun (tanning) is the result of a 2-step process. A physicochemical reaction occurs first, darkening the preexistent melanin and releasing it rapidly into the keratinocytes. In a second stage, the rate of melanin synthesis in the melanocytes accelerates, resulting in an increase in the amount of this pigment.

Melanocyte-stimulating hormone (α- and β-MSH), produced in the intermediate lobe of the pituitary, has a marked influence on melanophores of amphibia, promoting centrifugal migration of their pigment in their long cytoplasmic processes and an increase in the number of melanin granules in keratinocytes. Its action in humans is less dramatic. Lack of cortisol from the adrenal cortex causes overproduction of ACTH and probably MSH, both of which increase the pigmentation of the skin, as in Addison's disease (a disease due to dysfunction of the adrenal glands). The action of MSH is mediated through α-adrenergic receptors; the action of catecholamines is mediated through β-adrenergic receptors. Substances like ammoniated mercury may lighten the skin by exerting a mild peeling effect. Hydroquinone and its derivatives may inhibit the synthesis of melanin, with consequent depigmentation. Conversely, other substances such as dihydroxyacetone, when applied to the skin, react with the proteins of the keratin layer, darkening it promptly.

The Langerhans Cells

These star-shaped cells, morphologically similar to melanocytes, are found mainly in the stratum spinosum of the epidermis. After impregnation with gold chloride, they are delineated sharply against an unstained background. In the electron microscope they have an indented nucleus and a clear cytoplasm with no tonofilaments in their cytoplasm and no desmosomes in the plasma membrane. They present characteristic rodlike inclusions in their cytoplasm. Although their functional significance is still obscure, evidence suggests that they may be of dermal origin and exhibit an immune or macrophagic activity.

The Merkel Cell

The Merkel cells, generally present in the thick skin of palms and soles, somewhat resemble the epidermal epithelial cells but have in their cytoplasm small dense granules similar to those present in catecholamine-containing cells. Free nerve endings forming an expanded terminal disk are present at the base of the Merkel cells. Merkel cells may serve as sensory mechanoreceptors, although they have also been implicated as having APUD cell-like activity.

DERMIS

The dermis is composed of the connective tissue that supports the epidermis and binds it to the subjacent layer, the subcutaneous tissue (hypodermis). According to the region of the body, its thickness varies up to a maximum of 3 mm on the soles of the feet. The external surface of the dermis is very irregular and presents many outgrowths that interdigitate with infoldings of the epidermis (Fig 19–1). These structures are more numerous in skin subject to frequent pressure and are believed to increase and reinforce the dermo-epidermal junction. During embryonic development, dermis acts as the determinant of the developing pattern of the overlying epidermis. Dermis obtained from the sole always induces the formation of a heavily keratinized epidermis irrespective of the site of origin of the epithelial cells.

The distinctive dermo-epidermal junction is seen in histologic sections of the human skin, and this understructure of the epidermis is unique in each part of the body. A PAS-positive basement membrane always follows the surface of the basal cells of the stratum germinativum facing the dermis.

Two layers with rather indistinct boundaries have been described in the dermis. They are the outermost papillary layer and the deeper reticular layer (Fig 19–1). The **papillary layer** is thin and is composed of loose connective tissue. Besides fibroblasts, other connective tissue cells are present, the most abundant being the mast cells and macrophages. Extravasated leukocytes are also seen. The papillary layer is so called because it penetrates into the papillae. From this layer, type III collagen fibers insert into the basal lamina and extend perpendicularly into the dermis. They are thought to have a special function, binding the dermis to the epidermis, and are thus called **anchoring fibers** (Fig 4–3). The **reticular layer** is thicker, composed of irregular dense connective tissue (mainly type I collagen), and therefore has more fibers and fewer cells than the papillary layer. Both layers have many elastic fibers, which are in part responsible for the elasticity and firmness of the skin. The acid mucopolysaccharide content of the dermis varies in different regions. The principal glycosaminoglycans in the skin are dermatan sulfate, chondroitin sulfate A and C, and hyaluronate.

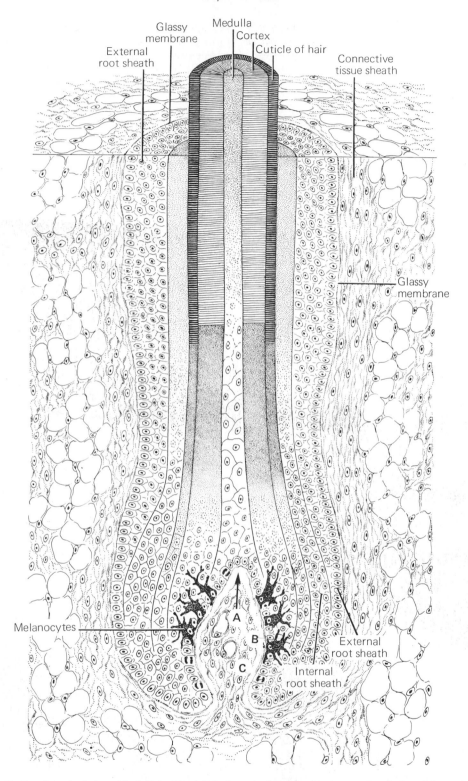

Figure 19–9. Drawing of a hair and its follicle. The follicle has a bulbous terminal expansion that contains a dermal papilla, which contains capillaries and is covered by cells that form the hair root and develop into the hair shaft. The central cells *(A)* indicated by the arrow produce large, vacuolated, poorly cornified cells that form the medulla of the hair. The cells that produce the cortex of the hair are located laterally *(B)*. Cells forming the hair cuticle originate in the next layer *(C)*. The peripheral epithelial cells develop into the internal and external sheaths. The external sheath continues with the epidermis, while the cells of the internal sheath disappear at the level of the openings of the sebaceous gland ducts.

Age changes in the dermis can be observed histologically and biochemically. Collagen fibers thicken and collagen synthesis decreases with age. Elastic fibers steadily increase in number and thickness, so that the elastin content of human skin increases approximately 5-fold from fetal to adult life. In old age, extensive cross-linking of the collagen and loss of elastic fibers causes the skin to become more fragile, lose its suppleness, and assume many wrinkles.

The dermis has a rich network of blood and lymph vessels. In certain areas of the skin, blood can pass directly from arteries to veins through the arteriovenous anastomoses or shunts. They play a very important role in temperature and blood pressure regulation, since skin can accommodate about 4.5% of the blood volume. A rich capillary network in the papillary region surrounds the epidermal ridges and functions in regulating body core temperature.

Besides these components, the dermis also contains some epidermal derivatives, the hair follicles and the sweat and sebaceous glands. A rich supply of nerves is found in the dermis, and the effector nerves to the skin are postganglionic fibers of the ganglia of the paravertebral chain. The afferent nerve endings form a superficial dermal nerve network with free nerve endings, a hair follicle network, and the encapsulated end organs, Meissner and pacinian corpuscles.

SUBCUTANEOUS TISSUE

This layer consists of loose connective tissue that binds the skin loosely to the subjacent organs, making it possible for the skin to slide over them. The hypodermis often contains fat cells, varying in number according to the area of the body and in size according to the nutritional status of the individual.

HAIRS

The hairs are thin keratinized structures derived from an invagination of the epidermal epithelium. Their color, size, and disposition are variable according to race, age, sex, and the region of the body. They are present almost everywhere on the surface of the body. Hairs grow discontinuously and have periods of growth followed by periods of rest. This growth does not occur synchronously in all regions of the body or even in the same area. This type of growth is known as **growth in mosaic.** The duration of the growth and rest periods also varies according to the region of the body. Thus, in the scalp, the growth periods may last for several years, whereas the rest periods average 3 months. Hair growth of certain regions of the body such as the

scalp, face, and pubis is strongly influenced not only by sex hormones—especially androgen—but by adrenal and thyroid hormones also. Hair growth is not affected by frequency of cutting or shaving.

Each hair derives from an epidermal invagination, the **hair follicle,** which presents during its growth period a terminal dilatation called the hair bulb. At the base of the **hair bulb,** a dermal papilla can be observed (Figs 19–9 and 19–10). The dermal papilla is invested with a capillary network, which is vital in sustaining the hair follicle. The loss of blood flow or vitality of dermal papilla will result in death of the follicle. The epidermal cells covering this dermal papilla form the hair root that produces and is continuous with the hair shaft that protrudes beyond the skin.

During periods of growth, the epithelial cells that cover the hair bulb are equivalent to those in the stratum germinativum of the skin. They divide constantly and differentiate into the following cell types:

(1) In certain types of thick hairs, the cells of the central region of the root at the apex of the

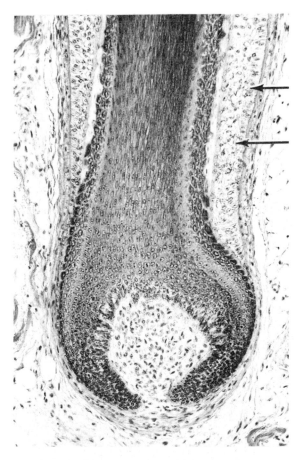

Figure 19–10. Photomicrograph of a section of hair follicle from a human lip. Observe the papilla and the outer root sheath (arrows), surrounded by a connective tissue sheath. H&E stain, × 118.

dermal papilla produce large vacuolated and moderately keratinized cells which form the **medulla** of the hair (Fig 19–9A).

(2) The cells located around the central region of the root (Fig 19–9B) multiply and differentiate into heavily keratinized, compactly grouped fusiform cells forming the **hair cortex.**

(3) Farther peripherally are the bulb cells (Fig 19–9C) that produce the **hair cuticle,** a layer composed of cells which, midway up the bulb, are cuboidal, then become tall and columnar, and, higher up, change from horizontal to vertical, at which point they form a layer of flattened, heavily keratinized cells disposed as shingles covering the cortex. The cuticle cells are the last cell line in the hair follicle to differentiate.

(4) Finally, the most peripheral cells give rise to the **internal root sheath,** which completely surrounds the initial part of the hair shaft. The internal sheath is a transient structure whose cells degenerate and disappear above the level of the sebaceous glands. The **outer** or **external root sheath** is the downgrowth of epidermal cells, and near the surface it shows all the layers of epidermis. Near the dermal papilla it is composed of cells corresponding to the stratum germinativum of the epidermis.

Separating the hair follicle from the dermis is a noncellular hyaline membrane, the **glassy membrane** (Fig 19–9), which represents a thickening of the basement membrane. The dermis that surrounds the follicle is denser, forming a special sheath of connective tissue. Bound to this sheath and connecting it to the papillary layer of the dermis are bundles of smooth muscle cells disposed in an oblique direction (Fig 19–11). Their contractions promote erection of the hair shaft into a more vertical position—commonly called "gooseflesh" in humans. These muscles are called the **arrector pili** muscles.

Hair color is due to the activity of melanocytes located between the papilla and the epithelial cells of the hair root that produce the pigment present in the medullary and cortical cells of the hair shaft (Fig 19–9). These melanocytes probably produce and transfer melanin to the epithelial cells by a mechanism similar to that described for the epidermis.

Although the keratinization processes in the epidermis and hair appear to be similar, they differ in the following ways:

(1) The epidermis produces relatively soft, keratinized outer layers of dead cells that adhere slightly to the skin and desquamate continuously. In the hair the opposite occurs, with the production of a hard and compact keratinized structure.

(2) Whereas in the epidermis keratinization occurs continuously and all over, in the hair it is intermittent and present only in the hair root. The hair papilla has an inductive action on the covering epithelial cells, promoting their proliferation and differentiation. Thus, injuries to the dermal papillae promote the loss of hair.

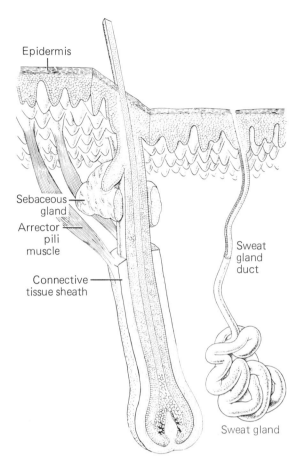

Figure 19–11. Diagram of the relations between the skin, hair follicle, arrector pili muscle, and sebaceous and sweat glands. The arrector pili muscle inserts itself in the papillary layer of the dermis and in the connective tissue sheath of the hair follicle.

(3) Contrary to what happens in the epidermis, where all cells differentiate in the same direction, giving rise to the final keratinized layer, in the hair root the cells differentiate into various cell types that differ in ultrastructure, histochemistry, and function. Mitotic activity in hair follicles and sebaceous glands is under the influence of androgens.

NAILS

The nails are cornified plates present on the dorsal surfaces of the terminal phalanges of the toes and fingers (Fig 19–12). The **nail beds** are thickened epithelial surfaces of the phalanges on which the nail plate rests. Seen from above, the nail body shows near the root a white, crescent-shaped area called the **lunula.** There is no generally accepted explanation for its presence. The proximal part of

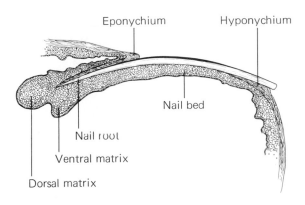

Figure 19–12. The nail and its components.

the nail, hidden in the nail groove, is the **nail root**. Processes of epithelial proliferation and differentiation that gradually produce the nail are localized in the nail root. The nail plate consists of a compact layer of highly adherent and keratinized epithelial cells. The nails grow in a distal direction, sliding over the skin of the nail bed, the **hyponychium**, which is continuous with the epidermis that covers the ventral surface of the digits. This underlying skin normally does not participate in the process of nail formation, and its main function is to act as a support. The horny epidermal extension of the tip of the proximal nail fold is the **eponychium** or **cuticle.**

GLANDS OF THE SKIN

Sebaceous Glands

Sebaceous glands are found embedded in the dermis almost all over the body except in areas lacking hairs. They are acinar glands that usually have various acini opening into a short duct. This duct usually ends in the upper portion of a hair follicle (Fig 19–11), but in certain regions, such as the glans penis, glans clitoridis, and lips, it opens directly onto the epidermal surface. The acini consist of a basal layer of undifferentiated flattened epithelial cells that rests on the basement membrane. These cells proliferate and differentiate, filling the acini with rounded cells containing abundant fat droplets in their cytoplasm (Fig 19–13). Their nuclei gradually shrink, and the cells simultaneously become filled with fat droplets and burst. The product of this process is the secretion of the sebaceous gland, which is gradually moved to the surface of the skin. This is a typical example of a holocrine gland, for its product of secretion, the **sebum**, is released with remnants of dead cells. This product is composed of a complex mixture of lipids that contains triglycerides, free fatty acids, and cholesterol and its esters. The primary controlling factor of sebaceous glands in men is testicular tes-

tosterone; in women, it is a combination of ovarian and adrenal androgens. The flow of sebaceous glands is continuous, and a disturbance in the normal secretion and flow of sebum is one of the reasons for the development of acne. The preen glands of certain aquatic birds are modified sebaceous glands, and their product is spread by the bird on its feathers, rendering them impermeable to water.

Sweat Glands

The sweat glands are widely distributed in the skin. Certain regions such as the glans penis are exceptions.

The sweat glands are simple, coiled, tubular glands (Fig 19–11). Their ducts do not divide and are thinner in diameter than the secretory portion (Fig 19–14). This secretory part of the gland is embedded in the dermis, measures approximately 0.4 mm in diameter, and is surrounded by myoepithelial cells (described in Chapter 4). Contraction of these cells is believed to help to discharge the secretion. A fairly thick basement membrane lies on the outside of the secretory portion of the glands. Two cell types have been described in the secretory portion of these glands: (1) a **dark cell,** with characteristics of a serous cell having an abundant granular endoplasmic reticulum and secretory granules containing glycoprotein; and (2)

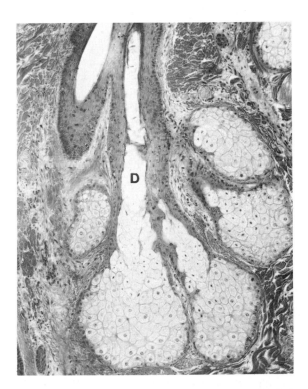

Figure 19–13. Photomicrograph of a sebaceous gland. It consists of various acini, which are limited externally by proliferating, flattened epithelial cells that give rise to the fat-filled round cells of the acinar center. D, duct. H&E stain, × 100.

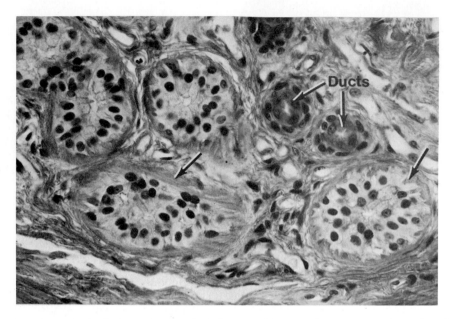

Figure 19–14. Photomicrograph of a human sweat gland. At upper right are 2 ducts transversely sectioned. Observe the myoepithelial cells, which form a sheath around the gland (arrows). H&E stain, × 360.

a **clear cell,** devoid of secretory granules, with a small amount of endoplasmic reticulum and presenting frequent invaginations of the plasma membrane in its basal portion. As explained in Chapter 4, this morphologic aspect is characteristic of cells that transport ions and water.

Ducts are lined by stratified cuboidal epithelium (Fig 19–14).

The fluid secreted by these glands is not viscous and contains little protein. Its main components are water, sodium chloride, urea, ammonia, and uric acid. Its sodium content of 85 mEq/L is distinctly below that of blood (144 mEq/L), and the cells present in the sweat ducts are responsible for sodium reabsorption. The fluid in the lumen of the secretory portion of the gland is an ultrafiltrate of the blood plasma. This ultrafiltrate is derived from a network of capillaries that intimately envelop the secretory region of each gland. Following its release on the surface of the skin, the expelled sweat evaporates and leads to a cooling of the surface. In the underlying dermis, blood in the extensive capillary loops encircling the dermal papillae is subsequently cooled as its heat is conducted into the overlying epidermis. The elimination of catabolites suggests that the sweat glands might have an excretory function.

Besides these **merocrine** sweat glands, another type of modified sweat gland—the **apocrine** gland—is present in the axillary, areolar, and anal regions. Apocrine glands are much larger (3–5 mm in diameter) than merocrine glands. They are embedded in the subcutaneous tissue and open into hair follicles. They produce a viscous secretion and in females undergo histologic changes during the menstrual cycle. While the apocrine glands are innervated by adrenergic nerve endings, the merocrine glands receive cholinergic fibers.

The glands of Moll in the margins of the eyelids and the ceruminous glands of the ear are modified sweat glands.

VESSELS & NERVES OF THE SKIN

The arterial vessels which nourish the skin form 2 plexuses, one located between the papillary and reticular layers and one between the dermis and the subcutaneous tissue. Thin branches leave these plexuses and vascularize the dermal papillae. Each papilla has only one arterial ascending and one venous descending branch. The veins are disposed in 3 plexuses, 2 of them in the position described for the arterial vessels and the third in the middle of the dermis. Arteriovenous anastomoses with glomera (see Chapter 12) are frequent in the skin. The lymphatic vessels begin as blind sacs in the papillae of the dermis and converge to 2 plexuses as in the arterial vessels.

One of the most important functions of the skin is to receive stimuli from the environment, and it is therefore richly innervated. Besides free nerve endings in the epidermis and cutaneous glands, receptors are present in the dermis and subcutaneous tissue, being more frequently found in the dermal papillae (see Chapter 10). The hair follicles possess a rich network of nerve endings essential in the processing of tactile impressions from the environment.

• • •

References

Briggaman RA, Dalldorf FG, Wheeler CE: Formation and origin of basal lamina and anchoring fibrils in adult human skin. J Cell Biol 51:384, 1971.

Bullough WS: Mitotic and functional homeostasis: A speculative review. Cancer Res 25:1683, 1965.

Cohen J, Szabó G: Study of pigment donation in vitro. Exp Cell Res 50:418, 1968.

Cummins H: Dermatoglyphics. In: *Dermatology in Medicine.* Fitzpatrick TB & others (editors). McGraw-Hill, 1971.

Epstein WL, Maibach HI: Cell renewal in human epidermis. Arch Dermatol 92:462, 1965.

Fitzpatrick TB, Breathnach AS: Das epidermale Melanin-Einheit-System. Dermatol Wochenschr 147:481, 1963.

Fitzpatrick TB, Szabó G: The melanocyte: Cytology and cytochemistry. J Invest Dermatol 32:197, 1959.

Fraser RDB, MacRae TP, Rogers CE: *Keratins: Their Composition, Structure, and Biosynthesis.* Thomas, 1972.

Frenk E, Schellhorn JP: Zur morphologie der epidermalen Melaninheit. Dermatologica 21:339, 1969.

Fukuyama K, Epstein WL: Protein synthesis studied by autoradiography in the epidermis of different species. Am J Anat 122:269, 1968.

Guevedo WC Jr: Epidermal melanin units: Melanocyte-keratinocyte interactions. Am Zool 12:35, 1972.

Halprin KM: Epidermal "turnover time": A reexamination. J Invest Dermatol 86:14, 1972.

Hashimoto K: Cementosome: A new interpretation of the membrane-coating granule. Arch Dermatol 240:349, 1971.

Laidlaw GG: The dopa reaction in normal histology. Anat Rec 53:399, 1932.

Lavker RM, Matoltsy AG: Formation of horny cells. J Cell Biol 44:501, 1970.

Masson P: Pigment cells in man. In: *The Biology of Melano-somes.* Miner RW, Gordon M (editors). Ann NY Acad Sci 4:15, 1948.

Matoltsy AG: Mechanism of keratinization. In: *Fundamentals of Keratinization.* Butcher EO, Sognnaes RF (editors). Publication No. 70. American Association for the Advancement of Science, 1962.

Menton DN, Eisen AZ: Structure and organization of mammalian stratum corneum. J Ultrastruct Res 35:247, 1971.

Mier PD, Cotton DWK: *Molecular Biology of Skin.* Blackwell, 1976.

Montagna W: *The Structure and Function of Skin,* 3rd ed. Academic Press, 1974.

Munger BL: The cytology of apocrine sweat glands. 2. Human. Z Zellforsch Mikrosk Anat 68:837, 1965.

Rowden G: Immuno-electron microscopic studies of surface receptors and antigens of human Langerhans cells. Br J Dermatol 97:593, 1977.

Snell RS: An electron microscopic study of the dendritic cells in the basal layer of guinea-pig epidermis. Z Zellforsch Mikrosk Anat 66:457, 1965.

Snell RS: An electron microscopic study of keratinization in the epidermal cells of the guinea pig. Z Zellforsch Mikrosk Anat 65:829, 1965.

Snell RS: The fate of epidermal desmosomes in mammalian skin. Z Zellforsch Mikrosk Anat 66:471, 1965.

Squier CA, Rooney L: The permeability of keratinized and nonkeratinized oral epithelium to lanthanum in vivo. J Ultrastruct Res 54:286, 1976.

Terzakis JA: The ultrastructure of monkey eccrine sweat glands. Z Zellforsch Mikrosk Anat 64:493, 1964.

Winkelmann RK: The Merkel cell system and a comparison between it and the neurosecretory or APUD cell system. J Invest Dermatol 69:41, 1977.

Zelickson AS: *Ultrastructure of Normal and Abnormal Skin.* Lea & Febiger, 1967.

20 | Urinary System

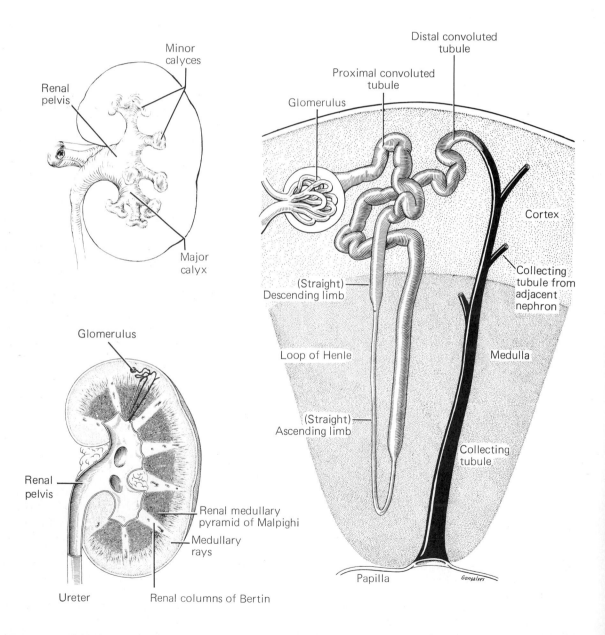

Figure 20–1. *Left:* The general organization of the kidney. *Right:* The cortical or medullary localization of nephron segments and collecting tubules (the latter shown in black).

The urinary system consists of the kidneys, ureters, bladder, and urethra and contributes to the maintenance of homeostasis by producing the urine, in which various metabolic waste products are eliminated. The kidneys also regulate the fluid balance of the body and are the site of production of renin and erythropoietin. The urine produced in the kidneys passes through the ureters to the bladder and is released to the exterior through the urethra.

THE KIDNEYS

Each kidney resembles a bean, with one concave border with a large indentation, the **hilum**— an area where nerves and blood and lymph vessels enter and leave—and a convex surface on the opposite side (Fig 20–1). In the hilum, the calyces unite to form the renal pelvis, which is the superior dilated part of the ureter. The kidney, covered by the **renal capsule** composed of dense connective tissue, has an outer **cortex** and an inner **medulla** (Figs 20–1 and 20–2).

In humans, the renal medulla is composed of 10–18 conical or pyramid-shaped structures, the **malpighian** or **medullary pyramids,** whose bases and sides are within the cortical zone and whose vertices protrude into the renal calyces (Fig 20–1). These protrusions are the **renal papillae.** The surface of each papilla is perforated by 10–25 orifices, the openings of the **collecting ducts,** forming the **area cribrosa.**

From the base of the medullary pyramid, 400–500 elongated parallel arrays of tubules, called the **medullary rays,** penetrate the cortex (Fig 20–1). Each medullary ray consists of a straight collecting duct surrounded by numerous parallel tubular portions of the **nephron,** the filtering unit of the kidney.

The cortex occupies the space between the **malpighian** pyramids and between the bases of the pyramids and the renal capsule. The cortical tissue in the areas between the pyramids constitutes the **renal columns of Bertin.** In sections of fresh kidney, the cortex shows small red dots corresponding to special vascular complexes called the **renal corpuscles** or **corpuscles of Malpighi.**

The renal cortex consists mainly of nephrons; in the medulla, collecting tubules—structures that differ from the nephrons in morphology, physiology, and embryologic origin—are most conspicuous.

In some mammals, the kidney is composed only of one medullary pyramid and associated cortical base. The apex of the pyramid enters the ureter. This type of organization represents a lobe of kidney tissue, and such kidneys are unilobar. In other mammals, including humans, the kidney is composed of many lobes (multilobar kidneys), each with a medullary pyramid and its corresponding cortical tissue. The **renal lobule** consists of a single medullary ray and the cortical tissue that surrounds it. Each renal lobule contains the collecting duct and all filtering nephron units that drain into that duct. In the adult human, the renal lobes and lobules are not always clearly visible.

Many aspects of renal histology and physiology have been discovered using the technic of dissociation, which consists of macerating the organ in dilute acid and subsequently separating its components, with the aid of fine needles, under a stereoscopic microscope. The acid attacks the delicate connective tissue that supports and binds the renal tubules, permitting their isolation with relative ease.

Nephrons

Each kidney is composed of 1–4 million functional filtering units called **nephrons.** Each nephron consists of (1) a dilated portion, the **renal corpuscle** or **malpighian corpuscle;** (2) the **proximal convoluted tubule;** (3) the **thin** and **thick portions of the loop of Henle;** and (4) the **distal convoluted tubule** (Fig 20–1). The **collecting duct,** which is of different embryologic origin from the nephron, represents the excretory duct of the system, although in some areas it is actively involved in water transport across its cells.

The components of the nephron are invested by a basal lamina continuous with the limited amount of connective tissue of the organ.

The **renal corpuscle** consists of a tuft of capillaries, the **glomerulus,** surrounded by a double walled epithelial capsule called **Bowman's capsule** (Figs 20–1, 20–2, and 20–3). The internal leaflet of the capsule envelops the capillaries of the glomerulus and is called the visceral layer, whereas the external leaflet forms the outer limit of the renal corpuscle and is called the parietal layer of Bowman's capsule (Figs 20–2 and 20–3). Between the 2 leaflets of Bowman's capsule is the **capsular space,** which receives the liquid filtered through the capillary wall and the internal leaflet. There is a relation between total glomerular volume and kidney weight expressed in a straight line on a logarithmic scale. In most mammals, including humans, development of renal corpuscles stops at birth.

Each renal corpuscle has a **vascular pole,** where the **afferent arteriole** enters and the **efferent arteriole** leaves, and a **urinary pole,** where the proximal convoluted tubule begins (Fig 20–3).

After entering the renal corpuscle, the afferent arteriole usually divides into 2–5 primary branches each of which subdivides into a capillary network. Whether the capillary loops originating from the same branch of the afferent arteriole anastomose only with each other and not with those of other branches, or whether the capillary tuft is in fact an unrestricted network with numerous anastomoses

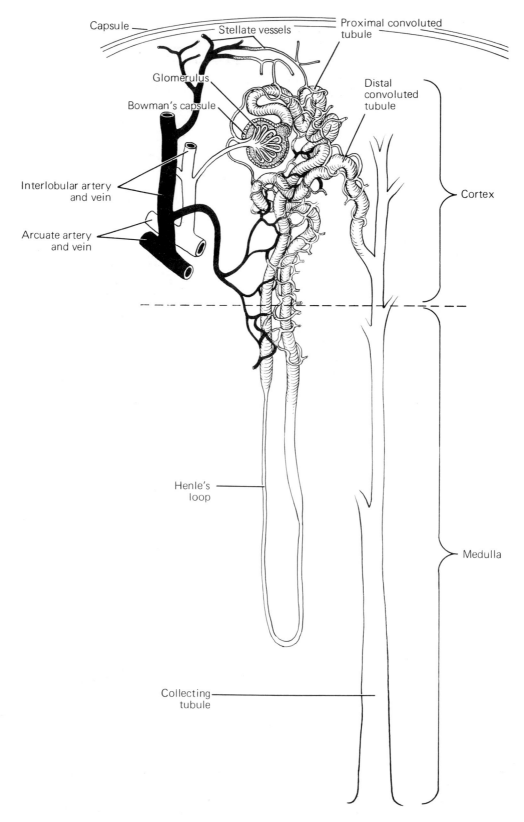

Figure 20–2. Vascular supply of the nephron in the outer zone of the cortex.

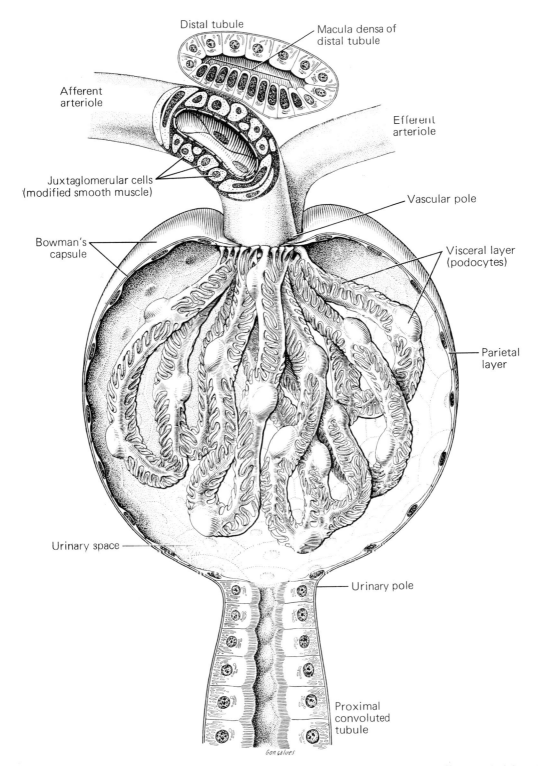

Distal tubule

Macula densa of
distal tubule

Afferent
arteriole

Efferent
arteriole

Juxtaglomerular cells
(modified smooth muscle)

Vascular pole

Bowman's
capsule

Visceral layer
(podocytes)

Parietal
layer

Urinary space

Urinary pole

Proximal
convoluted
tubule

Goncalves

Figure 20 –3. The renal corpuscle. The upper part shows the vascular pole, with afferent and efferent arterioles and the macula densa. Note the juxtaglomerular cells in the wall of the afferent arteriole. Podocytes cover glomerular capillaries. Their nuclei protrude on the cell surface while their processes line the outer surface of the capillaries. Note the flattened cells of the parietal layer of Bowman's capsule. The lower part of the drawing shows the urinary pole and the proximal convoluted tubule.

is not yet clear. Direct connections (shunts) between afferent and efferent arterioles, by which blood can circulate without passing through the glomerulus, have also been described.

The hydrostatic pressure of the arterial blood contained in the glomerular capillaries may be regulated by the efferent arteriole. The wall of this arteriole contains a considerable amount of smooth muscle and is thus capable of changing luminal diameter, whereas the lumens of the afferent arterioles probably remain constant in diameter, since their encircling smooth muscle cells play more of a secretory (ie, renin secretion) than a contractile role. (aff.)

The **parietal** layer of Bowman's capsule consists of simple squamous epithelium supported on a basal lamina and a thin layer of reticular fibers that anastomose with the reticular framework around the tubules of the organ. At the urinary pole, the epithelium changes into that of the proximal tubule.

Whereas epithelium of the parietal layer remains unchanged, the internal or visceral layer is modified during embryonic development, acquiring a peculiar character. The cells of the internal layer, called **podocytes** (Figs 20–4 and 20–5), present a cell body from which arise several primary processes. Each primary process gives rise to numerous secondary processes (Figs 20–3 and 20–4) that embrace capillaries of the glomerulus. The secondary (foot) processes, at a regular distance of 25 nm from each other, are in direct contact with the basal lamina of the capillaries, but most of the cellular bodies of the podocytes and their primary processes do not touch the basal lamina (Figs 20–4 and 20–5). The foot processes from one epithelial cell embrace more than one capillary. The foot processes contain few or no organelles, but microfilaments and microtubules are numerous.

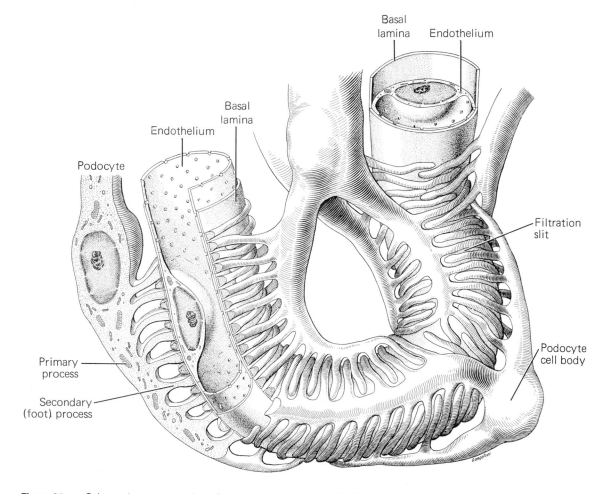

Figure 20 –4. Schematic representation of a glomerular capillary, with the visceral layer of Bowman's capsule (formed by podocytes). In this capillary, endothelial cells are fenestrated; however, the basal lamina on which they rest is continuous. At left is a podocyte shown in partial section. As viewed from the outside, the nuclei of the podocytes protrude into Bowman's capsule. Each podocyte has many primary processes from which arise an even greater number of secondary processes. The secondary processes are in contact with the basal lamina of the capillary wall. (Redrawn and modified after Gordon. Reproduced, with permission, from Ham AW: *Histology,* 6th ed. Lippincott, 1969.)

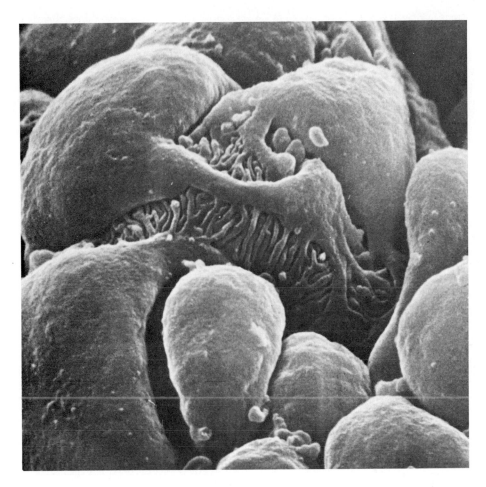

Figure 20 –5. Scanning electron micrograph of a renal glomerulus from a newborn rat. The round structures are podocytes seen in surface views. Primary and secondary processes are apparent. × 12,000. (Reproduced, with permission, from Miyoshi M, Fujita T, Tokunaga J: Arch Histol Jpn 33:161, 1971.)

The secondary processes of the podocytes interdigitate, delimiting elongated spaces—the filtration slits—between them. Spanning adjacent processes (and, therefore, bridging the filtration slits), a thin membrane has been described (Fig 20–6) that is about 6 nm thick and comparable to the diaphragm encountered in the pores of endothelial cells. The cytoplasm of the podocytes contains numerous free ribosomes, microtubules, and microfilaments (Fig 20–6). In spite of extensive study, the exact physiologic role of these cells is still not well understood. The glomerular capillaries are of the fenestrated type (Fig 20–6).

Between fenestrated endothelial cells of the capillaries and podocytes that cover their external surface is an unusually thick but otherwise typical basal lamina. This membrane is the only continuous structure separating the blood contained in the capillary from the capsular space. With the aid of the electron microscope, one can distinguish a central electron-dense layer and on each side a more electron-lucent layer. Histochemical methods are providing evidence that the 2 electron-lucent zones have different biochemical compositions from the denser central zone.

The endothelial cells of the glomerular capillaries have a thin cytoplasm that is thicker around the nucleus where most of the organelles are clustered. The pores of these cells are larger and more numerous than in the fenestrated capillaries of other organs, and they do not usually have the thin diaphragm commonly observed spanning the pores of other fenestrated capillaries.

Besides endothelial cells and podocytes, the glomerular capillaries have **mesangial cells** adhering to their walls in places where the basal lamina forms a sheath that is shared by 2 or more capillaries (Fig 20–7). The mesangial cells sometimes lie between the endothelial cells and their ensheathing basal lamina.

The mesangial cells possess short extensions and are covered by a layer of amorphous material. Little is known about their cytophysiology, but possibly they are supporting elements for the capil-

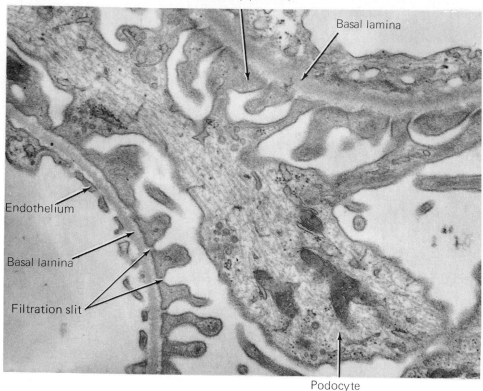

Figure 20–6. Electron micrograph of a glomerular capillary wall. Note the processes of the podocytes, the glomerular basal lamina, and the endothelium of the capillaries. × 36,000. (Courtesy of T de Brito.)

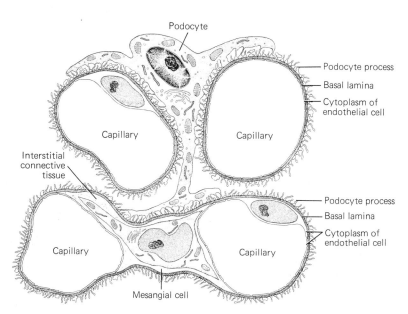

Figure 20–7. Mesangial cells of glomerular capillaries. They are located between 2 capillary lumens, enveloped by the basal lamina.

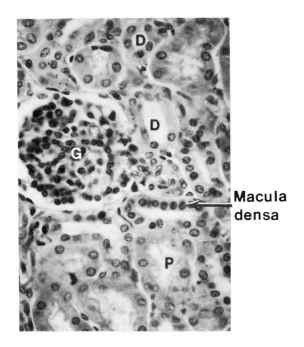

Figure 20–8. Photomicrograph of kidney cortical layer. Observe the glomerulus (G), a proximal convoluted tubule (P), and a distal convoluted tubule (D). H&E stain, × 250.

laries and constitute a pericytelike population. After the injection of ferritin (an electron-scattering, iron-containing protein easily identified with the electron microscope), the cytoplasm of the mesangial cells appears to be loaded with this protein. These cells may act as macrophages and serve to clean the basal lamina of particulate matter that accumulates in the matrix during filtration of the blood fluids.

Proximal Convoluted Tubule

This structure comprises an initial tortuous segment of the nephron that arises at the urinary pole of the renal corpuscle and subsequently becomes the descending straight segment that penetrates the medulla for a short distance, continuous with that part of the nephron called **Henle's loop** (Figs 20–1 and 20–2). It is longer and larger than the distal convoluted tubule that constitutes the terminal portion of the nephron.

The proximal convoluted tubule, found in the cortex usually in cross sections, is lined by simple cuboidal epithelium (Fig 20–8). The cells of this epithelium have a strongly acidophilic cytoplasm as a result of the presence of abundant elongated mitochondria. The cell apex exposed to the lumen of the tubule exhibits abundant microvilli about 1 μm in length that form the so-called **brush border** described long ago by the light microscopists (Fig 20–9). Because these cells are large, each transverse section of proximal tubule contains only 3 or 4

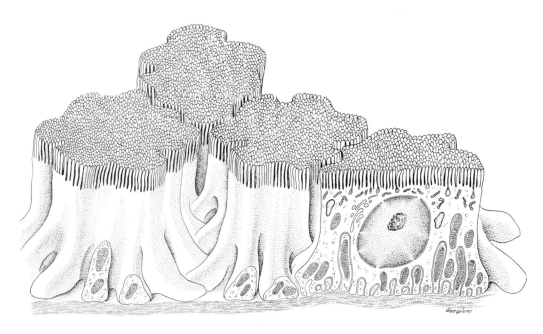

Figure 20–9. Schematic drawing of proximal convoluted tubule cells. These cuboidal cells show abundant microvilli constituting the brush border of their apical surfaces. They have 2 types of lateral processes: some along the whole side of the cell and others only in the basal half of the cell. The latter are longer than the former and penetrate deeply among the neighboring cells. In order to make the drawing more easily understandable, artificial spaces have been shown among the cells. (Modified from a figure [5] by Bulger R: Am J Anat 116:237, 1965.)

spherical nuclei, usually located in the center of the cell (Fig 20–8). A well-developed, PAS-positive basal lamina is seen around the proximal tubule.

In the normal living animal, proximal convoluted tubules have wide lumens and flattened cells with a clear cytoplasm. The tubules are separated from each other by large interstitial spaces. Their lumens become wider as they approach the medulla. This has been shown through observation in living kidneys or in preparations carefully fixed by freezing in situ or by special fixation for examination with the electron microscope. In the usual preparations, however, the tubular lumens frequently appear greatly reduced or collapsed.

The outer surface of the microvillar brush border is lined by a PAS-positive **cell coat** (a structure adherent to the glycocalyx), which presumably aids in absorption of materials (eg, peptides and glucose) lost from the blood during filtration. Related to resorption activity, the apical cytoplasm of the cells has numerous canaliculi arising from the base of the microvilli. Their membranes are continuous with the cytoplasmic membrane. Close to the canaliculi are small vesicles that originated from the canaliculi

as a result of pinching off during pinocytosis. The basal portion of these cells presents abundant lateral extensions that interdigitate profusely with analogous extensions of the neighboring cells (Fig 20–9). This process considerably increases the contact surface between neighboring cells and intercellular space. The mitochondria are concentrated at the base of the cell (Fig 20–10) and arranged parallel to the long axis of the cell. This mitochondrial location and the increase in surface area of the cell membrane at the base of the cell through which the sodium pump operates are characteristics of cells engaged in ion transport (see Chapter 4). Because of the extensive interdigitation of the lateral membranes, no discrete cell margins can be observed with the light microscope between cells of the proximal tubule.

Loop of Henle

The more numerous renal corpuscles located close to the medulla, the **juxtamedullary glomeruli,** have longer loops of Henle that penetrate more deeply into the medulla than those located next to the capsule that do not descend far into the me-

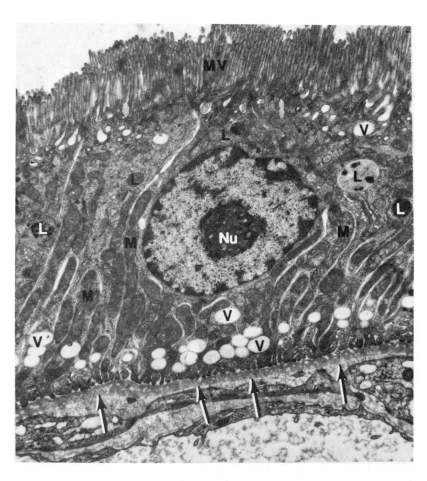

Figure 20–10. Electron micrograph of a proximal convoluted tubule wall. Observe the microvilli (MV), the lysosomes (L), the vacuole (V), the nucleolus (Nu), and the mitochondria (M). The arrows point to the basal lamina. × 10,500.

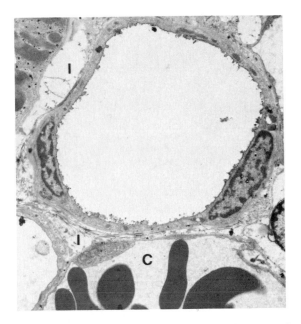

Figure 20–11. Electron micrograph of the thin part of Henle's loop composed entirely of squamous cells. Note fenestrated capillaries (C), the interstitium (I) with bundles of collagen filaments, and the basal lamina. Reduced from × 4000. (Courtesy of J Rhodin.)

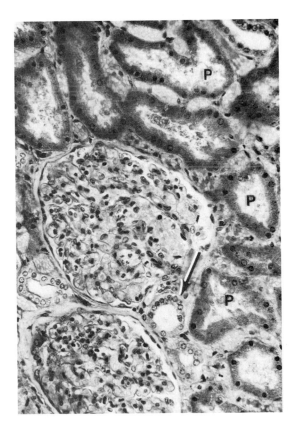

Figure 20–12. Photomicrograph of a kidney cortex showing a macula densa (arrow). P indicates proximal convoluted tubules. H&E stain, × 360.

dulla. Each loop of Henle is U-shaped and presents a thin segment followed by a thick one. In long loops, the turn occurs always in the thin part; in short loops, this happens in the thick part. Most of the thin portion is descending and most of the thick portion is ascending (Figs 20–1 and 20–2).

The thin part of the loop of Henle, which is a continuation of the proximal convoluted tubule, has an external diameter of about 12 μm, but the lumen is wide because its wall consists of flattened squamous cells whose nuclei protrude into the lumen (Fig 20–11). The thin part of Henle's loop resembles a blood capillary, with which it may be confused; differences in content, appearance of nuclei, and width of the lumen are the main criteria used for differentiation.

The transition between the proximal convoluted tubule and the loop of Henle may be abrupt or gradual. In the latter case, flat cells are interspersed between cuboidal cells with brush borders.

The thick ascending loop of Henle is similar in structure to the distal convoluted tubule.

Distal Convoluted Tubule

When the thick part constituting the **ascending limb** of the loop of Henle penetrates the cortex, it preserves its histologic structure but becomes tortuous and then becomes the distal convoluted tubule, which is the last segment of the nephron (Figs 20–1 and 20–8). This tubule is lined by simple cuboidal epithelium.

In histologic sections, the distinction between the proximal and distal convoluted tubules, both found in the cortex and having cuboidal epithelium, is based on the following characteristics: The cells of the proximal tubules are larger, have brush borders, and are more acidophilic because of their abundance of mitochondria (Fig 20–12). The lumens of the distal tubules are larger, and, because the distal tubule cell is flatter and smaller than that of the proximal tubule, more cells and more nuclei are seen in the distal tubule wall than in the proximal tubule wall on the same section. The distal tubule cells are less acidophilic than the proximal tubule cells, and they do not show brush borders or large numbers of microvilli. Cells of the distal convoluted tubule have lateral extensions, as described in the basal region of the proximal tubule cells, and the tubules show a basal lamina. As with the proximal tubule, no lateral cell margins are observed in the light microscope between adjacent distal tubule cells.

Along its path in the cortex, the distal convoluted tubule establishes contact with the vascular pole of the renal corpuscle of its own nephron, close to the afferent and efferent arteriole. At this point of close contact, the distal tubule shows modifications along with the afferent arteriole. Its cells usually become columnar, and their nuclei are closely packed together. Most of these cells have a Golgi apparatus in the basal region. This modified segment of the wall of the distal tubule, which appears darker in microscopic preparations (because of the close proximity of its nuclei), is called the **macula densa** (Figs 20–3 and 20–12). The exact functional significance of the macula densa, although not clear, may be related to the transmission to the glomerulus of data on the osmolarity of the fluid in the distal tubule.

Collecting Tubules

The urine passes from the distal convoluted tubules to the collecting tubules, which join each other, forming larger straight ducts, the **papillary ducts of Bellini,** which widen gradually as they approach the papillae. The collecting tubules, which constitute one of the major elements in the medulla, follow a straight path (Fig 20–1).

The smaller collecting tubules are lined with cuboidal epithelium and have a diameter of approximately 40 μm. As they penetrate deeper into the medulla and approach the papillae, their cells become taller until they are columnar cells. The diameter of the collecting duct reaches 200 μm near the papillae.

Along their entire extent, the collecting tubules are composed of cells that stain weakly by the usual stains and frequently exhibit a halo of less staining cytoplasm around the nucleus. The intercellular limits are clearly visible under the light microscope since there are no interdigitations between the lateral margins of adjacent cells (Figs 20–13 and 20–14). Each large collecting duct is joined at right angles by several generations of smaller collecting tubules draining each medullary ray. Many nephrons are united with the straight collecting ducts through their arched collecting tubules.

Juxtaglomerular Apparatus

Next to the renal corpuscle, the media of the afferent arteriole is modified and consists of cells having the appearance of epithelioid cells instead of smooth muscle. These cells, called **juxtaglomerular (JG) cells** (Fig 20–3), have cigar-shaped nuclei and a cytoplasm full of granules that stains darkly by special technics (PAS-positive). The macula densa of the convoluted tubule is usually located next to the region of the afferent arteriole containing the juxtaglomerular cells, forming, with this portion of the arteriole, the **juxtaglomerular apparatus.** Also part of the juxtaglomerular apparatus are some lightly staining cells whose functions are not well understood. They are variously called **extraglomerular mesangial cells, lacis cells,** or **polkissen** ("pole cushions"). In the area of the juxtaglomerular cells, the internal elastic membrane of the afferent arteriole disappears.

When examined with the electron microscope, the juxtaglomerular cells present characteristics of secretory cells, including an abundant granular endoplasmic reticulum, a highly developed Golgi apparatus, and secretory granules. The recently

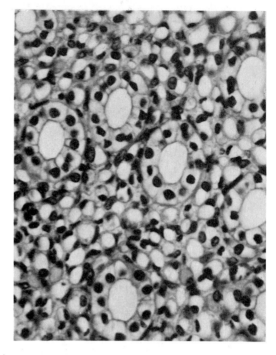

Figure 20–13. Photomicrograph of the medulla of the kidney, close to the papilla. There are several collecting tubules whose walls are composed of cuboidal cells. H&E stain, × 250.

formed secretory granules measure around 10–40 nm and join in clumps that appear to constitute the mature form of the secretory material (Fig 20–3).

The juxtaglomerular cells produce the enzyme **renin,** and the amount of renin present in a kidney is proportionate to the number of secretory granules in these cells; furthermore, fluorescent antibody (antirenin) has been shown to react specifically with the juxtaglomerular cells. Renin is known to act on a plasma protein called **angiotensinogen,** producing an inactive decapeptide called **angiotensin I.** This substance, as a result of the action of converting enzyme presumably present in the lung, loses 2 amino acids, becoming an octapeptide called **angiotensin II.**

The main physiologic effect of angiotensin II is to increase the secretion of the hormone aldosterone by the adrenal cortex, thus influencing blood pressure. Aldosterone acts on the cells of the renal tubules (mostly the distal tubules), increasing the reabsorption of sodium and chloride. Sodium deficiency is known to be a stimulus for the liberation of renin, which indirectly accelerates the secretion of aldosterone, which in turn leads to a resorption of sodium and consequently inhibits its excretion. Inversely, an excess of sodium in the blood depresses the secretion of renin with the consequent inhibition of the production of aldosterone and in this way increases the concentration of urinary sodium. Thus, the juxtaglomerular apparatus

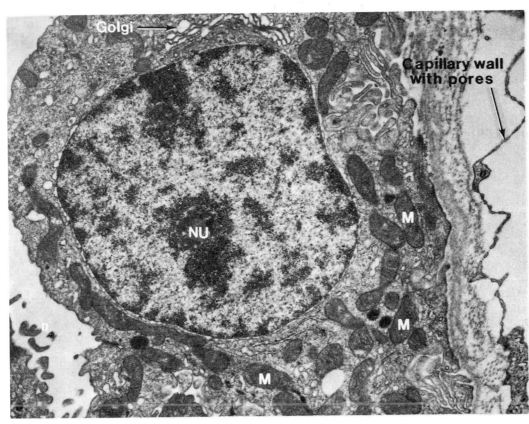

Figure 20–14. Electron micrograph of a collecting tubule wall. Note the mitochondria (M), Golgi apparatus, and the nucleolus (Nu). × 15,000.

has an important homeostatic role in the control of ionic balance.

Blood Circulation

Each kidney receives blood from its renal artery, which, at the level of the hilum and before entering this organ, usually divides into 2 branches: one in the anterior part of the kidney and the other in the posterior part. While still in the hilum, these branches give rise to fine arteries that further branch to form the **interlobar arteries** located between the renal pyramids of Malpighi (Fig 20–15). At the level of the base of the pyramids, the interlobar arteries form the **arcuate arteries,** which follow a path parallel to the capsule of the organ along the corticomedullary junction. Arcuate arteries originating from one interlobar artery do not communicate with vessels from other interlobar arteries. Thus, these arteries are terminal arteries. From the arcuate artery, the **interlobular arteries** branch off at right angles and regular intervals and follow a course in the cortex perpendicular to the renal capsule. The interlobular arteries are situated between the medullary rays, which, with the adjacent cortex, form the lobules of the kidneys (Fig 20–15). From the interlobular arteries arise the **afferent arterioles** of the glomeruli, which supply the blood to the capillaries of the glomeruli. From there the blood passes into the **efferent arterioles** of the glomeruli, which at once branch again to form a peritubular capillary network that will nourish the proximal and distal tubules of the renal cortex. However, the efferent arterioles derived from glomeruli located deeper in the juxtamedullary cortex and near the medullary region form long and thin vessels that follow a deep straight path into the medulla; these vessels are the **arteriolae rectae,** or straight arterioles, and some arise directly from arcuate arteries, probably as a consequence of glomerular degeneration.

In the medulla, one can observe the **venulae rectae,** from which blood flows back up to the arcuate veins. The straight venules are situated very close and parallel to the straight arteries, with which they form a loop. In the kidney medulla, these loops are physiologically important and are called collectively the **vasa recta** of the kidney. These vessels, containing mainly blood which has been filtered through the glomeruli, play a prominent role in maintaining a high osmolarity in the interstitial tissue of the medulla.

The capillaries of the outer cortex and of the capsule of the kidney converge to form the **stellate veins** (so called because of their configuration when

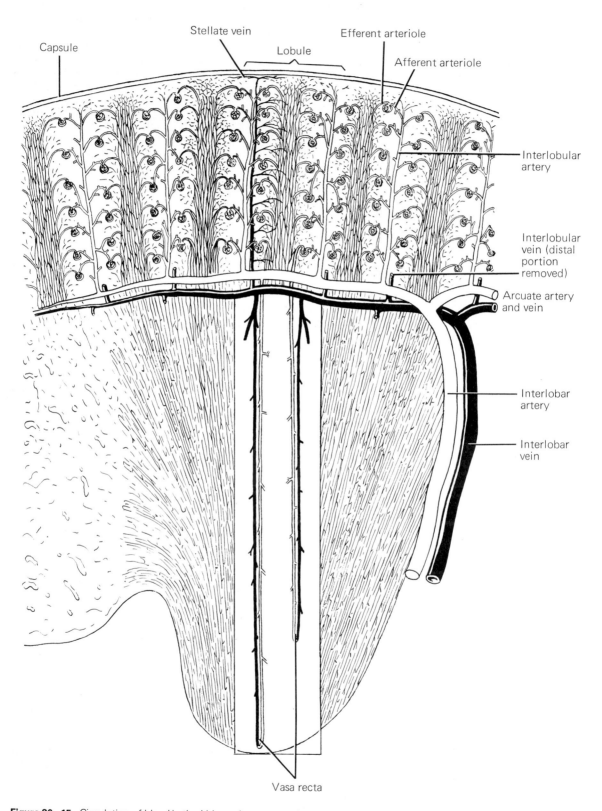

Figure 20–15. Circulation of blood in the kidney. Arcuate arteries are seen in the border between the cortical and medullary zones.

seen from the surface of the kidney), which empty into the interlobular veins.

The veins follow the same course as the arteries. Blood from the **interlobular veins** flows into the **arcuate** and from there to the **interlobar veins.** The interlobar veins form the **renal vein** through which the blood leaves the kidney.

HISTOPHYSIOLOGY OF THE KIDNEY

The kidney regulates the chemical composition of the internal environment by a complex process that involves **filtration, active absorption, passive absorption,** and **secretion.** Filtration takes place in the glomerulus, where an ultrafiltrate of blood plasma is formed. The tubules of the nephron, primarily the proximal convoluted tubule, reabsorb from this filtrate the substances that are useful for body metabolism, thus maintaining the homeostasis of the internal environment. They also transfer from blood to the tubular lumen certain waste products that are eliminated with the urine. The collecting tubules absorb water, thus contributing to the concentration of urine, which in general is hypertonic in relation to blood plasma. In this way the organism controls its water, intercellular fluid, and osmotic balance.

The 2 kidneys produce about 125 mL of filtrate per minute; of this amount, 124 mL are absorbed and only 1 mL is released into the calyces as urine. Every 24 hours, about 1500 mL of urine are formed.

Filtration

The blood flow in the 2 kidneys of an adult amounts to 1.2–1.3 L of blood per minute, which means that all of the circulating blood in the body passes through the kidneys every 4–5 minutes. The glomeruli are composed of arterial capillaries whose hydrostatic pressure is higher than that in other capillaries. This pressure is about 75 mm Hg— about 70% of the hydrostatic pressure in the aorta.

The glomerular filtrate is formed in response to the hydrostatic pressure of blood, to which the following forces are opposed: (1) osmotic pressure of plasma colloids (30 mm Hg); (2) pressure of the liquid contained in the tubular part of the nephron (10 mm Hg); and (3) interstitial pressure in the interior of the renal parenchyma (10 mm Hg), which acts on Bowman's capsule and is transmitted to the capsular liquid.

Since the hydrostatic pressure is 75 mm Hg and the forces that oppose it total 50 mm Hg, the resulting **force of filtration** is approximately 25 mm Hg.

The glomerular filtrate has a chemical composition similar to that of blood plasma but has almost no proteins because macromolecules do not cross the glomerular wall. The largest protein molecules that succeed in crossing the glomerular capillary walls have a molecular weight of about 70,000, and some plasma albumin fractions appear in very small amounts in the filtrate.

The endothelial cells of the glomerular capillaries are fenestrated with numerous pores mainly without diaphragms, so that the endothelium is easily permeated. According to most authors, filtration occurs at the basal lamina. Injections of larger molecules, such as ferritin (MW 460,000), show that they pass through the endothelial cells but are concentrated at the basal lamina. The filtration slits between the secondary processes of the podocytes also play a role in retaining molecules that pass through both the pores of the endothelial cells and the matrix of the basal lamina.

Proximal Convoluted Tubule

The glomerular filtrate formed in the renal corpuscle passes into the proximal convoluted tubule, and the process of resorption and excretion then begins. The site of resorption of diverse substances can be precisely identified, and the points of resorption of various substances are different. Various amino acids are absorbed in different parts of the tubule. The proximal convoluted tubule absorbs all of the glucose and about 85% of the sodium chloride and water contained in the filtrate. The resorption of glucose is maximal near the renal corpuscle. Glucose, chloride, and sodium are absorbed by the tubular cells through an active process involving expenditure of energy. Water diffuses passively, following the osmotic gradient. When the amount of glucose in the filtrate is excessive, it exceeds the absorbing capacity of the proximal tubule and the urine becomes more abundant and contains glucose.

The proximal convoluted tubule also absorbs, by an active process, all of the amino acids, ascorbic acid, and proteins present in the filtrate. Absorption of the proteins takes place by pinocytosis, which occurs at the base of the microvilli, and most of the products are eventually transferred from the filtrate into the interstitial tissue. The absorbed proteins appear first in the pinocytotic vesicles, which are later joined by primary lysosomes, forming secondary lysosomes. In these, the proteins are digested and the resultant amino acids are reutilized by the tubular cells or returned to the blood to be used by other cells.

Besides these activities, the proximal convoluted tubule transfers creatinine and excretes substances foreign to the organism such as para-aminohippuric acid, phenol red, and iodopyracet (an iodinated organic compound used as an x-ray contrast medium) from the interstitial plasma to the filtrate. This is an active process referred to in this organ as tubular excretion.

Loop of Henle

Although the filtrate that leaves the loop of Henle is hypotonic, this segment of the nephron is mainly responsible for the formation of a final hypertonic urine, and only animals with a loop of Henle in their kidneys are capable of producing hypertonic urine. The loop of Henle creates a gradient of hypertonicity in the medulla that influences the concentration of the urine as it flows in the collecting tubule.

The descending part of the loop of Henle is quite permeable, permitting the free passage of water, Na^+, and Cl^-. Since the interstitial fluid of the kidney medulla is hypertonic, sodium and chloride enter and water leaves the glomerular filtrate in the descending part of the loop.

The ascending part is impermeable to water and is highly active in transporting chloride to the interstitial fluid. It is directly responsible for the hypertonicity of the interstitial fluid of the medullary region. As a consequence of the loss of sodium and chloride, the filtrate that reaches the distal convoluted tubule is hypotonic.

Distal Convoluted Tubule

In the distal convoluted tubule, there is an ion exchange site at which, if aldosterone is acting, sodium is reabsorbed and potassium ions are excreted—ie, it is the site of the mechanism for the control of total salt and water in the body mentioned

above in the discussion of the juxtaglomerular apparatus. The distal tubule also secretes hydrogen ions and ammonium ion into tubular urine. This activity is essential for maintenance of the acid-base balance of the blood.

Collecting Tubules

Beginning in the distal tubule but becoming more important in the collecting tubules is the antidiuretic hormone (ADH)-dependent mechanism for final dilution or concentration of urine. The walls of the distal tubules and the collecting tubules are freely permeable to water if large amounts of ADH are present.

Formation of Hypotonic or Hypertonic Urine

The loop of Henle forms a multiplying countercurrent system that concentrates the filtrate by repetitive transfer of relatively small amounts of sodium along the length of the loop (Fig 20–16).

The ascending part of the loop of Henle is impermeable to water; in this part, chloride is transferred actively ("chloride pump") to the intercellular space of the kidney medulla (Fig 20–16). The interstitial fluid of the pyramid shows a gradient of hypertonicity increasing toward the papillae (Fig 20–16). Part of the chloride and sodium

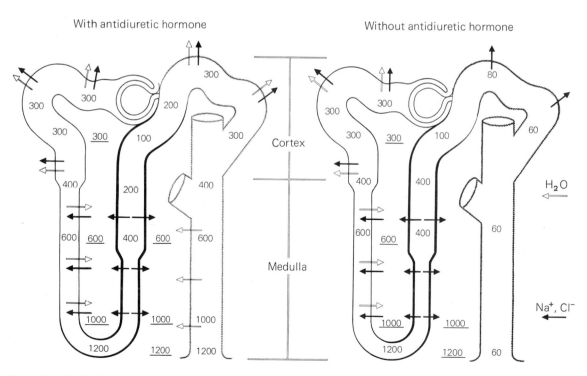

Figure 20–16. Multiplying countercurrent system formed by the loop of Henle. The segment of Henle's loop impermeable to water is represented by thick lines. The distal convoluted tubule and the collecting tubules, which are sensitive to antidiuretic hormone (ADH), are indicated by serrated lines. *Left:* Under the influence of ADH, the urine formed is hypertonic. *Right:* With very low levels of ADH or none at all, a great quantity of hypotonic urine is formed. The numbers in the tubules and interstitial spaces indicate the local concentration in mOsm/L. (Redrawn and reproduced, with permission, from Pitts RF: *Physiology of the Kidney and Body Fluids,* 2nd ed. Year Book, 1968.)

transferred to the intertubular environment by the ascending part of the loop is transferred passively to the filtrate by the descending part and passes again through the chloride pump present in the cells of the ascending part of the loop of Henle (Fig 20–16).

The hypotonic or isotonic urine present in the collecting tubules of the medulla (the interstitial fluid of the cortex is isotonic) will lose water into the interstitium if there is enough ADH to make the tubules permeable to water. A hypertonic urine is formed. When ADH is lacking, the walls of the collecting tubules are impermeable to water, so that concentration of the urine does not occur and the kidneys produce abundant hypotonic urine (Fig 20–16).

The permeability of the distal convoluted tubule to water depends on ADH, but this tubule, being located in the cortex, where the interstitial fluid is isotonic, cannot contribute appreciably to urine concentration. The urine that leaves the distal convoluted tubule is at most isotonic (as a result of equilibration with the interstitial fluid of the region).

The vasa recta or straight vessels of the medullary region are situated so that blood circulation does not disturb the osmotic gradient created by the chloride pump of the loop of Henle, and they form a countercurrent exchange system as shown in Fig 20–17.

The straight arterioles and veins are very thin vessels whose walls are similar to those of capillaries. Each straight vessel—an arterial and a venous part—forms a loop whose branches run side by side. While moving through the straight arterioles toward the inner medulla, the blood loses water and gains sodium because in the medulla the interstitial fluid gradually becomes more and more hypertonic. Returning in the opposite direction, blood is again exposed to the same gradient—now decreasing—and loses sodium and gains water. The water lost by the descending vessel is gained by the ascending one, and the sodium that enters the descending vessel is recovered by the ascending one.

The function of the osmotic changes in the blood of the straight vessels is to keep constant the osmotic gradient existing in the kidney medulla. These movements of water and sodium are passive, taking place without utilization of energy.

Hormonal Effects

As explained above, water balance is controlled in part by the posterior lobe of the pituitary, which releases ADH. When there is a high intake of water, production of ADH is inhibited, the walls of the distal tubules and collecting tubules become impermeable to water, and water is not reabsorbed. The result is the formation of large amounts of hypotonic urine with excess water eliminated while the ions necessary for the osmotic balance are retained. When small amounts of water are ingested or when a great loss of water occurs (eg, by excessive

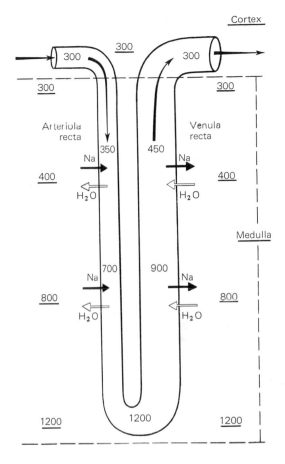

Figure 20–17. The countercurrent exchange system formed by the straight vessels of the kidney. The number 300 in the cortical segment of the arteriole and venule represents blood osmolarity (more precisely, 285–295 mOsm/L). The sodium and water exchanges between these straight vessels and the interstitium are passive, depending on the osmotic gradient formed by the loop of Henle.

sweating), the walls of the distal and collecting tubules become permeable to water, which is reabsorbed, and the formed urine is hypertonic.

Steroid hormones of the adrenal cortex, mainly **aldosterone,** increase the tubular absorption of sodium from the glomerular filtrate and thus decrease sodium elimination by the urine. Aldosterone facilitates the elimination of potassium and hydrogen. This hormone is critical in maintaining ionic equilibrium in the body. Aldosterone deficiency in adrenalectomized animals and in humans with Addison's disease produces an excessive loss of sodium by the urine.

BLADDER & URINARY PASSAGES

The bladder and the urinary passages store the urine formed in the kidneys and conduct it to the exterior. The calyces, pelvis, ureter, and bladder have the same basic histologic structure. The walls of the ureters become gradually thicker with increasing proximity to the bladder.

The mucosa of these organs consists of **transitional epithelium** and a lamina propria of loose or dense connective tissue. Surrounding the lamina propria of these organs is a dense, woven sheath of smooth muscle (Fig 20–18).

The superficial cells of the transitional epithelium, **facet cells,** are responsible for the osmotic barrier between urine and tissue fluids. They have a special membrane of thick plates separated by narrow bands of thinner membrane. When the bladder contracts, the membrane folds along the thinner regions, and the thicker plates invaginate to form fusiform cytoplasmic vesicles. This luminal membrane is assembled in the Golgi apparatus and has an unusual chemical composition; cerebroside is the major component of the polar lipid fraction.

The muscular layers in the calyces, renal pelvis, and ureters have a helical arrangement. As the ureteral muscle cells reach the bladder, they become longitudinal; therefore, the intravesical part of the ureter is composed of longitudinal fibers which then fan out distally to form the superficial trigone whose muscles continue dorsally to the verumontanum in the male and the external urethral meatus in the female.

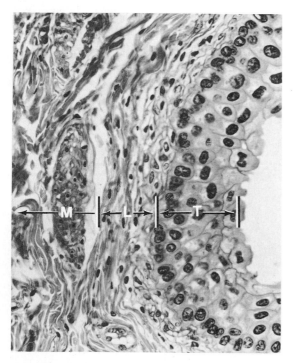

Figure 20–18. Photomicrograph of the urinary bladder wall. The transitional epithelium (T), with overlying facet cells, lies on a thin lamina propria (L). A thick, woven muscularis consists of helically wound bundles of smooth muscle (M). H&E stain, reduced from × 320.

Beginning 2–3 cm proximal to the bladder, Waldeyer's sheath or muscle is found on the outer surface of the ureter. It extends to the ureteral meatus, below which it fans out to form the deep trigone, which ends at the bladder neck.

The muscle fibers of the bladder run in every direction (without distinct layers) until they approach the bladder neck, where 3 distinct layers can be identified: (1) The internal longitudinal layer, which, distal to the bladder neck, becomes circular around the prostatic urethra and the prostatic substance in the male. It extends to the external meatus in the female. Its fibers form the true involuntary urethral sphincter. (2) The middle layer, which ends at the bladder neck. (3) The outer longitudinal layer, which continues to the end of the prostate and to the external urethral meatus in the female.

The ureters pass through the wall of the bladder obliquely, so that a valve is formed that prevents the backflow of urine. The intravesical ureter has only longitudinal muscle fibers.

The urinary passages are covered externally by an adventitial membrane—except for the upper part of the bladder, which is covered by (serous) peritoneum.

Urethra

The urethra is a tube that carries the urine from the bladder to the exterior. In the male, sperm also pass through it during ejaculation. In the female, the urethra is exclusively a urinary organ.

A. Male Urethra: The male urethra consists of 4 parts: a **prostatic part,** a **membranous part,** a **bulbous part,** and a **pendulous part.**

The prostate (see Chapter 23) is situated very close to the bladder, and the initial part of the urethra passes through it. Ducts that transport the secretions of the prostate open into the prostatic urethra.

In the dorsal and distal part of the prostatic urethra, there is an elevation, the **verumontanum,** which protrudes into its interior. In the tip of the verumontanum opens a blind tube called the prostatic utricle, which has no known function. On the sides of the verumontanum open the ejaculatory ducts through which the seminal fluid enters the posterior urethra to be stored just prior to ejaculation. The prostatic urethra is lined by transitional epithelium.

The membranous urethra extends for only 1 cm and is lined with pseudostratified columnar epithelium. Surrounding this part of the urethra there is a sphincter of striated muscle, the **external sphincter** of the urethra.

The voluntary external striated sphincter adds further closing pressure to that exerted by the involuntary urethral sphincter formed by the continuation of the internal longitudinal muscle of the bladder.

The bulbous and pendulous parts of the urethra are located in the **corpus spongiosum** of the penis. Distally, the urethral lumen dilates, forming the **fossa navicularis.** The epithelium of this portion of the urethra is mostly pseudostratified and columnar, with areas that are squamous and stratified.

The glands of Littré are mucous glands found along the entire length of the urethra but mostly in the pendulous part. The secretory portions of some of these glands are directly linked to the epithelial lining of the urethra; others possess excretory ducts.

B. Female Urethra: The female urethra is a tube 4–5 cm long, lined with squamous stratified epithelium with areas of pseudostratified columnar epithelium. The mid part of the female urethra is surrounded by an external striated voluntary sphincter.

• • •

References

Anderson WA: The use of exogenous myoglobin as an ultrastructural tracer: Reabsorption and translocation of protein by the renal tubule. J Histochem Cytochem 20:672, 1972.

Arakawa M, Tokunaga J: Further scanning electron microscope studies of the human glomerulus. Lab Invest 31:436, 1974.

Barajas L: The ultrastructure of the juxtaglomerular apparatus as disclosed by 3-dimensional reconstruction from serial sections. J Ultrastruct Res 33:116, 1970.

Barger AC, Herd JA: The renal circulation. N Engl J Med 284:482, 1971.

Bing J, Karimierczac J: Renin content of different parts of the juxtaglomerular apparatus. Acta Pathol Microbiol Scand 54:80, 1962.

Boudeau JE, Carone FA, Ganote CE: Serum albumin uptake in isolated perfused renal tubules. J Cell Biol 54:382, 1972.

Brenner BM, Rector FC Jr: *The Kidney.* Vol 1. Saunders, 1976.

Brenner BM, Troy JL, Daugharty TM: The dynamics of glomerular ultra-filtration in the rat. J Clin Invest 50:1776, 1971.

Bulger RE & others: Human renal ultrastructure. 2. The thin limb of Henle's loop and the interstitium in healthy individuals. Lab Invest 16:124, 1967.

Dirks JH, Clapp JR, Berliner RW: The protein concentration in the proximal tubule of the dog. J Clin Invest 43:916, 1964.

Ericsson JLE, Trump BF: Electron microscopic studies of the epithelium of the proximal tubule of the rat kidney. 1. The intracellular localization of acid phosphatase. Lab Invest 13:1427, 1964.

Ganong WF: Formation and excretion of urine. In: *Review of Medical Physiology,* 9th ed. Lange, 1979.

Ganote CE & others: Ultrastructural studies of vasopressin: Effect on isolated, perfused, renal collecting tubules of the rabbit. J Cell Biol 36:355, 1968.

Hartroft PM, Sutherland LE, Hartroft WS: Juxtaglomerular cells as the source of renin: Further studies with the fluorescent antibody technique and the effect of passive transfer of antirenin. Can Med Assoc J 90:163, 1964.

Hatt PI: The juxtaglomerular apparatus. In: *Ultrastructure of the Kidney.* Dalton AJ, Haguenau F (editors). Academic Press, 1967.

Hicks RM: The mammalian urinary bladder: An accommodating organ. Biol Rev 50:215, 1975.

Kriz W, Lever AF: Renal countercurrent mechanisms: Structure and function. Am Heart J 78:101, 1969.

Latta H: The glomerular capillary wall. J Ultrastruct Res 32:526, 1970.

Latta H, Maunsbach AB, Osvaldo L: The fine structure of renal tubules in cortex and medulla. In: *Ultrastructure of the Kidney.* Dalton AJ, Haguenau F (editors). Academic Press, 1967.

Maul CG: Structure and formation of pores in fenestrated capillaries. J Ultrastruct Res 36:768, 1971.

Maunsbach AB: Observations of the ultrastructure and acid phosphatase activity of the cytoplasmic bodies in rat kidney proximal tubule cells, with a comment on their classification. J Ultrastruct Res 16:197, 1966.

Menefee MG, Mueller CB: Some morphological considerations of transport in the glomerulus. In: *Ultrastructure of the Kidney.* Dalton AJ, Haguenau F (editors). Academic Press, 1967.

Michielsen P, Creemers J: The structure and function of the glomerular mesangium. In: *Ultrastructure of the Kidney.* Dalton AJ, Haguenau F (editors). Academic Press, 1967.

Miller F, Palade GE: Lytic activities in renal protein absorption droplets: An electron microscopical cytochemical study. J Cell Biol 23:519, 1964.

Miyoshi M, Fujita T, Tokunaga J: The differentiation of renal podocytes: A combined scanning and transmission electron microscope study in rats. Arch Histol Jpn 33:161, 1971.

Murakami T, Miyoshi M, Fujita T: Glomerular vessels of the rat kidney with special reference to double efferent arterioles: A scanning electron microscopic study of corrosion casts. Arch Histol Jpn 33:179, 1971.

Oliver C, Essner E: Protein transport in mouse kidney utilizing tyrosinase as an ultrastructural tracer. J Exp Med 136:291, 1972.

Osvaldo L, Latta H: The thin limb of the loop of Henle. J Ultrastruct Res 15:144, 1966.

Post RS: The distribution of normal serum proteins within rat and human renal tubule cytoplasm as demonstrated by immunofluorescence. J Lab Clin Med 67:189, 1966.

Rodewald R, Karnovsky MJ: Porous substructure of the glomerular slit diaphragm in the rat and mouse. J Cell Biol 60:423, 1974.

Spinelli F: Structure and development of the renal glomerulus as revealed by scanning electron microscopy. Int Rev Cytol 39:345, 1974.

Staehelin LA, Chlapowski FJ, Bonneville MA: Luminal plasma membrane of the urinary bladder. 1. Three-dimensional reconstruction from freeze-etch images. J Cell Biol 53:73, 1972.

Straus W: Occurrence of phagosomes and phagolysosomes in different segments of the nephron in relation to the reabsorption, transport, digestion and extrusion of intravenously injected horseradish peroxidase. J Cell Biol 21:295, 1964.

21 | Pituitary & Hypothalamus

In the evolutionary development of the metazoans, multicellularity led to a division of labor wherein cells carrying out particular functions assembled into coherent associations known as tissues. The integration and coordination of the activities of various tissues are under the control of chemical messengers, the **hormones,** synthesized and released by cells of the **endocrine system.** The products of endocrine glands are not secreted through ducts but are released directly into the connective tissue or vascular network.

A hormone is an organic chemical liberated at a specific time in small amounts by endocrine cells into the tissue fluids or vascular system. In general, the hormones exert their effects at a distance from the site of their secretion. The tissues and organs the hormones act on are called **target organs.** The endocrine and nervous systems, both of which have the function of integrating the activities of diverse parts of the organism, are clearly coordinated in function. The hormones of many endocrine glands have an effect on the nervous system, and several endocrine organs are stimulated or inhibited by neural mechanisms. Fig 21–1 illustrates several situations in which endocrine function is controlled by the nervous system. Most biologic phenomena

are under the overlapping authority of both systems. This interlocking mechanism is so remarkable that its nervous and endocrine elements are regarded as constituting a single **neuroendocrine system.**

The structure, histophysiology, and cytophysiology of the endocrine glands comprise the subject matter of this and the following chapters.

PITUITARY
(Hypophysis)

The **pituitary gland** or **hypophysis** weighs about 0.5 g, and its normal dimensions in humans are about $10 \times 13 \times 6$ mm. It lies in a bony cavity at the base of the brain below the hypothalamus, with which it has important anatomic and functional relations.

During embryogenesis, the pituitary develops partly from oral ectoderm and partly from nerve tissue. An evagination from the floor of the diencephalon grows caudally as a stalk, without detaching itself from the brain. An outpocketing of ec-

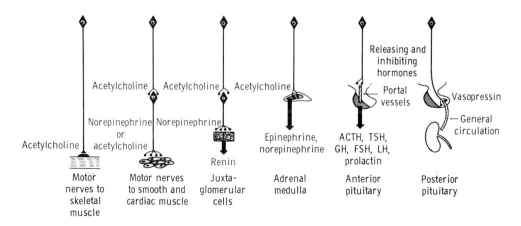

Figure 21–1. Diagrammatic representation of 6 situations in which humoral substances are released by neurons. The last 2 are examples of neurosecretion. (Reproduced, with permission, from Ganong WF: *Review of Medical Physiology,* 9th ed. Lange, 1979.)

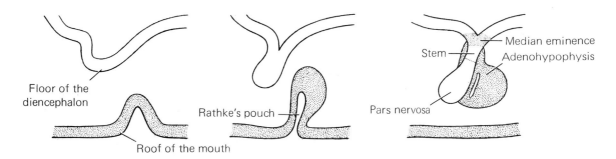

Figure 21–2. Diagram of the development of the adenohypophysis and neurohypophysis. The ectoderm of the roof of the mouth and its derivatives is stippled (lower portion). In the upper portion is the neural ectoderm from the floor of the diencephalon.

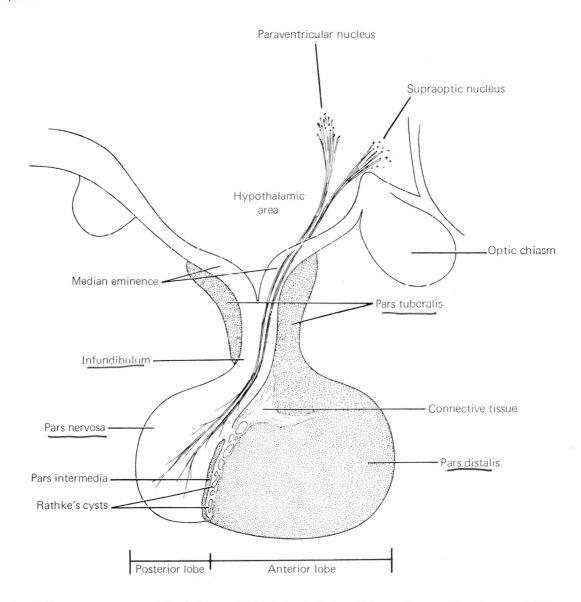

Figure 21–3. The component parts of the pituitary and their relation to the hypothalamus. The pars tuberalis, pars distalis, and pars intermedia form the adenohypophysis. The infundibulum and pars nervosa form the neurohypophysis. (Modified, redrawn, and reproduced, with permission, from the *Ciba Collection of Medical Illustrations,* by Frank H. Netter, MD.)

toderm from the roof of the primitive mouth of the embryo grows cranially, forming a cavity called **Rathke's pouch.** Later, a constriction at the base of this pouch separates it from the oral cavity. Its anterior wall thickens at the same time, so that the lumen of Rathke's pouch is reduced to a small fissure (Fig 21–2).

The part of the pituitary that develops from nerve tissue is the **neurohypophysis.** It consists of a large portion, the **pars nervosa** or **infundibular process,** and the smaller **infundibulum** or **neural stalk** (Fig 21–3). The infundibulum is composed of the **stem** and **median eminence.** The infundibulum

is continuous with the hypothalamus and connects the pituitary with the central nervous system. Through the infundibulum pass important nerve tracts and substances that act upon the anterior lobe of the pituitary.

The part of the pituitary that arises from oral ectoderm is known as the **adenohypophysis** and is subdivided into 3 portions: a large part, the **pars distalis** or **anterior lobe;** a cranial part, the **pars tuberalis,** which surrounds the infundibulum; and the **pars intermedia,** which lies between the neurohypophysis and the pars distalis, separated from the latter by the remaining fissure of the primi-

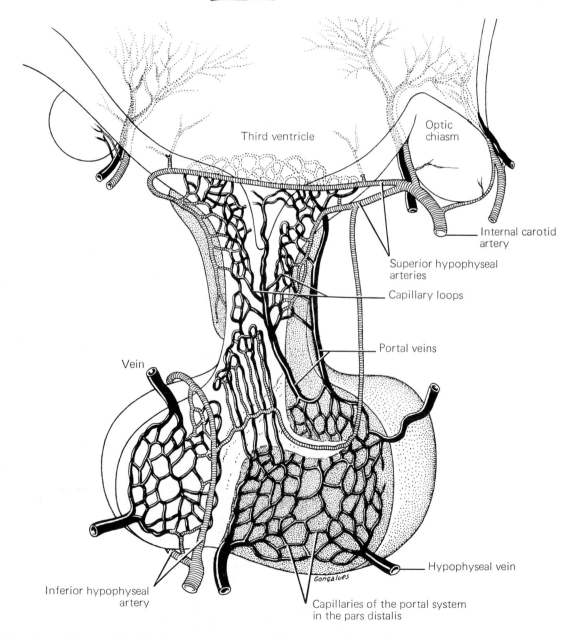

Figure 21 –4. Diagram of the blood circulation in the pituitary, including the portal system. (Redrawn and reproduced, with permission, from the *Ciba Collection of Medical Illustrations,* by Frank H. Netter, MD.)

tive cavity of Rathke's pouch, the residual cleft (Fig 21–3). The **posterior lobe** of the pituitary consists of the pars nervosa and the pars intermedia. The gland is covered by a connective tissue capsule and is situated in a depression of the sphenoid bone known as the **sella turcica.** Loose connective tissue with abundant venous drainage is found between the periosteum of the sphenoid bone and the capsule of the pituitary gland.

Blood Supply

The blood supply of the pituitary derives from 2 groups of blood vessels: from above, the right and left **superior hypophyseal arteries** supply the median eminence and the infundibulum; from below, the right and left **inferior hypophyseal arteries** mainly provide for the neurohypophysis and a small supply to the stalk. The superior hypophyseal arteries supply mainly the more cranial portion of the pituitary stalk, where they branch, and they also supply branches to the hypothalamus and the caudal portion of the pituitary stalk. The capillaries thus formed join again, giving rise to veins which arborize once again in the pars distalis, forming sinusoid capillaries and constituting, in this way, a **portal system** (Fig 21–4).

This vascular disposition makes possible the transport of hormones from the cranial portion of the pituitary stalk to the cells of the pars distalis. There are 2 **lower hypophyseal arteries** running

alongside the gland and supplying the posterior lobe of the pituitary. Blood from both pituitary lobes drains into the cavernous sinus through a number of venous channels (Fig 21–4).

The nerve supply of the anterior lobe is derived from the carotid plexus, which accompanies the arteriolar branches. These nerves appear to have a vasomotor function and do not directly affect the cells of the anterior lobe.

ADENOHYPOPHYSIS

Pars Distalis

As opposed to the neurohypophysis, which retains some characteristics of nerve tissue, the part of the pituitary that arises from oral ectoderm presents the typical appearance of an endocrine gland composed of cells grouped in cords and follicles. Its sinusoid capillaries were classically considered to be part of the macrophage system, although it has been verified that its lining cells do not have the capacity of phagocytosis.

Two types of cells have been described in this region: chromophobe and chromophil cells. **Chromophobe cells** are so called because they have no affinity for the usual dyes used in histology (Figs 21–5 and 21–9). When observed in the light mi-

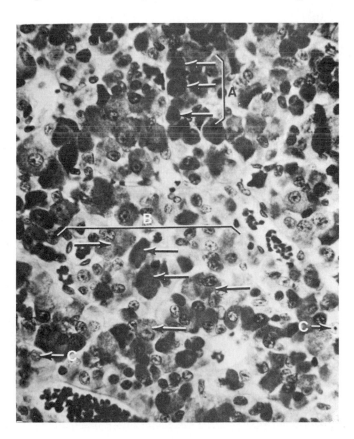

Figure 21 –5 (at right). Photomicrograph of a section of the pars distalis of the pituitary. At (A), acidophilic cells stain orange-red; at (B), basophilic cells (lower arrows) stain blue. At left and right, note unstained chromophobe (C) cells. Mallory stain, reduced from × 200.

croscope, these cells present no visible secretory granules and were once thought to be undifferentiated or resting cells without secretory activity. Electron microscopic examination shows, however, that most of them have small secretory granules and therefore could be active glandular cells. At present, only a small percentage of chromophobe cells are considered to be undifferentiated nonsecretory cells, and most of them are probably partially degranulated chromophil cells.

Another group of chromophobes are the **follicular cells,** which are star-shaped cells with multiple, long cytoplasmic processes that interconnect, forming a network that seems to constitute bridges between the capillaries. They have been described in several species, including humans. They have a clear perinuclear cytoplasm with few organelles and few, if any, secretory granules. They probably form part of the supporting stroma of the glandular cells. They appear to function as macrophages in that they are involved with the digestion of waste materials from other cells.

Chromophil cells contain specific cytoplasmic granules that have great affinity for some dyes (Figs 21–5 and 21–9). They are generally found near the capillaries. These cells are classified as **acidophils** or **basophils** according to the affinity of their granules for acidic or basic dyes. It is known, however, that both acidophils and basophils can be classified in subgroups according to other histochemical and staining affinities. Most of these cells present the characteristics described in Chapter 4 for cells that synthesize, store, and export proteins. In the glycoprotein-producing cells (gonadotropic and thyrotropic cells), the carbohydrate portion of the hormone molecules is probably added to the protein moiety both in the endoplasmic reticulum and in the Golgi complex. The extrusion of the storage granules occurs by a process of exocytosis. The slow mitotic cycle of these cells is controlled by the same factors that influence their secretory activity. Such factors include hypothalamic hormones, the influence of target cells and organs, bioamines, and cAMP.

The gradual discovery of various hormones synthesized by the pars distalis led investigators to try to correlate each hormone with a different cell type responsible for its production. Several staining and histochemical methods have been applied to the adenohypophysis, and the diverse results obtained in the different species has confused rather than clarified the issues. The recent application of histochemical, immunofluorescent, and electron microscopic technics has facilitated the study of the sites of hormone production in the adenohypophysis. Since these hormones are polypeptides or glycoproteins, it is possible to purify them and to produce specific antibodies for use in immunocytochemical studies (Fig 21–6). The human adenohypophysis contains approximately 50% chromophobes, 40% acidophils, and 10% basophils, varying within certain limits according to several factors such as age, pregnancy, thyroidectomy, hyperthyroidism, and the functional status of the gonads. Distribution of various types of cells in the gland is not homogeneous. Acidophils predominate at the periphery, whereas chromophobes and basophils show a preference for the most central part of the gland.

Cells of the Pituitary Gland

The cells of the pituitary can be classified on the basis of the hormone secreted and staining characteristics (Table 21–1).

A. Somatotropic Cells: The association of acidophilic tumors of the pituitary with acromegaly or gigantism has linked these cells with growth hormone production and secretion in the normal

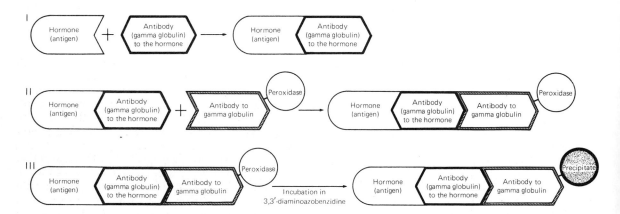

Figure 21–6. Intracellular detection of pituitary hormones by means of immunocytochemistry. *First stage:* The sections are treated by a solution containing an antibody to the hormone to be studied. The antibody binds itself to the hormone. *Second stage:* The section is incubated in a solution containing an antiantibody labeled by coupling it to peroxidase. This antiantibody binds itself to the antibody. *Third stage:* The section is incubated in an adequate substrate (3,3'-diaminoazobenzidine plus H_2O_2) that forms a brown precipitate in the sites that contain the hormone.

Table 21–1. Hormone-secreting cells in the human anterior pituitary. PAS, periodic acid–Schiff reaction. (Courtesy of C. Ezrin.)*

Cell Type	Hormone Secreted	Staining Reactions		
		General	Orange G	PAS
Somatotropic	Growth hormone	Acidophil	+	–
Mammotropic	Prolactin	Acidophil	+	–
Corticotropic	ACTH	Basophil	–	+
FSH gonadotropic	FSH	Basophil	–	+
LH gonadotropic	LH	Basophil	–	+
Thyrotropic	TSH	Basophil	–	+

*Reproduced, with permission, from Ganong WF: *Review of Medical Physiology*, 9th ed. Lange, 1979.

pituitary. Immunofluorescent studies of human pituitary tissue support this conclusion. The acidophilic granules are easily seen in the light microscope. The somatotropic cells are easily recognized in the electron microscope by their numerous dense (300–350 nm) secretory granules, central nucleus, and large Golgi apparatus.

B. Mammotropic Cells: These cells contain eosinophilic granules and can be distinguished from somatotropic cells, which also contain acidophilic granules, by their preferential affinity for erythrosin or carmine stains. They are located in a small zone in the lateral acidophilic wings of the pituitary. In the electron microscope they have large, dense, pleomorphic secretory granules, 550–600 nm in diameter. These cells secrete **prolactin,** and their numbers and size increase during pregnancy and lactation. Lysosomes and their derivatives are more numerous when secretion is inhibited, and they are believed to function in the regulation of secretion by degrading the unused secretory granules.

C. Gonadotropic Cells: There are 2 different cells in this classification. One produces **follicle-stimulating hormone (FSH)** and has a large, round cell body with dense secretory granules about 200 nm in diameter. The Golgi apparatus is well developed, and the granular endoplasmic reticulum is composed of distended vesicular elements.

The second type of gonadotropic cell secretes **luteinizing hormone (LH),** which, in males, is called interstitial cell–stimulating hormone (ICSH). These are small, round cells with uniform dense granules about 250 nm in diameter—larger than those that produce FSH. The Golgi complex is not as extensive, and the endoplasmic reticulum is composed of some flattened elements, in contrast to the dilated sacs of the FSH-producing cell.

In humans, both types of gonadotropic cells are distributed singly throughout the pituitary, and both belong to the basophilic subgroup.

D. Thyrotropic Cells: These cells produce **thyroid-stimulating hormone (TSH;** also called **thyrotropin)** and are located mainly in the central wedge of the adenohypophysis. They are large, polyhedral, and easily identified in the electron

microscope by their small granules, which are only 120–200 nm in diameter. They belong in the basophilic subgroup. These last 3 cells (FSH-, LH-, and TSH-producing) have a positive periodic acid–Schiff (PAS) reaction owing to the fact that these 3 hormones are glycoproteins.

E. Corticotropic and Melanotropic Cells: The corticotropic cells produce **adrenocorticotropic hormone (corticotropin, ACTH),** and the melanotropic cells produce **melanocyte-stimulating hormone (MSH).** Human corticotropic pituitary cells can be identified by immunostaining with an antiserum that is specific for corticotropin. They are found mostly in the medial wedge of the pituitary, some in the lateral portion and some in the pars tuberalis. ACTH seems to be produced in chromophobe cells in rats and in basophilic cells in humans. They contain granules about 100–200 nm in diameter and are not as abundant as in the other cell types.

Antisera raised against melanocyte-stimulating hormone react with the cells of the pars intermedia and with the corticotropic cells of the pituitary. Secretion of both hormones by a single cell would explain why their secretion changes in parallel in a number of diseases of the adrenal glands. They are polygonal in shape, with round eccentric nuclei, a well-developed Golgi apparatus, and granular endoplasmic reticulum that tends to be more elongated and at the periphery of the cell.

Histophysiology of the Pars Distalis

The hormones synthesized by this region are capable of exerting several kinds of effects. Some have a general metabolic action on the whole organism, whereas others act on specific structures known as "target organs"; the latter include nearly all of the other endocrine glands. Secretory granules appear in the human fetal pituitary at the end of the first trimester of pregnancy. The time at which hormonal secretion is initiated and controlled by feedback mechanisms is unknown in humans. The following are the hormones synthesized by the pars distalis and their main effects (Fig 21–7):

A. Growth Hormone (Somatotropin, STH): Human growth hormone is a protein which has a molecular weight of 21,700 and 191 amino acids in its straight chain structure. It influences many metabolic processes, but its most marked effect is on the epiphyseal cartilage of long bones, stimulating their growth. This is not a direct action, for somatotropin acts on the liver and kidney to elicit the production of a peptide called **somatomedin** that acts on the epiphyseal cartilage. An excess of somatotropin production in children and adolescents produces gigantism. If this excess occurs in adults, in whom no epiphyseal disks are present, only growth of the extremities of the body (mandible, nose, fingers, etc) takes place, producing the condition known as **acromegaly.** Deficient secretion of growth hormone during childhood causes **hypopituitary**

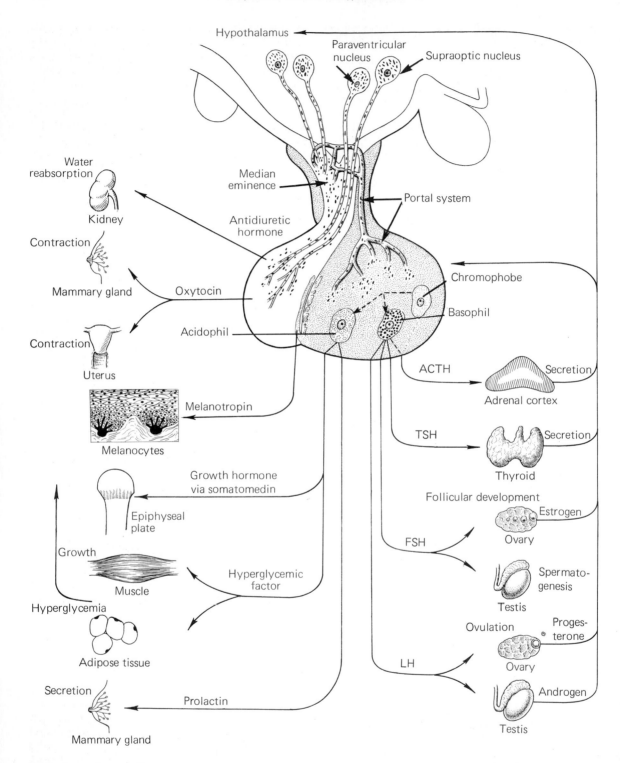

Figure 21–7. Drawing illustrating the effects of various pituitary hormones on target organs. Observe that several of the hormones produced by the target organs can act on the pituitary or hypothalamus to regulate their activity.

dwarfism, mainly as a result of incomplete growth of the long bones.

B. Prolactin (Lactogenic Hormone; Luteotropic Hormone, LTH): This protein hormone has a molecular weight of 22,500 and contains 198 amino acids. It triggers the secretion of milk by the mammary glands and maintains it in association with other hormones after birth. In addition to its effect on mammary development, prolactin also stimulates maternal behavior. The role of this hormone in males, if any, is unknown.

C. Thyrotropin (Thyroid-Stimulating Hormone, TSH): This hormone is a glycoprotein with a molecular weight of 26,600. Thyrotropin stimulates the synthesis and liberation of thyroid hormones. In experimental animals, thyrotropin preparations have a number of extrathyroidal effects.

D. Follicle-Stimulating Hormone (FSH): FSH is a glycoprotein (MW 32,000) with 236 amino acids. It stimulates early follicular development in the ovary and gametogenesis in the testis.

E. Luteinizing Hormone (LH; Interstitial Cell-Stimulating Hormone, ICSH): This glycoprotein hormone has a molecular weight of about 30,000 with 2 amino acid chains: an α chain made up of 96 amino acids and a β chain with 119 amino acids. LH is responsible for the final maturation and rupture of the graafian follicles and consequently ovulation, and for the development of the corpus luteum in the ovary, maintaining the production of progesterone. It helps to maintain the interstitial cells of the testis and stimulates their secretion of androgens.

F. Adrenocorticotropic Hormone (ACTH; Corticotropin): ACTH has a molecular weight of 4500 and is made up of 39 amino acids. It stimulates the production of corticosteroid hormones and sex hormones from the cortex of the adrenal gland.

G. Lipotropins: Two polypeptides having 90 and 58 amino acid residues and respectively called β and γ lipotropins have been isolated from the anterior pituitary. The name derives from their capacity to mobilize fat in some species but not in rats, dogs, and humans. Beta lipotropin may be a precursor of endorphin, a polypeptide that binds to opiate receptors. The physiologic significance of the lipotropins is so far unknown.

Study of the blood supply to the pituitary reveals that its portal system can transport to the pars distalis substances produced in the hypothalamus and accumulated in the infundibular and tuberal region of the hypothalamus. These **releasing** or **inhibiting factors** have the capacity to simulate or inhibit release of the hormones produced by cells of the pars distalis. The following factors have been extracted to date from the mammalian hypothalamus: **growth hormone-releasing factor (GRF), growth hormone-inhibiting factor (GIF;** also called somatostatin), **prolactin-inhibiting factor (PIF), prolactin-releasing factor (PRF),**

thyrotropin-releasing factor (TRF), follicle-stimulating hormone-releasing factor (FRF), luteinizing hormone-releasing factor (LRF), and **corticotropin-releasing factor (CRF).** These hypothalamic polypeptide hormones are synthesized in the body of as yet unidentified hypothalamic or extrahypothalamic neurons and transported by their axons to a specific region of the hypothalamus—the **median eminence** (Figs 21–3 and 21–7). In this region, these factors accumulate in the form of secretory granules in bulblike dilatations at the ends of the axons. These axonal terminals containing the releasing factors are in close proximity to the primary capillary loops of the pituitary portal system. In this arrangement, the portal system permits the rapid transport of micro amounts of active polypeptides released from the median eminence to the pars distalis. Control of function of the glands influenced by the hormones of the pars distalis is one of the most important features of pituitary physiology and is accomplished by a feedback mechanism (Fig 21–8) of which an example follows:

The pars distalis is known to synthesize a hormone, **thyrotropin** (thyroid-stimulating hormone, TSH), which acts on the thyroid, stimulating the production and secretion of thyroxine and triiodothyronine. In addition to affecting the organism as a whole, thyroxine acts on the pituitary, inhibiting the cells which synthesize thyrotropin. Thyroxine may act directly on the hypothalamus, inhibiting the nerve cells encountered there which produce TRF (thyrotropin-releasing factor), a hormone that stimulates liberation of thyrotropin by the pituitary. In this way, a sensitive double control mechanism is established by which the concentration of a hormone in the blood regulates its own secretion through the secretory activity of the hypothalamus and pituitary (Fig 21–8). These control mechanisms play an important role in the adaptation of the organism to its environment. A great number of physical and psychologic stimuli that reach the central nervous system are reflected at the level of the hypothalamus, which by means of the hypothalamic factors modifies the secretions of the pituitary and consequently of the "target organs," thus enabling them to respond efficiently to stimuli.

Pars Tuberalis

This funnel-shaped region surrounds the infundibulum of the neurohypophysis (Fig 21–3). Microscopically, it appears highly vascularized, for it is reached by the superior hypophyseal arteries that terminate there as the initial part of the hypophyseal portal system. Its cells, whose function is unknown, differ in structure and histochemistry from those in the pars distalis. They are arranged in cords alongside the blood vessels. Small follicles filled with an amorphous substance and lined with these cells are sometimes observed.

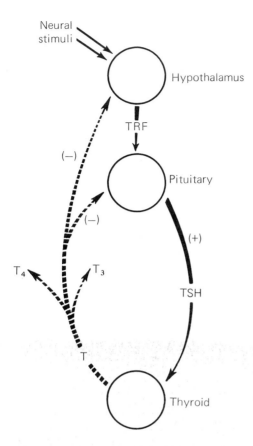

Figure 21–8. Relationships between the hypothalamus, the pituitary, and the thyroid. Thyrotropin-releasing factor (TRF) promotes secretion of thyrotropin (TSH) and acts to regulate the synthesis and secretion of the target organ hormones T_3 and T_4. These hormones, besides their effect on the peripheral tissues, regulate TSH and TRF secretion from the pituitary and the hypothalamus by a negative feedback mechanism. T, thyroid hormones. Solid arrows indicate stimulation; dashed arrows, inhibition.

Pars Intermedia

In humans, the pars intermedia is a rudimentary region made up of cords of weakly basophilic cells that present small secretory granules (200–300 nm) hardly visible in the light microscope. The fissure that results from Rathke's pouch is rarely found in adults, and follicles lined by cuboidal epithelium containing colloid and known as Rathke's cysts appear in its place (Fig 21–3).

The pars intermedia synthesizes a polypeptide, **melanocyte-stimulating hormone (MSH, intermedin)**, which in amphibia acts on the melanophores, causing dispersion of the melanin granules in these cells and darkening of the animal's skin. Recent evidence suggests that this region of the pituitary also secretes a large protein that splits into ACTH and lipotropin. The functions of the pars intermedia in humans are not well understood.

NEUROHYPOPHYSIS

The neurohypophysis consists of the **pars nervosa** or **neural lobe** and the **infundibulum.** The latter joins the gland with the hypothalamus. As opposed to the adenohypophysis, which presents epithelial characteristics, the neurohypophysis consists of about 100,000 unmyelinated axons of **secretory nerve cells.** The cell bodies of these neurons are not in the pituitary but lie primarily in the **supraoptic** and **paraventricular nuclei** (Figs 21–3 and 21–7).

The fibers (unmyelinated axons) of the secretory neurons converge, forming the **hypothalamohypophyseal tract.** They proceed to the neurohypophysis where they terminate blindly in close relation to a rich capillary plexus. The neurosecretory material produced in the neuronal perikaryon moves along these axons into the neural lobe, where it is stored at the terminal dilated blind endings of the axons and released as needed. The neural lobe is a depot for the storage of hormones and not an endocrine gland since its secretions originate elsewhere.

Neurosecretory Cells

The secretory neurons and their branches have all the constituents typical of nerve structures in general but have more developed Nissl bodies related to the production of the neurosecretory material. In addition, the axons and the cell bodies contain a granular substance that can be studied by specific technics such as staining with Gomori's chrome hematoxylin stain. The hormones of the neurohypophysis are contained in these granules.

The electron microscope reveals that these neurosecretory granules have a diameter of 100–200 nm, are surrounded by a membrane, and are more numerous in the dilated terminal parts of the axons that are closely related to fenestrated blood capillaries. Here they form accumulations visible with the light microscope and known as **Herring corpuscles.**

In addition to the secretory granules, the terminal parts of the neurohypophyseal axons contain vesicles that are morphologically similar to those of the synaptic vesicles. The function of these vesicles is still not known.

Neurosecretion is believed to be elaborated in the granular endoplasmic reticulum (Nissl bodies) of the cell bodies of the neurons and then to pass to the Golgi apparatus. It then moves along the axons of the hypothalamohypophyseal tract and is discharged around blood vessels in the pars nervosa.

The differential centrifugation technic has permitted the isolation of these secretory granules. The granules were found to contain either the **oxytocin** or **vasopressin** hormones, ATP, and the binding protein **neurophysin.** There is one neurophysin for binding oxytocin and another for vasopressin. Neurophysins are so specific in their binding of neurohypophyseal hormones that they can be used in separating these hormones from other peptides in pituitary extracts. Although it is not clear whether neurohypophyseal hormones exist as free peptides or as peptide-neurophysin complexes in the blood plasma, neurophysins have been identified in the peripheral blood, where they are measurable by radioimmunoassay. These proteins may act as carriers, and there may be more than two. Vasopressin and oxytocin are stored in the posterior pituitary and released into the blood by impulses in the nerve fibers from the hypothalamus. Although there is some overlap, the fibers from supraoptic nuclei are concerned with vasopressin secretion, while those from the paraventricular nuclei are concerned with oxytocin secretion.

Neurohypophyseal Cells

The neurohypophysis consists mainly of axons from hypothalamic neurons. To a lesser extent, however, it also presents connective tissue cells and a specific type of cell called a **pituicyte** (Fig 21–9).

The pituicytes have an irregular shape and, at times, numerous branches. The cytoplasm of these cells may contain lipid droplets or pigment. The pituicytes do not have ultrastructural characteristics typical of secretory cells, and it is believed that their role is similar to that of neuroglia. Many of the cytoplasmic processes of the pituicytes end in perivascular spaces.

Histophysiology

The neurohypophysis of all mammals except members of the pig family has 2 hormones, both cyclic peptides made up of 8 different amino acids. These hormones are **arginine vasopressin**—also called **antidiuretic hormone (ADH)**—and **oxytocin**. These hormones are present in different secretory granules. In large doses, vasopressin promotes the contraction of smooth muscle of blood vessels, raising the blood pressure. It acts mainly on the muscle layers of small arteries and arterioles. It is doubtful if endogenous vasopressin is secreted in an amount sufficient to exert any appreciable effect on blood pressure homeostasis. The main effect of vasopressin is to increase the permeability to water of the distal convoluted tubules and collecting tubules of the kidney. As a result, water is reabsorbed by these tubules and urine becomes hypertonic. Thus, vasopressin helps to regulate the osmotic balance of the internal milieu. Vasopressin increases the permeability of the collecting ducts to urea and decreases blood flow in the renal medulla. It increases the permeability to water of the toad bladder and the skin of the frog. This hormone is secreted whenever the osmotic pressure of the blood increases. In this case, the blood acts on osmoreceptor cells in the anterior hypothalamus, stimulating the secretion of this hormone from supraoptic neurons. Sections of the neurohypophysis of animals previously given injections of hypertonic solutions do not contain the neurosecretory material usually present in control animals. Vasopressin secretion is increased when extracellular fluid vol-

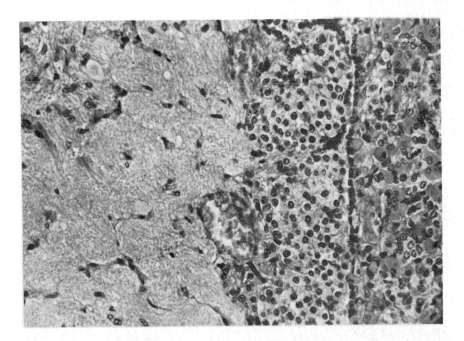

Figure 21 –9. Section of pituitary showing (from left to right) the neurohypophysis, the pars intermedia, and the pars distalis. Between the pars intermedia and the pars distalis is the pituitary cleft. Chromophilic and chromophobic cells are apparent in the pars distalis. The pars intermedia consists of cords of one cell type. Mallory stain, × 340.

ume is low and vice versa. A variety of stimuli in addition to these increase vasopressin secretion, eg, pain, trauma, emotional upsets, and drugs such as morphine and nicotine. Circulating vasopressin is rapidly inactivated (its half-life in humans is about 18 minutes), mainly in the liver and kidneys, and acts on its target organ by increasing intracellular cyclic adenosine-3',5'-monophosphate (cyclic AMP, cAMP).

Lesions of the hypothalamus, which destroy the neurosecretory cells, cause diabetes insipidus, a disease characterized by loss of renal capacity to concentrate urine. Consequently, an individual suf-

fering from this disease may excrete up to 20 liters of urine per day (polyuria) and will drink enormous quantities of liquids.

Oxytocin promotes contraction of the smooth muscle of the uterine wall during copulation and childbirth and the contraction of the myoepithelial cells which surround the alveoli and alveolar ducts of the mammary glands. The secretion of oxytocin is stimulated by distention of the vagina or of the uterine cervix and by nursing. This occurs via nerve tracts which act on the hypothalamus. The neurohormonal reflex triggered by nursing is called the **milk ejection reflex** (Fig 21–7).

•   •   •

References

Baker BL & others: Differentiation of growth hormone and prolactin-containing acidophils with peroxidase-labeled antibody. Anat Rec 164:163, 1969.

Baker BL & others: Identification of the corticotropin cell in rat hypophyses with peroxidase-labeled antibody. Anat Rec 166:557, 1970.

Bancroft FC, Tashjian AH Jr: Growth in suspension culture of rat pituitary cells which produce growth hormone and prolactin. Exp Cell Res 64:125, 1971.

Bodian D: Cytological aspects of neurosecretion in opossum neurohypophysis. Bull Johns Hopkins Hosp 113:57, 1963.

Daniel PM: The blood supply of the hypothalamus and pituitary gland. Br Med Bull 22:202, 1966.

Dierickx K, Vandesande F: Immunocytochemical localization of the vasopressinergic and oxytocinergic neurons in the human hypothalamus. Cell Tissue Res 184:15, 1977.

Farquhar MG: Processing of secretory products by cells of the anterior pituitary gland. Mem Soc Endocrinol (Cambridge) 19:79, 1971.

Ganong WF: *Review of Medical Physiology,* 9th ed. Lange, 1979.

Green JD: The comparative anatomy of the portal vascular system and of the innervation of the hypophysis. In: *The Pituitary Gland.* Vol 1. Harris GW, Donovan BT (editors). Univ of California Press, 1966.

Guillemin R: The adenohypophysis and its hypothalamic control. Annu Rev Physiol 29:313, 1967.

Guillemin R, Burgus R: The hormones of the hypothalamus. Sci Am 227:24, Nov 1972.

Harris GW, Reed M: Hypothalamic releasing factors and the control of anterior pituitary function. Br Med Bull 22:266, 1966.

Herbert DC, Hayashida T: Prolactin localization in the primate pituitary by immunofluorescence. Science 169:378, 1970.

Kurosumi K: Functional classification of cell types of the anterior pituitary gland accomplished by electron microscopy. Arch Histol Jpn 29:329, 1968.

Li CH: Hormones of the adenohypophysis. Proc Am Philos Soc 116:365, 1972.

Nakane PK: Classification of anterior pituitary cell types with immunoenzyme histochemistry. J Histochem Cytochem 18:9, 1970.

Nakayama I, Nickerson PA, Skelton PR: An ultrastructural study of the adrenocorticotropic hormone-secreting cell in the rat adenohypophysis during adrenal cortical regeneration. Lab Invest 21:169, 1969.

Pantic VR: The specificity of pituitary cells and regulation of their activities. Int Rev Cytol 40:153, 1975.

Phifer RF, Spicer SS: Immunohistologic and immunopathologic demonstration of adrenocorticotropic hormone in the pars intermedia of the adenohypophysis. Lab Invest 23:543, 1970.

Phifer RF, Spicer SS, Orth DN: Specific demonstration of the human hypophyseal cells which produce adrenocorticotropic hormone. J Clin Endocrinol 31:347, 1970.

Siperstein ER: Identification of the adrenocorticotrophin producing cells in the rat hypophysis by autoradiography. J Cell Biol 17:521, 1963.

Smith RE, Farquhar MG: Lysosome function in the regulation of the secretory process in cells of the anterior pituitary gland. J Cell Biol 31:319, 1966.

Vila-Porcile E: Le réseau des cellules folliculo-stellaires et les follicules de l'adenohypophyse du rat (Pars distalis). Z Zellforsch Mikrosk Anat 129:328, 1972.

Adrenals, Islets of Langerhans, Thyroid, Parathyroids, & Pineal Body | 22

THE ADRENAL (SUPRARENAL) GLANDS

The adrenal glands are paired organs that lie near the anterior poles of the kidneys embedded in adipose. They are flattened structures with a half-moon shape. In the human, they are about 4–6 cm long, 1–2 cm wide, and 4–6 mm thick, and all together weigh about 15 g, but their weight and size vary depending upon the age and physiologic condition of the individual. Examination of a fresh section of adrenal gland shows it to be covered by a capsule of dense collagenous connective tissue and to consist of 2 concentric layers: a yellow peripheral layer, the **adrenal cortex;** and a reddish-brown central layer, the **adrenal medulla** (Figs 22–1 and 22–5). Cortical and medullary tissue may sometimes also occur at other sites as shown in Fig 22–2.

These 2 layers may be considered as 2 mor-phologically and functionally distinct organs that become united during embryologic development. They derive from different tissues. The cortex arises from celomic intermediate mesoderm and therefore is of mesodermal origin. The medulla consists of cells derived from the neural crest from which the sympathetic ganglion cells also originate. In fact, one might consider the medulla to be a modified sympathetic ganglion whose postganglionic neurons lost their branches during development and became secretory cells. The general histologic appearance is typical of an endocrine gland wherein cells of both cortex and medulla are grouped in cords along capillaries and sinusoids (see Chapter 4).

The collagenous connective tissue capsule that covers the gland sends thin septa to the interior of the gland as trabeculae. The stroma consists mainly of a rich network of reticular fibers that supports the secretory cells.

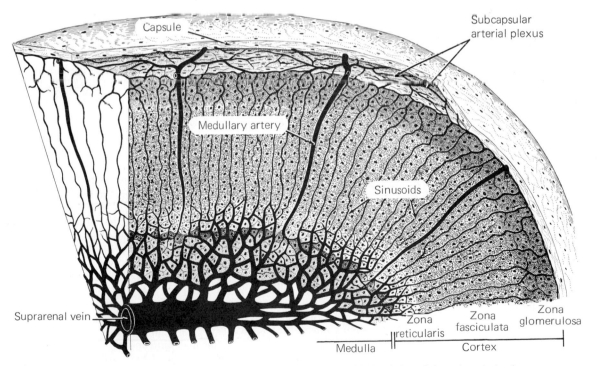

Figure 22–1. Diagram of the general architecture and blood circulation of the adrenal gland.

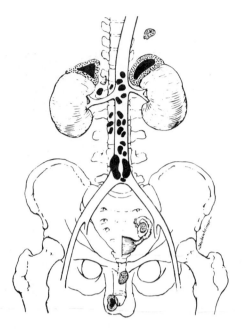

Figure 22 –2. Human adrenal glands. Adrenocortical tissue is stippled; adrenal medullary tissue is black. Note location of adrenals at superior pole of each kidney. Also shown are extra-adrenal sites at which cortical and medullary tissue is sometimes found. (Reproduced, with permission, from Forsham in: *Textbook of Endocrinology,* 4th ed. Williams RH [editor]. Saunders, 1968.)

Blood Supply

The adrenals are supplied by a number of arteries that enter at various points around their periphery (Fig 22–1). The 3 main groups of arteries are the **superior suprarenal** artery, arising from the inferior phrenic artery; the **middle suprarenal** artery, arising from the aorta; and the **inferior suprarenal** artery, arising from the renal artery. The various arterial branches that reach the organ provide for a subcapsular plexus which arborizes and forms capillaries running throughout the cortex (Fig 22–1). The cortical arteries arise from this capsular plexus and distribute blood to the anastomosing network of sinusoids associated with the cords of cortical cells. At the corticomedullary junction, the sinusoids drain into medullary sinusoids since there is no venous system in the cortex. Some branches, called **medullary arteries,** leave the capsule and bypass the cortex by traversing through connective tissue trabeculae. These vessels, which do not supply branches to the cortex, terminate in a rich capillary network around the cells of the medullary cords. This dual vascular supply provides the medulla with both arterial (via medullary arteries) and venous (via cortical arteries) blood. As this blood passes into the medulla, it has a profound effect upon the physiology of the medullary cells because of the glucocorticoids secreted into the cortical arteries. These capillaries, together with those that

supply the cortex, form the medullary veins that join to constitute the **adrenal** or **suprarenal veins** (Fig 22–1). The adrenal cortical capillaries are considered to be sinusoids, for their lumens are large. The endothelium is extremely attenuated and interrupted by small fenestrae closed by a very thin diaphragm. A continuous basal lamina is seen beneath the endothelium in the capsule and medulla; however, it may be discontinuous beneath endothelial cells of the cortex. It has been reported that endothelial cells were phagocytic since they take up colloidal vital dyes, but more recent studies with the electron microscope have failed to reveal evidence of phagocytosis by the endothelium. Observations in the former studies were related to the fact that selected dyes were apparently binding to the endothelial cell surface. Macrophages present in the subendothelial space probably were the only cells participating in phagocytosis. In the adrenal glands of some animals, including humans, there is a subendothelial space between the endothelial cells of the capillaries and glandular cells in which the microvilli of the latter are observed.

The Adrenal Cortex

Because of the different disposition and appearance of its cells, the adrenal cortex can be subdivided into 3 concentric layers which, in humans, are usually not sharply defined (Figs 22–1 and 22–3A): the **zona glomerulosa** (Fig 22–3B), the **zona fasciculata** (Fig 22–3C), and the **zona reticularis** (Fig 22–3D). The zona glomerulosa secretes the mineralocorticoids, primarily aldosterone, which are involved with maintenance of electrolyte (eg, sodium and potassium) and water balance. The zona fasciculata and probably the zona reticularis secrete the glucocorticoids cortisone and cortisol or, in some animals, corticosterone, which are concerned with the regulation of carbohydrate, protein, and fat metabolism. Estrogens and androgens are produced in small amounts in these 2 zones (Fig 22–5).

The cells of the adrenal cortex have the characteristics of steroid-synthesizing cells described in Chapter 4. The glomerulosa, fasciculata, and reticularis zones occupy, respectively, 15%, 50%, and 7% of the total volume of the adrenals.

The layer immediately beneath the connective tissue capsule is the **zona glomerulosa,** in which the columnar or pyramidal cells are arranged in closely packed, rounded, or arched clusters surrounded by capillaries (Fig 22–3A). Glomerulosa cells have a spherical nucleus, a well-developed nucleolus, and an acidophilic cytoplasm containing basophilic granules and lipid droplets (Fig 22–3B). The cell contour is smooth except near the subendothelial space, where the plasma membrane is thrown up into folds and microvilli. A prominent feature of the cell is the extensive smooth endoplasmic reticulum that forms an anastomosing tubular network (Fig 22–4). There are a few short segments of granular endoplasmic reticulum and some free cytoplasmic

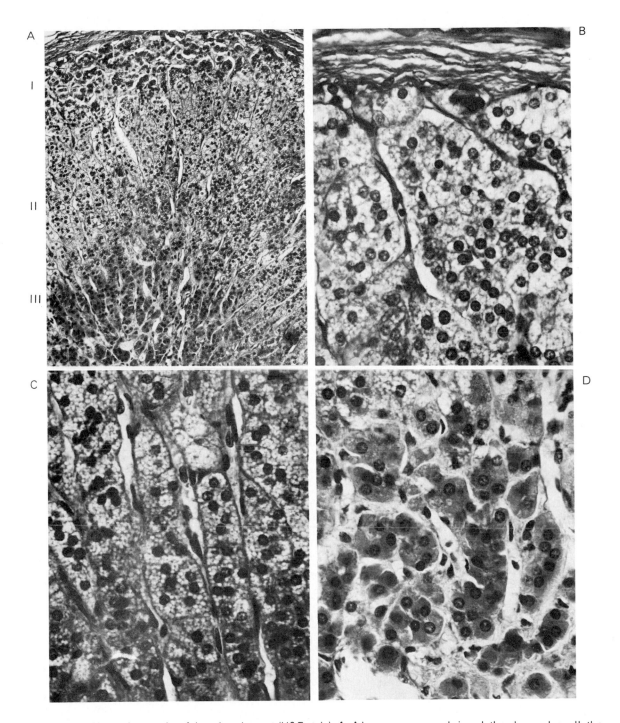

Figure 22 –3. Photomicrographs of the adrenal cortex (H&E stain). *A:* A low-power general view. I, the glomerulosa; II, the fasciculata; III, the reticularis. × 80. *B:* The capsule and the zona glomerulosa. × 330. *C:* The zona fasciculata. × 330. *D:* The zona reticularis. × 330.

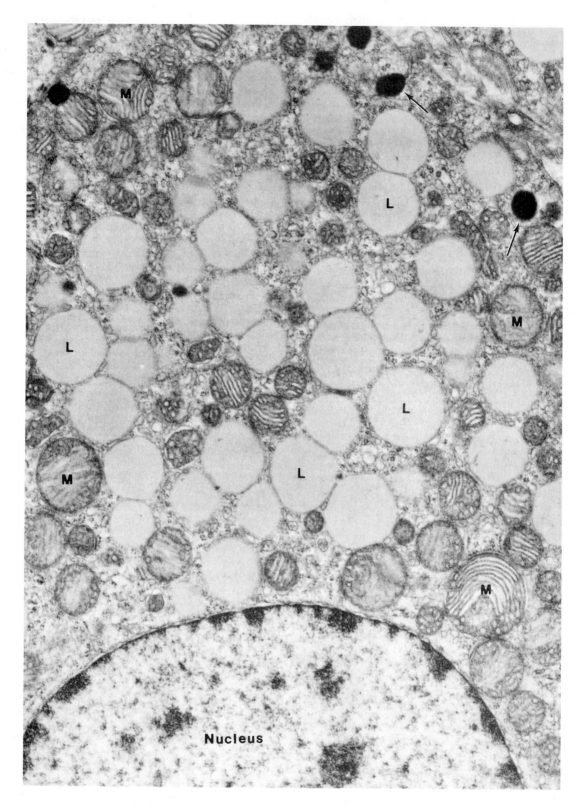

Figure 22–4. Fine structure of an adrenal gland cell involved in the synthesis and secretion of steroid hormones. The clear vacuoles are lipid droplets (L), and the dense granules (arrows) are lysosomes. The abundant mitochondria (M) exhibit the characteristic tubular cristae of a steroidal cell. In the background are numerous circular profiles of smooth endoplasmic reticulum. × 15,000.

ribosomes. The abundant mitochondria are spherical or ovoid and exhibit tubular cristae. The smooth endoplasmic reticulum sometimes occurs in close relationship to the lipid droplets. A well-developed Golgi apparatus is present. The localization of the enzymes participating in aldosterone synthesis has been determined by the differential centrifugation technic. The synthesis of cholesterol from acetate takes place in smooth endoplasmic reticulum, whereas the conversion of cholesterol to pregnenolone takes place in the mitochondria. The enzymes associated with the synthesis of progesterone and deoxycorticosterone from pregnenolone are found in smooth endoplasmic reticulum; those enzymes that convert deoxycorticosterone → corticosterone → 18-hydroxycorticosterone → aldosterone are located in the mitochondria.

The next layer of cells is known as the **zona fasciculata** because the cells are arranged in straight cords, one or 2 cells thick (Fig 22–3C), that run at right angles to the surface of the organ and have capillaries between them. The cells of the zona fasciculata are polyhedral, with a central nucleus, and their cytoplasm is slightly basophilic. Microvilli extend into the subendothelial space. The cells contain a great number of lipid droplets in their cytoplasm. As a result of dissolution of the lipids during the dehydration steps in tissue preparation, the fasciculata cells appear highly vacuolated in common histologic preparations (Fig 22–3C). The smooth endoplasmic reticulum is even more fully developed in the zona fasciculata than in the zona glomerulosa, and the granular endoplasmic reticulum, which is more abundant in this zone, is responsible for the observed basophilia.

The innermost layer of the cortex, between the zona fasciculata and the medulla, contains cells disposed in irregular cords forming an anastomosing network and is called the **zona reticularis** (Fig 22–3D). These cells are smaller than those of the other 2 layers. The cells have many of the features of the cells in the zona fasciculata, but they differ in the structure of the mitochondria, which are more often elongated. In addition, the lipofuscin pigment granules in these cells are large and quite numerous. Their cytoplasm is acidophilic and contains a few lipid droplets and, at times, glycogen. Irregularly shaped cells with pyknotic nuclei—suggesting cellular degeneration—are often found in this layer (Fig 22–3D).

Histophysiology

The function of the adrenal cortex is to produce steroids, lipids that contain the cyclopentanoperhydrophenanthrene nucleus. Chemical radicals are added to or removed from this nucleus during the process of hormone biosynthesis, resulting in various substances with different physiologic activities. The steroids secreted by the cortex may be divided into 3 groups according to their main physiologic actions: **glucocorticoids,** **mineralocorticoids,** and **17-ketosteroids (sex hormones)** (Fig 22–5).

The **glucocorticoids,** mainly cortisol and corticosterone, exert a profound effect upon the metabolism of carbohydrates, as well as on proteins and lipids. In the liver, glucocorticoids promote the uptake and usage of fatty acids (energy source), amino acids (enzyme synthesis), and carbohydrates (glucose synthesis) that are utilized in gluconeogenesis and in glycogen assembly (glycogenesis). In fact, these hormones can stimulate the synthesis of so much glucose that the resulting high levels of this sugar that enter the blood produce a condition similar to diabetes. However, outside of the liver, glucocorticoids induce an opposite, or catabolic, effect on peripheral organs (eg, skin, muscle, adipose tissue). In these structures, these steroid hormones not only decrease synthetic activity, but they also promote protein and lipid degradation. The by-products of degradation, amino and fatty acids, are removed from the blood and utilized by the synthetically active hepatocytes.

Glucocorticoids also repress the immune response by decreasing the amount of circulating eosinophils by accelerating their sequestration in the lungs and spleen. Circulating lymphocytes are reduced as a result of an increased destruction of these cells and inhibition of mitotic activity in lymph-forming organs. Patients receiving organ transplants are frequently provided with massive doses of these steroid hormones because of their ability to suppress the immune response.

The **mineralocorticoids,** of which aldosterone is the most important, act mainly on the distal renal tubules (and perhaps also on the proximal tubules) as well as the gastric mucosa and the salivary and sweat glands, stimulating the reabsorption of sodium. They may increase the concentration of potassium and decrease that of sodium in muscle and brain cells.

Dehydroepiandrosterone is the only sex hormone secreted in significant physiologic quantities by the adrenal cortex. It has masculinizing and anabolic effects, but it is less than one-fifth as potent as testicular androgens. For this reason, and because it is secreted in small quantities—21 mg/d in males and 16 mg/d in females—it produces a negligible physiologic effect under normal conditions. When a congenital enzyme defect exists whereby the gland produces this hormone in abundance, this may result in precocious puberty in males or virilism in females.

The basic function of the adrenal gland is to maintain essential homeostatic mechanisms, eg, the chemical constitution of the intercellular and extracellular fluids. This is easily understood when one considers the total effects of the hormones of this gland. A wide variety of physiologic stimuli as well as pathologic states—stress, fasting, temperature changes, infections, drugs, exercise, hemorrhage, etc—affect the central nervous system and,

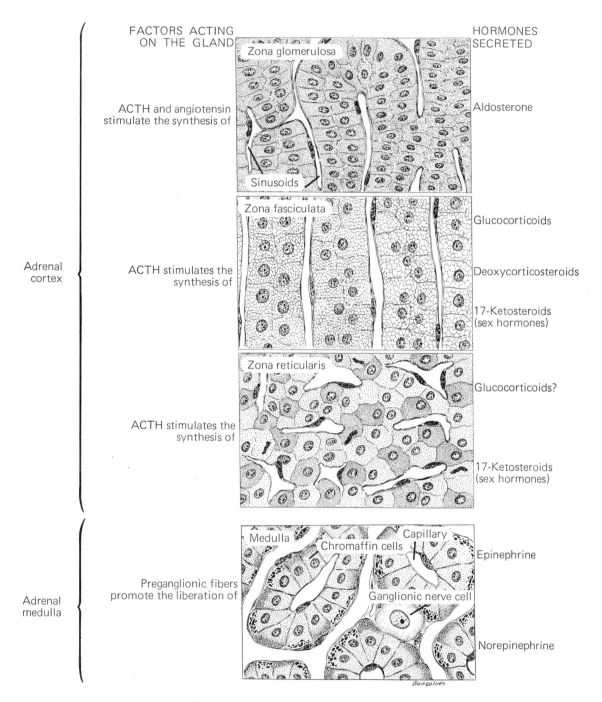

Figure 22–5. Structure and histophysiology of the adrenal gland. *Left:* Factors acting on the gland. *Right:* The hormones secreted.

FACTORS ACTING
ON THE GLAND

GLAND
REACTION

Hypophysectomy causes

Cortical atrophy

Stress → Hypothalamus →
Pituitary → ACTH, causing

Cortical hypertrophy

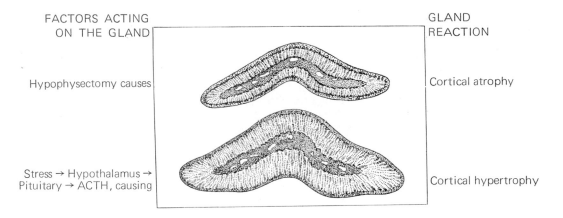

Figure 22–6. Effects of decreased and increased stimulation on the structure of the adrenal gland.

by stimulating hypothalamic secretion of corticotropin-releasing factor, cause an increase in the production of ACTH by the pituitary (Fig 22–7). The consequent increase in production of adrenal hormones permits the organism to counterbalance the effects of such stimuli. Since the organism is continuously receiving such stimuli, the adrenal gland and other homeostatic mechanisms are continually functioning, either in concert or in opposed balance, in order to maintain the equilibrium of the internal milieu.

In hypophysectomized animals, the effects of glucocorticoid deficiency can be observed while their ionic equilibrium is found to be essentially normal, so the secretion of aldosterone is not completely affected. In the morphologic study of the adrenal glands of these animals, cortical thinning is noticeable—mainly as a result of the atrophy of the zona fasciculata and zona reticularis—while the zona glomerulosa remains unaltered or may even be hypertrophic (Fig 22–6). Another argument in support of the theory that mineralocorticoid production occurs mainly in the glomerulosa is that in sodium deficiency the glomerulosa hypertrophies considerably, and this change is accompanied by a severalfold increase in aldosterone production. The presence only in the zona glomerulosa of the 18-hydroxylating enzyme necessary for the synthesis of aldosterone is another indication that synthesis of this hormone occurs in the zona glomerulosa.

The administration of ACTH to a hypophysectomized animal normalizes the secretion of glucocorticoids, demonstrating the dependence of these hormones on the pituitary hormones (Fig 22–5). The secretion of sex hormones is also controlled by ACTH. ACTH acts via the cAMP system, promoting an increase in the uptake of cholesterol and its conversion to pregnenolone by the mitochondria. It is now believed that ACTH does promote a weak aldosterone secretion but that this secretion is regulated primarily via the renin-angiotensin system in a feedback fashion. Renin is

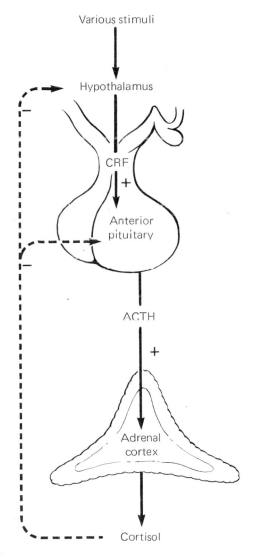

Figure 22–7. Feedback mechanism of ACTH-glucocorticoid secretion. Solid arrows indicate stimulation; dashed arrows, inhibition.

produced by the juxtaglomerular cells that surround the renal afferent arterioles as they enter the glomeruli (see Chapter 20) and is liberated in response to several types of stimuli, eg, decrease of sodium concentration in the blood, decrease of the volume of circulating blood, and constriction of the renal artery. Once secreted, renin acts as an enzyme on a circulating α_2 globulin (angiotensinogen), causing the liberation of angiotensin I, a decapeptide that is converted by a "converting enzyme" present in abundant amounts in the lungs into angiotensin II, an octapeptide that in turn acts on the adrenal gland to stimulate the secretion of aldosterone.

The Fetal or Provisional Cortex

In humans and some other animals, the adrenal gland of the newborn is larger than that of the adult. At this early age, a layer known as **fetal cortex** or **provisional cortex** is present between the thin adrenal cortex and the medulla. This layer is fairly thick, and its cells are disposed in cords. After birth, the provisional cortex undergoes involution, while the permanent cortex—the initially thin layer—develops, differentiating into the 3 layers described above. A major function of this fetal adrenal is secretion of sulfate conjugates of androgens, which are converted in the placenta to active androgens and estrogens that enter the maternal circulation.

Adrenal Medulla

The adrenal medulla is composed of polyhedral epithelioid cells arranged in cords, forming a compact network surrounded by capillaries and venules and a few sympathetic ganglion cells (Fig 22–8). They are regarded as modified postganglionic neurons. The nerve fibers that reach these cells are found on the side of the capillary. The secretory product accumulates at the cellular pole facing the vein into which it is released. The function of the medulla is to secrete the catecholamines epinephrine and norepinephrine, and this seems to be controlled largely by neural mechanisms. Norepinephrine is the chemical mediator of the postganglionic endings of the sympathetic nervous system. Histochemical studies in which the cells are reacted with oxidizing agents such as potassium bichromate or ferric chloride lead to a specific coloration of the secretory granules known as the **chromaffin reaction.** The specific staining characteristics of these granules, due to the presence of **catecholamines,** has led to the identification of these cells as **chromaffin cells.** In addition to catecholamines, the granules also contain ATP, specific proteins (chromogranins), and dopamine β-hydroxylase, an enzyme that converts dopamine to norepinephrine. On the basis of observed differences in the structure of the granules and the results of histochemical studies, it is apparent that epinephrine and norepinephrine are secreted by 2 different types of cells in the medulla. Epinephrine-secreting cells are similar in structure to those cells that contain norepinephrine and differ only in the composition and structure of the granules. The chromaffin cells of the adrenal medulla have the following 3 characteristics: they are derived from neuroectoderm; they secrete catecholamines; and they are innervated by preganglionic cholinergic fibers. In humans, 80% of the catecholamine output of the adrenal vein is epinephrine.

In tissue fixed in glutaraldehyde and osmium, the granules of norepinephrine-containing cells, which average 200 nm in diameter, present a very dense core, and a halo occurs between the granule

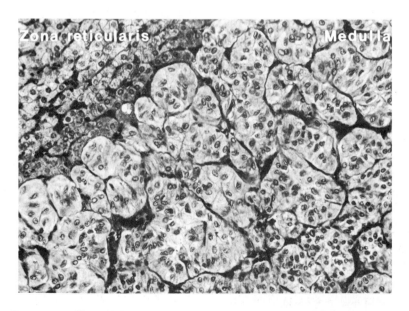

Figure 22 –8. Photomicrograph of a section of adrenal medulla. H&E stain, × 200.

and the enclosing membrane. The granules of the epinephrine-containing cells are less dense and have a relatively homogeneous content. Granule release is triggered by acetylcholine released from the preganglionic neurons that innervate the medullary cells. The separate liberation of these 2 hormones into the bloodstream suggests that the 2 types of cells are influenced by different factors. The enzyme phenylethanolamine-N-methyltransferase, which is required in the conversion of norepinephrine to epinephrine, is induced by glucocorticoids. The vascular connections between the cortex and medulla, wherein the cortical sinusoids drain into the medullary sinusoids, facilitate this action of the glucocorticoids.

The **paraganglia** are groups of cells found near the thoracic and abdominal sympathetic ganglia that have the same embryologic origin as the cells of the adrenal medulla and also present the **chromaffin reaction.** The chromaffin system consists of the paraganglia and the cells of the adrenal medulla. Chromaffinlike cells are also found in the kidney, ovary, testis, liver, heart, and gastrointestinal tract.

Unlike the cortex, which secretes its products continuously into the bloodstream, cells of the medulla accumulate them and store them in granules. During normal activity, only small quantities are continuously secreted by the medulla. However, epinephrine and norepinephrine are generally secreted in large quantities as a response to intense emotional reactions (eg, fright). The secretion of these substances is mediated by the preganglionic fibers that reach the chromaffin cells of the adrenal medulla. Vasoconstriction, hypertension, changes in heart rate, and metabolic effects such as blood glucose elevation result from secretion of these substances into the bloodstream. These effects are part of the organism's defense reaction to stress.

Adrenal Dysfunction

A common disorder of the adrenal medulla is a tumor of chromaffin cells known as **pheochromocytoma** that causes hyperglycemia and transient elevations of blood pressure.

Disorders of the adrenal gland may be classified as **hyperfunction** or **hypofunction.** Adrenal malfunction may result in undersecretion or oversecretion of only one hormone or of several hormones simultaneously.

Hyperfunction of the adrenal cortex may result in excessive production of glucocorticoids or of aldosterone. Excessive production of sex hormones by adrenal glands causes **adrenogenital syndrome,** which may also occur with an increase of glucocorticoids. This condition is caused by enzymatic abnormalities in the biosynthesis of these hormones.

Hypofunction of the adrenal cortex affects mainly the glucocorticoids and may have 2 causes. The first is due to a fault in the gland itself; the other is due to reduced pituitary secretion of ACTH.

THE ISLETS OF LANGERHANS

The islets of Langerhans constitute the endocrine portion of the pancreas and appear as rounded clusters of cells embedded within exocrine pancreatic tissue.

The islets, which appear to be randomly dispersed throughout the exocrine portion of the pancreas, are apparently more numerous in the tail region of this gland. The number of endocrine cells varies in the islets, and in many instances, individual endocrine cells are interspersed among the pancreatic exocrine cells. Recent evidence reveals that there are 2 types of islets in regard to constituent cells. The differences are related to the fact that the pancreas develops from the fusion of two primordia. Islets in the dorsal primordium are richer in α cells, while the ventral primordium gives rise to glucagon-poor islets.

Each islet consists of polygonal or rounded cells arranged in cords separated by a network of sinusoidlike blood capillaries (Fig 22–9). A fine capsule of reticular fibers surrounds each islet, separating it from the remaining pancreatic tissue. The islets constitute about 1.5% of the total pancreatic volume, and there are about 1–2 million in the human pancreas.

The cells in these islets stain by hematoxylin and eosin less heavily than pancreatic acinar cells. This explains their light appearance when observed with the light microscope.

Using special staining methods, 3 different types of cells—α, β, and δ—have been described in the islets.* The β cells are most numerous and tend to be concentrated in the center of the islet (Fig 22–9); they constitute about 60–80% of the cells found in human pancreatic islets. These cells are small and contain in their cytoplasm granules that stain blue with Gomori's chrome hematoxylin and phloxine technic. The α cells are larger and less numerous (20%), are found usually at the periphery, and are characterized by the presence of secretory granules that stain red with Gomori stain. The least numerous δ cells are small and do not stain heavily.

The ultrastructure of the α, β, and δ cells is that of cells synthesizing polypeptides, for they have a relatively diffuse granular endoplasmic reticulum, free polysomes, Golgi apparatus, and secretory granules (Fig 22–10). These characteristics are typical of the cells from the APUD series studied in Chapter 4. There is much less granular endoplasmic reticulum in these cells than in the acinar cells of the exocrine pancreas. This is in accord with the less intense protein synthesis that occurs in these cells as compared to this activity in the acinar cells. The islets weigh approximately 1 g

*The α, β, and δ cells are sometimes referred to as A, B, and D cells in other texts.

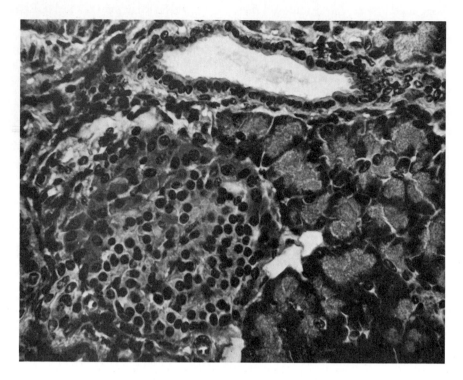

Figure 22 –9. Photomicrograph of a section of the pancreas of a guinea pig. Observe the islet of Langerhans, where the α cells appear mainly in the periphery as large cells with a dark cytoplasm. The remaining cells are mostly β cells. Masson's stain, × 400.

and produce about 2 mg of insulin per day. This amount is about 20% of the weight of all of the protein produced per unit weight by the acinar cells, as determined by administration of radioactive amino acids and quantitation of silver granules that appear over the acinar cells and islet cells in radioautographs.

Fine structural studies reveal significant differences in the appearance of granules in the α and β cells (Fig 22–10). While the morphology of granules in α cells is consistent among species, β cell granule appearance varies among different species.

The rounded β cell secretory granules are membrane-bound and in some species, including humans, composed of one or more dense crystals surrounded by an electron-lucent halo. At high magnification, these crystals have a periodic internal substructure.

The granules of α cells are slightly larger than those of the β cells and consist of a dense central spherical core and an outer halo of low density between the core and the membrane (Fig 22–10).

β Cells are the source of **insulin,** a polypeptide molecule (MW 5734) that produces a decreased blood glucose as a consequence of increased glucose uptake and glycogen synthesis by the liver. α Cells secrete the hormone glucagon, a smaller polypeptide that is antagonistic to insulin and has a glycogenolytic effect of raising blood glucose.

The δ cells also exhibit membrane-bound granules although their contents differ from α and β cells in that they appear as homogeneous granules with moderate to low electron density. A fourth cell type, the C cell, has been described in some species. These cells exhibit no granules and have an organellar-poor cytoplasm. Both δ and C cells have been considered to be morphological variants of the α or β cells.

In addition to insulin and glucagon, some pancreatic cells (probably α and δ) secrete **gastrin,** a hormone that effects acid release by parietal cells in the fundic stomach. The synthesis of excessive gastrin, related to a pancreatic tumor, is the basis for excessive acid secretion in the Zollinger-Ellison syndrome. A peptide that inhibits the release of growth hormone by the adenohypophysis, **somatostatin,** has also been implicated with the pancreatic δ cell.

Insulin is formed as a single polypeptide chain, **proinsulin,** containing 81–86 residues depending on the species. The conversion of proinsulin to insulin occurs by proteolytic cleavage, producing one molecule of insulin and one of C-peptide, and takes place at the time of transport of proinsulin to the Golgi apparatus, or soon after, where it is packaged into granules (Fig 22–11). Since the granules contain insulin and C-peptide in the same amounts, packaging presumably occurs first, followed by

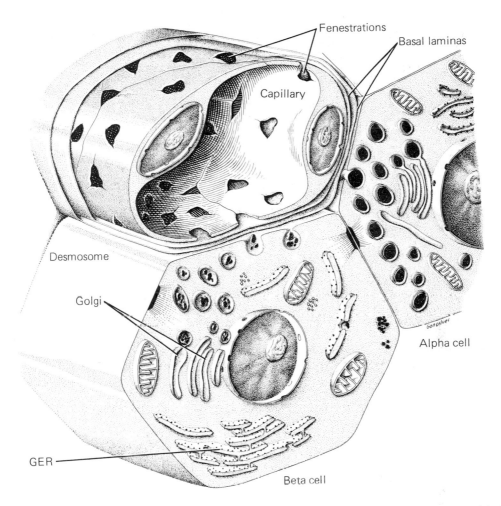

Figure 22–10. Schematic drawing of the α and β cells, showing the morphology of the secretory granules and their relation to blood vessels. The β cell has irregular granules, while the granules are round and uniform in the α cells. GER, granular endoplasmic reticulum.

cleavage. Insulin is stored as a zinc complex. The β cell granules contain lipids and, in some species, monoamines.

The earliest change in the insulin release process, after a stimulus is applied, is margination of the cytoplasmic granules to the plasma membrane of the β cell. Their membranes fuse with plasma membrane of the cell and rupture, and the contents are then liberated into the extracellular space. They then rapidly disappear by a process of dissolution. With the disappearance of the granules, microvilli remain, and they have been shown to increase in number in proportion to the rate of release of the β granules. Evidence has been presented of the existence of microtubules and microfilaments in β cells and of their participation in transport of the secretory granules to the plasma membrane and extrusion of the hormone (Fig 22–11).

Immunofluorescence technics support the view that α cells synthesize and accumulate the hyperglycemia-inducing polypeptide called **glucagon** (MW 3485) (Fig 22–12). A synthetic sequence analogous to that in the β cell occurs in the δ cell—ie, synthesis in the endoplasmic reticulum, transport to the Golgi apparatus, and packaging for release as granules.

The islets have a doubly sensitive regulating mechanism capable of increasing or decreasing blood glucose content. Secretion of the β cells is controlled to a large extent by the level of blood glucose because when an isolated pancreas is perfused with blood rich in glucose, the secretion of insulin is increased.

Terminations of nerve fibers on islet cells can be observed by light or electron microscopy. Both sympathetic and parasympathetic nerve endings have been found in close (synaptic?) association with α, β, and δ cells. These nerves function as part of the insulin and glucagon control system.

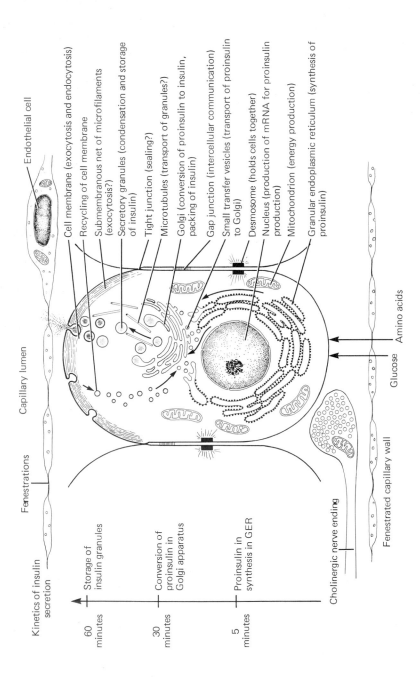

Figure 22–11. The physiology of the β cell of the pancreatic islet. Observe the complex secretory processes, which have been simplified elsewhere in this book for teaching purposes. The process begins with the entrance of blood amino acids into the cell, probably aided by an active amino acid pump present in the cell membrane. The amino acids are polymerized to proinsulin by the polysomes present on the surface of the granular endoplasmic reticulum, and the polypeptide chain is injected through the membrane of the GER into the cisternae. The proinsulin is then transferred to small vesicles by a process of budding that occurs in the cisternae close to the Golgi apparatus. In this region, no polysomes cover the endoplasmic reticulum. The small vesicles are transported by an unknown mechanism and fuse to the Golgi apparatus. In the Golgi apparatus, proinsulin is converted enzymatically by a protease to insulin plus a peptide. This material is then packed into secretory granules by the Golgi apparatus, and the contents gradually condense to form the mature secretory granule. Microtubules may play a role in the transport of these granules to the cell apex. Granule extrusion occurs when the cell membrane fuses with the membrane of the granule and the contents of the granule empty into the extracellular space. In this region, the contents of the granule dissolve and move to a blood vessel. Evidence has been presented suggesting that a submembranous net of microfilaments participates in mechanical support for the extrusion process.

The used granule membrane is incorporated into the cell membrane and is probably recycled by the cell by means of small endocytotic vesicles (upper left). The control of the secretory processes of the β cell is regulated mainly by the blood glucose level and by auxiliary nerve endings. GER, granular endoplasmic reticulum. (Based on data presented by Orci L: Diabetologica 10:163, 1974.)

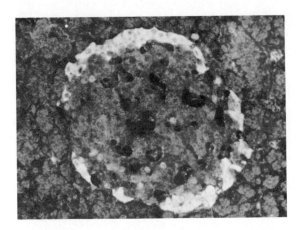

Figure 22–12. Photomicrograph of an immunofluorescent preparation of a rat islet of Langerhans, obtained with anti-glucagon. The glucagon is produced by the α cells located in the periphery of the islet in this species. In this figure, the fluorescent α cells appear light against the dark background. (Courtesy of S Ito.)

THYROID

In early embryonic life, the thyroid is derived from the cephalic portion of the alimentary canal endoderm. Its function is to synthesize the hormones thyroxine and triiodothyronine, which stimulate the metabolic rate.

The thyroid gland is located in the cervical region, in front of the larynx, and consists of 2 lobes united by an isthmus (Fig 22–13). Thyroid tissue is composed of **follicles** consisting of a simple epithelial sphere whose lumen contains a gelatinous substance, the **colloid** (Fig 22–14). In typical sections, follicle cells range from squamous to low columnar cells. Follicles may reach a diameter of 0.9 mm. The gland is covered by a loose connective tissue capsule that sends septa into the parenchyma. These septa become gradually thinner and reach all of the follicles, separating one from another by fine irregular connective tissue composed mainly of reticular fibers. The thyroid is an extremely vascularized organ, presenting an extensive blood and lymphatic capillary network surrounding the follicles. Endothelial cells of these capillaries are fenestrated, as in other endocrine glands. This configuration facilitates the passage of the hormone into the blood capillaries.

Innervation of the thyroid, via the sympathetic and parasympathetic systems, serves an essentially vasomotor function. Recent ultrastructural and radioautographic studies have shown a network of adrenergic fibers terminating near the basal membrane of the follicular cells. These findings, together with evidence that adrenergic and other amines influence thyroid iodine metabolism in isolated thyroid cells and in vivo, indicate that the

neurogenic stimuli can influence thyroid function through a direct effect on the epithelial cells. However, in many respects, thyroid-stimulating hormone (TSH; thyrotropin), which is secreted by the anterior pituitary, can be considered to be the major regulator of the anatomic and functional state of the thyroid gland.

The morphologic aspect of the thyroid follicles varies (polymorphism) according to the region of the gland and its functional activity. Thus, in the same gland, larger follicles full of colloid and having a cuboidal or squamous epithelium are found alongside smaller ones lined by prismatic epithelium. In spite of this variation, when the average composition of these follicles is squamous, the gland is considered hypoactive. When drugs capable of stimulating the synthesis of thyroid hormone are administered, a marked increase in the height of the follicular epithelium is observed. This phenomenon is accompanied by a decrease in quantity of the colloid and size of the follicles (Fig 22–14).

The thyroid epithelium always rests on a basal lamina. The ultrastructure of the follicular epithelium presents all of the characteristics of a cell which at the same time synthesizes, secretes, reabsorbs, and digests proteins. The basal part of these cells is rich in granular endoplasmic reticulum. The nucleus is generally round and situated in the center of the cell. The apical pole presents a discrete

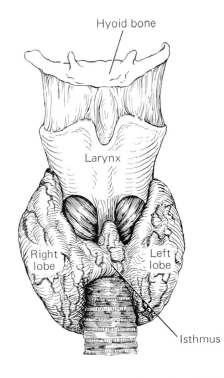

Figure 22–13. The human thyroid. (Reproduced, with permission, from Ganong WF: *Review of Medical Physiology,* 9th ed. Lange, 1979.)

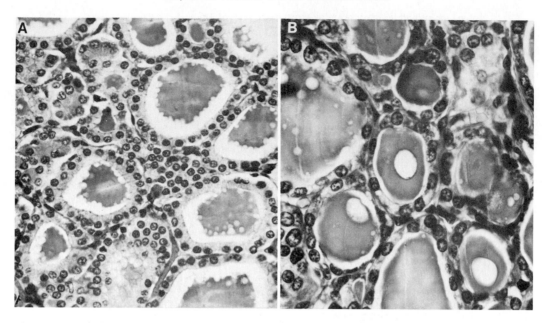

Figure 22 – 14. Photomicrographs of sections of thyroid glands. The higher epithelial cells and the vesicular aspect of the colloid strongly indicate that the section on the left is from a more active gland. H&E stain, × 200 *(A)* and 400 *(B)*.

Golgi apparatus and secretory granules with the staining characteristics of follicular colloid. Abundant lysosomes, 0.5–0.6 μm in diameter, and some (usually) large phagosomes containing a clear fluid are found in this region. The cell membrane of the apical pole contains a moderate number of microvilli. Mitochondria, distended cisternae of rough endoplasmic reticulum, and ribosomes are dispersed throughout the cytoplasm.

Small isolated clusters of light cells are frequently found between the thyroid follicles. These are **parafollicular cells** or **C cells (clear cells)** (Fig 22–15). These cells, which are functionally equivalent to APUD cells (described in Chapter 4), stain

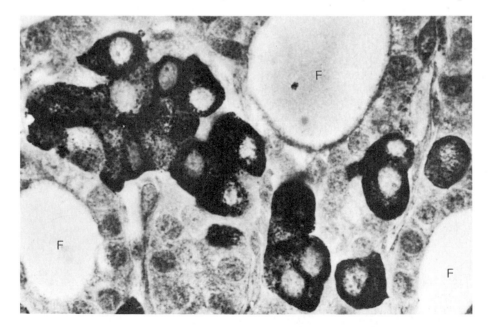

Figure 22 –15. Photomicrograph of a dog's thyroid showing its parafollicular cells. F indicates the follicular lumen. Silver impregnation. In this preparation, the aspect observed is the reverse of what is seen in a hematoxylin-eosin –stained slide, for the clear or parafollicular cells appear black against a light background owing to the silver precipitate. × 800. (Courtesy of F Kameda.)

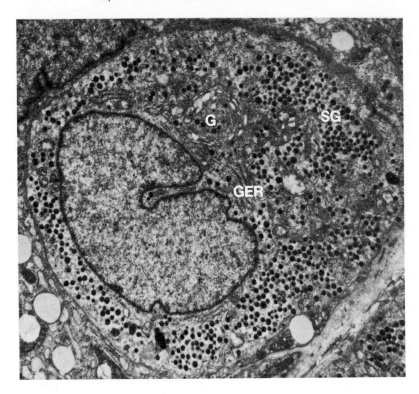

Figure 22 –16. Electron micrograph of a calcitonin-producing cell. Observe the small secretory granules (SG) and the scarcity of granular endoplasmic reticulum (GER). G, Golgi region. × 5000.

palely, although silver impregnation technics intensely stain their catecholamine-containing secretion granules. These cells are responsible for the synthesis and secretion of the hormone **calcitonin**, a polypeptide consisting of 32 amino acids that promotes a reduction in the concentration of calcium in the blood, primarily by inhibiting bone resorption. The following observations support this statement: (1) cytologic alterations of the parafollicular cells occur when experimental hypercalcemia is induced, and (2) there is selective binding of a fluorescent antibody (anticalcitonin) to the parafollicular cells.

The C cells have the characteristics of the polypeptide-secreting cells and their ultrastructure is illustrated in Fig 22–16. Regulation of the secretion of these cells depends exclusively on the calcium blood level and is independent of thyroid, parathyroid, and pituitary functions. In humans, calcitonin is found also in the thymus.

Histophysiology

The thyroid is the only endocrine gland whose secretory product is stored in great quantity. This accumulation is unusual in that it occurs in the extracellular colloid. In humans, there is sufficient hormone within the follicles to supply the organism for up to 10 months. Thyroid colloid is composed mainly of a glycoprotein (thyroglobulin) of high molecular weight (680,000). The staining affinity of

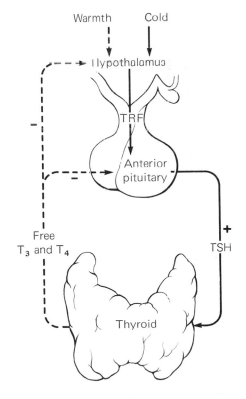

Figure 22 –17. Regulation of TSH secretion. Solid arrows indicate stimulation; dashed arrows, inhibition.

the follicular colloid varies greatly; it may be either acidophilic or basophilic. When the colloid is strongly basophilic, the follicle containing it is in a stage of intense metabolic activity—as opposed to follicles containing acidophilic colloid. In active follicles, following fixation and staining, the colloid appears irregular and vesiculated in the portion alongside the follicular cells. This is due to ingestion of thyroglobulin by these cells.

The activity of the follicular cells of the thyroid is controlled by the circulating level of thyrotropin, which acts via cAMP of the cells. A rise in the circulating free thyroid hormones in turn inhibits the synthesis of thyrotropin, and when the thyroid hormone level drops the secretion of TSH by the adenohypophysis is stimulated, establishing in this way a homeostatic balance that maintains an adequate quantity of thyroxine and triiodothyronine within the organism. TSH secretion is also increased by exposure to cold in animals and humans and is depressed by heat and stressful stimuli. The negative feedback effect of thyroid hormones on TSH secretion may be exerted in part at the hypothalamus but to a greater extent upon the anterior pituitary. A tripeptide has been isolated from the hypothalamus (thyrotropin-releasing factor, TRF) that stimulates TSH secretion (Fig 22–17). The level of iodine also controls thyroid function. High concentrations of intrathyroidal iodine inhibit the rate of release of thyroidal iodine. In addition, the magnitude of the organic iodine pool inversely affects the iodide transport mechanism and the response to TSH.

Synthesis & Accumulation of Hormones by the Follicular Cells

This process takes place in 4 stages, as follows: synthesis of thyroglobulin, uptake of iodide from the blood, activation of the iodide, and iodination of the tyrosyl radicals of thyroglobulin.

These stages are exemplified in Fig 22–18. They take place in the following manner:

(1) The **synthesis of thyroglobulin** occurs in a manner typical of other protein exporters (described in Chapter 4). This process has been studied by means of radioautographic technics with the use

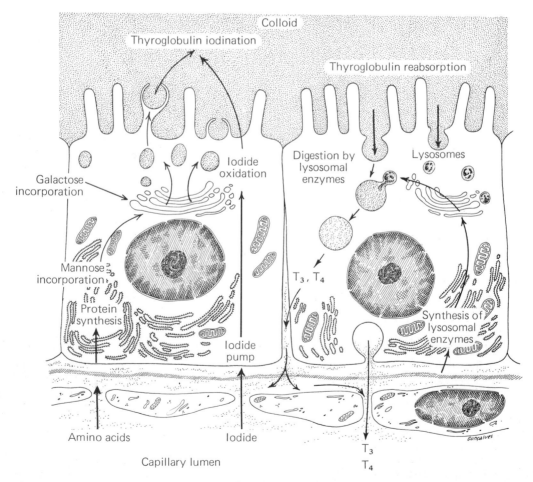

Figure 22–18. Diagram showing the processes of synthesis and iodination of thyroglobulin *(left)* and its reabsorption and digestion *(right)*. These events occur in the same cell.

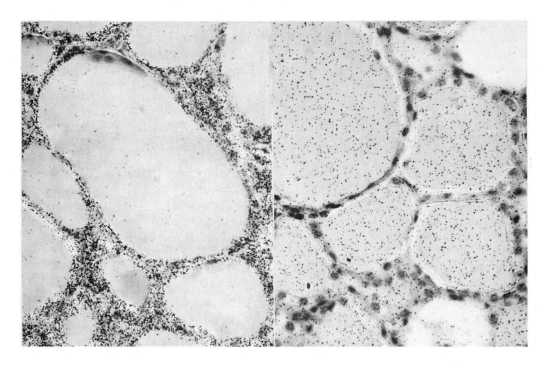

Figure 22 –19. Radioautographs of the thyroid glands of rats previously injected with radioactive leucine. ***Left:*** The tracer was injected 30 minutes before the animal was killed. Observe the radioactivity (dark dots) concentrated mainly over the cells. ***Right:*** The amino acid was injected 45 days before the animal was killed, and all radioactivity is in the colloid (thyroglobulin). × 385.

of tritiated leucine, an amino acid abundant in thyroglobulin (Fig 22–19). Briefly, the secretory pathway is as follows: synthesis of protein in the endoplasmic reticulum, addition of polysaccharide in the endoplasmic reticulum and the Golgi apparatus, and release from formed vesicles at the apical surface of the cell into the follicles.

Radioautographic studies performed with the electron microscope show that the synthesis of the carbohydrate fraction of thyroglobulin occurs both in the endoplasmic reticulum and the Golgi apparatus. Mannose is incorporated within the endoplasmic reticulum, whereas galactose is added to thyroglobulin at the Golgi apparatus.

(2) The **uptake of circulating iodide** is accomplished in the thyroid by a mechanism of active transport, utilizing the iodide pump, located next to or on the cytoplasmic membrane of the basal region of the follicular cells. This pump also exists in other organs—the salivary and mammary glands, the stomach, etc—although in these places, the synthesis of thyroid hormone does not occur. This pump is readily stimulated by thyrotropin. The uptake of iodide can be inhibited by certain drugs such as perchlorate and thiocyanate, which act by competing with iodide. Another case in which the uptake of iodide is prevented is known to be a genetically determined disease in which the iodide pump does not function. In these cases, the same deficiency is observed in the other organs that have

an active iodide transport.

(3) During the phase of **oxidation of iodide**, iodide is transformed into iodine, which in turn combines in the colloid with the tyrosyl radicals of thyroglobulin. An enzyme, peroxidase, which has been identified in the thyroid by biochemical and histochemical methods, is responsible for the oxidation of iodide inside the follicular cells. This process can be blocked by drugs (eg, propylthiouracil and carbimazole) that inactivate the peroxidase. It is now agreed that the main function of these compounds is to inhibit the coupling of iodotyrosines into T_3 or T_4 and that the influence on the formation of monoiodotyrosine (MIT) and diiodotyrosine (DIT) is secondary. Thyroid dysfunction may also occur as a result of a genetically determined deficiency of peroxidase.

(4) In contrast to the processes described above, **iodination of the tyrosyl radicals** bound to thyroglobulin takes place not inside the follicular cells but in the portion of colloid in contact with the membrane of the apical region of the cells. This process has been extensively studied by means of radioautography using [125]I (Fig 22–19). Initially, a monoiodine compound, MIT, is formed, followed by the production of the diiodine compound, DIT. Two diiodotyrosine molecules are then united, releasing an amino acid, alanine, and forming the tetraiodine compound tetraiodothyronine (T_4), also known as thyroxine, which is the main thyroid hor-

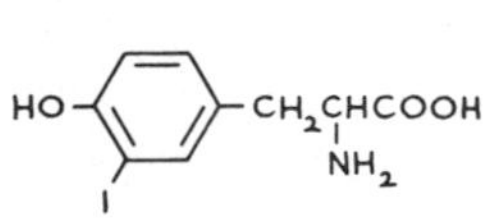

HO—⟨⟩—CH$_2$CHCOOH | NH$_2$

3-Monoiodotyrosine (MIT)

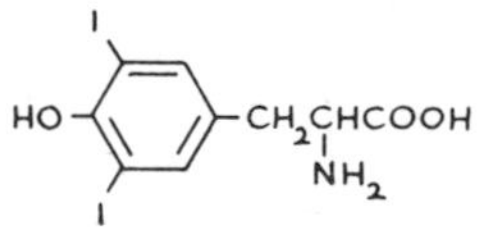

HO—⟨⟩—CH$_2$CHCOOH | NH$_2$

3,5-Diiodotyrosine (DIT)

HO—⟨⟩—O—⟨⟩—CH$_2$CHCOOH | NH$_2$

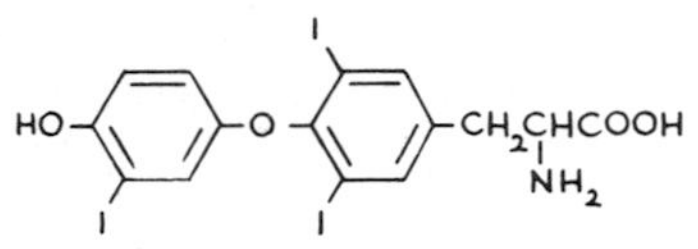

3,5,3'-Triiodothyronine (T$_3$)

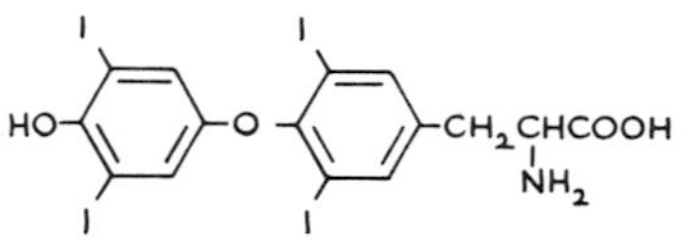

HO—⟨⟩—O—⟨⟩—CH$_2$CHCOOH | NH$_2$

3,5,3',5'-Tetraiodothyronine
(T$_4$, thyroxine)

Figure 22–20. Formulas of 3-monoiodotyrosine (MIT) and 3,5-diiodotyrosine (DIT). The condensation of 2 molecules of DIT with the elimination of an alanine residue results in the formation of tetraiodothyronine (T$_4$; thyroxine). The condensation of one molecule of MIT and one molecule of DIT with the elimination of one alanine residue results in the formation of triiodothyronine (T$_3$).

mone. Another hormone produced, although on a much smaller scale, is triiodothyronine (T$_3$), probably by condensation of monoiodotyrosine with diiodotyrosine. (See Fig 22–20.) The condensation reaction is an aerobic, energy-requiring one. It is postulated that the union of the iodinated tyrosines is catalyzed by an enzymatic mechanism. For this process to occur normally, thyroglobulin must present the correct spatial configuration. When disease causes the production of abnormal thyroglobulin, this process is blocked, resulting in deficient synthesis of thyroid hormone.

Liberation of T$_3$ & T$_4$

The thyroid hormones remain in the inactive bound form with thyroglobulin until secreted. Although some believed that proteases were secreted into the colloid, most of the evidence now supports the hypothesis that the thyroid cells ingest the colloid by pinocytosis, where the colloid merges with lysosomes. It has been shown that the injection of TSH promotes the appearance of abundant lamellapodia on the surface of thyroid cells, which precedes the increased uptake of colloid by these cells. The peptide bonds between the iodinated residues and the thyroglobulin are broken by the proteases in the lysosomes, and thyroxine, triiodothyronine, diiodotyrosine, and monoiodotyrosine are liberated into the cytoplasm. The free thyroxine and triiodothyronine then cross the cell membrane and are discharged into the capillaries. Tetraiodothyronine (thyroxine) is the most abundant of these compounds, constituting 90% of the circulating thyroid hormone, although T$_3$ acts more rapidly and is more potent than T$_4$. In humans, 80 μg/d of free T$_4$ and 50 μg/d of T$_3$ are secreted by the thyroid cells into the capillaries.

Apparently, the contents of some of the vesicles containing thyroglobulin are not digested, for this protein occurs normally in the lymph that drains from the thyroid.

Thyroxine stimulates mitochondrial respiration and oxidative phosphorylation. Since this effect is blocked by actinomycin D, it is consequently dependent on RNA synthesis.

T$_3$ and T$_4$ increase both the number of mitochondria and the number of their cristae. Mitochondrial protein synthesis is increased, while degradation of their proteins is decreased in those tissues studied.

Most of the effects of thyroid hormones are secondary to calorigenic action, although they influence body growth and the development of the nervous system during fetal life; increase the absorption of carbohydrates from the intestine; and help to regulate lipid metabolism. Monoiodotyrosine and diiodotyrosine are not secreted into the blood since their iodine is removed as a result of the intracellular action of **iodotyrosine dehalogenase.** The products of this enzymatic reaction, iodine and tyrosine, are probably reused by the follicular cells.

Factors That Affect the Synthesis of Thyroid Hormone

A diet that contains less than 10 μg/d of iodine hinders the synthesis of thyroid hormones. Thyroid hypertrophy as a result of increased TSH secretion causes the disorder known as **iodine deficiency goiter,** which occurs widely in some regions of the world.

The syndrome of adult hypothyroidism is called **myxedema** and may be the result of a number of diseases of the thyroid gland or may be secondary to pituitary or hypothalamic failure. Children who are hypothyroid from birth are called **cretins.**

Hyperthyroidism or thyrotoxicosis may be caused by a variety of thyroid diseases, but the most common form is **Graves' disease** or **exophthalmic goiter.** The levels of TSH are subnormal, and the thyroid hyperfunction in this disease is due to a circulating gamma globulin which exerts effects resembling those of TSH.

THE PARATHYROID GLANDS

The parathyroids are 3 or more (often 4) small glands—3×6 mm—with a total weight of less than 0.2 g. They are situated behind the thyroid gland, one at each end of the upper and lower poles, usually in the capsule that covers the lobes of the thyroid (Fig 22–21). Sometimes they are found embedded in the thyroid gland. They may be found in the mediastinum, lying beside the thymus since the parathyroid glands and the thymus originate from the closely contiguous pharyngeal pouch.

The parathyroid glands are derived from pharyngeal pouches—the superior glands from the fourth pouch and the inferior glands from the third.

Histology

Each parathyroid gland is contained within a connective tissue capsule. These capsules send septa to the inside of the gland, where they merge with the reticular fibers supporting elongated cordlike clusters of secretory cells.

The parenchyma of the parathyroid glands consists of 2 types of cells: the chief or principal cells and the oxyphil cells (Fig 22–22). In hyperplasia, however, a third cell type, the water clear cell, is also seen. Adipose tissue cells are frequently found inside the human parathyroid gland.

The **chief cells** are the most numerous. In most mammals, they are the only cells found in the

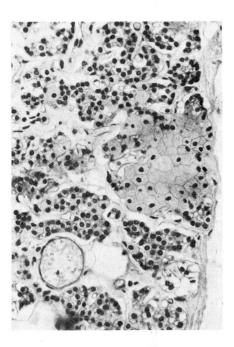

Figure 22–22. Photomicrograph of a section of the parathyroid gland. Observe a group of large, acidophilic, oxyphil cells at the middle right portion. (Courtesy of J James.)

parathyroid gland. They are polygonal, with a vesicular nucleus and a pale-staining, slightly acidophilic cytoplasm. Electron microscopy shows irregularly shaped granules 200–400 nm in diameter in the cytoplasm of the chief cells. They are believed to be secretory granules containing parathyroid hormone, which in the active form is a polypeptide with a molecular weight of 9500. These granules, the number of which varies from one cell to another, are distributed throughout the cytoplasm, but sometimes they are more numerous at the vascular pole of the cell. A prominent Golgi apparatus is situated adjacent to the nucleus. Granular endoplasmic reticulum and free ribosomes are found. Small ovoid or spherical mitochondria and lipofuscin pigment bodies are also evident. Masses of glycogen granules occur and are especially large in resting or inactive chief cells.

In humans, the **oxyphil cells** begin to appear at about age 7 and increase in number with age. They too are polygonal in shape, but they are larger than chief cells and their cytoplasm contains many acidophilic granules. The electron microscope reveals that these granules are mitochondria with abundant cristae. The function and importance of such a large concentration of mitochondria in these cells are unknown (Fig 22–22).

Cells with structural characteristics intermediate between chief and oxyphil cells are also seen, suggesting that they are transitions of a single cell type. With increasing age, replacement of se-

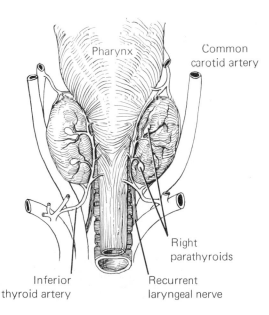

Figure 22–21. The human parathyroid glands, viewed from behind. (Redrawn and reproduced, with permission, from Nordland: The larynx as related to surgery of the thyroid based on an anatomical study. Surg Gynecol Obstet 51:449, 1930; and from *Gray's Anatomy of the Human Body,* 29th ed. Goss CM [editor]. Lea & Febiger, 1973.)

cretory cells by adipocytes occurs. Adipose can constitute over 50% of the gland in older individuals.

Histophysiology

Parathyroid glands are essential for life. They secrete parathyroid hormone, which controls the concentration of calcium and phosphate ions in the blood. A plasma calcium level of about 10 mg/dL is normal. If calcium levels are lowered, neuromuscular transmission is severely affected.

Decrease in blood calcium stimulates the parathyroid gland to secrete its hormone. Magnesium appears to have a similar direct effect. In turn, parathyroid hormone acts on the cells of bone tissue, increasing the number of osteoclasts and promoting in this way the absorption of the calcified bone matrix and the release of calcium into the blood. Increase in the concentration of calcium in the blood probably suppresses the production of this hormone. Calcitonin also influences the osteoclasts by inhibiting their resorptive action on bone and liberation of calcium; thus calcitonin lowers blood calcium and increases osteogenesis.

In addition to increasing the concentration of calcium, parathyroid hormone reduces the concentration of phosphate in the blood. This effect is a consequence of an increase in the excretion of phosphate in urine. Parathyroid hormone diminishes the absorption of phosphate from the glomerular filtrate at the level of the kidney tubules. There is also strong evidence that parathyroid hormone increases absorption of calcium from the gastrointestinal tract and that vitamin D is necessary for this effect. The actions of parathyroid hormone involve activation of adenylate cyclase, with consequent increased formation of cAMP in the affected cells.

In hyperparathyroidism, blood phosphate is low and blood calcium is increased. This frequently promotes a pathologic deposit of calcium in several organs such as the kidneys and arteries. Bones are decalcified and become subject to fractures. The bone disease caused by hyperparathyroidism is characterized by multiple bone cysts and is known as **osteitis fibrosa cystica.**

Hypoparathyroidism causes an increase in the concentration of phosphate and a decrease in the concentration of calcium in the blood. The bones become denser and more mineralized. This condition causes spastic contractions of the skeletal muscles and generalized convulsions (also called tetany). These symptoms are due to the exaggerated excitability of the nervous system caused by the lack of calcium ions in the blood. The endogenous administration of calcium or of parathyroid hormone terminates the convulsions—the former much more rapidly.

The secretion of the parathyroid cells is regulated by the blood calcium level and apparently is not directly affected by other endocrine glands or the nervous system.

THE PINEAL BODY

The pineal body is also known as the epiphysis or pineal gland. In the adult, it is a flattened, cone-shaped organ measuring approximately 5–8 mm in length and 3–5 mm in its greatest width and weighing about 120 mg. It is found in the posterior extremity of the third ventricle, above the roof of the diencephalon, to which it is connected by means of a short stalk.

The pineal is covered by pia mater. Connective tissue septa containing blood vessels and unmyelinated nerve fibers originate in the pia mater and enter the pineal tissue to surround, along with blood capillaries, the cellular cords and follicles, forming irregular lobules.

The pineal body consists of several types of cells but principally **pinealocytes** and interstitial cells. Pinealocytes have a slightly basophilic cytoplasm with large irregular or lobate nuclei and sharply defined nucleoli. They are also known as cells of the pineal parenchyma. When impregnated with silver salts (Del Rio Hortega's method), the pinealocytes appear to have long and tortuous branches reaching out to the vascular connective tissue septa where they end as flattened dilatations. The pineal itself is surrounded by cerebrospinal fluid. The cytoplasm of the pinealocytes contains a great number of free ribosomes and a small amount of granular endoplasmic reticulum. The Golgi apparatus and the mitochondria are poorly developed. In addition, one also finds lipid droplets and structures similar to lysosomes. Two distinctive features of the cytoplasm are the presence of large numbers of microtubules and an extensive smooth endoplasmic reticulum.

The **interstitial cells** of the pineal body are a specific type of cell characterized by elongated nuclei which stain more heavily than those of parenchymal cells. They are observed between the cords

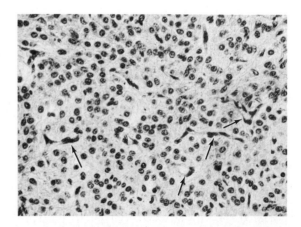

Figure 22–23. Section of a pineal gland. The arrows indicate blood vessels that surround the cellular cords.

of pinealocytes and perivascular areas. These cells have long cytoplasmic processes containing a large number of fine filaments 5–6 nm in diameter and of moderate length. Interstitial cells resemble the fine structure of astrocytes and may be a type of glial cell.

In addition to the above-mentioned cell types, cells frequently encountered in the pineal body are the glia and mast cells. Mast cells are probably responsible for the high histamine content of this organ.

Age causes an increase in the amount of connective tissue in the pineal body and the formation of calcified bodies (**brain sand**) in the parenchyma of this organ. These calcified bodies are used as a reference point in skull radiology for they appear clearly in x-rays.

Innervation

Silver impregnation reveals nerve fibers throughout the pineal body. When these nerve fibers penetrate the organ, they lose their myelin sheath, the unmyelinated axons ending among pinealocytes (Fig 22–24), and some actually form synapses. A great number of small vesicles 40 nm in diameter containing norepinephrine are observed in these nerve endings. Serotonin is present also, both in the pinealocytes and in sympathetic nerve terminals. The pineal body is mainly innervated by postganglionic sympathetic fibers derived from the superior cervical sympathetic ganglion. In primates, there are also parasympathetic fibers.

Histophysiology

In spite of the great quantity of research on the pineal gland, its role as an endocrine gland is still a subject of controversy. It is thought to be capable of participating in some endocrine functions.

The pineal has been claimed at one time or another to be a source of (1) a gonadotropin-releasing hormone; (2) a gonadotropin-inhibiting principle having a structure similar to that of arginine vasotocin; (3) a growth-inhibiting factor; (4) a thyrotropin-releasing hormone; (5) a substance that inhibits the onset of puberty; (6) melatonin, which may inhibit gonadotropin release, and causes lightening of the skin; and (7) factors that antagonize the secretion of ACTH and regulate the secretion of aldosterone.

The hypothesis that has received the widest acceptance is that the pineal acts on the gonads. Whether it secretes hormones into the blood, the cerebrospinal fluid, or both has not been clearly determined.

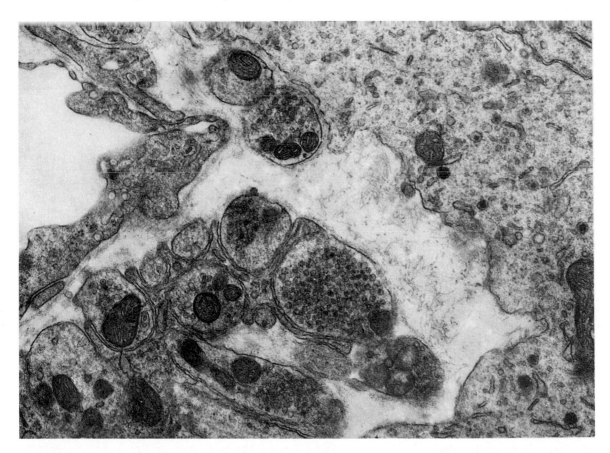

Figure 22 –24. Electron micrograph of adrenergic nerve endings in the pineal body. × 32,000. (Courtesy of S Matsushima.)

Melatonin

Melatonin is an indolic compound, isolated from the pineal body of mammals, that induces the aggregation of pigment granules in the melanophores of amphibia. This substance, synthesized only in the pineal, has a 100,000 times stronger effect on melanophores than norepinephrine, which has a similar effect. From this organ has been isolated an enzyme called hydroxyindole-O-methyltransferase, which is capable of methylating N-acetyl-5-hydroxytryptamine and transforming it into melatonin.

The quantity of melatonin and serotonin in the pineal body of rats and humans undergoes diurnal rhythmicity according to the alternations of light and dark periods. A diminished activity of hydroxyindole-O-methyltransferase and a consequent inhibition of melatonin synthesis are observed if the rats are maintained in constant illumination.

The first evidence that the pineal body might affect the function of the gonads was the observation that an individual suffering from a destructive tumor of this organ developed precocious puberty and hypertrophy of the gonads. However, the precise role of this organ remains an open question. The mammalian pinealocytes are neuroendocrine transducers since they respond to a neurotransmitter (ie, norepinephrine) released from their sympathetic neurons by synthesizing a group of biologically active compounds that modify the function of different endocrine organs.

●   ●   ●

References

Adrenal Gland

Christy NP (editor): *The Human Adrenal Cortex.* Harper & Row, 1971.

Eisenstein AB: *The Adrenal Cortex.* Little, Brown, 1967.

Ganong WF: *Review of Medical Physiology,* 9th ed. Lange, 1979.

Giacomelli F, Wiener J, Spiro D: Cytological alterations related to stimulation of the zona glomerulosa of the adrenal gland. J Cell Biol 26:499, 1965.

Mortimore GE: The adrenal medulla. In: *Best and Taylor's Physiological Basis of Medical Practice,* 9th ed. Brobeck JR & others (editors). Williams & Wilkins, 1973.

Rhodin JAG: The ultrastructure of the adrenal cortex of the rat under normal and experimental conditions. J Ultrastruct Res 34:23, 1971.

Islets of Langerhans

Baetens D & others: Endocrine pancreas: Three-dimensional reconstruction shows two types of Islets of Langerhans. Science 206:1323, 1979.

Caramia F, Munger BL, Lacy PE: The ultrastructural basis for the identification of cell types in the pancreatic islets. 1. Guinea pig. Z Zellforsch Mikrosk Anat 67:533, 1965.

Falkner S, Hellman B, Taljedal IB: *The Structure and Metabolism of the Pancreatic Islets.* Pergamon Press, 1970.

Ganong WF: *Review of Medical Physiology,* 9th ed. Lange, 1979.

Gomez-Acebo J, Parilla R, Candela JLR: Fine structure of the A and D cells of the rabbit endocrine pancreas in vivo and incubated in vitro. 1. Mechanism of secretion of the A cells. J Cell Biol 36:33, 1968.

Ichikawa A: Fine structural changes in response to hormonal stimulation of the perfused canine pancreas. J Cell Biol 24:369, 1965.

Like AA: The ultrastructure of the islets of Langerhans in man. Lab Invest 16:937, 1967.

Munger BL, Caramia F, Lacy PE: The ultrastructural basis for the identification of cell types in the pancreatic

islets. 2. Rabbit, dog and opossum. Z Zellforsch Mikrosk Anat 67:776, 1965.

Thyroid Gland

Anast CS: Thyrocalcitonin: A review. Clin Orthop 47:179, 1966.

Bradley AS, Wissig SL: The anatomy of secretion in the follicular cell of the thyroid gland. 3. The acute effect in vivo of thyrotropic hormone on amino acid uptake and incorporation into protein by the mouse thyroid gland. J Cell Biol 30:433, 1966.

Bussolati G, Pearse AGE: Immunofluorescence localization of calcitonin in the C cells of pig and dog's thyroid. J Endocrinol 37:205, 1967.

Dumont E: The action of thyrotropin on thyroid metabolism. Vitam Horm 29:289, 1971.

Fujita H: Fine structure of the thyroid cell. Int Rev Cytol 40:197, 1975.

Haddad A & others: Radioautographic study of in vivo and in vitro incorporation of fucose-^{3}H into thyroglobulin by rat thyroid follicular cells. J Cell Biol 49:856, 1971.

Heimann P: Ultrastructure of the human thyroid: A study of normal thyroid, untreated and treated toxic goiter. Acta Endocrinol 53 (Suppl 110):5, 1966.

Ibrahim MS, Budd GC: An electron microscopic study of the site of iodine binding in the rat thyroid gland. Exp Cell Res 38:50, 1965.

Klinck GH, Oertel JE, Winship I: Ultrastructure of normal human thyroid. Lab Invest 22:2, 1970.

Nunez EA, Gershon MD: Cytophysiology of thyroid parafollicular cells. Int Rev Cytol 52:1, 1978.

Sterling K, Lazarus JH: The thyroid and its control. Annu Rev Physiol 39:349, 1977.

Strum JM, Karnowsky MJ: Cytochemical localization of endogenous peroxidase in the thyroid follicular cells. J Cell Biol 44:655, 1970.

Wetzel BK, Spicer SS, Wollman SH: Changes in fine structure and acid phosphatase localization in rat thyroid cells following thyrotrophin administration. J Cell Biol 25:593, 1965.

Whur P, Herscovics A, Leblond CP: Radioautographic

visualization of the incorporation of galactose-^{3}H and mannose-^{3}H by rat thyroid in vitro in relation to the stages of thyroglobulin synthesis. J Cell Biol 43:289, 1969.

Parathyroid Gland

Gaillard PJ, Talmage RV, Budy AM (editors): *The Parathyroid Glands.* Univ of Chicago Press, 1965.

Gray JK, Cooper CW, Munson PL: Parathyroid hormone. Thyrocalcitonin and the control of mineral metabolism. In: *Endocrine Physiology.* McCann SM (editor). Butterworth, 1974.

Mecca CE, Martin GP, Goldhaber P: Alterations of bone metabolism in tissue culture in response to parathyroid extract. Proc Soc Exp Biol Med 113:538, 1963.

Tremblay G, Cartier GE: Histochemical study of oxidative enzymes in the human parathyroid. Endocrinology 60:658, 1961.

Wong ET, Lindall AW: Subcellular location of human parathyroid hormone immunoreactive peptides and preliminary evidence for a precursor to human PTH. Proc Soc Exp Biol Med 148:387, 1975.

Pineal Body

Altschule MD (editor): *Frontiers of Pineal Physiology,* MIT Press, 1975.

Pelham RW & others: Twenty-four hour cycle of melatonin-like substance in the plasma of human males. J Clin Endocrinol Metab 37:341, 1973.

Reiter RJ: Comparative physiology: Pineal gland. Annu Rev Physiol 35:305, 1973.

Tapp E, Huxley M: The histological appearance of the human pineal gland from puberty to old age. J Pathol 108:137, 1972.

23 | The Male Reproductive System

The male reproductive system is composed of the testes, genital ducts, accessory glands, and penis. The **testis** is a compound tubular gland which has 2 functions—reproductive and hormonal. It is surrounded by a thick, resistant capsule of collagenous connective tissue, the **tunica albuginea.** The tunica albuginea has a thickening in its posterior region, the **mediastinum testis,** from which fibrous septa project into the gland, dividing it into about 250 pyramidal compartments called the **testicular lobules** (Fig 23–1). These septa are not complete, and intercommunications frequently exist between the lobules. Each lobule is occupied by 1–4 seminiferous tubules immersed in a web of

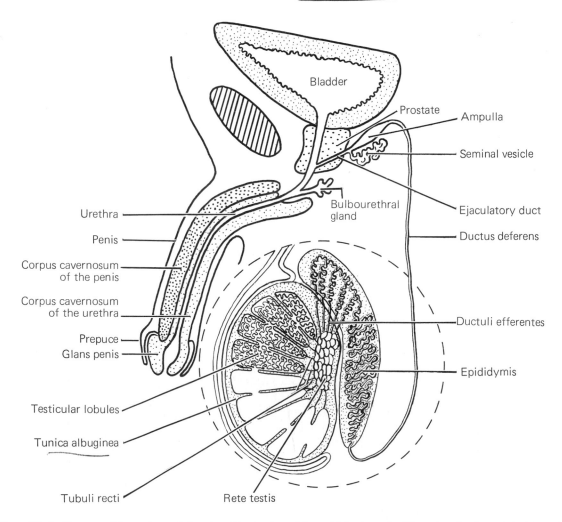

Figure 23 –1. Diagram of the male genital system. The testis and the epididymis are in different scales from the other parts of the reproductive system. Observe the communication between the testicular lobules.

loose connective tissue rich in vessels and nerves (Fig 23–1).

The testes develop in the dorsal wall of the peritoneal cavity and later are suspended in the scrotum outside the abdominal cavity at the ends of the spermatic cords, each carrying with it a serous sac derived from the peritoneum called the **tunica vaginalis.** This tunic consists of an outer parietal and an inner visceral layer, covering the tunica albuginea on the anterior and lateral sides of the testis. The scrotal sacs have an important role in maintaining the testicles at a temperature below intra-abdominal temperature.

Seminiferous Tubules

Seminiferous tubules, lined with a complex stratified epithelium, are about 150–250 μm in diameter and 30–70 cm long. The convoluted tubules form a network, wherein individual tubules are either blind-ended or branched. At the apical termination of each tubule, the lumen narrows and the epithelial lining abruptly changes into a simple cuboidal layer the cells of which possess a single flagellum. These short segments, known as **straight tubules** or **tubuli recti,** connect the seminiferous tubules to an anastomosing labyrinth of epithelial-lined channels, the **rete testis.** The rete, present in the connective tissue of the mediastinum, is connected to the cephalic portion of the **epididymis** by from 10 to 20 **ductuli efferentes** (Fig 23–1).

The seminiferous tubules consist of the following components (Figs 23–2 and 23–3): (1) a tunic of fibrous connective tissue; (2) a well-defined basal lamina; and (3) a complex **germinal** or **seminiferous epithelium.**

The fibrous **tunica propria** enveloping the seminiferous tubule consists of several layers of fibroblasts. The innermost layer adhering to the connective tissue side of the basal lamina consists of squamous epitheliumlike **myoid cells,** which exhibit smooth muscle characteristics.

The epithelium consists of 2 types of cells: **Sertoli** or **supporting cells** and cells that constitute the **spermatogenic** or **seminal lineage.** The cells of spermatogenic lineage are stacked in 4–8 layers that occupy the space between the basal membrane and the lumen of the tubule. These cells reproduce several times and finally differentiate, producing spermatozoa. They represent various stages in the continuous process of differentiation of the male primitive germ cells. This phenomenon from start to finish is called **spermatogenesis** and can be divided into 3 phases: (1) **spermatocytogenesis,** during which spermatogonia divide, producing successive generations of cells that finally give rise to **spermatocytes;** (2) **meiosis,** during which the spermatocyte goes through 2 successive divisions, with reduction by half of the number of chromosomes and amount of DNA per cell, producing **spermatids;** and (3) **spermiogenesis,** during which the spermatids go through an elaborate process of cytodifferentiation, producing **spermatozoa.**

The process of spermatogenesis begins with a primitive germ cell, the **spermatogonium,** situated next to the basal lamina. It is a relatively small cell, and its nucleus contains irregular chromatin, forming rough clusters (Fig 23–3). At sexual maturity, this cell undergoes a series of successive mitoses, and the newly formed cells can follow one of 2 paths: they can continue, after one or more mitotic divisions, in the same way as the mother cell (the

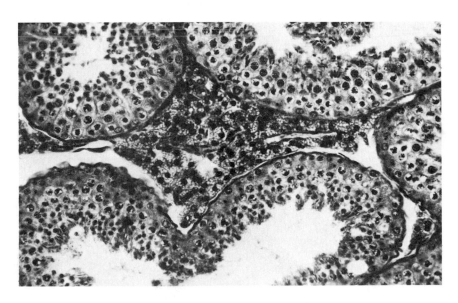

Figure 23–2. Photomicrograph of the testis of a monkey. The interstitial cells in the middle of the field present vacuoles resulting from the dissolution of lipid droplets during preparation. H&E stain, × 400.

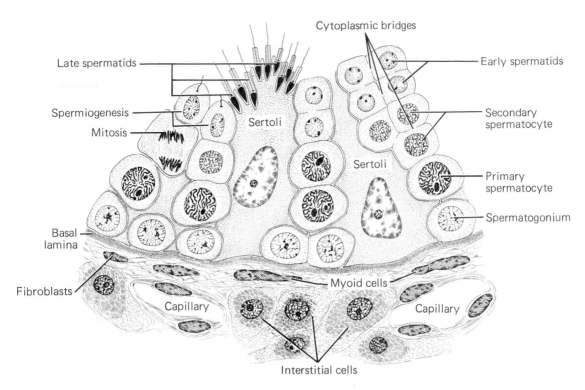

Late spermatids

Spermiogenesis

Mitosis

Basal lamina

Fibroblasts

Cytoplasmic bridges

Early spermatids

Sertoli

Sertoli

Secondary spermatocyte

Primary spermatocyte

Spermatogonium

Myoid cells

Capillary

Capillary

Interstitial cells

Figure 23 –3. Diagram of the structure of a part of a seminiferous tubule and interstitial tissue. This figure does not show the lymphatic vessels frequently found in the connective tissue.

spermatogonium), and thus **spermatogonia A** cells become a continuous source of spermatogonia; or they can divide and grow, thus becoming larger than the mother spermatogonium, in which case they are called **spermatogonia B.** The spermatogonia B give rise to the **primary spermatocytes.** Soon after their formation, they enter the prophase of the first meiotic division. At the beginning of the prophase of the first meiotic division, the primary spermatocyte has 46 (44 + XY) chromosomes and 4N amount of DNA. In this prophase, the cell passes through 4 stages—leptotene, zygotene, pachytene, and diplotene—and reaches the stage of diakinesis, resulting in the separation of the chromosomes. During these stages of meiosis, crossing over of genes of the chromosomes occurs. Thereafter, the cell enters the metaphase, and in the following anaphase the chromosomes move toward each pole. Since the prophase of this division takes a long time (about 22 days), the majority of cells seen in sections will be in this phase; their chromatin will be coiling to form the chromosomes. The primary spermatocytes are the largest cells of spermatogenic lineage and are characterized by the presence of chromosomes in different stages of their coiling process within their nuclei. From this first meiotic division there result smaller cells called **secondary spermatocytes** (Fig 23–3) with only 23 chromosomes (22 + X or 22 + Y). This decrease in number (from 46 to 23) is followed by a reduction in

the amount of DNA per cell (from 4N to 2N). Secondary spermatocytes are difficult to observe in sections of the testicle because they remain in interphase very briefly and enter quickly into the second meiotic division, thus being short-lived cells. Division of the secondary spermatocytes results in **spermatids,** cells that contain 23 chromosomes. In this second division, the amount of DNA per cell is reduced by half, forming haploid (1N) cells. This happens because no S phase (DNA synthesis) occurs between the first and second mitosis of the spermatocytes.

The meiotic process therefore results in formation of cells with a haploid number of chromosomes. With fertilization, they return to the normal diploid number. It is the meiotic process which, because of the reductional process of cell division, guarantees a constant (fixed) number of chromosomes for the species.

Spermatids are cells resulting from the division of the secondary spermatocytes. They can be distinguished by their small size, nuclei with areas of condensed chromatin, and near-central location within the seminiferous tubules (Fig 23–3). With the appearance of the spermatids, spermatocytogenesis ends. Thereafter, the spermatids undergo a complex process of differentiation called **spermiogenesis,** which results in the transformation of the spermatids into spermatozoa. Spermatids exhibit variable morphologic characteristics

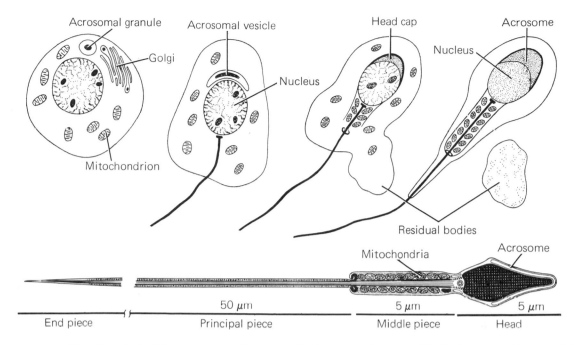

Figure 23 –4. *Top:* The principal changes occurring in spermatids during spermiogenesis. The basic structural feature of the spermatozoon is the head, which consists primarily of condensed nuclear chromatin. The reduced volume of the nucleus permits the greater mobility of the sperm and may protect the genome from damage while in transit to the egg. The rest of the spermatozoon is structurally arranged to provide a motor function. *Bottom:* The structure of a spermatozoon.

depending upon the phase of spermiogenesis in which they are observed. This process of spermiogenesis can be summarized in the following changes illustrated in Figs 23–4 and 23–5:

(1) In the Golgi apparatus, formation of proacrosomal granules rich in carbohydrates occurs first. These discrete granules coalesce into a single large granule, the acrosomal granule, contained within a membrane called the **acrosomal vesicle.** This vesicular structure, moving along with the Golgi complex in the direction of the nucleus, attaches itself to the outer part of the nuclear envelope at the future anterior end of the sperm. This is called the **Golgi phase.** The limiting membrane of the acrosomal vesicle extends as a thick fold on the surface of the nucleus. The vesicle finally covers half or two-thirds of the nucleus with a hood called the **head cap.** This is followed by a redistribution of the acrosomal substance within the head cap, thus constituting the **acrosomal cap** (or **acrosome**), rich in carbohydrates and having a characteristic shape and size in different species. The acrosome contains several hydrolytic enzymes such as hyaluronidase, neuraminidase, acid phosphatase, and a protease having trypsinlike activity. Thus, the acrosome serves as a specialized type of lysosome. These enzymes are known to separate the cells of the corona radiata of the ova and digest the zona pellucida, structures that surround recently ovulated eggs (Fig 24–3). When spermatozoa abut ova, the acrosome is partially lysed, liberating its enzyme content. This pro-

cess, the **acrosome reaction,** facilitates fertilization. Spermatid nuclei elongate and pass through the final maturation phase of spermiogenesis until they assume their final shape, ie, a dense homogeneous nuclear mass.

(2) Simultaneously, the centrioles migrate to the posterior pole of the spermatid; from one centriole a flagellum emerges perpendicular to the surface of the cell to form the tail of the spermatozoon (Figs 23 4 and 23 5). The other centriole migrates to form a collar around the initial part of its tail.

(3) At the same time, the cytoplasm shifts toward the flagellum and covers part of it. As the process evolves, parts of the cytoplasm not utilized in the formation of the spermatozoon are cast off from the cell as **residual bodies** that are phagocytosed and digested by Sertoli cells (Figs 23–4 and 23–10).

(4) Concomitantly, the mitochondria gradually move toward the flagellum. They arrange themselves as a spiral around the initial part of the tail, known as the **middle piece** of the spermatozoon. This disposition of the mitochondria is another example of a concentration of these organelles in sites related to cell movement and high energy consumption. The flagellum of the spermatozoon has a motor function, and the mitochondria are related to the production of energy for this movement. Flagellar structure and function are described in the section on the cell (see Chapter 3). Movement of the flagellum is related to the interac-

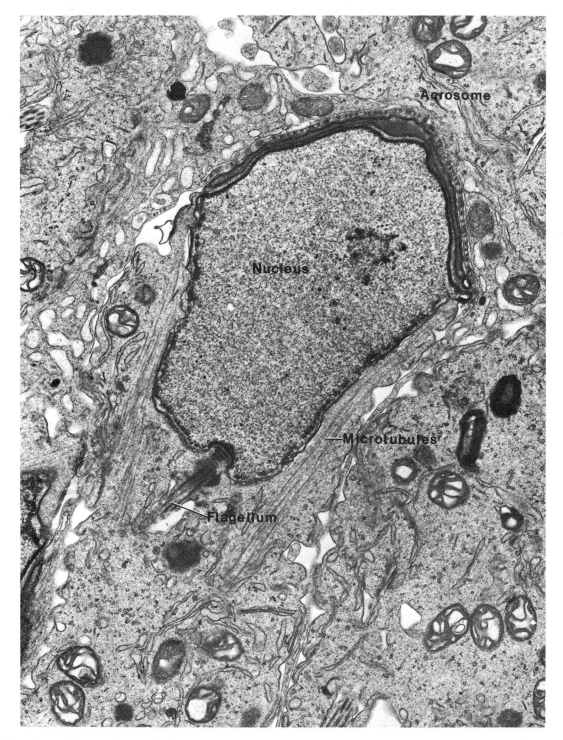

Figure 23–5. Electron micrograph of a mouse spermatid. In the center is its nucleus, covered by the acrosomal head cap. The flagellum can be seen emerging in the lower region below the nucleus. A cylindric bundle of microtubules, the manchette (M), limits the cell laterally. Reduced from × 32,500. (Courtesy of KR Porter.)

tion among microtubules, ATP, and a protein called **dynein.** Kartagener's syndrome, characterized by immotile spermatozoa and consequent sterility, has been described as being due to lack of dynein in the patient's spermatozoa. This disorder is usually coincident with chronic respiratory infections, since a similar deficiency may exist in the ciliary axonemes of the respiratory epithelial cells. Carbohydrates produced by the associated glands of the male seminal system and secreted in the seminal fluid are the source of energy for sperm motility. Among these carbohydrates, the most abundant is the monosaccharide fructose.

(5) The nuclear chromatin condenses and becomes a homogeneous dense mass without visible substructure. The **manchette,** a cylindric band of microtubules associated with the posterior margin of the acrosomal cap, forms around the nucleus (Fig 23–5). The manchette appears to play a role in the

subsequent elongation and flattening of the spermatid nucleus.

As a result of the processes described above, the mature spermatozoa have the structure illustrated in Figs 23–4 and 23–7.

During division of the spermatogonia, the resulting cells do not separate completely but remain held together by cytoplasmic bridges. This concept is illustrated in Fig 23–6. The intercellular bridges provide communication between every primary and secondary spermatocyte and spermatid derived from a single spermatogonium. By permitting the interchange of information from cell to cell, these bridges play an important role in coordinating the sequence of events in spermatogenesis. This detail may be of importance in understanding the processes involved in the seminiferous epithelium cycle (described below). When the process of spermatogenesis is completed, the sloughing off of the

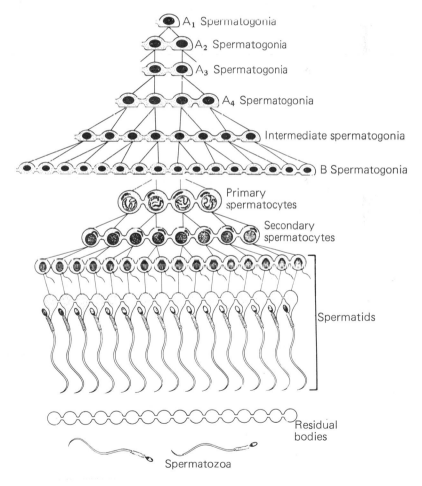

Figure 23–6. Diagram showing the clonal nature of the germ cells. Only the initial spermatogonia divide and produce separate daughter cells. Once committed to differentiation, the cells of all subsequent divisions present intercellular cytoplasmic bridges. Only after they are separated from the residual bodies can the spermatozoa be considered isolated individuals. The actual number of cells is larger than shown in this figure. See the text for the functional implication of the intercellular bridges. (Reproduced, with permission, from Bloom W, Fawcett DW: *A Textbook of Histology,* 10th ed. Saunders, 1975.)

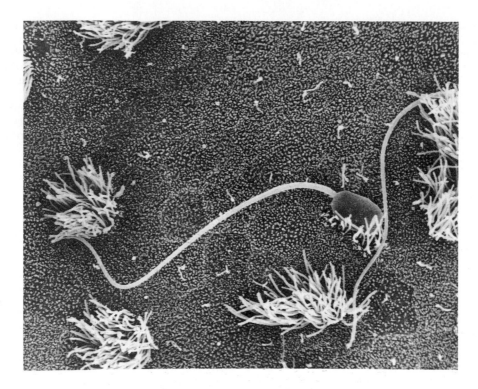

Figure 23 –7. Spermatozoon in the uterine cavity of a rodent as seen using scanning electron microscopy. The tufts are ciliated cells. (Courtesy of KR Porter.)

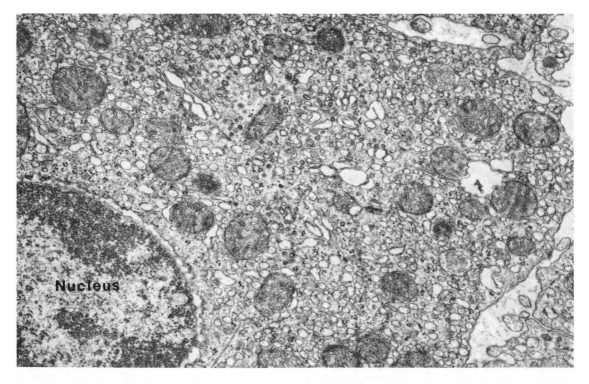

Figure 23 –8. Electron micrograph of a section of an interstitial cell from the testis of a rat. There are abundant mitochondria and smooth endoplasmic reticulum. × 12,000.

cytoplasm and cytoplasmic bridges as residual bodies leads to a separation of the spermatids.

Experimental injection of tritiated thymidine into the testicles of volunteers shows that, in men, the changes that occur between the spermatogonia stage and the formation of the spermatozoa take about 64 days. Besides being a slow process, spermatogenesis occurs neither simultaneously nor synchronously in all of the seminiferous tubules. The process occurs in wavelike fashion, which explains the irregular appearance of the tubules, where each region exhibits a different phase of spermatogenesis. This is why spermatozoa are encountered in some regions of the seminiferous tubules and only spermatids in others. The **cycle of the seminiferous epithelium** refers to the sequence of maturation changes occurring in a given area of the germinal epithelium between 2 successive appearances of a given cell stage. Each cycle in the human lasts 16 ± 1 days and spermatogenesis ends 4 cycles or about 64 ± 4.5 days later. The seminiferous cycle is clearly seen in rodents, in which 12 different stages have been described. In men, 6 stages are known to occur, but the presence is not as clear-cut. Fig 23–9 shows the sequence of stages in the human testis.

The **nutrient** or **Sertoli cells** are elongated pyramidal cells that interdigitate with cells of the spermatogenic series. The bases of the Sertoli cells adhere to the basal lamina, while their apical ends frequently extend into the lumen of the seminiferous tubule. In the light microscope, Sertoli cell cytoplasm appears poorly defined; it is barely visible, and the cells are irregularly shaped (Fig 23–3). Electron microscopic studies reveal that these cells contain abundant smooth endoplasmic reticulum, some rough endoplasmic reticulum, a well-developed Golgi apparatus, and numerous mitochondria and lysosomes. The elongated nucleus is often triangular in outline, possesses numerous infoldings, and exhibits little visible chromatin. The characteristic well-developed nucleolus has a central oval nucleolonema flanked by 2 basophilic masses of chromatin.

The margins of the Sertoli cells are bound with occluding junctions; consequently, these cells form a continuous sheath surrounding the lumen of the seminiferous tubule. Beneath the Sertoli cells lies the basal lamina and the **extratubular space** containing the blood vessels and lymphatics. The spermatogonial cells lie in the extratubular space between the Sertoli cells and the basal lamina (Fig 23–10). During spermatogenesis, progeny of the spermatogonia traverse the Sertoli cell occluding junctions and subsequently reside in the lumenal or **intratubular space.** Spermatocytes and spermatids lie within deep clefts (invaginations) of the lateral and apical margins of the Sertoli cells. Consequently, the Sertoli cells exhibit an irregular morphology. As the flagellar tails of the spermatids develop, they appear as tufts extending from the apical end of the Sertoli cells (Figs 23–3 and 23–10). Sertoli cells are also connected with gap junctions that provide ionic and chemical coupling of the cells, and this may be important in coordinating the cycle of the seminiferous epithelium described above.

Sertoli cells have at least 3 main functions: **(1) Support, protection, and nutritional regulation of the developing spermatozoa.** As mentioned above, the cells of the spermatogenic series are interconnected with cytoplasmic bridges. This network of cells is physically supported by extensive cytoplasmic ramifications of the Sertoli cells. Because spermatocytes, spermatids, and spermatozoa are isolated from the blood supply by the intervening Sertoli cell sheath, these spermatogenic cells depend upon the Sertoli cells to mediate the exchange of nutrients and metabolites. The Sertoli cell barrier also protects the developing sperm cells from immunologic attack (discussed below). **(2) Phagocytosis.** During spermiogenesis, excess spermatid cytoplasm is shed as residual bodies. These cytoplasmic fragments are phagocytosed, broken down, and subsequently resorbed by Sertoli cell lysosomes. **(3) Secretion.** Sertoli cells continuously secrete into the seminiferous tubules a fluid that flows in the direction of the genital ducts and is utilized for sperm transport. Secretion of an androgen-binding protein by Sertoli cells is under the control of FSH and testosterone and serves to concentrate testosterone in the seminiferous tubule, where it is utilized in spermatogenesis. Sertoli cells may secrete steroid hormones (estrogens), although this function has yet to be verified.

Sertoli cells in humans and other animals do not divide during the reproductive period. They are extremely resistant to adverse conditions such as infection, malnutrition, or x-ray irradiation and survive these insults much better than cells of the spermatogenic lineage.

The gonadotropic hormone produced in the human placenta and eliminated in the urine of pregnant women, when injected into male frogs, stimulates the vacuolization of the apical cytoplasm of the Sertoli cells and liberates the spermatozoa held there (Fig 23–11). This action explains why frog spermatozoa are eliminated after the injection of urine from pregnant females—a phenomenon on which the Galli Mainini test for the diagnosis of pregnancy was based. In mammals, however, this process is not observed, and the release of spermatozoa probably occurs as a result of cellular movements, with the probable participation of microtubules and microfilaments in the cell apex.

Interstitial Tissue

The spaces between the seminiferous tubules in the testicle are filled with accumulations of connective tissue, nerves, blood, and lymphatic vessels. Testicular capillaries are of the fenestrated type and permit the free passage of macromolecules

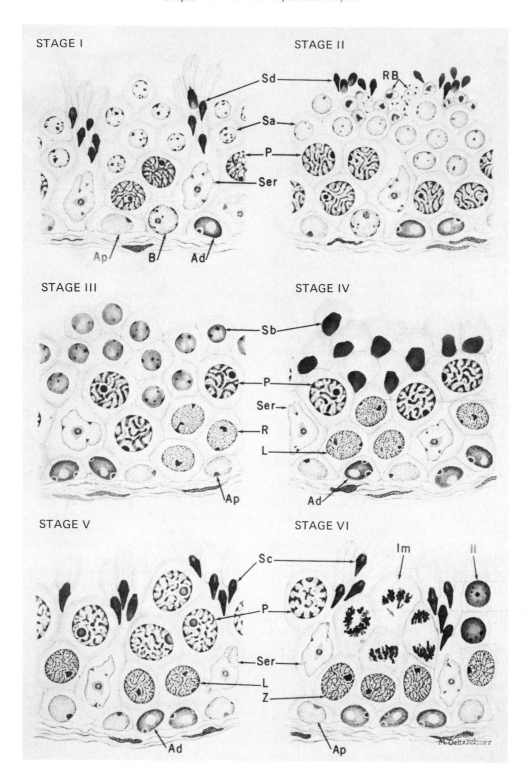

Figure 23 –9. Diagrammatic representation of the 6 recognizable cell associations corresponding to the stages of the cycle of the human seminiferous epithelium. Ser, Sertoli cell; Ad and Ap, dark and pale type A spermatogonia; B, type B spermatogonia; R, resting primary spermatocyte; L, leptotene spermatocyte; Z, zygotene spermatocyte; P, pachytene spermatocyte; Im, primary spermatocyte in division; II, secondary spermatocyte in interphase; Sa, Sb, Sc, Sd, spermatids in various stages of differentiation; RB, residual bodies of Regnaud. (Reproduced, with permission, from Clermont Y: Am J Anat 112:35, 1963.)

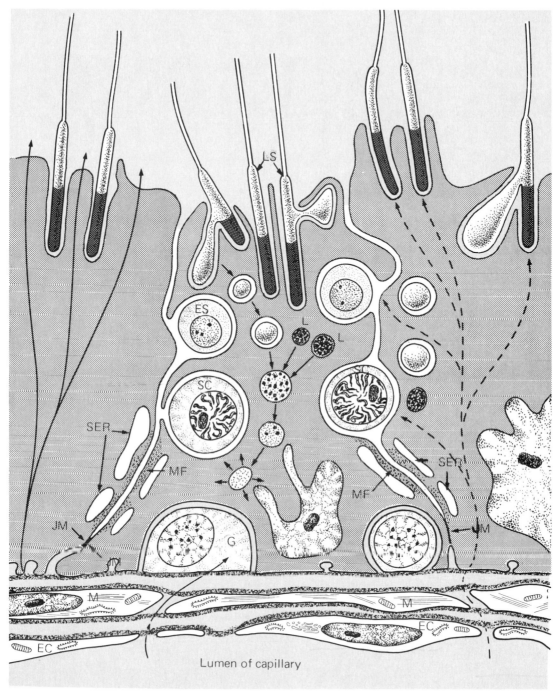

Figure 23–10. The position and functions of the Sertoli cells. These cells are bounded by their lateral walls and divide the seminiferous tubules into 3 compartments. The lower part is extratubular and comprises the lumen of the blood vessels, the interstitial space, and the regions occupied by the spermatogonia (G). The central dark part comprises the intracellular space of the Sertoli cells. The third (upper) part represents the lumen of the seminiferous tubules. The arrows pointing to the occluding junctional membrane (JM) show the zones where the membranes converge and impede the passage of substances from the first to the third compartment. Above these zones appear specialized regions characterized by the presence of circularly disposed microfilaments (MF) and of cisternae of the smooth endoplasmic reticulum (SER). The 3 main functions of the Sertoli cells are also portrayed. In the cell at left, the arrows indicate the secretion of testicular fluid. In the middle cell, cytoplasmic residual bodies from the forming spermatids are captured and digested by lysosomes (L). In the cell at right, the dotted arrows indicate the transport of metabolites from the extracellular space to the spermatocytes (SC), and the early (ES) and late (LS) spermatids. Observe that the transport of material from the extratubular compartment to the lumen and spermatogenic cells passes through the Sertoli cells. Note also the myoid cells (M) and the endothelial cell (EC)

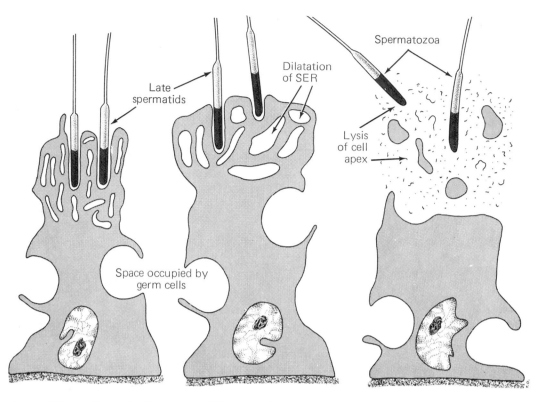

Figure 23–11. Diagram illustrating the process of liberation of spermatozoa in amphibia. At left is a Sertoli cell containing mature spermatids. After the injection of luteinizing hormone in amphibians, the smooth endoplasmic reticulum (SER) swells (center cell) and promotes the lysis of the cell apex with liberation of spermatozoa (right). (Redrawn and reproduced, with permission, from Vitale-Calpe R, Burgos MH: J Ultrastruct Res 31:394, 1970.)

such as the blood proteins. An extensive network of lymphatic vessels is present in the interstitial space, and this explains the similarity of composition between the interstitial fluid and lymph collected from this organ. The connective tissue consists of various cell types, including fibroblasts, undifferentiated connective cells, mast cells, and macrophages. After puberty, an additional cell type appears that is either rounded or polygonal in shape and has a central nucleus and an eosinophilic cytoplasm rich in small lipid droplets (Figs 23–3 and 23–8). These are the **interstitial** or **Leydig cells** of the testicle, which have the characteristics of steroid secretory cells described in Chapter 4. These cells produce the male hormone **testosterone,** responsible for the development of the secondary male sex characteristics. Thus, a direct correlation is observed between presence of interstitial cells and production of androgen by the testis. The presence in the interstitial cells of enzymes necessary for the synthesis of testosterone has been demonstrated using histochemical methods. Among these enzymes is 17β-hydroxysteroid dehydrogenase, which participates in transformation of androstenedione into testosterone. 17α-Hydroxylase is present, but 11- and 21-hydroxylase, found in the adrenal cortex, are absent. Pregnenolone is hy-

droxylated in the 17 position, then subjected to side chain cleavage to form 17-ketosteroids. These are converted to testosterone. Interstitial cell tumors can cause precocious puberty in the male.

Small amounts of estrogen are synthesized in the testes, although it is not clear whether they are products of the Leydig cells, the Sertoli cells, or both.

The activity and the quantity of the interstitial cells depend on hormonal stimuli. During human pregnancy, placental gonadotropic hormone passes from the maternal blood to the fetus, stimulating the abundant fetal testicular interstitial cells that produce androgenic hormone. The presence of the hormone is important for the embryologic differentiation of the male genitalia. The embryonic interstitial cells remain fully differentiated until up to 4½ months of gestation and then regress, with an associated decrease in testosterone synthesis. They then remain quiescent throughout the rest of the pregnancy and up to the prepuberal period, when they resume testosterone synthesis in response to the stimulus of luteinizing hormone (LH; also called **interstitial cell-stimulating hormone** [ICSH]) from the pituitary gland. This is the main factor controlling androgen secretion. The mechanism by which luteinizing hormone stimulates Leydig cells ap-

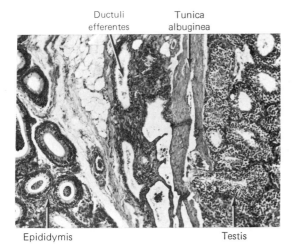

Figure 23 –12. Photomicrograph of a section of testis and epididymis showing the ductuli efferentes and the thick tunica albuginea. H&E stain, × 80.

pears to involve an increase in cAMP and protein synthesis.

Intratesticular Genital Ducts

These are the **tubuli recti** (straight tubules), the **rete testis**, and the **ductuli efferentes** (Fig 23–1). The transition from seminiferous tubules to **tubuli recti** is abrupt. In the initial portion, spermatogenic cells disappear, and only the Sertoli cells remain. The main portion of the straight tubule consists of cuboidal epithelium supported on a dense connective tissue sheath.

Straight tubules empty into the **rete testis**, contained within the mediastinum, a thickening of the tunica albuginea. It is lined with cuboidal epithelium.

From the rete testis extend 10–20 **ductili efferentes** (Fig 23–12). They have an epithelium composed of alternating groups of cuboidal and columnar cells, which are often ciliated. The rapid movement of the cilia impels the spermatozoa toward the **epididymis**. These ducts penetrate the cranial region of the epididymis, where they merge after a sinuous stretch.

Histophysiology of the Testis

Temperature is very important in the regulation of spermatogenesis, and this process generally occurs only in temperatures below that of the human body. This is why, with rare exceptions, the testicles of mammals are located outside the abdominal cavity and in the scrotal sacs, where the temperature is generally lower.

Testicular temperature is controlled by several mechanisms. A rich vascular plexus in the spermatic cord forms a countercurrent heat exchange system important in maintaining a low testicular temperature. Other factors are the evaporation of

sweat from the scrotum and contraction of the muscles of the spermatic cord that pulls the testicles into the inguinal canal, where their temperature can be increased.

Failure of descent of the testis (**cryptorchidism**) holds the testicles at a core temperature of 37 C, which inhibits spermatogenesis. In cases that are not too far advanced, spermatogenesis can occur normally if the testicle is moved surgically to the scrotum. Although germ cell proliferation is inhibited by abdominal temperature, testosterone synthesis is not. This explains why patients with cryptorchidism can be sterile but still remain potent and assume secondary male characteristics.

Malnutrition, alcoholism, and the action of certain drugs hinder spermatogenesis and lead to alterations in the cells of spermatogenic origin, with consequent decreased production of spermatozoa. Lack of vitamin E can produce—especially in the rat—total and irreversible destruction of spermatogenic cells, including the spermatogonia, thus resulting in permanent sterility. This has not been observed in men. X-ray radiation causes destruction of spermatogonia with irreversible sterility. Cadmium salts are quite toxic to the cells of spermatogenic lineage, causing death of those cells and sterility in animals. The drug busulfan acts on the germinal cells, and when administered to pregnant female rats it promotes the death of the germinal cells of their offspring. These animals are therefore sterile, and their seminiferous tubules contain exclusively Sertoli cells.

Without doubt, however, endocrine factors have by far the most important effect on spermatogenesis. Spermatogenesis depends on the action of the follicle-stimulating (FSH) and luteinizing (LH) hormones of the pituitary gland on the testicular cells. LH acts on the interstitial cells, stimulating the production of testosterone necessary for the normal development of cells of seminal lineage. FSH is known to act on the Sertoli cells, stimulating the adenylate cyclase and consequently increasing the presence of cAMP, and promoting the synthesis of the **androgen-binding protein** (ABP). This protein combines with testosterone and is secreted into the lumen of the seminiferous tubules (Fig 23–13). Spermatogenesis is inhibited by estrogens and progestogens. The mechanisms of endocrine control are shown in Fig 23–13.

The spermatozoa are transported to the epididymis in an appropriate medium called **testicular fluid** produced by the Sertoli cells and rete testis. This fluid contains steroids, proteins, ions, and a specific androgen-binding protein.

Blood-Seminiferous Tubule Barrier

The observation that few substances present in blood appear in the testicular fluid suggested the existence of a barrier between the blood and the interior of the seminiferous tubules. The testicular capillaries are of the fenestrated type and permit

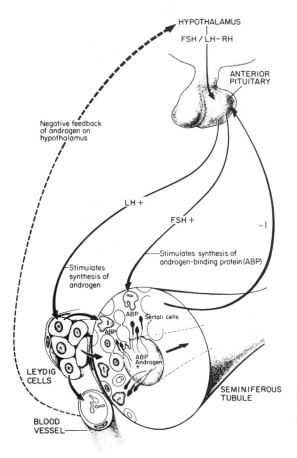

Figure 23 –13. Diagram of the hypophyseal control of male reproduction in which luteinizing hormone (LH) acts upon the Leydig cells and follicle-stimulating hormone (FSH) acts upon the seminiferous tubules. A testicular hormone called **inhibin** (I), still not well characterized but probably of protein nature, inhibits FSH secretion in the pituitary. (Modified and reproduced, with permission, from Bloom W, Fawcett DW: *A Textbook of Histology,* 10th ed. Saunders, 1975.)

free passage of large molecules. The occluding junctions between Sertoli cells are responsible for this barrier, which is of importance in protecting the seminal cells against blood-borne noxious agents.

Differentiation of spermatogonial cells leads to the appearance of sperm-specific proteins. Since sexual maturity occurs long after the development of immunocompetence, differentiating sperm cells could be recognized as "foreign" and provoke an immune response, which would destroy the germ cells. Consequently, the blood-testis barrier would eliminate any interaction between developing sperm and the immune system. This barrier prevents the passage of gamma globulins into the seminiferous tubule and would account for the absence of any impairment of fertility in patients whose serum possesses high levels of sperm antibodies. The Sertoli cell barrier therefore functions in protecting the seminiferous epithelium against an autoimmune reaction.

Excretory Genital Ducts

The ducts that transport the spermatozoa produced in the testis toward the surface of the body are the ductuli efferentes, the epididymis, the ductus deferens (vas deferens), and the urethra.

The **epididymis** consists of one long, highly tortuous tube about 4–6 meters in length. This long canal forms, with surrounding connective tissue, the body and tail of the epididymis. It is lined by pseudostratified columnar epithelium composed of rounded basal and columnar cells. These cells are supported on a basement membrane surrounded by smooth muscle cells, which probably help to move the sperm along the duct, and by loose connective tissue rich in blood capillaries (Fig 23–14).

The surface of the columnar cells is covered with cytoplasmic projections forming long and irregular microvilli, improperly called **stereocilia**. Stereocilia have neither basal bodies nor internal microtubules, whereas true cilia have both. When observed with an electron microscope, the cytoplasm of these cells is seen to be filled with granules of unknown nature. A morphologic appearance similar to that of pinocytosis and digestion of the engulfed material with the presence of polymorphous vesicles, lysosomes, etc is frequently observed in these cells. This aspect suggests that epididymal cells have more than one function, including, probably, intracellular digestion and secretion into the lumen. Little is known about their function, but it is probably a major one, for it is in the interior of the epididymis that the spermatozoa from the seminiferous tubules mature and become motile and fertile. This epithelium participates in the reabsorption and digestion of residual bodies that are eliminated during spermatogenesis. Most of the fluid leaving the testis is reabsorbed in the epididymis, and this activity is under hormonal control.

From the epididymis the **ductus (vas) deferens,** a straight tube with thick walls, continues toward the prostatic urethra and empties into it. It is characterized by a narrow lumen and a thick wall of smooth muscle (Fig 23–15). Its mucosa forms longitudinal folds and is covered along most of its extent by pseudostratified columnar epithelium with stereocilia. Its lamina propria is a layer of connective tissue rich in elastic fibers. The thick muscular layer consists of layers of spirally oriented smooth muscle cells. Along the ductus deferens and linked to it run the vessels and nerves which go to and come from the testicle. Before it penetrates the prostate, the ductus deferens dilates, forming a region called the **ampulla.** In this area, the epithelium becomes thicker, assuming a lacelike aspect. At the final portion of the ampulla, the seminal vesicles join. From there on, the ductus deferens enters the prostate, opening into the prostatic urethra. The segment entering the prostate is called the **ejaculatory duct** and presents a mucous layer similar to that of the ampulla but without the muscle layer.

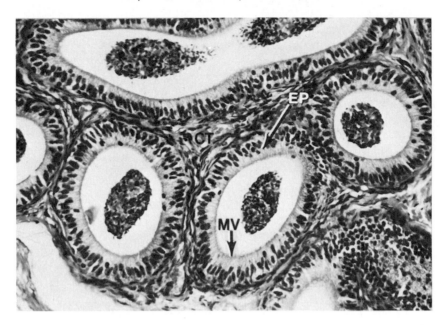

Figure 23 –14. Photomicrograph of a section of epididymis showing its structure. Note the epithelium (EP), the connective tissue (CT), and the microvilli (MV) (stereocilia). H&E stain, × 200.

Accessory Male Genital Glands

These are the seminal vesicles, the prostate gland, and the bulbourethral glands.

The **seminal vesicles** consist of 2 highly tortuous tubes 15 cm in length. On sectioning the organ, the same tube is observed sectioned in different orientations. It has a folded mucosa lined with pseudostratified columnar epithelium that exhibits great individual variations depending on age and other conditions. The epithelium consists of a discontinuous layer of spherical basal cells and a layer of longer superficial cuboidal or low columnar cells, rich in secretory granules. They present an ultrastructure characteristic of protein-synthesizing cells (see Chapter 4). The lamina propria of the seminal vesicles is rich in elastic fibers and sur-

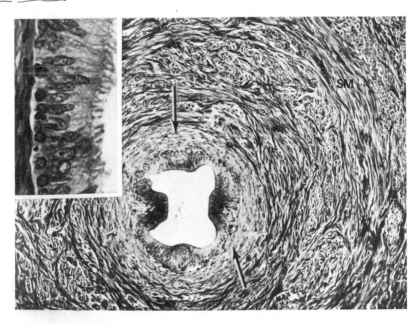

Figure 23 –15. Photomicrograph of a section of ductus deferens. The ductus has a thick wall formed by smooth muscle cells (SM). The arrows point to the thin tunica propria layer. × 16. Observe in the inset the details of the pseudostratified columnar epithelium showing stereocilia. Masson's trichrome stain, × 400.

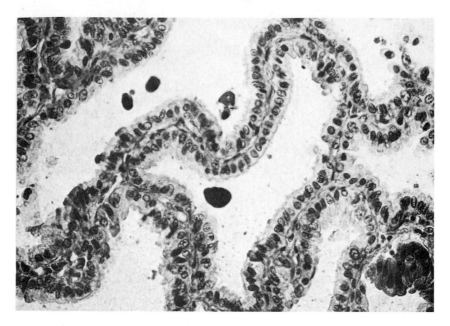

Figure 23 –16. Photomicrograph of a section of human seminal vesicle. Masson's trichrome stain, × 300.

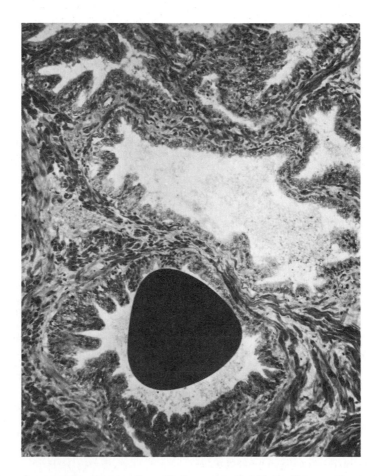

Figure 23 –17. Section of a prostate, showing its epithelium, smooth muscle fibers, and a typical lamellar prostatic concretion (corpus amylaceum). H&E stain, × 300.

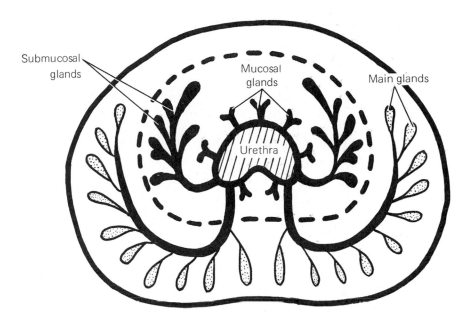

Figure 23–18. Diagram illustrating the position of the prostatic glands.

rounded by a thin layer of smooth muscle (Fig 23–16). The muscular wall of the seminal vesicles contains a plexus of nerve fibers and small sympathetic ganglia. The secretion of the seminal vesicles, which accumulates in the interior of this gland, is eliminated during ejaculation by the contraction of its smooth muscle. It contains globulin and is rich in vitamin C and fructose, metabolites that are of importance in the nutrition and motility of the spermatozoa. The height of the epithelial cells of the seminal vesicles and the degree of activity of the secretory processes are testosterone-dependent. In the absence of testosterone, the epithelium of the seminal vesicles atrophies. This atrophy can be reversed by the administration of testosterone. The function of the smooth muscle of the epididymis and of the glands of the male genital system is affected by the sex hormones.

The **prostate** is a collection of 30–50 branched tubulo-alveolar glands whose ducts empty into the prostatic urethra. The prostate produces prostatic fluid and stores it in its interior for expulsion during ejaculation.

The prostate is surrounded by a fibroelastic capsule rich in smooth muscle. This capsule emits septa that penetrate the gland. An exceptionally rich fibromuscular stroma is formed that surrounds the glands (Fig 23–17). The basal lamina is indistinct, and the epithelial cells rest upon a layer of connective tissue with much smooth muscle, a dense elastic fiber network, and blood capillaries. Its epithelium may be cuboidal or even squamous but in most places is columnar, with a few basal cells. Its cells secrete proteins and have the characteristics described for this type of cell in Chapter 4. These cells are rich in lysosomes and possess in-

tense acid phosphatase activity. This peculiarity is preserved in carcinoma of the prostate, which is characterized by the presence of this enzyme in high concentrations in the tumor and in the blood. Serum acid phosphatase is measured not only in the diagnosis but also in the follow-up of patients with this tumor.

The prostatic gland is divided into 3 types of structures—mucosal, submucosal, and main glands—arranged in 3 separate areas situated concentrically around the urethra as shown in Fig 23–18. The main glands contribute most to the volume of the prostatic secretion. For unknown reasons—often after age 40—the mucosal and submucosal glands begin to hypertrophy. This can lead to partial or total obstruction of the urethra. Carcinoma of the prostate, a frequent tumor in old men, usually starts in the main glands. The secretory process of the prostate depends, as in the seminal vesicles, on testosterone.

Small spherical bodies of glycoprotein composition less than 0.2 mm in diameter are frequently observed in the lumen of the prostate. They are called **prostatic concretions** (Fig 23–17). These bodies often form calculi. Their significance is not understood, but their number increases with age.

The **bulbourethral glands** are pea-sized formations located behind the membranous portion of the urethra and emptying into it. They are tubuloalveolar glands with a mucous type of epithelium. They have skeletal and smooth muscle cells in their septa which separate their lobes. Their secretion has a mucoid appearance.

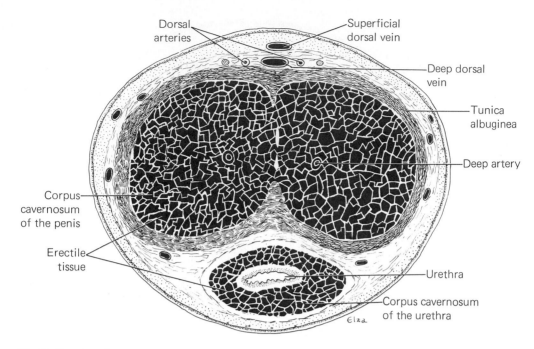

Dorsal arteries — Superficial dorsal vein — Deep dorsal vein — Tunica albuginea — Deep artery — Corpus cavernosum of the penis — Erectile tissue — Urethra — Corpus cavernosum of the urethra

Figure 23 –19. Drawing of a transverse section of the penis. (Redrawn and reproduced, with permission, from Leeson TS, Leeson CR: *Histology,* 2nd ed. Saunders, 1970.)

PENIS

The penis consists mainly of 3 cylindric masses of erectile tissue plus the urethra, surrounded externally by skin. Two of these cylinders—the **corpora cavernosa of the penis**—are placed dorsally. The other, ventrally located, is called the **corpus cavernosum of the urethra** and surrounds the urethra. At its end it dilates, forming the **glans penis** (Fig 23–1). The corpora cavernosa are covered by a resistant membrane of hard connective tissue, the **tunica albuginea.** Orifices are present in the area that separates the 2 corpora cavernosa of the penis, permitting communications between these 2 bodies (Fig 23–19). The corpora cavernosa of the penis and urethra are composed of a tangle of dilated blood vessels lined by endothelium.

The prepuce is a retractile fold of skin. It contains connective tissue with smooth muscle in its interior. Sebaceous glands are present in the internal fold and in the skin that covers the glans.

•   •   •

References

Afzelius BA & others: Lack of dynein arms in immotile human spermatozoa. J Cell Biol 66:225, 1975.

Bustos-Obregon E & others: Morphological appraisal of gametogenesis: Spermatogenetic process in mammals with particular reference to man. Andrologia 7:141, 1975.

Clermont Y: Renewal of spermatogonia in man. Am J Anat 118:509, 1966.

Clermont Y, Leblond CP: Spermiogenesis of man, monkey, ram and other mammals as shown by the "periodic acid–Schiff" technique. Am J Anat 96:229, 1955.

De Kretser DM: Changes in the fine structure of the human testicular interstitial cells after treatment with human gonadotrophins. Z Zellforsch Mikrosk Anat 83:344, 1967.

De Kretser DM: Ultrastructure features of human spermiogenesis. Z Zellforsch Mikrosk Anat 98:477, 1969.

Dym M: The fine structure of monkey Sertoli cells in the transitional zone at the junction of the seminiferous tubules with the tubuli recti. Am J Anat 140:1, 1974.

Dym M: The mammalian rete testes: A morphological examination. Anat Rec 186:493, 1976.

Dym M, Fawcett DW: The blood-testis barrier in the rat and physiologic compartment of the seminiferous epithelium. Biol Reprod 3:308, 1970.

Fawcett DW: The mammalian spermatozoon. Dev Biol 44:394, 1975.

Fawcett DW, Anderson WA, Phillips DM: Morphogenetic factors influencing the shape of the sperm head. Dev Biol 16:220, 1971.

Fawcett DW, Neaves WB, Flores MN: Comparative observations on intertubular lymphatics and the organization of the interstitial tissue of the mammalian testis. Biol Reprod 9:500, 1973.

Friend DS, Farquhar MG: Functions of coated vesicles during protein absorption in the rat vas deferens. J Cell Biol 35:357, 1967.

Hartree EF, Srivastava PN: Chemical composition of the acrosomes of ram spermatozoa. J Reprod Fertil 9:47, 1965.

Johnson AD, Gomes WR (editors): *The Testis.* Vols 1–4. Academic Press, 1970–1977.

Johnson MH: An immunological barrier in the guinea-pig testis. J Pathol 101:129, 1970.

Leeson TS, Leeson CR: The fine structure of cavernous tissue in the adult rat penis. Invest Urol 3:144, 1965.

Murota S, Shikita M, Tamaoki B: Intracellular distribution of the enzymes related to androgen formation in mouse testes. Steroids 5:409, 1965.

Nagano T, Suzuki F: Freeze-fracture observations on the intercellular junctions of Sertoli cells and of Leydig cells in the human testis. Cell Tissue Res 166:37, 1976.

Ross MH: The fine structure and development of the peritubular contractile cell component in the seminiferous tubules of the mouse. Am J Anat 121:523, 1967.

Ross MH: The Sertoli cell specialization during spermiogenesis and at spermeation. Anat Rec 186:79, 1976.

Stambough R, Buckley J: Identification and subcellular localization of the enzymes affecting penetration of the zona pellucida of rabbit spermatozoa. J Reprod Fertil 19:423, 1969.

Steinberger E: Hormonal control of mammalian spermatogenesis. Physiol Rev 51:1, 1971.

Wong PYD, Yeung CH: Hormonal regulation of fluid reabsorption in isolated rat cauda epididymis. Endocrinology 101:1391, 1977.

24 | The Female Reproductive System

The female reproductive system (Fig 24–1) consists of 2 ovaries, 2 uterine tubes (oviducts), the uterus, the vagina, and the external genitalia. Between menarche and menopause, the system undergoes cyclic changes in structure and functional activity. These modifications are controlled by neurohumoral mechanisms. **Menarche** is the time when the first menses appears; **menopause** is a variable period during which the cyclic changes become irregular and eventually disappear altogether. In the postmenopausal period there is a slow involution of the reproductive system. In this chapter we shall also study the mammary glands, though they do not belong to the genital system— being, in fact, cutaneous glands—for the reason that they undergo changes directly connected with the functional state of the reproductive system.

THE OVARY

The ovary is an almond-shaped body up to 5 cm in diameter, 1.5–3 cm in width, and 0.6–1.5 cm in thickness. It consists of a **medullary region,** con-

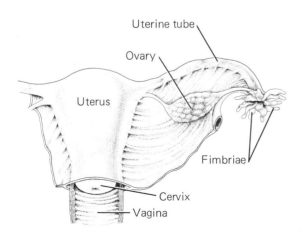

Figure 24 –1. Internal organs of the female reproductive system: ovary, fimbriae of infundibulum, uterine tube, uterus, cervix, and vagina.

taining several blood vessels and a small amount of loose connective tissue; and a **cortical region,** where ovarian follicles, containing the oocytes, predominate. There are no sharp limits between the cortical and the medullary regions (Fig 24–2). During embryonic life, germ cells migrate into the ovary and there are called **oogonia.** All germ cells present at birth are primary oocytes in the prophase of the first meiotic division.

The stroma of the cortical region is composed of characteristic spindle-shaped connective cells that respond in a different way to hormonal stimuli than connective cells of other organs. The surface of the ovary is lined by continuous simple squamous or cuboidal epithelium called **germinal epithelium.** Under the germinal epithelium, the stroma forms a layer of dense, poorly delineated connective tissue called the **tunica albuginea** of the ovary. The tunica albuginea is responsible for the whitish color of the ovary (Fig 24–2).

Ovarian Follicles

The ovarian follicles are embedded in the stroma of the cortex. Three types can be distinguished: **primordial follicles, growing follicles,** and **mature** or **graafian follicles.** Some histologists divide the growing follicles into 3 categories: (1) **primary follicles,** which are enveloped by a monolayer of cuboidal granulosa cells; (2) **secondary follicles,** showing a multiple compact layer of granulosa cells; and (3) **tertiary** or **vesicular follicles,** exhibiting fluid-filled cavities among the granulosa cells. The total number of follicles in the 2 ovaries of a normal young adult woman is estimated to be 400,000, but most of them will disappear by a degenerative process known as **atresia** during the reproductive years. This follicular regression takes place prior to birth and continues over the entire span of reproductive life. After menopause, only a small number of follicles remain. The regression may affect any type of follicle from primordial ones to those that are completely mature. Since, in general, only one oocyte is liberated by the ovaries in each menstrual cycle (average duration: 28 days) and the reproductive life of a woman lasts about 30–40 years, the total number of oocytes liberated is about 450. All of the other follicles, with their

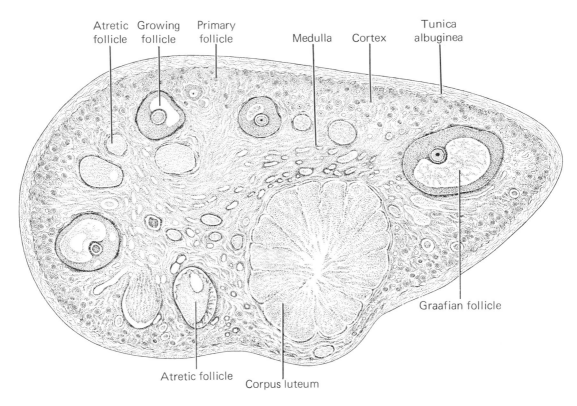

Atretic follicle · Growing follicle · Primary follicle · Medulla · Cortex · Tunica albuginea · Graafian follicle · Atretic follicle · Corpus luteum

Figure 24–2. Schematic drawing showing the main components of the ovary of an adult woman. (Redrawn and reproduced, with permission, from Copenhaver WM, Bunge RP, Bunge MTS: *Bailey's Textbook of Histology,* 16th ed. Williams & Wilkins, 1972.)

oocytes, fail to develop and degenerate, becoming atretic.

A. Primordial Follicles: The primordial follicles are the principal ones present before birth. Each consists of a primary oocyte enveloped by only one layer of flattened **follicular cells** (Fig 24–3).

The oocyte in the primordial follicle is a large cell measuring about 40 μm in diameter. Its nucleus is large, slightly eccentrically situated, and has finely dispersed chromatin and a large nucleolus. The electron microscope shows, in the cytoplasm of the oocytes—besides the usual elements—formations consisting of parallel lamellas and a great number of small vesicles. These 2 elements are more abundant in the oocytes of the growing and mature follicles. As soon as the oogonia are changed into primary oocytes, they enter the prophase of their first meiotic division and rest there. This takes place before birth.

B. Growing Follicles: Follicular growth comprises mainly the follicular cells but also the primary oocyte and the stroma surrounding the follicle (Figs 24–2, 24–3, and 24–4). The morphology and size of the growing follicles both vary greatly since these follicles range in age from those that are only starting to grow to very large ones that have almost reached maturity. As the oocyte grows, the single layer of follicular cells becomes cuboidal and then,

through mitotic division, increases into a stratified epithelium (Fig 24–3). The oocyte also becomes larger, and an acidophilic, homogeneous, and acellular layer called the **zona pellucida** appears around it (Figs 24–3 and 24–5). The zona pellucida becomes visible with the light microscope when the oocyte reaches 80 μm in diameter. With the electron microscope, its presence can be detected earlier. The zona pellucida contains glycoproteins and is PAS-positive. In its interior one can see—with the electron microscope—filopodia of the follicular cells and microvilli of the oocyte (Fig 24–5). The origin of the zona pellucida is not absolutely clear; it may be formed by the oocyte, by the follicular cells, or—the most widely held current opinion—by both.

While these modifications are taking place, the stroma immediately around the follicle modifies itself in order to form the **theca folliculi.** This layer subsequently differentiates into the theca interna and the theca externa (Fig 24–3). The cells of the theca interna are cuboidal and, when completely differentiated, present the same ultrastructural characteristics of the cells that produce steroids. Evidence suggests that these cells synthesize testosterone, which is converted into estrogen by cells of the granulosa. Like all organs of endocrine function, the theca interna is richly vascularized. The

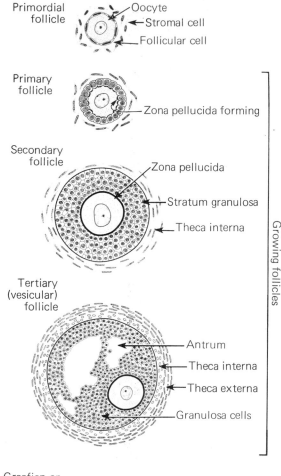

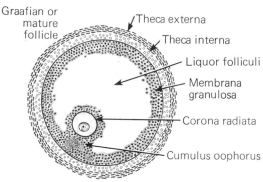

Figure 24–3. Schematic drawing of ovarian follicles, starting with the primordial follicle and ending with mature follicles.

theca externa consists mainly of connective tissue. Small vessels penetrate it and supply a rich capillary plexus in the secretory cells of the theca interna. In the granulosa cell layer there are no blood vessels during the stage of follicular growth. The boundary between the 2 thecas is not clear, and the same is true of the boundary between the theca externa and the ovarian stroma. The boundary between the

theca interna and the granulosa layer is well defined since their cells are morphologically different and there is a thick basal lamina between them. As the oocyte grows, changes occur in the distribution of its organelles. The single Golgi apparatus gives rise to multiple Golgi apparatuses dispersed in the ooplasm. The granular endoplasmic reticulum becomes more extensive, and more free ribosomes are found in the ooplasm. The number of small vesicles and multivesicular bodies also increases.

As the follicle grows—mainly because of the increase in number and in size of the granulosa cells—some accumulations of hyaluronic acid–rich fluid appear (**follicular liquid**). The cavities that contain liquid converge and finally form only one cavity, the **follicular antrum** (Figs 24–3 and 24–4). The cells of the granulosa layer are more numerous at a certain point on the follicular wall, forming a dense cell mass, the **cumulus oophorus,** which contains the oocyte. The cumulus oophorus protrudes toward the interior of the antrum (Fig 24–4). The oocyte grows no more thereafter.

C. Mature Follicles: The mature follicle is about 1 cm in diameter and can be seen as a transparent vesicle which protrudes from the surface of the ovary. As a result of the accumulation of liquid, the follicular cavity increases greatly and the oocyte adheres to the wall of the follicle through a pedicle formed by granulosa cells. Since the granulosa cells do not multiply in proportion to the accumulation of liquid, the granulosa layer becomes thinner.

The granulosa cells forming the first layer around the oocyte—and, therefore, in close contact with the zona pellucida—become elongated and form the **corona radiata,** which accompanies the oocyte when it leaves the ovary. The corona radiata is still present when the spermatozoon fertilizes the oocyte and is retained for some time during the passage of the ovum through the tube.

Ovulation

Ovulation is a process that consists of rupture of the mature follicle with liberation of the oocyte which will be caught by the dilated end of the uterine tube. In the human female, only one oocyte is usually liberated by the ovary at a time, but 2 or more oocytes can be expelled at the same time. In the latter case, if 2 or more of the liberated oocytes are fertilized, there may be more than one fetus (fraternal twins).

Ovulation takes place approximately in the middle of the menstrual cycle, ie, around the 14th day of a 28-day cycle. Under the pressure of the mature follicle, the superficial part of the ovary undergoes ischemia before ovulation, which contributes to weakening of the tissues and facilitates the extrusion of the oocyte.

It has been demonstrated with the electron microscope that there are smooth muscle cells in the theca externa of the follicular walls of several species of mammals. It is possible that contraction

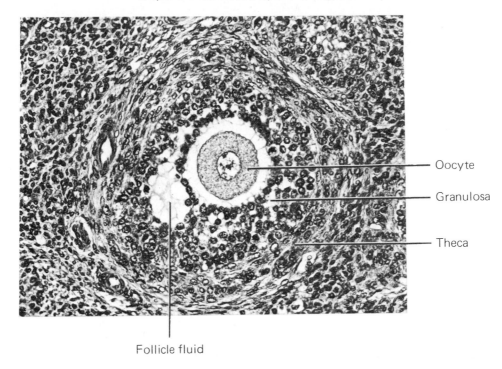

Oocyte

Granulosa

Theca

Follicle fluid

Figure 24 –4. Developing ovarian follicle. In the center of the follicle is an oocyte with a lightly staining nucleus. The limits between the 2 theca layers are not clear.

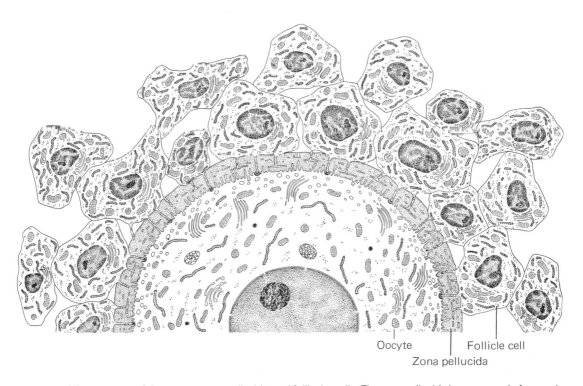

Oocyte

Follicle cell

Zona pellucida

Figure 24 –5. Ultrastructure of the oocyte, zona pellucida, and follicular cells. The zona pellucida is composed of amorphous material, penetrated by oocyte microvilli and by longer processes from follicular cells. In the oocyte cytoplasm there are several arrays of parallel smooth membranes. The nucleus is in prophase of the first meiotic division.

of these cells participates in the process of ovulation. A number of hypotheses with supporting data have been advanced to account for ovulation. These include the above-mentioned intrafollicular increase in pressure, the enzymatic dissolution of the connective tissue, and mechanical rupture. In any event, a midcycle surge of luteinizing hormone (LH) appears to be indispensable to the occurrence of rupture.

Before ovulation, the oocyte—together with the cells of the corona radiata—detaches itself from the wall of the follicle and floats in the follicular liquid. The first maturation division is completed after an increase in LH secretion but before the exit of the oocyte from the follicle. An indication of impending ovulation is the appearance on the surface of the follicle of the **macula pellucida** or **stigma,** in which the flow of blood ceases, resulting in a local change in color and translucency of the follicular wall. The germinal epithelium in this area becomes discontinuous, and the stroma becomes thinner. The cone then ruptures and the oocyte is extruded from the ovary together with the follicular liquid and blood.

The extremity of the uterine tube that faces the ovary is fringed with fimbriae and funnel-shaped. At the moment of ovulation, this end is very close to the surface of the ovary and receives the oocyte. By the action of the fimbriae, ciliated cells, and muscular contraction, the oocytes enter the infundibulum of the uterine tube where they are fertilized. Once fertilized, the oocyte, called the ovum, begins to undergo cleavage and is transported to the uterus, a trip that lasts about 3 days. If the oocyte is not fertilized within the first 24 hours after ovulation, the egg begins to degenerate.

Follicular Atresia

Most ovarian follicles undergo an involutional process called **follicular atresia** by which the follicles are said to become atretic. This is a degenerative process characterized by cessation of mitosis in the granulosa cells, separation of granulosa cells from the basal lamina, and death of the oocyte. Although follicular atresia takes place from the time of birth until a few years after the menopause, there are moments in which it is particularly intense. Follicular atresia is quite accentuated just after birth, when the effect of maternal hormones ceases, and also during puberty and pregnancy, ie, when marked qualitative and quantitative hormonal modifications take place.

The process of atresia may take place during any stage in the development of a follicle.

When atresia starts in a primordial follicle, the outline of the oocyte becomes irregular and the follicular cells become smaller, separating from one another. The oocyte and the follicular cells start to autolyze, finally leaving a space that is immediately occupied by cells of the ovarian stroma so that no vestige is left.

In growing follicles the degenerative process is basically the same. The zona pellucida is very resistant, becoming wavy and pleated at the onset of the atretic process as a result of the collapse of the follicle, but its material persists longer than the cells of the follicle.

When a follicle in the late stage of growth undergoes atresia, a large quantity of degenerative material is produced which elicits the formation of macrophages from monocytes carried in the blood by vessels that invade the area of atresia. While removal of the remnants of the follicle in atresia takes place, cells of the ovarian connective tissue that invade the area produce a small amount of collagenous matrix—similar to a cicatricial process. Later, all vestiges of the follicle disappear since the collagen is reabsorbed and replaced by typical ovarian stroma, but the theca cells persist as part of the ovarian stroma.

Interstitial Glands

Although granulosa cells and the oocytes undergo degeneration during atresia of the follicles, the theca interna cells frequently persist and in fact become quite active steroid secretors. These active thecal cells are called **interstitial cells** and actually constitute the **interstitial glands.** These glands, which are present from childhood through menopause, may be the source of ovarian testosterone.

Origin & Maturation of Oocytes

Oocytes are formed during intrauterine life, and their number does not increase after birth. The cells which are precursors of the oocytes are called **primordial germ cells** and originate in the endoderm of the yolk sac. Primordial germ cells migrate to the genital ridge and into the developing ovary.

Primary follicles as well as growing follicles contain primary oocytes equivalent to primary spermatocytes of the seminiferous tubules (see Chapter 23). These oocytes are in the prophase of the first meiotic division.

The first meiotic division is completed just before ovulation. The chromatin is equally divided between the daughter cells, but one of the secondary oocytes has almost all of the cytoplasm. The other becomes the first polar body, a very small cell containing the nucleus and a minimal amount of cytoplasm.

Immediately after expulsion of the first polar body, and while still in the cortical region of the ovary, the nucleus of the secondary oocyte starts the second meiotic division, which stops in metaphase and will only be completed when fertilization has taken place. Fertilization consists of penetration into the oocyte of the body of the spermatozoon but not the tail. The fertilized oocyte is called an **ovum.**

The secondary oocyte remains viable for an estimated maximum of 24 hours. Penetration of the sperm cell head reconstitutes the diploid number of

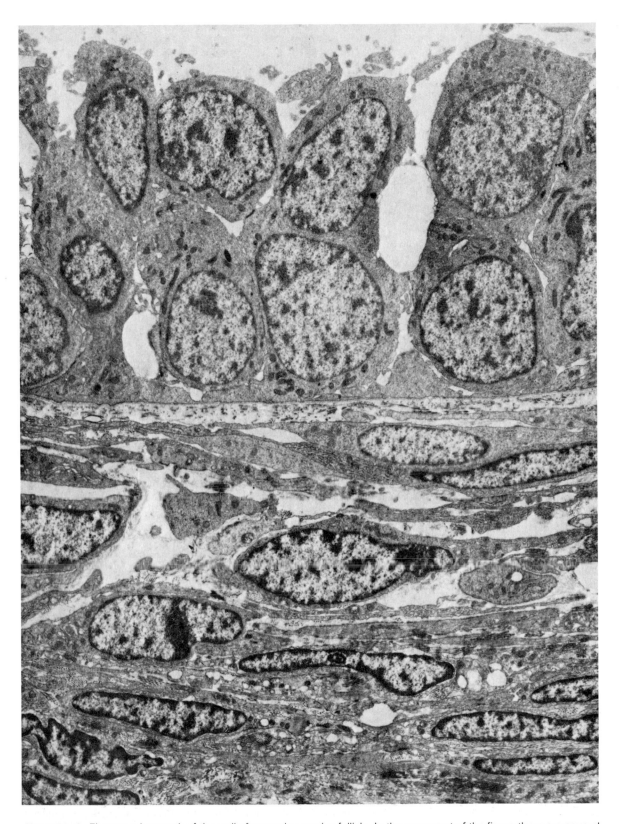

Figure 24 –6. Electron micrograph of the wall of a growing ovarian follicle. In the upper part of the figure there are several cuboidal follicular cells. A basement membrane separates these cells from the flattened cells of the theca interna. × 6400.

chromosomes typical of the species and serves as a stimulus for the ovum to complete the second meiotic division and cast off the second polar body. When fertilization does not take place, the secondary oocyte undergoes autolysis in the uterine tube without completing the second maturation division.

Corpus Luteum

After ovulation, the granulosa cells and those of the theca interna (Fig 24–6) that remain in the ovary form a temporary endocrine gland called the corpus luteum (yellow body) (Fig 24–7). The corpus luteum is localized in the cortical region of the ovary and secretes progesterone and estrogens. Progesterone prevents the development of new ovarian follicles and ovulation.

When the follicular liquid is ejected under pressure, it results in collapse of the follicle's wall so that it becomes pleated. Some blood flows out to the follicular cavity, where it coagulates and later is invaded by connective tissue cells that originate in the ovarian stroma. This connective tissue, with remnants of blood clot that are gradually removed, remains as the most central part of the corpus luteum.

The granulosa cells do not divide after ovulation. However, they increase greatly in volume and

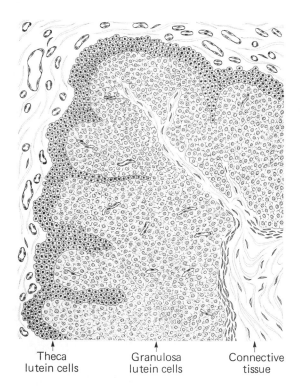

Figure 24–7. Drawing of a small portion from a corpus luteum. Lutein cells derived from the granulosa layer are larger and less darkly stained than the paralutein cells, which derive from the stroma, with some contribution likely from the theca interna.

Theca lutein cells   Granulosa lutein cells   Connective tissue

assume the characteristics of cells that secrete steroid hormones, thus becoming **granulosa lutein cells** (Fig 24–7). These cells contain lipid droplets in their cytoplasm, which, as a consequence of leaching out during dehydration, appears vacuolated in common preparations. The cytoplasm of granulosa lutein cells contains **lipochrome,** a pigment that is soluble in lipids and is responsible for the yellow color of the corpus luteum when examined in the fresh ovary.

The cells of the surrounding stroma and perhaps of the theca interna also contribute to the formation of the corpus luteum by giving rise to the **theca lutein (paralutein) cells** (Fig 24–7). These cells are similar to the lutein cells of the granulosa layer, but they are smaller, stain more darkly, and are localized at the periphery of the corpus luteum.

The granulosa lutein and the theca lutein cells show the ultrastructural organization typical of steroid-secreting cells. In humans, these cells characteristically show parallel arrays of large amounts of smooth endoplasmic reticulum, mitochondria with tubular cristae, and some flat cisternae of the granular endoplasmic reticulum (Fig 24–8).

The blood capillaries and lymphatics of the theca interna grow into the interior of the corpus luteum and form the rich vascular network of this structure.

The corpus luteum is formed by the stimulus of luteinizing hormone synthesized by the pars distalis of the pituitary under hypothalamic control. The stimulating effect of LH on progesterone secretion by the corpus luteum has been shown to be via increased formation of cAMP. In mice and rats, it was shown that prolactin (luteotropic hormone, LTH), also secreted by the pars distalis, stimulates the secretion of progesterone by the corpus luteum, but in humans this activity has not been observed. Since the progesterone produced by the corpus luteum has an inhibiting effect on the production of LH, the corpus luteum will soon degenerate unless it receives a stimulus from another source. This inhibiting effect of progesterone on luteinizing hormone production is indirect and mediated through the hypothalamus (Figs 24–9 and 24–10).

Both the brain and the pituitary may be responsive to ovarian hormones and may be either stimulated or inhibited independently during different stages of the cycle.

When pregnancy does not occur, the corpus luteum lasts only 10–14 days, ie, it persists during the second half of the menstrual cycle. After this period, as a result of the lack of luteinizing hormone, it degenerates and disappears. This is the **menstrual yellow body** or **corpus luteum spurium.**

When pregnancy occurs, the **chorionic gonadotropin** produced by the placenta will stimulate the corpus luteum, which maintains itself for about 6 months and then gradually declines but does not disappear completely and continues to

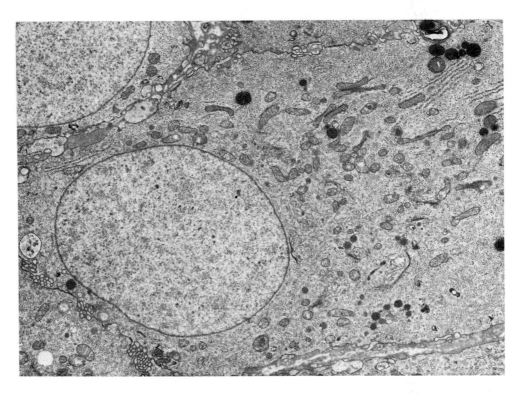

Figure 24 –8. Electron micrograph of a human luteal cell. The nucleus contains finely dispersed chromatin, without a visible nucleolus in this section. Observe the marked development of the smooth endoplasmic reticulum. There are also many elongated mitochondria. (Reproduced, with permission, from Adams EC, Hertig AT: J Cell Biol 41:696, 1969.)

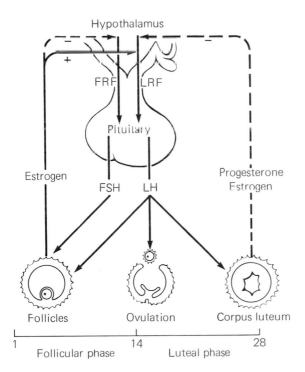

Figure 24 –9. Diagram showing the relationships of the hypothalamus, pituitary, and ovaries in the feedback mechanism regulating the secretion of hormones produced during the menstrual cycle.

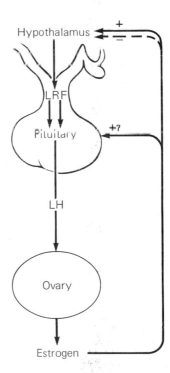

Figure 24 –10. Diagram showing the relationships of the hypothalamus, pituitary, and ovaries in the feedback mechanism regulating the secretion of luteinizing hormone and estrogen.

secrete progesterone until the end of pregnancy. This is the **gravidic yellow body** or **corpus luteum verum.** The corpus luteum of pregnancy is larger than the corpus luteum spurium, reaching a diameter of 5 cm.

The cells of the gravidic or menstrual corpus luteum that undergo degeneration disappear by autolysis, and their cellular remnants are phagocytosed by macrophages. The site is occupied by a scar of dense connective tissue forming a **corpus albicans.** The corpus albicans remains for a variable period and is gradually resorbed by the stroma. The absorption process of a corpus albicans may take months or even years and is dependent upon the size of the preexisting corpus luteum.

UTERINE TUBE
(Oviduct)

The uterine tube (oviduct or fallopian tube) is a musculomembranous tube (Fig 24–1) of great mobility measuring about 12 cm in length. One of its extremities opens into the peritoneal cavity next to the ovary; the other crosses the wall of the uterus and opens into the interior of this organ.

The oviduct is divided into 4 segments, some of which do not have clear limits. The first segment, the intramural portion (**pars interstitialis**), is situated in the interior of the uterine wall. The second segment, or **isthmus,** is formed by the portion of the tube that is adjacent to the uterus. The third is the **ampulla,** which is more dilated than the isthmus. The fourth segment, the **infundibulum,** is funnel-shaped and situated near the ovary. The free (larger) extremity of the infundibulum presents fringed extensions called **fimbriae** (Fig 24–1).

Histologic Structure

The wall of the oviduct is composed of 3 layers: a mucosa, a muscular layer, and a serosa represented by the peritoneum (Fig 24–11).

The mucosa has long longitudinal folds that are numerous in the ampulla. In cross sections, the lumen of the ampulla resembles a labyrinth (Fig 24–11). These folds become smaller in the segments of the tube that are closer to the uterus. In the intramural portion, the folds are reduced to small bulges in the lumen, so that its outline is almost regular.

The epithelium lining the mucosa is simple columnar and contains 2 types of cells. One is provided with cilia and the other is devoid of cilia and

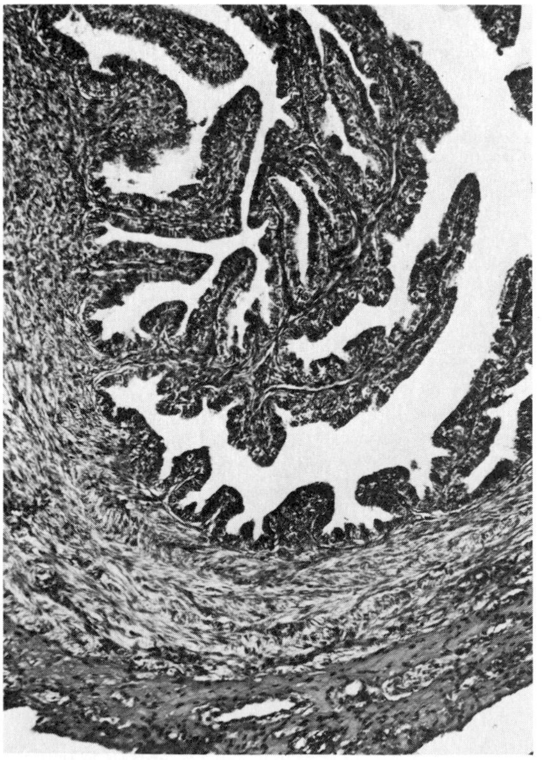

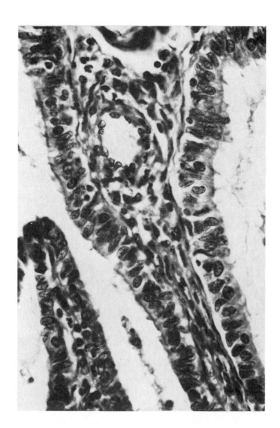

Figure 24–11. Photomicrograph of a cross section through the ampulla of the oviduct. The mucosa projects many folds into the lumen. H&E stain, × 31.

Figure 24–12. Photomicrograph of mucosa of oviduct. The section was made at the level of the ampulla. Masson's stain, × 320.

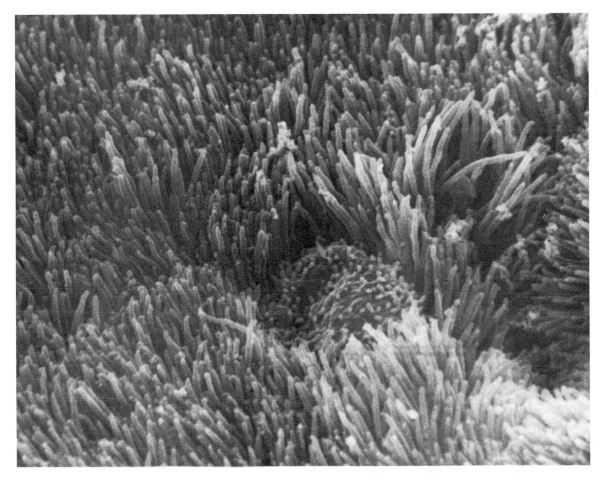

Figure 24 –13. Scanning electron micrograph of the lining of an oviduct. Observe the abundant cilia. In the middle is the apex of a secretory cell covered by short microvilli. (Courtesy of KR Porter.)

appears to be secretory (Figs 24–12 and 24–13). The 2 types of epithelial cells may be different functional states of a single cell type. Most of the cilia beat toward the uterus, causing movement of the viscous liquid film that covers its surface. This liquid consists mainly of products of secretory cells interspersed between ciliated cells. Movement of the film that covers the mucosa of the tube, in conjunction with contractions of the external muscle layer, helps to transport the oocyte or the embryo toward the uterus and hampers the passage of microorganisms from the uterus to the peritoneal cavity. However, cinematographic films of the uterine lining reveal that some cilia do beat toward the ovary. It is believed that this flow facilitates the movement of the sperm toward the unfertilized egg.

The lamina propria of the mucosa is composed of loose connective tissue. In cases of abnormal nidation, in which the embryo implants itself in the tube (ectopic pregnancy), the lamina propria reacts as the endometrium, forming numerous decidual cells.

The muscle layer is composed of smooth muscle fibers disposed in crisscrossing groups separated by abundant loose connective tissue.

Histophysiology

The oviduct receives the oocyte expelled by the ovary and carries it toward the uterus. Its lumen represents an environment adequate for fertilization, and its secretions contribute to the nutrition of the embryo during the early phases of development.

At the time of ovulation, the oviduct exhibits active movement. The fimbriae of the infundibulum move closer to the surface of the ovary, and the funnel shape of the infundibulum portion of the oviduct facilitates the recovery of the liberated oocyte.

The oviduct presents waves of rhythmic contractions, generated by its external musculature, which start at the infundibulum and are directed toward the uterus. These waves seem to be important in the movement of the ovum toward the uterus.

The wall of the oviduct is richly vascularized, and its vessels become dilated at the time of ovulation. This gives rigidity and distention to the organ, facilitating its approximation to the ovary.

Fertilization usually takes place at the ampullar-isthmic junction.

UTERUS

The uterus is a pear-shaped organ with a dilated portion, the **body,** whose upper part is the **fundus of the uterus;** and a lower cylindric part that opens into the vagina—**cervix** or **uterine neck.** The cervix bulges into the lumen of the vagina.

The wall of the uterus is relatively thick and is formed by 3 layers: in different parts of the uterus either the outer **serosa** (connective tissue and mesothelium) or **adventitia** (connective tissue); the **myometrium,** a tunic of smooth muscle; and the **endometrium,** or mucosa of the uterus.

Myometrium

Myometrium is the thickest tunic of the uterus, being composed of bundles of smooth muscle fibers separated by connective tissue. The bundles of smooth muscle form 4 layers that are not well defined. The first and the fourth are composed mainly of fibers disposed longitudinally, ie, parallel to the long axis of the organ.

During pregnancy, the myometrium goes through a period of great growth; after childbirth, it regresses to its former size. The growth is due to an increase in the number of smooth muscle fibers through division of existing smooth muscle cells and through redifferentiation of intercellular connective tissue cells into new muscle fibers as well as to hypertrophy of existing smooth muscle fibers. During pregnancy, many smooth muscle fibers have ultrastructural characteristics of protein-secreting cells and actively incorporate collagen precursors (^{3}II-proline).

After pregnancy, there is destruction of some smooth muscle fibers, reduction in size of others, and enzymatic degradation of the collagen. The uterus is reduced in size almost to its prepregnancy dimensions. The connective tissue consists of collagen fibers, fibroblasts, macrophages, and mast cells. An elastic network and some reticular fibers are also present.

Endometrium

The endometrium consists of epithelium and lamina propria containing simple tubular glands that sometimes branch in their deeper portions (near the myometrium). Its epithelial cells are simple columnar and are a mixture of ciliated and secretory cells. The epithelium of the uterine glands is similar to the superficial epithelium, but ciliated cells are more rare in the glands.

The connective tissue of the lamina propria is rich in cells and contains abundant amorphous intercellular material. Connective tissue fibers are rare, which makes this tissue somewhat similar to mesenchyme. Special **coiled arteries** nourish the endometrium.

The endometrial layer can be subdivided into 2 zones: (1) the **functionalis,** which constitutes that portion sloughed off at menstruation and replaced during each menstrual cycle; and (2) the **basalis,** that portion of the endometrium retained during menstruation which subsequently provides new epithelium and lamina propria for the renewal of the endometrium. The bases of the uterine glands, which lie deep within the basalis, are the source of the stem cells that divide and provide for the new epithelial lining of the uterus after menstruation.

The Menstrual Cycle

The action of ovarian hormones (estrogens and progesterone) under the stimulus of the anterior lobe of the pituitary causes the endometrium to undergo cyclic structural modifications that constitute the menstrual cycle. Duration of the menstrual cycle is variable but averages 28 days.

Menstrual cycles start usually between 12 and 15 years of age and continue until about age 45–50. Since menstrual cycles are a consequence of ovarian modifications related to the production of ova, the female is fertile only during the years when she is having menstrual cycles. This does not mean that sexual activity is terminated by menopause—only that fertility ceases.

For practical purposes, the beginning of the menstrual cycle is taken as the day when menstrual bleeding appears. The menstrual discharge consists of endometrium that is partially destroyed and desquamated and mixed with blood from the degenerating vessels. The **menstrual phase** is defined as the first to the fourth days of the cycle; the **proliferative phase** is the fifth to the 14th days; and the **secretory phase** is the 15th to the 28th days. The duration of each phase is variable, and the intervals given are only estimates.

The functional sequence of the menstrual cycle will be described in the following order: proliferative phase, secretory or luteal phase, and menstrual phase.*

A. Proliferative Phase: After the menstrual phase, the uterine mucosa is reduced to a small band of connective tissue containing the basal portion of the glands but without their upper part and the epithelial lining. This residual part of the endometrium, which does not peel off during menstruation, is the **basal layer;** the portion that is destroyed and renewed in each cycle is the **functional layer.**

The proliferative phase is the **estrogenic phase**

---

*The structural changes that occur during the menstrual cycle are gradual; the clear division of the phases implied in the text has mainly teaching value.

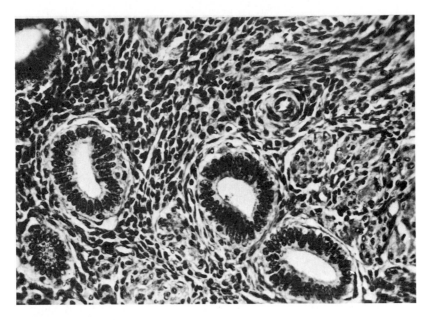

Figure 24–14. Endometrium in the proliferative phase. The epithelial cells of the gland are usually organized as a simple columnar lining, although during the active proliferation phase, the lining may assume a pseudostratified appearance. H&E stain, × 320.

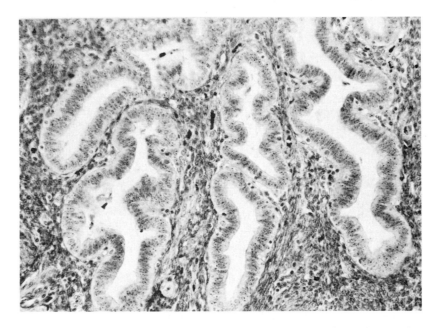

Figure 24–15. Endometrium in the secretory phase (21st day of the menstrual cycle). Uterine glands are tortuous, with lumens dilated by accumulation of secretory material. H&E stain, × 224.

because it coincides with development of ovarian follicles and with production of estrogens.

The cells in the fundi of the glands proliferate and reconstitute the glands and epithelial lining of the endometrium. Cellular proliferation continues during the entire proliferative phase, and mitoses are observed both in the cells of the epithelial lining and in the glands (Fig 24–14). Proliferation of the connective cells of the lamina propria also occurs, with consequent growth of the endometrium as a whole.

At the end of the proliferative phase, the glands appear straight, with narrow lumens, and their cells begin to accumulate glycogen in a subnuclear position. The coiled arteries are elongated and convoluted.

B. Secretory or Luteal Phase: This phase starts after ovulation and depends upon the formation of corpus luteum, which secretes progesterone. Acting upon the glands already developed by the action of the estrogens, the progesterone stimulates the gland cells to secrete.

The glands become tortuous as the lumens are dilated by the secretion that accumulates in their interiors. In this phase, the endometrium reaches its maximum thickness (5 mm) as a result of the accumulation of secretions and edema of the stroma. Mitoses are rare during the secretory phase (Fig 24–15). The elongation and convolution of the coiled arteries continue and extend into the superficial portion of the endometrium.

C. Menstrual Phase: When fertilization of the ovum expelled by the ovary fails to occur, nidation does not occur and the levels of estrogens and progesterone in the blood fall suddenly. The endometrium developed in response to the stimulus of these hormones undergoes involution and is partially destroyed.

At the end of the secretory phase, the walls of the coiled arteries contract, closing off blood flow and producing ischemia, which leads to death (necrosis) of the endothelium. At this stage, desquamation of the endometrium and rupture of blood vessels above the constrictions take place and bleeding begins.

The endometrium becomes partially detached. The amount lost is variable in different women and even in the same woman at different times. At the end of the menstrual phase, the endometrium is almost always reduced to nothing but the basal layer, containing the blind ends of the endometrial glands. At that time, the surface of the endometrium is entirely deprived of its lining. Proliferation of the gland cells and their migration to the surface begin the proliferative phase, restarting the cycle.

Uterine Cervix

As previously noted, the **cervix** is the lower, cylindric part of the uterus. This portion differs in histologic structure from the rest of the uterus. It has few smooth muscle fibers and a large quantity of connective tissue.

The mucosa of the cervix contains the mucous **cervical glands,** which are extensively branched. This mucosa does not desquamate during menstruation, although its glands undergo small variations in their structure during the menstrual cycle. When blocking of the ducts of these glands occurs, the retained secretion causes a dilatation that gives rise to **nabothian cysts.**

During pregnancy, the cervical mucous glands proliferate and secrete a more viscous and more abundant mucus.

The external aspect of the cervix that bulges into the lumen of the vagina is lined by stratified squamous epithelium.

Cervical secretions play a significant role in fertilization of the oocyte. During ovulation, the mucous secretions are watery and allow penetration of sperm into the uterus. In the luteal phase or in pregnancy, the progesterone levels influence the mucous secretions so that they become more viscous and prevent the passage of microorganisms, as well as sperm, into the body of the uterus. As a consequence, the cervical secretions are able to provide a barrier to the passage of materials into the uterus.

IMPLANTATION

The human oocyte is fertilized at the ampullar-isthmic junction of the oviduct, and cleavage of the ovum occurs as it moves passively toward the uterus. Through successive mitoses, a compact collection of cells, the **morula,** covered by the zona pellucida is formed (Fig 24–16). Formation of this structure is followed by the appearance on the surface of special regions where the cells come into contact with each other. These regions are smoother than the rest of the surface, which continues to be covered with microvilli. During this period, the fertilized ovum does not increase in size (Fig 24–16) and is contained by the zona pellucida. The cells that result from segmentation of the fertilized ovum are called **blastomeres.**

A cavity at the central part of the morula appears as a result of the gradual accumulation of liquid transferred from the lumen of the oviduct; the cells form a fluid-filled sphere, the **blastocyst.** The blastomeres separated by this liquid arrange themselves in a peripheral layer (**trophoblast**) that is thickened at one point where a collection of cells remains (**inner cell mass**) and bulges into the cavity. This is the phase of the blastocyst and corresponds approximately to the fourth or fifth day after ovulation. At this time, the embryo reaches the uterus. For 1 or 2 days, the blastocyst remains in the lumen of the uterus and comes into contact with the surface of the endometrium, immersed in the secretion of the endometrial glands.

In the blastocyst phase, the zona pellucida becomes thinner and disappears, allowing cells of the trophoblast, which have the capacity to invade the mucosa, to come into direct contact with the endometrium. Immediately thereafter, the cells of the trophoblast begin to multiply, thus ensuring, with the help of the endometrium, the nourishment of the embryo. The inner cell mass, from which the body of the embryo will originate, grows slightly during this phase.

Implantation or **nidation** involves penetration through the uterine epithelium, with little sign of necrosis (Fig 24–17). This type of **interstitial** implantation occurs exclusively in humans and some other animals. The process starts around the sixth

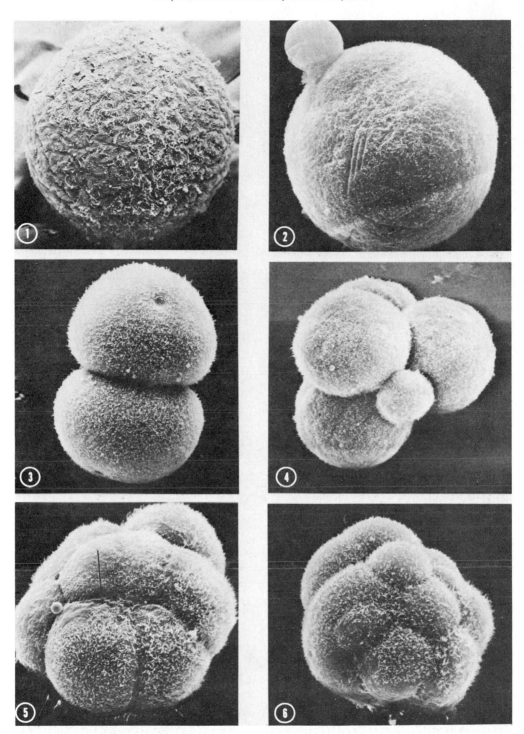

Figure 24 –16. Scanning electron microscopic photographs of the surface of an oocyte after fertilization and up to the stage of a morula. The zona pellucida has been digested with pronase. *(1)* The primary oocyte of the mouse shortly after its release from an ovarian follicle. The oocyte has an intact germinal vesicle at this stage. × 1380. *(2)* Fertilized egg. Note the microvillous surface of the egg and the smooth surface of the first polar body. × 1300. *(3)* Two-cell stage evenly covered with microvilli. × 1320. *(4)* Four-cell stage with microvillous second polar body. × 1870. *(5)* Eight-cell stage. Note smoother regions of membrane where cells come into contact (arrow). × 1400. *(6)* Morula of the mouse. Microvilli are quite numerous, particularly in the area of cell contact. × 1540. (Reproduced, with permission, from Calarco P: Mammalian preimplantation development. In: *Scanning Electron Microscopy Atlas of Mammalian Reproduction.* Hafez ESE [editor]. Igaku Shoin Ltd, 1975.)

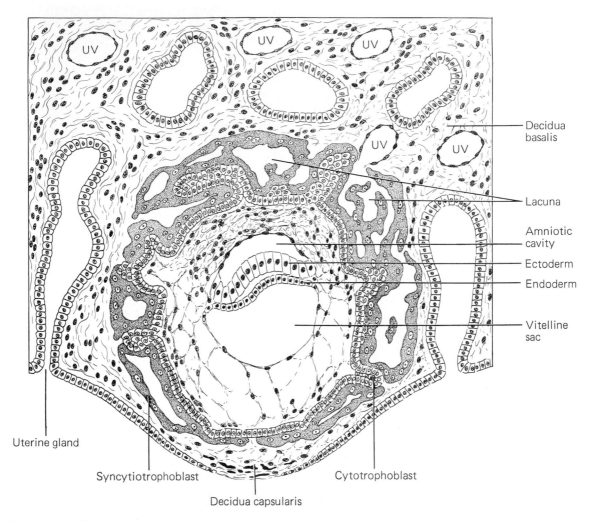

Uterine gland

Syncytiotrophoblast

Decidua capsularis

Cytotrophoblast

Decidua basalis

Lacuna

Amniotic cavity

Ectoderm

Endoderm

Vitelline sac

Figure 24–17. Schematic drawing of a human embryo at 12 days, showing the relationships between the embryo and the endometrium (which after implantation is called the decidua). UV, uterine vessels, one of which opens into a lacuna, filling those spaces with blood.

day, and on about the ninth day after ovulation the embryo is totally submerged in the endometrium from which it will receive protection and nourishment during pregnancy.

Implantation takes place when the endometrium is in the secretory phase. The uterine glands contain glycoproteins and glycogen. The vessels are dilated and the lamina propria slightly swollen. The endometrium at that point is 5 mm thick.

During implantation, the trophoblast differentiates into 2 layers, the **syncytiotrophoblast** and the **cytotrophoblast** (Figs 24–17 and 24–18). The former, an external layer, has many large nuclei as a result of the fusion of mononucleated cytotrophoblasts; and its cytoplasm is continuous, forming a syncytium. The cytotrophoblast consists of an irregular layer of mononucleated ovoid cells immediately under the syncytiotrophoblast.

The surface of the syncytiotrophoblast contains irregular microvilli, and the superficial cytoplasm contains several vesicles delimited by smooth membranes. This suggests the existence of an intense process of pinocytosis in the syncytiotrophoblast, possibly related to the transference of material from the maternal circulation to the fetus. More deeply, the cytoplasm of the syncytiotrophoblast shows an abundance of both granular and smooth endoplasmic reticulum, a developed Golgi apparatus, and numerous mitochondria. These ultrastructural characteristics are consistent with the role presently attributed to the syncytiotrophoblast in the secretion of chorionic gonadotropin (a glycoprotein hormone), placental lactogen (a protein hormone), and estrogen and progesterone (steroids). The syncytiotrophoblast contains lipid droplets whose composition (as determined by cytochemical methods) is compatible with the presence of steroids.

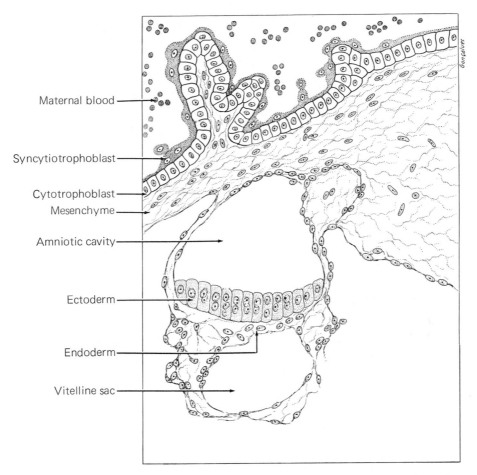

Figure 24–18. Human embryo at 15 days. At upper left is shown a chorionic villus protruding into a lacuna containing maternal blood.

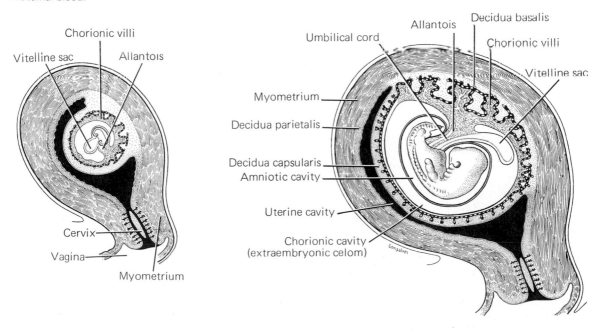

Figure 24–19. Schematic drawings showing formation of the 3 regions of decidua and the chorionic villi.

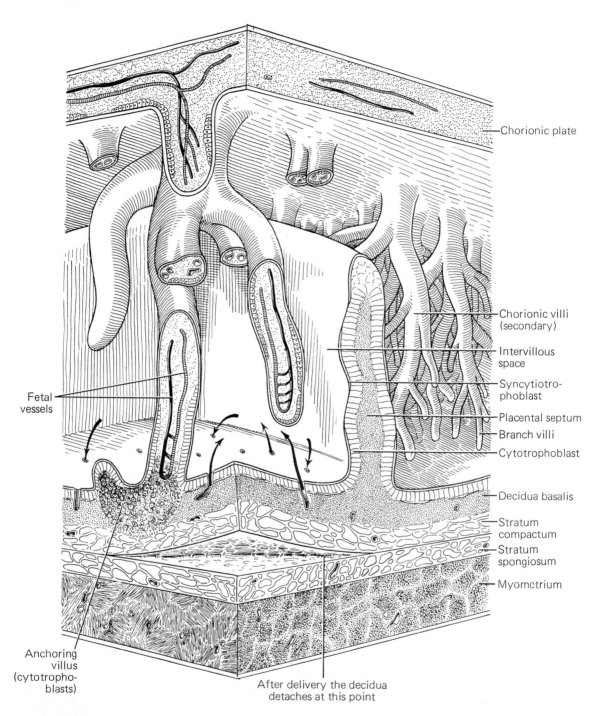

Chorionic plate

Chorionic villi
(secondary)

Intervillous
space

Syncytiotro-
phoblast

Placental septum

Branch villi

Cytotrophoblast

Decidua basalis

Stratum
compactum

Stratum
spongiosum

Myometrium

Fetal
vessels

Anchoring
villus (cytotropho-
blasts)

After delivery the decidua
detaches at this point

Figure 24 –20. Schematic drawing of placental structure. Arrows indicate the blood flow from decidual arteries to intervillous space and back to decidual veins. This direction is determined by the difference in pressure between arterial and venous blood. (Redrawn and reproduced, with permission, from Duplessis GDT, Haegel P: *Embryologie.* Masson, 1971. [English edition © Springer-Verlag, 1972; Chapman & Hall, 1972; Masson, 1972.])

The syncytiotrophoblasts delineate extracytoplasmic cavities. These cavities increase in size and communicate with one another, conferring a spongy structure (Fig 24–17). Thus, **lacunas** are formed, lined with syncytiotrophoblast. On the other hand, the lytic activity of the syncytiotrophoblast causes the rupture of both arterial and venous blood vessels, with overflow of blood into these lacunar spaces. The direction of blood flow in the lacunar spaces is due to the difference in pressure between arterial and venous vessels. Blood flows from the arterial vessels to these spaces and from there to the veins.

After implantation of the embryo, the endometrium goes through profound changes and is called **decidua;** and cells of the stroma become enlarged and polygonal. The decidua can be divided into **decidua basalis,** situated between the embryo and the myometrium; **decidua capsularis,** between the embryo and the lumen of the uterus; and **decidua parietalis,** which is the remainder of the decidua (Fig 24–19).

The trophoblast in contact with the decidua capsularis develops only to a slight extent since its nutrition is deficient. Growth of the trophoblast in the part of the embryo facing the myometrium is assured by the maternal blood, and its growth is exuberant. From this part of the trophoblast, elongated projections, **primary villi,** are formed. Their main characteristic is that they are composed only of internal cytotrophoblasts and an external syncytiotrophoblast lining early in pregnancy. During this stage of embryonic development, an extraembryonic mesenchyme appears before the intraembryonic one and contributes to the formation of the fetal membranes and placenta. The extraembryonic mesenchyme plus the trophoblast form the **chorion.** On the side of the **decidua capsularis,** the chorion develops to a very slight extent (**smooth chorion** or **chorion laeve**); on the side of the decidua basalis, the chorion grows extensively and forms the **chorion frondosum.** The layers of the chorion (beginning at the surface) are (1) syncytiotrophoblast, (2) cytotrophoblast, and (3) extraembryonic mesenchyme.

The mesenchyme, when it penetrates into the primary villi, transforms them into **secondary villi** (Fig 24–20). Within the villi, vessels are formed gradually and later will join those formed in the body of the embryo, establishing a circulation and thus allowing exchange of substances and gases between the fetal and maternal blood (Fig 24–20).

PLACENTA

The placenta is a temporary organ found only in eutherian mammals at the site where the physiologic exchanges between the mother and the fetus occur. It consists of a fetal part (chorion) and a maternal part (decidua basalis).

The placenta is the only organ composed of cells derived from 2 different individuals.

Fetal Part

The fetal part of the placenta consists of the chorion. It has a **chorionic plate** at the point where

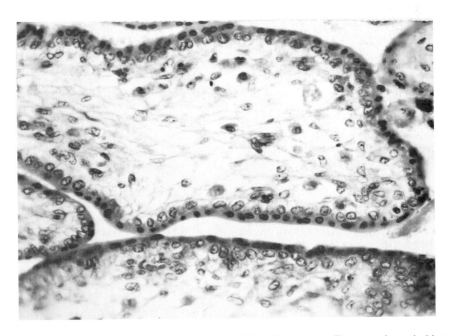

Figure 24–21. Photomicrograph of a chorionic villus in the second half of pregnancy. The syncytiotrophoblast is continuous. H&E stain, × 320.

the **chorionic villi** start—the secondary villi already described. These villi consist of a connective tissue core derived from the extraembryonic mesenchyme surrounded by the syncytiotrophoblast and the cytotrophoblast (Fig 24–21). The syncytiotrophoblast remains until the end of pregnancy, but the cytotrophoblast disappears gradually during the second half of pregnancy. The cytotrophoblasts undergo extensive proliferation and concomitant fusion during early placentation. However, in the second half of pregnancy, proliferation slows down, yet fusion continues, which results in a loss of the cytotrophoblasts since they contribute their cell mass to the growing syncytium.

The chorionic villi can be either free or anchored into the decidua basalis. Both have the same structure, but the free ones do not reach the decidua, whereas the anchored chorionic villi become embedded within the decidua basalis. The surface of the villi is bathed with blood from the lacunas of the basal decidua and is the site where the exchange of substances between fetal and maternal blood occurs.

Maternal Part

The maternal part of the placenta—the decidua basalis—supplies arterial blood for the lacunas situated between the secondary villi and receives venous blood from these lacunas. Although the maternal blood vessels are opened during implantation, the fetal vessels contained in the secondary villi remain intact. Fetal blood and maternal blood do not mix except occasionally at the end of pregnancy, when the cytotrophoblast is no longer continuous, the capillaries of the villi are close to the surface, and a very slight exchange of blood cells may occur. At that time, the walls of the fetal capillaries are separated from the maternal blood only by the syncytiotrophoblast. Ruptures of the capillaries are not rare at this time, with a consequent mixture of fetal and maternal blood.

In the borderlines of the placenta, the decidua basalis is firmly united to the chorion by the **marginal zone.** This zone follows the outline of the placenta.

During pregnancy, cells from the connective tissue of the decidua basalis and a lesser number of cells from the decidua parietalis form the **decidual cells.** These large cells have a vacuolated cytoplasm that contains glycogen and lipids and a clear nucleus with a prominent nucleolus. Decidual cells are more numerous during the first half of pregnancy. Although they represent a substantial population, the function of the decidual cells is unknown.

At the end of pregnancy, the placenta has the shape of a disk. The umbilical cord usually starts from the center of the placenta and forms a communication between the fetal and placental circulations.

Histophysiology

Fetal venous blood reaches the placenta through the 2 umbilical arteries, which branch and continue with the vessels of the chorionic villi. In these villi, the fetal blood is oxygenated, loses its CO_2, and returns to the fetus through the umbilical vein.

Since the chorionic villi are submerged in maternal blood, the fetal blood remains isolated by the following structures that form the **placental barrier:** (1) the walls of the fetal capillaries, (2) the basal lamina of the capillaries and of the trophoblast, (3) the mesenchyme in the interior of the villus, (4) the cytotrophoblast (during the first half of pregnancy), and (5) the syncytiotrophoblast.

The placenta is permeable to several substances, and normally it transfers oxygen, water, electrolytes, carbohydrates, lipids, proteins, vitamins, hormones, antibodies, and some drugs from maternal blood to fetal blood. From the fetal blood to the maternal blood it transfers CO_2, water, hormones, and residual products of metabolism.

The placenta is also an endocrine organ that elaborates chorionic gonadotropin, estrogen, progesterone, one or possibly 2 substances with thyrotropic activity, renin, and relaxin. It also secretes a protein hormone called human placental lactogen (HPL), which has lactogenic and growth-stimulating activity. All of these hormones seem to be synthesized by the syncytiotrophoblast. Even the gonadotropin, whose synthesis was attributed to the cytotrophoblast—because at the end of pregnancy the level of gonadotropin decreases when the cells of the cytotrophoblast almost disappear—is today considered to be a product of the syncytiotrophoblast. Examination of sections of placenta treated with fluorescent antigonadotropin antibody shows fluorescence in the syncytiotrophoblast but not in cytotrophoblasts.

Radioautographic studies after injection of radioactive thymidine show that the cells of the cytotrophoblast multiply actively and incorporate themselves into the syncytiotrophoblast. This indicates that the syncytiotrophoblast grows as a result of growth and mitotic activity of the cytotrophoblast.

VAGINA

The wall of the vagina is devoid of glands and presents 3 layers: a **mucosa,** a **muscular layer,** and a **fibrous layer.** The mucus found in the lumen of the vagina comes from the glands of the uterine cervix.

The epithelium of the mucous layer is stratified squamous and has a thickness of 150–200 μm. Its cells may contain a certain amount of keratohyalin. However, intense keratinization with change of the cells into keratin plates, as in typical keratinized

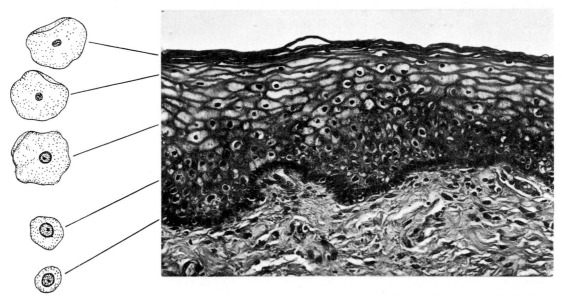

Figure 24 –22. Photomicrograph of a section of vaginal mucosa and drawings of the cells found in various epithelial layers. Masson's stain, × 250.

epithelia, does not occur (Fig 24–22). Under the stimulus of estrogen, the vaginal epithelium synthesizes and accumulates a large quantity of glycogen, which is thrown into the lumen of the vagina when the vaginal cells desquamate or peel off. Bacteria in the vagina metabolize glycogen and form lactic acid, which is responsible for the usually low pH of the vagina.

The lamina propria of the vaginal mucosa is composed of loose connective tissue that is very rich in elastic fibers. Among the cells present, one can find lymphocytes and neutrophils in relatively large quantities. During certain phases of the menstrual cycle, these 2 types of leukocytes usually invade the epithelium and pass into the lumen of the vagina. The glandless lamina propria exhibits a rich vascularization which is the source of the fluid exudate that seeps through the squamous epithelium during sexual stimulation. The vaginal mucosa is virtually devoid of sensory nerve endings, and the few naked nerve endings that do exist are probably pain fibers.

The muscular layer of the vagina is composed mainly of longitudinal bundles of smooth muscle fibers. There are some circular bundles, especially in the innermost part (next to the mucosa).

Outside the muscular layer, a coat of dense connective tissue, the **adventitial coat,** rich in thick elastic fibers, unites the vagina with the surrounding tissues. The great elasticity of the vagina is related to the large number of elastic fibers in the connective tissues of its wall. In this connective tissue are an extensive venous plexus, nerve bundles, and groups of nerve cells.

EXTERNAL GENITALIA

The female external genitalia or vulvae consist of the **clitoris, labia minora, labia majora,** and certain glands that open into the vestibulum, a space enclosed by the labia minora.

The urethra and the ducts of the vestibular glands open into this portion of the vagina. The 2 **glandulae vestibulares majores,** or **glands of Bartholin,** are situated one on each side of the vestibulum; the **glandulae vestibulares minores** are more numerous and scattered, occurring with greater frequency around the urethra and clitoris. All of the glandulae vestibulares are of the mucous type.

Both in embryonic origin and in histologic structure, the clitoris can be thought of as a rudimentary and incomplete penis. It is formed by 2 erectile bodies ending in a rudimentary **glans clitoridis** and a prepuce. The clitoris is lined by stratified squamous epithelium.

The labia minora are folds of skin with a core of spongy connective tissue permeated by elastic fibers. The stratified squamous epithelium which lines them has cells with melanin and has a thin keratinized layer on the surface, and sebaceous and sweat glands are present on both surfaces.

The labia majora are folds of skin and contain a large quantity of adipose tissue and a thin layer of smooth muscle. Their inner aspect has a histologic structure similar to that of the labia minora. The external surface is covered by skin and coarse, curly hair. Sebaceous and sweat glands are numerous on both surfaces.

The external genitalia are abundantly supplied

with sensory tactile nerve endings including Meissner and pacinian corpuscles, which contribute to the physiology of sexual arousal.

ENDOCRINE INTERRELATIONSHIPS

Female reproductive function is regulated through certain nuclei of the hypothalamus. Nerve cells in the hypothalamus produce and introduce into the blood specific polypeptides that act on the anterior lobe of the pituitary and liberate gonadotropins; these gonadotropins in turn stimulate the secretion of ovarian hormones (estrogens and progesterone) (Fig 24–23). The hypothalamic localization of the ovarian hormone control mechanism might explain why strong, nonspecific cerebral stimuli occasionally affect reproductive function— "boarding school amenorrhea," pseudocyesis, etc. Similar results have been obtained experimentally.

The developing ovarian follicle synthesizes es-

trogens, and the corpus luteum synthesizes estrogens and progesterone. The main source of the estrogens in the developing follicle seems to be the cells of the theca interna. Recent evidence suggests that these cells release testosterone, which is subsequently modified by the granulosa cells that convert this steroid into estradiol.

The principal estrogen isolated from the ovary is estradiol-17β; in the blood, estrone is the predominant circulating hormone, secreted directly in small amounts by the ovary and accumulated in the circulation by metabolism of estradiol and androstenedione. Estrone is further metabolized to estriol, probably in the liver. Estradiol is the most potent estrogen of the three.

The pituitary gonadotropins, follicle-stimulating hormone (FSH) and luteinizing hormone (LH), are produced under the control of "releasing factors" liberated by the hypothalamus. FSH stimulates the growth of the ovarian follicles and the formation of estrogens. It is important to note that at any particular time in the cycle, the ovary possesses follicles in all stages of growth. The release of FSH

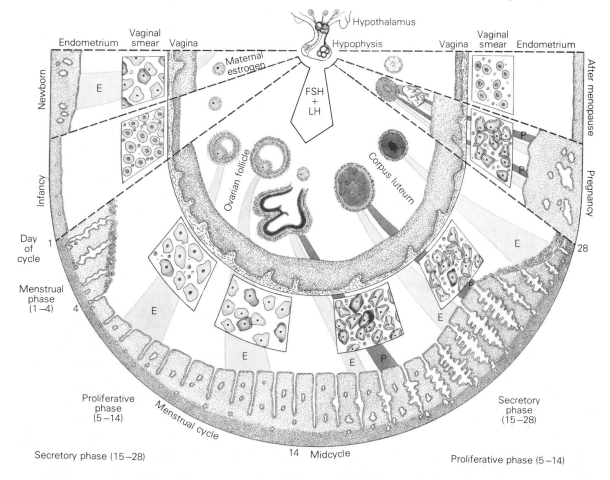

Figure 24 –23. Functional changes relating to the hypothalamus, pituitary, ovary, vaginal epithelium, and endometrium. E, estrogen; P, progesterone. (Modified and redrawn from FH Netter, MD.)

does not promote the formation of a graafian follicle from a primordial follicle during one cycle. The most immediate effect of FSH is probably the maturation of existing late secondary or tertiary follicles. LH promotes the formation of the corpus luteum through differentiation of granulosa cells that remain in the follicle after expulsion of the oocyte (Fig 24-23).

The ovary also acts on the pituitary directly and through the hypothalamus. Estrogen appears to inhibit the secretion of FSH and stimulate the secretion of LH. The production of LH is inhibited by progesterone. Just prior to mid cycle, estrogen secretion reaches a peak and causes a brief surge of LH. Luteinizing hormone promotes ovulation, maturation of the oocyte, and formation of the corpus luteum. In most mammals other than humans, **prolactin (luteotropic hormone, LTH)** is necessary for the maintenance of corpus luteum. As the secretion of LH is inhibited by progesterone produced by the corpus luteum, this structure is soon deprived of the pituitary stimulus (LH) necessary for its functioning and consequently degenerates.

When fecundation and nidation occur, the chorion synthesizes the chorionic gonadotropins that stimulate and maintain the function of the corpus luteum during pregnancy.

In rats and mice, the corpus luteum is sensitive to prolactin. In these species, prolactin stimulates the secretion of an already formed corpus luteum. There is no evidence that prolactin has any influence on human corpus luteum. In humans, prolactin initiates and maintains milk secretion by mammary glands already stimulated by estrogen, progesterone, corticosteroids, and insulin.

The Menstrual Cycle

The menstrual cycle is under the control of ovarian and pituitary hormones. The proliferative phase corresponds to the period during which—under the action of follicle-stimulating hormone—the developing follicle is synthesizing estrogens that stimulate the growth of the uterine mucosa. The secretory phase of the menstrual cycle occurs when the ovary is secreting both estrogens and progesterone (Fig 24-23).

Data now available allow us to assume that menstruation is a consequence of the decline of estrogens and progesterone. There are 2 peaks in the production of estrogens during the menstrual cycle; on the 13th and on the 21st days of the cycle. The former, which is reached after a gradual elevation in the level of estrogen, can be explained by the growth of the follicle that reaches its maximum on the 13th day. The latter is due to the production of estrogens by the corpus luteum. The production of progesterone increases gradually after ovulation as a consequence of formation of the corpus luteum; it then declines around the 26th day of the cycle.

EXFOLIATIVE CYTOLOGY

Exfoliative cytology is the study of the characteristics of cells that normally desquamate from various surfaces of the body. Cytologic examination of vaginal mucosa gives important data on hormonal balance and allows early detection of some types of cancer of the female genital system.

The cells to be examined are taken from the vagina with the secretion contained there; they are spread on a slide, fixed, and stained by special technics such as the Shorr trichrome technic, acridine orange, etc. Cells from the epithelium of the vagina predominate in this type of preparation.

In the fully mature vaginal mucosa, 5 types of cells are easily identifiable: (1) cells of the internal portion of the basal layer (called basal cells), (2) cells of the external portion of the basal layer (called parabasal cells), (3) cells of the intermediate layers, (4) precornified cells, and (5) cornified cells (Figs 24-22 and 24-23).

Under the stimulus of estrogens, the vaginal epithelium becomes thicker, with a larger number of cellular layers. Partial keratinization of the most superficial cells also occurs. The superficial keratinized cells are characterized by a dense, shrunken (pyknotic) nucleus and an acidophilic cytoplasm (keratin is an acidophilic protein). These cells predominate in the smears of estrogen-stimulated vaginal secretions. They have the shape of a plate since they represent the most superficial elements of stratified squamous epithelium. This aspect is so characteristic of the action of the estrogens that the percentage of acidophilic cells in a smear is a reliable index of estrogenic stimulation. Cytologic smears reveal not only quantitative changes in estrogen but also the effect of progesterone. In the normal menstrual cycle, by day 6 most of the cells are from the intermediate layer, polygonal in shape, and contain basophilic cytoplasm. At the time of ovulation, under the influence of estrogen, most of the cells are from the precornified layer but 20% or more are fully cornified cells. By day 20, the influence of progesterone in addition to estrogen can be clearly noted. There is an increased number of desquamated cells of the intermediate type. In contrast to the clearly outlined and separated cells of the proliferative phase, during the secretory phase a loss of cellular outline and clumping can be seen. Almost all of the cells have again become basophilic.

The above characteristics of the progesterone effect are more prominent during pregnancy.

Hormonal deficiency during menopause causes the vaginal epithelium to be thin, with no keratinized cells. The vaginal smear cells are mainly spherical, basal or parabasal cells with basophilic cytoplasm whose large nuclei present dispersed chromatin. The same type of vaginal smear is obtained during the prepubertal state.

Internal basal cells—those from the deepest layer of the vaginal epithelium—rarely peel off. This does happen after childbirth but is not due to the trauma caused by expulsion of the fetus, as one might suppose, because it occurs as well in women who have had abdominal deliveries (cesarean operation). The internal basal cells appear on the smear as a result of the intense peeling off of the vaginal epithelium that occurs after delivery, which in turn is a consequence of the sudden decline of the hormonal levels of the placenta and ovaries. These cells are small, spherical, and basophilic and present large nuclei with dispersed chromatin (Fig 24–22).

MAMMARY GLANDS

Each mammary gland comprises 15–25 irregular lobes of the compound tubulo-alveolar type whose function is to secrete milk to nourish newborns (Fig 24–24). Each lobe is separated from the others by dense connective tissue and much adipose tissue and is really a gland in itself with its own excretory duct. These excretory **lactiferous**

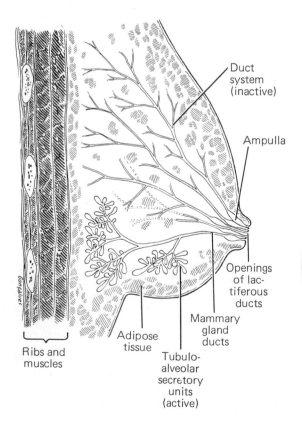

Figure 24 –24. Schematic drawing of female breast showing the mammary glands with ducts that open in the nipple.

ducts, 2–4.5 cm long, emerge independently in the **mammary papilla,** or nipple, which has 15–25 openings, each about 0.5 mm in diameter.

The interlobar connective tissue penetrates each lobe, dividing it into lobules. This connective tissue also surrounds and supports each secretory unit.

The histologic structure of the mammary glands varies according to sex, age, and physiologic status.

Embryonic Breast Development

The mammary gland appears in a human embryo of 8 mm as a thickening of the epidermis, the "milk line." It continues to thicken and becomes the mammary fold. In the course of time, these epithelial thickenings become spherical or club-shaped, with cylindric and polyhedral cells. By continuing to multiply, they form projections with swellings at their ends. These projections gradually grow in the direction of the connective tissue and become the mammary ducts. Most of the "milk line" degenerates subsequently.

In newborns of both sexes, the glands have a diameter of 3.5–9 mm and contain distinct alveoli. Differentiation and secretion of milk by neonatal alveoli is not unusual since these glands are affected by placental and maternal estrogens. In females, the development continues and, with the onset of sexual maturity, increases in intensity and quantity.

Breast Development During Puberty

Before puberty, the mammary glands are composed of lactiferous sinuses and ramified lactiferous ducts that have small cellular aggregates in their extremities.

The development of mammary glands in females during puberty constitutes one of the secondary sex characteristics. During this period, the mammary glands increase in size and develop a prominent nipple. In males, they remain flattened.

Breast enlargement during puberty is the result of 2 growth processes: (1) increase in volume of the lactiferous ducts, promoted by cell proliferation; and (2) accumulation of adipose tissue in both interlobar and interlobular connective tissue. Proliferation of the lactiferous ducts and accumulation of fat are due to an increase in the amount of ovarian hormones during puberty. During this stage, the formation of small tubulo-alveolar structures can be observed in the extremities of the ducts.

Breast Development in Adult Women

The adult mammary glands are composed of **lactiferous ducts** and tubulo-alveolar secretory glands. Near the opening of the papilla, the lactiferous ducts dilate to form the **lactiferous sinuses** or **ampullae** (Fig 24–24).

The lactiferous ducts are lined by squamous stratified epithelium near their external openings. Deeper in the gland the epithelium becomes progressively thinner, with fewer cell layers, until there are only 2 layers of cuboidal or low columnar cells. Closer to the secretory portions of the gland—the alveolar ducts and alveoli—the epithelium becomes simple cuboidal, resting on a basal lamina and a discontinuous layer of myoepithelial cell processes. In the connective tissue surrounding the alveoli are large numbers of lymphocytes and plasma cells. At the time of lactation, the plasma cell population increases significantly and is responsible for the synthesis and release of immunoglobulins (IgA) that are released into the milk and confer passive immunity to the newborn.

During the menstrual cycle, small alterations in the histologic structure of these glands are observed, ie, proliferation of the ducts and the secretory parts at about the time of ovulation. This coincides with the period during which circulating estrogen is at its peak. Growth of adipocytes because of increased lipid accumulations and greater hydration of connective tissue in the premenstrual phase produce breast enlargement. Division of the mammary glands into lobules is also accentuated.

The mammary papilla or nipple has a cylindroconical shape. In color it may be light brown, dark brown, or black. Externally, it is covered by keratinized stratified squamous epithelium which is continuous with that of the adjacent skin.

The epithelium of the mammary papilla rests on a layer of connective tissue rich in smooth muscle fibers. These fibers are disposed in circles around the lactiferous ducts and parallel to them where they cross the papilla and open separately in the apex of the papilla.

During puberty, the mammary papillae become more prominent.

The skin around the papilla constitutes the areola. The color of the areola changes from rose to dark brown during pregnancy owing to a local accumulation of melanin. After delivery, it may become lighter in color but never returns to its original shade.

The Breasts During Pregnancy

The mammary glands undergo intense growth during pregnancy as a result of proliferation and ramification of the lactiferous ducts with a consequent active production of secretory tubules and alveoli. The connective stroma and the adipose tissue decrease considerably. Despite this great growth process, there are no visible signs of secretion until late in pregnancy (Fig 24–25).

Growth of the mammary glands during pregnancy occurs as a result of the synergistic action of several hormones, mainly estrogen, progesterone, prolactin, and placental mammotropic hormone. The estrogen acts upon the lactiferous ducts, stimulating their growth by increasing the number of mitoses and causing ramification to occur. Progesterone stimulates the growth of the secretory parts of the mammary glands.

During pregnancy, the quantity of estrogen increases since this hormone is also produced by the placenta. The amount of progesterone also increases, as this steroid is produced first by the corpus luteum (which remains during pregnancy) and later by the placenta.

In hypophysectomized animals, estrogen and progesterone have no effect upon the mammary glands. The pituitary glands of animals can be removed when pregnancy is advanced without impairing growth of the mammary glands, which continue to enlarge as long as the placenta remains

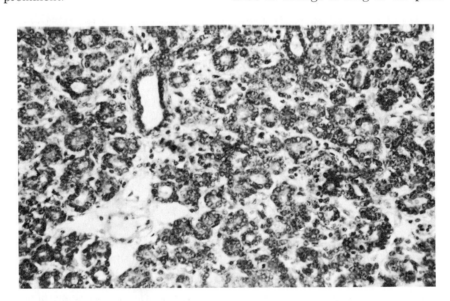

Figure 24–25. Photomicrograph of a mammary gland during pregnancy. There is intense proliferation of the gland alveoli. No secretion is seen. H&E stain, × 200.

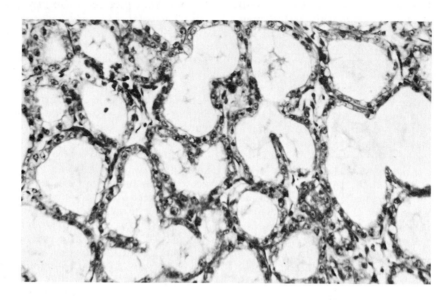

Figure 24 –26. Photomicrograph of a lactating mammary gland. The alveoli are distended by the secretion (milk) accumulated in their lumens. H&E stain, × 200.

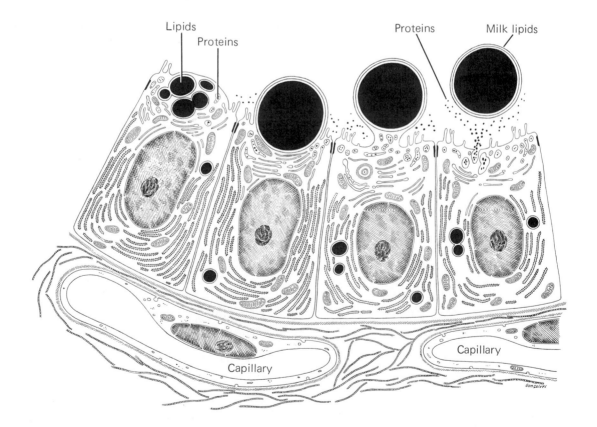

Figure 24 –27. Schematic drawing of secretory epithelium from the mammary gland. Observe from left to right the accumulation and extrusion of milk lipids and proteins. The proteins are released through merocrine secretion, while lipid extrusion involves apocrine secretion.

functioning. Prolactin is essential for the early phase of growth of the mammary glands but not for continuation of growth.

Although estrogen, progesterone, and prolactin are the main hormones responsible for the growth of mammary glands during pregnancy, other hormones such as thyroxine, corticosteroids, and growth hormone also play a role in this process.

The Breasts During Lactation

Milk is produced inside the epithelial cells of the secretory portions of the glands and accumulates in their lumens and inside the lactiferous ducts (Fig 24–26). The secretory cells become small and cuboidal or squamous. Their cytoplasm contains spherical vacuoles of various sizes containing lipids. These vacuoles have a continuous smooth surface membrane. They pass out of the cells into the lumen with this membrane intact (Fig 24–27). The lipids constitute 4% of human milk.

Besides the lipid vacuoles, which are at the apical pole of the secretory cells, one can see protein granules. The synthesis of milk proteins occurs at the level of the granular endoplasmic reticulum, which is abundant in the basal part of this cell, passing then through the Golgi apparatus and accumulating at the apical portion. Contrary to what occurs with the vacuoles of lipids, the smooth membrane that involves the granules of protein is not eliminated with the protein that appears free in the lumen of the secretory portions (Fig 24–27).

Proteins constitute approximately 1.5% of human milk.

Lactose, the third important component of milk, is synthesized from glucose. Lactose constitutes about 7% of human milk.

The first milk to appear after birth is called **colostrum.** It contains less fat and more proteins than regular milk and is rich in antibodies (predominantly IgA) that provide some degree of passive immunity to the newborn, especially within gut lumen.

Sections of mammary gland from a lactating woman show several alveoli in different phases of secretion. Large cells filled with secretion and small cuboidal cells with almost no secretion in their interiors can be seen.

When a woman is breast feeding, the suction of the child stimulates tactile receptors, which are abundant around the nipple, resulting in liberation of the posterior pituitary hormone oxytocin. This hormone causes contraction of myoepithelial cells in the gland, and ejection of milk occurs. Emotional and genital stimuli also can result in the liberation of oxytocin, forcing milk to appear in the nipples.

Senile Involution of the Breasts

After menopause, involution of the mammary gland is characterized by reduction in size and atrophy of its secretory portion and partly also of the excretory ducts. Striking atrophic changes occur also in the interstitial connective tissue.

•   •   •

References

Adams EC, Hertig AT: Studies on guinea pig oocytes. 1. Electron microscopic observations on the development of cytoplasmic organelles in oocytes of primordial and primary follicles. J Cell Biol 21:397, 1964.

Adams EC, Hertig AT: Studies on the human corpus luteum. J Cell Biol 41:696, 1969.

Anderson E, Beams HW: Cytological observations on the fine structure of the guinea pig ovary with special reference to the oogonium, primary oocyte and associated follicle cells. J Ultrastruct Res 3:432, 1960.

Baker TG: A quantitative and cytological study of oogenesis in the rhesus monkey. J Anat 100:761, 1966.

Banarjee MR: Responses of mammary cells to hormones. Int Rev Cytol 47:1, 1976.

Bjersing L, Cajander S: Ovulation and the role of surface epithelium. Experientia 31:605, 1975.

Blanchette EJ: Ovarian steroid cells. 2. The lutein cell. J Cell Biol 31:517, 1966.

Boyd JD, Hamilton WJ: Electron microscopic observations on the cytotrophoblast contribution to the syncytium in the human placenta. J Anat 100:535, 1966.

Brandes D, Anton E: An electron microscopic cytochemical study of macrophages during uterine involution. J Cell Biol 41:50, 1969.

Dirksen ER, Satir P: Ciliary activity in the mouse oviduct as studied by transmission and scanning electron microscopy. Tissue Cell 4:389, 1972.

Enders AC, Lyon WR: Observations on the fine structure of lutein cells. 2. The effects of hypophysectomy and mammotrophic hormones in the rat. J Cell Biol 22:127, 1964.

Ferenczy A & others: Scanning electron microscopy of the human Fallopian tube. Science 175:783, 1972.

Fredricsson B, Björkman N: Studies on the ultrastructure of the human oviduct epithelium in different functional states. Z Zellforsch Mikrosk Anat 58:387, 1962.

Guraya SS: Recent advances in the morphology, histochemistry and biochemistry of the developing mammalian ovary. Int Rev Cytol 51:49, 1977.

Hertig AT, Adams EC: Studies on the human oocyte and its follicle. 1. Ultrastructural and histochemical observations on the primordial follicle stage. J Cell Biol 34:647, 1967.

Jones RE (editor): The Vertebrate Ovary. Plenum Press, 1978.

McNatty KP & others: The production of progesterone, androgens, and estrogens by granulosa cells, thecal tissue, and stromal tissue from human ovaries in vitro. J Clin Endocrinol Metab 49:687, 1979.

Moseman HW: Comparative Morphology of the Mammalian Ovary. Univ of Wisconsin Press, 1973.

Motta P, Van Blerkom J: A scanning electron microscope study of the luteo-follicular complex. 1. Follicle and oocyte. J Submicrosc Cytol 6:297, 1974.

Nemanic MK, Pitelka DR: A scanning electron microscope study of the lactating mammary gland. J Cell Biol 48:410, 1971.

Ross R, Klebanoff SJ: Fine structural changes in uterine smooth muscle and fibroblasts in response to estrogens. J Cell Biol 32:27, 1967.

Segal SJ: The physiology of human reproduction. Sci Am 231:52, Sept 1974.

Tersakis J: The ultrastructure of normal human first trimester placenta. J Ultrastruct Res 9:268, 1963.

Villee DB: Development of endocrine function in the human placenta and fetus. N Engl J Med 281:473, 1969.

Vorherr H: The Breast: Morphology, Physiology and Lactation. Academic Press, 1974.

Wellings SR, Phelp JR: The function of the Golgi apparatus in lactating cells of the BALB/c Crgl mouse: An electron microscopic and autoradiographic study. Z Zellforsch Mikrosk Anat 61:871, 1964.

Yoshida Y: Ultrastructure and secretory function of the syncytial trophoblast of human placenta in early pregnancy. Exp Cell Res 34:305, 1964.

Zamboni L: Modulations of follicle cell–oocyte association in sequential stages of mammalian follicle development and maturation. In: Ovulation in the Human. Proceedings of the Serono Symposia. Vol 8. Crosignani PG, Mishell DR (editors). Academic Press, 1976.

Index

Thymus (cont'd)
development and involution of, 295
grafting of, 299
hormones acting on, 299
zones of, 293
Thymus-dependent antigens, 297
Thymus-dependent areas of lymphoid
organ, 297
Thymus-dependent lymphocytes, 262,
289, 304
Thyroglobulin, 435
synthesis of, 436
Thyroid, 433
colloid of, 433
follicles of, 433
Thyroid-stimulating hormone, 415, 417,
433
Thyrotropic cells, 415
Thyrotropin, 417, 433
Thyrotropin-releasing factor, 417
Thyroxine, 417, 437, 438
Tissue(s)
adipose, **115–120**
brown, 116, 119
yellow, 116
adrenal medullary, 422
adrenocortical, 422
connective, **89–114**
epithelial, **62–88**
biology of, 74
characteristics of, 62
ciliated pseudostratified, 70
covering, 71
diagrams of, 70
nutrition and innervation of, 74
photomicrographs of, 63
pseudostratified columnar ciliated,
63
simple ciliated columnar, 70
simple cuboidal, 70
simple squamous, 70
stratified nonkeratinized squamous,
63
stratified squamous, 70
stratified squamous keratinized, 63
transitional, 63, 70
interstitial, 451
muscle, **217–235**
nerve, **152–185**
reticular, 112
subcutaneous, 378, 387
Tissue culture cell, electron micrograph of, 49
Tissue fluid, 89, 108
Tissue sections, problems in interpretation of, 9
TnC, 220
TnI, 220
TnT, 220
Tomes fibers, 310, 311
Tongue, 307
papillae of, 307
fungiform and circumvallate, 189, 307
Tonofibrils, 379, 381
Tonofilaments, 47
Tonsil(s), 290
lingual, 290, **291**
palatine, 290, **291**
pharyngeal, 290, **291**
Touch, sense of, 186
Trabecular arteries, 301
Trabecular veins, 301

Trachea, 362, 364
Tracheal mucosa, photomicrograph
of, 362
Transfer vesicles, 37
Transplantation, organ, 299
Transport component, 287
Transverse tubule system, 224
TRF, 417
Triad, 224, 227
Triglyceride lipase, 118
Trigona fibrosa, 247
Triiodothyronine, 438
Trophoblast, 474
Tropocollagen, 91, 92
Tropomyosin, 220
Troponin, 220
Trypanosoma cruzi infection, 313
Trypsinogen, 341
Tryptophan, 20
TSH, 415, 417, 418, 433
secretion of, regulation of, 435
Tubule(s)
seminiferous, structure of, 446
straight, 445
transverse, system of, 224
Tubuli recti, 445, 455
Tubulin, 43
Tubulo-alveolar secretory glands, 484
Tubulovesicles, 316, 317
Tubulovesicular structures, 316
Tunic
internal, 240
middle, 240
Tunica
adventitia, 242
albuginea, 444, 460, 462, 463
fibrosa, of eye, 192
intima, 240
media, 240
propria, **445**
vaginalis, 445
Turnover, of gastric mucosa, 321
Tympanic membrane, 209
Type I cell, **371**, 375
Type II cell, **371**, 375
Tyrosinase, 384
Tyrosine, 20, 384
Tyrosyl radicals, iodination of, 437

Unit membrane, 29
Unitarian theory, 267, 275
Unitary smooth muscles, 234
Unmyelinated axons, 166
Unmyelinated fibers, 164, **166**
Unmyelinated nerve fiber, 169
Ureter, 392
Urethra, 408, 456
corpus cavernosum of, 460
external sphincter of, 408
female, 409
male, 408
Urinary bladder, section of, 231
Urinary passages and bladder, 407
Urinary system, **392–409**
Urine, hypotonic or hypertonic, forma-
tion of, 406
Urogastrone, 327
Uronic acid, 107
Uterine cervix, 474
Uterine neck, 472
Uterine tube, 462, **470**

Uterus, 462, 472
endometrium of, 472
myometrium of, 472
Utricle, 210, 211
Uveal tract, 192
Uvula, 307

Vagina, 462, 480
Vaginal mucosa, photomicrograph of,
481
Vagus nerve, 365
Valves, cardiac, 247
Vas deferens, 456, 457
Vasa vasorum, 242
Vascular feet of neuroglia, 161
Vasomotor nerves, nonmyelinated,
242
Vasopressin, 418
Vein(s), 236, **245**
central, 344, 345
centrolobular, 345
distributing, 345
large, 245, 246
small or medium-sized, 245
of spleen, 301
sublobular, 345
trabecular, 301
valves of, 247
vortex, 193
Venules, 243, 245
inlet, 345
portal, 345
postcapillary, 290
Vermis, 182
Verumontanum, 408
Vesicles
secretory, 82
seminal, 457, 458
synaptic, 159
transfer, 37
Vesicular follicles, 462
Vessel(s), blood
general structure of, 240
oxygen content of, 252
pulmonary, 375
Vestibular function, 213
Vestibular membrane, 212, 213
Vestibule, 363
auditory, 210, 211
histophysiology of, 213
nasal, 363
Vestibulocochlear apparatus, 209
Vestibulum, 481
Vibrissae, 363
Villi
chorionic, 477, 479, 480
primary, 479
secondary, 479
Visceral sensitivity receptors, 186
Visceral smooth muscles, 234
Vision, process of, 203
Visual purple, 202
Vitamin A, 146
Vitamin B_{12}, 317
Vitamin C, 146
deficiency, 113
Vitamin D, 145
Vitamin E, lack of, 455
Vitelline sac, 476
Vitreous, 192, 193, 194, 200
Vitreous space, 192